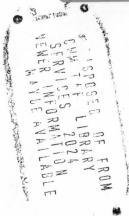

Sobotta
Atlas of Human Anatomy
Vol. 1

# Sobotta Atlas of Human Anatomy

Edited by

HELMUT FERNER and JOCHEN STAUBESAND

Vol. 1: Head, Neck, Upper Extremities

10th English Edition with Nomenclature in English
Translated and Edited by WALTHER J. HILD
614 Illustrations, most in color

1983

Urban & Schwarzenberg · Baltimore–Munich

This book was founded by Johannes Sobotta, former Professor of Anatomy and Director of the Anatomical Institute of the University of Bonn,
followed by Hellmut Becher, former Professor of Anatomy and Director of the Anatomical Institute of the University of Münster.

Address of the English translator and editor:

Walther J. Hild, M.D., Professor and Chairman, Department of Anatomy, The University of Texas Medical Branch, Galveston, Texas 77550

Addresses of the German Editors:

Professor emerit. Dr. med. Helmut Ferner, I. Anatomische Lehr-kanzel der Universität Wien
Währingerstraße 13, A-1090 Wien

Professor Dr. med. Jochen Staubesand, Direktor des Anatomi-schen Instituts (Lehrstuhl I) der Albert-Ludwigs-Universität, Freiburg
Albertstraße 17, 7800 Freiburg i. Br.

This atlas consists of two separate volumes:

Vol. 1: Head, Neck, Upper Extremities

Vol. 2: Thorax, Abdomen, Pelvis, Lower Extremities, Skin

**Library of Congress Cataloging in Publication Data**

**Sobotta, Johannes, 1869–1945.**
  Sobotta's Atlas of human anatomy.

  Translation of: Atlas der Anatomie des Menschen.
18th ed. 1982.
  Includes indexes.
  Contents: v. 1. Head, neck, upper extremities -- v. 2.
Thorax, abdomen, pelvis, lower extremities, skin.
  1. Anatomy, Human--Atlases    I. Hild, Walther J.
II. Title.  III. Title: Atlas of human anatomy.
[DNLM: 1. Anatomy--Regional--Atlases.    QS 17 S677a]
QM25.S676    1983    611'.0022'2    82-13604
  ISBN 0-8067-1710-6 (U.S. : v. 1)
  ISBN 0-8067-1720-3 (U.S. : v. 2)

German Editions:

1. Edition: J. F. Lehmanns Verlag, München 1904
2.–11. Edition: J. F. Lehmanns Verlag, München 1913–1944
    since 12. Edition: Urban & Schwarzenberg, 1948
13. Edition: 1953
14. Edition: 1956
15. Edition: 1957
16. Edition: 1967 (ISBN 3-541-02816-5)
17. Edition: 1972 (ISBN 3-541-02817-3)
18. Edition: 1982 (ISBN 3-541-02818-1)


Foreign Editions:

English Edition (with nomenclature in English)
Urban & Schwarzenberg

English Edition (with nomenclature in Latin)
Urban & Schwarzenberg

French Edition
Urban & Schwarzenberg

Turkish Edition
Urban & Schwarzenberg

Arabic Edition
Al Ahram, Cairo/Egypt

Italian Edition
USES, Florence, Italy

Greek Edition
Gregory Parisianos, Athens, Greece

Japanese Edition
Igaku-Shoin Ltd., Tokyo, Japan

Portuguese Edition
Editora Guanabara Koogan, Rio de Janeiro, Brazil

Spanish Edition
Ediciones Toray, Barcelona, Spain

Printed in Germany by Kastner & Callwey, München
© Urban & Schwarzenberg 1983

ISBN 0-8067-1710-6 Baltimore

ISBN 3-541-71710-6 Munich

# Preface

The Sobotta Atlas of Human Anatomy has been a success by any standard.

For generations it has been indispensable to anatomists and artists, as well as an important reference for the practicing physician. Thoughts of changing such an integral part of the medical literature have not come easily. However, the teaching and learning of anatomy have changed dramatically, and the time has come for the Sobotta Atlas to do the same. This new edition reflects those changes, undertaken with the greatest care, and we are pleased to have had a part in the "remaking" of Sobotta.

The most important modification is that of organization. The Sobotta Atlas is now arranged in a regional format and follows the usual sequence of anatomic study. All information related to a specific area of the body – from the skin surface to the underlying organs to the skeleton – can now be found together in one volume. And, because this regional/topographical completeness is applied consistently throughout, it has been possible to reduce the three volumes of former editions to the two now available.

Another important change in this edition of Sobotta involves the illustrations. To make the leap into the modern era complete, many older illustrations have been repainted in more vivid color, a large number of the formerly black and white illustrations now appear in full color, and new radiographs have been added throughout both volumes. All of this has proved to be expensive, and we are especially grateful to the publishers for their enthusiastic support.

A new appendix (by Dr. F. Platz, Freiburg i. Br.) on the areas of arterial blood supply has been added.

The recommendations found in the 4th edition of Nomina Anatomica were followed whenever it was thought they were justified.

The editors would like to thank their many colleagues who supported them with help and advice. These include Prof. Dr. J. Altaras (Gießen), Prof. Dr. G. Kaufmann (Freiburg i. Br.) and Dr. S. Rau, lecturer (Freiburg i. Br.), who supplied us with radiographs and xeroradiographs; Prof. Dr. H. Roskamm (Bad Krozingen) who provided angiocardiographs of the ventricles; Prof. Dr. A. Kappert (Bern) who let us use originals from his "Leitfaden und Atlas der Angiologie" *(Textbook and Atlas of Angiology),* and Prof. Dr. R. May (Innsbruck) who made original illustrations of perforating veins in the foot and lower leg available to us. Dr. T. Grimm (Würzburg) supplied us with new material on the pattern of the dermal ridge of the finger and palm, as well as a revised text. We would also like to thank Dr. L. Wicke for a number of X-ray photographs from his "Atlas of Radiologic Anatomy" (Second Edition, Urban & Schwarzenberg, Baltimore–Munich, 1982) and Dr. R. Unsöld (Freiburg i. Br.) for computer tomograms with explanatory texts.

Our thanks are also due to our closest co-workers for their constant and reliable assistance and support. Dr. H. Schmiebusch and Frau M. Engler in particular helped in the great amount of editing required for the figures and texts. Dr. S. Zuleger took special interest in the chapter on the heart. Dr. H. Schmiebusch revised and extended the glossary.

The editors can look back at a long period of intensive and productive cooperation with Mr. Michael Urban, the managing partner of the Urban & Schwarzenberg publishing house, and his colleagues. Without their whole-hearted cooperation, the understanding they showed for our requests, and their technical expertise, the work for this new edition of the Sobotta Atlas could never have been completed on schedule.

Vienna and Freiburg i. Br.,      H. FERNER
May 1982      J. STAUBESAND

# American Editor's Preface to the 10th English Edition

The new two-volume edition of the Sobotta Atlas of Human Anatomy has been rearranged in a regional format. This will enhance its usefulness as a reference work, and it can be consulted in the dissecting laboratory more efficiently in conjunction with various dissecting manuals. The anglicized nomenclature as used in North America has been consistently applied. A new and simplified index will facilitate rapid orientation.

I would like to thank various faculty members of the Department of Anatomy at UTMB for valuable advice. I am indebted to Mr. Braxton D. Mitchell and Ms. Nan Curtis Tyler of Urban & Schwarzenberg in Baltimore for their cooperation in every phase of translating and editing. Special thanks are due to my secretary, Ms. Phyllis Fletcher, whose superior typing and proofreading skills were essential for the completion on schedule of this English Edition.

Galveston, Texas, February 1983      WALTHER J. HILD

# Table of Contents

page

General Terms of Direction and Position . . . . . . . . . . VII

Short Explanation Concerning Derivation, Significance
   and Pronunciation of Anatomical Names . . . . . . . . VIII

## Illustrations

Osteology . . . . . . . . . . . . . . . . . . . . . . . . . . . . . .   1

Brain, Meninges, Blood Vessels . . . . . . . . . . . . . .  33

Spinal Cord, Spinal Nerves, Sympathetic Trunk . . . . . . 117

Superficial and Deep Facial Region . . . . . . . . . . . . . . 133

Nose, Nasal Cavity, Paranasal Sinuses . . . . . . . . . . . . 149

Oral Cavity, Teeth, Masticatory System* . . . . . . . . . . 161

\* ERRATUM: Due to a technical error, x-ray 263, p. 170, is inverted.

page

Pharynx . . . . . . . . . . . . . . . . . . . . . . . . . . . . . . . . 189

Larynx . . . . . . . . . . . . . . . . . . . . . . . . . . . . . . . . . 197

Eye and Orbit . . . . . . . . . . . . . . . . . . . . . . . . . . . . 211

Organ of Hearing and Equilibrium . . . . . . . . . . . . . . 243

Neck and Nuchea . . . . . . . . . . . . . . . . . . . . . . . . . . 263

Upper Extremity . . . . . . . . . . . . . . . . . . . . . . . . . . 299

Hand . . . . . . . . . . . . . . . . . . . . . . . . . . . . . . . . . . . 349

## Appendix

Etymology of Anatomical Terms . . . . . . . . . . . . . . . . 369

Index . . . . . . . . . . . . . . . . . . . . . . . . . . . . . . . . . . 375

# Abbreviations

| | | | | | | | |
|---|---|---|---|---|---|---|---|
| ant. | = anterior | int. | = interior | sup. | = superior | | |
| a. or aa. | = artery or arteries | inteross. | = interosseous | superf. | = superficial | | |
| art. | = articulation | lat. | = lateral | surf. | = surface | | |
| br. | = branch | lig. or ligg. | = ligament or ligaments | sut. | = suture | | |
| caud. | = caudal | m. or mm. | = muscle or muscles | transv. | = transverse | | |
| cran. | = cranial | med. | = medial | tuberc. | = tubercle | | |
| dist. | = distal | n. or nn. | = nerve or nerves | tuberos. | = tuberosity | | |
| dors. | = dorsal | obl. | = oblique | v. or vv. | = vein or veins | | |
| ext. | = external | post. | = posterior | vent. | = ventral | | |
| exten. | = extensor | prot. | = protuberance | vert. | = vertebra | | |
| flex. | = flexor | prox. | = proximal | | | | |
| inf. | = inferior | r. or rr. | = ramus or rami | | | | |

# General Terms of Direction and Position

The following terms designate the position of organs and parts of the body in their relationship to each other, sometimes irrespective of the position of the body in space. These designations are used not only in human anatomy, but also in medical practice and in comparative anatomy.

## General designations

*Anterior – posterior* = in front – behind (e.g., anterior and posterior tibial arteries)

*ventral – dorsal* = toward the belly – toward the back

*superior – inferior* = above – below

*cranial – caudal* = toward the head – toward the tail

*dexter – sinister* = right – left (e.g., right and left common iliac arteries)

*internal – external* = located inside – located outside

*superficial – deep* = located superficially – located deeply (e.g., superficial and deep flexores digitorum muscles)

*medius* or *intermedius* = middle (in the middle between two other structures) (e.g., the middle nasal concha is located between the superior and inferior nasal concha)

*medianus* = located in the midline, median (e.g., median fissure of the spinal cord)
   A "median sagittal section" divides the body into two mirror image-like portions.

*medial – lateral* = located toward the middle of the body – located toward the side of the body (e.g., medial and lateral inguinal fossae)

*frontal* = located in a frontal plane, also located toward the forehead (e.g., frontal process of maxilla)

*longitudinal* = parallel to the long axis (e.g., superior longitudinal muscle)

*sagittal* = in a plane perpendicular to the frontal plane (e.g., sagittal suture of the cranium)

*transversal* = in a transversal plane, at right angles to the long axis of the body or organ (e.g., transversus abdominis muscle)

*transverse* = running transversely (e.g., transverse process of a thoracic vertebra)

## Designations for Directions and Positions of the Extremities

*proximal – distal* = located toward the root of the extremity – located toward the free end of the extremity (e.g., proximal and distal radioulnar joints)

For the upper extremity:

*radial – ulnar* = on the radial side – on the ulnar side (e.g., ulnar and radial arteries)

For the hand:

*palmar – dorsal* = toward the palm of the hand – toward the back of the hand (e.g., palmar aponeurosis)

For the lower extremity:

*tibial – fibular (peroneal)* = on the tibial side – on the fibular side

For the foot:

*plantar – dorsal* = toward the sole of the foot – toward the upper surface of the foot (e.g., lateral and medial plantar arteries, dorsal artery of the foot)

# Short Explanation Concerning Derivation, Significance and Pronunciation of Anatomical Names

## General

The Basle Anatomical Names (B.N.A.), adopted by the Anatomische Gesellschaft in 1895 and revised in 1955 as Paris Anatomical Names (P.N.A.), which are internationally used (Int. Anatomical Nomenclature Comm.: Nomina Anatomica; 4th ed. Excerpta Medica Amsterdam, Oxford 1977), have, for the most part, been used since antiquity. Only a relatively few names have been added over time. The large majority of the official names used today are derived from Latin, and many are derived from Greek and later Latinized to a greater or lesser degree. Occasionally, names are derived from oriental languages (Arabic, Aramaic). However, they have been Latinized in their grammatical form to such a degree that their original derivation can hardly be recognized.

Since the Greek alphabet differs markedly from the Latin, Greek names are written in Latin letters.

## Spelling and Pronunciation of Names of Greek Derivation

The Greek Kappa (K) is changed to c, the Chi (ch) to ch, the Phi (ph) to ph, the Psi (ps) to ps, the Xi (X) to x, the Theta (th) to th, the so-called Spiritus asper to h. Gamma (g) before Gamma, Kappa (K), Chi (ch), and Xi (x) is pronounced as n (e.g. aggeion = angeion, agkos = ankos). Since Greek words that begin with Rho (r) carry the Spiritus asper over the Rho, they are spelled in Latin with rh, e.g. rhomboideus etc. Of the vowels and diphthongs of the Greek language the Omega (long O) and the Omikron (short O) are both spelled as O, the (short) Epsilon as well as the (long) Eta are both E; Ypsilon, Alpha, and Jota are spelled as in Greek. The diphthong Epsilon-Jota in its Latinized form (as in modern Greek) is pronounced i, e.g., Aristeides (gr.) Latinized = Aristides. Occasionally it is also pronounced as e as in tracheia (gr.) Latinized = trachea. The diphthong Omicron-Jota is spelled and pronounced as oe (oikos gr. = oecus lat., e.g. oeconomia), Alpha-Jota is changed to ae, Alpha-Ypsilon to au, Omikron-Ypsilon to u, Epsilon-Ypsilon to eu. The endings of nouns and adjectives are Latinized; e.g. sternon to sternum, isthmos to isthmus, and the adjective of thorax (thorakikos) to thoracicus. As a rule, the Latin declension is used (less frequently the Greek declension: e.g. hypophysis, gen. hypophyseos). Frequently, as was common in Roman times, Greek nouns are provided with Latin adjectival endings (e.g., centralis, derived from Latinized centrum, gr. kentron). Pronunciation and accentuation of Latinized names derived from Greek follow the Latin rule. The old rule of accentuation, vocalis ante vocalem brevis est (a vowel before a vowel is short), is generally valid and is neglected only if the vowel is derived from a Greek diphthong and therefore long. (Macron over the vowel = length; breve over the vowel = shortness; accent = accentuation; the Greek vowel Epsilon is given as e, Eta as ē).

## A note regarding the color figures

The multicolor figures presented here are based on didactic considerations. Contrasts have been intensified to enhance the recognition of areas that are naturally difficult to discern. Hence, the colors used for various tissues (e.g., tendons, cartilage, bones, musculature) and pathways (arteries, veins, lymphatic vessels, nerves) are different from those found in living or dead bodies or in a preserved cadaver.

Any deviations in the tint or intensity of the colors found in this edition (e.g., in illustrations of muscles, blood vessels and nerves) exist primarily because the various illustrations were made over a long period of time. In addition to the artists who prepared the illustrations with Prof. Sobotta, later with Prof. Becher for the original collection (K. HAJEK, Prof. E. LEPIER, H. v. EICKSTEDT, W. WOHLSCHLEGEL), the following artists worked on the 18th edition: Elisabeth ALTHAUS: Figs. 462, 463, 464, 465, 466, 476, 477, 480; Ulrike BRUGGER: Figs. 59, 60, 99, 131, 132, 212, 216, 217, 289, 291, 292, 358, 380, 382, 409, 417, 418, 426, 427, 428, 429, 430, 431, 437, 439, 443, 444, 445, 448, 457, 467, 473, 481, 483; Marie Anne ERHARD: Figs. 182, 184a; Luitgard KELLNER: Figs. 135, 136, 234, 235, 295, 296, 373, 378, 379; Li KÖRNER: Figs. 198a−c; Ingrid VON MARCHTALER: Fig. 16; Barbara G. RUPPEL: Fig. 583; Horst RUSS: Figs. 214, 221, 223, 224; Christiane SCHAEFFER: Figs. 263b, 264b; Hanna SCHIMEK: Figs. 314, 471; Lothar SCHNELLBÄCHER: Figs. 304, 501, 504; Ingo WEGERL: Figs. 19, 65, 80, 82, 138, 229, 232, 254, 255, 309, 310, 311, 312, 315, 316, 317, 318, 327, 328, 331, 347, 348, 474, 507, 508, 517, 518, 539, 540, 541, 542, 548, 549, 552, 553, 554, 555, 556, 587, 588, 594, 595, 597, 598; David WILLIAMS: Figs. 64, 94, 349, 350, 351, 352, 353, 364, 365, 366, 367, 368, 369, 371, 374, 375, 376, 377, 381; G. ZEH-KOSANKE: Figs. 515, 516, 521, 533, 534, 535, 536, 537, 538, 546, 550, 551, 557, 558, 559, 589, 590.

# Osteology

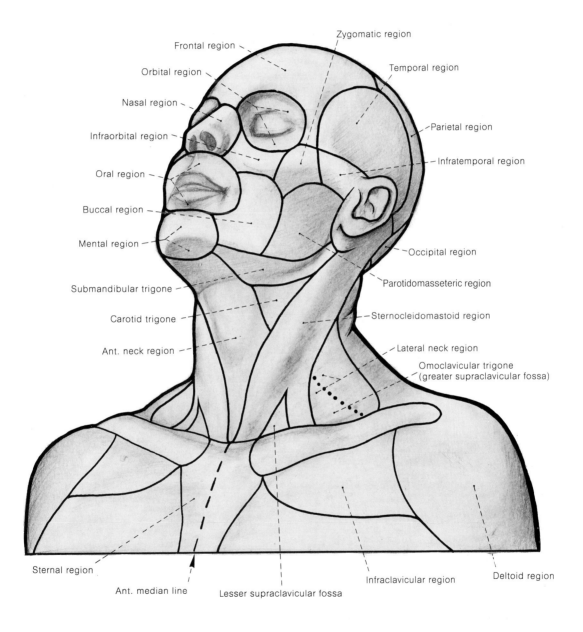

**Fig. 1.** Regions of head and neck. Anterior view.

Zygomatic region

Frontal region

Temporal region

Orbital region

Nasal region

Parietal region

Infraorbital region

Infratemporal region

Oral region

Buccal region

Mental region

Occipital region

Submandibular trigone

Parotidomasseteric region

Carotid trigone

Sternocleidomastoid region

Ant. neck region

Lateral neck region

Omoclavicular trigone
(greater supraclavicular fossa)

Sternal region

Infraclavicular region

Deltoid region

Ant. median line

Lesser supraclavicular fossa

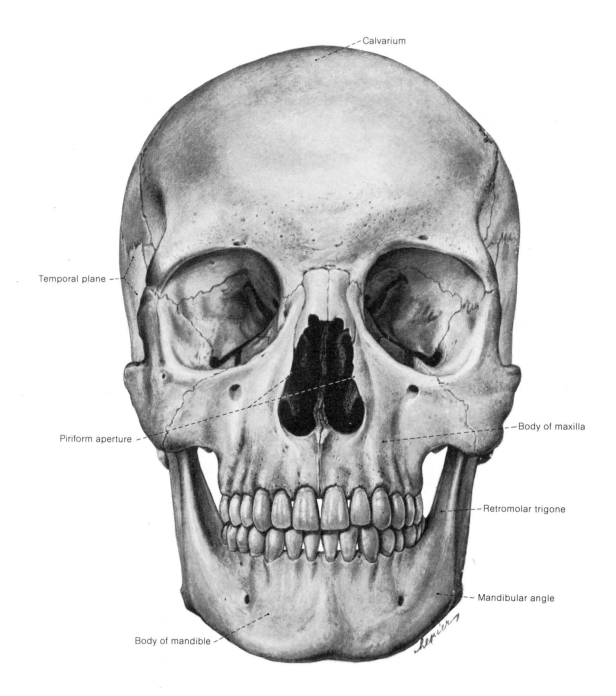

**Fig. 2.** The skull; anterior view. Centric occlusion.

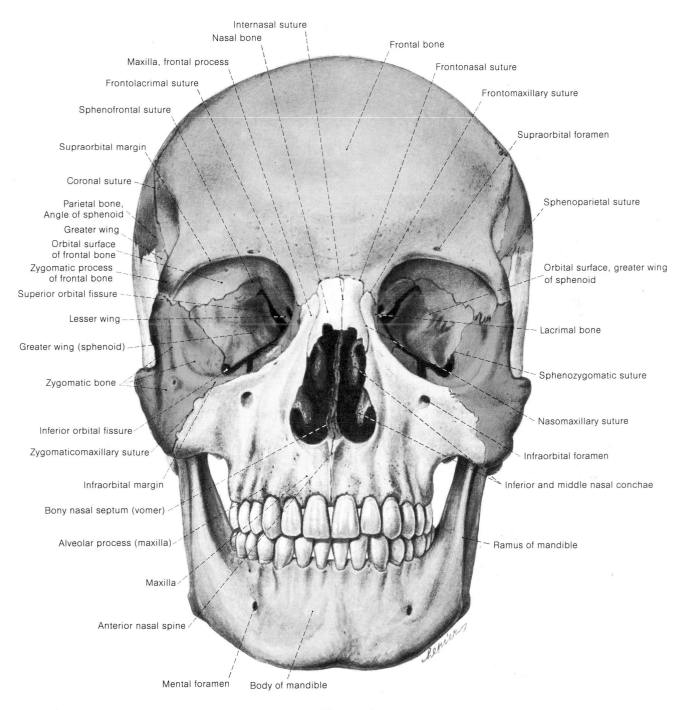

Internasal suture

Nasal bone

Frontal bone

Maxilla, frontal process

Frontonasal suture

Frontolacrimal suture

Frontomaxillary suture

Sphenofrontal suture

Supraorbital margin

Supraorbital foramen

Coronal suture

Parietal bone, Angle of sphenoid

Sphenoparietal suture

Greater wing

Orbital surface of frontal bone

Zygomatic process of frontal bone

Orbital surface, greater wing of sphenoid

Superior orbital fissure

Lesser wing

Lacrimal bone

Greater wing (sphenoid)

Zygomatic bone

Sphenozygomatic suture

Inferior orbital fissure

Nasomaxillary suture

Zygomaticomaxillary suture

Infraorbital foramen

Infraorbital margin

Inferior and middle nasal conchae

Bony nasal septum (vomer)

Alveolar process (maxilla)

Ramus of mandible

Maxilla

Anterior nasal spine

Mental foramen    Body of mandible

**Fig. 3.** The skull. Anterior aspect. The bones are set apart by different colors.

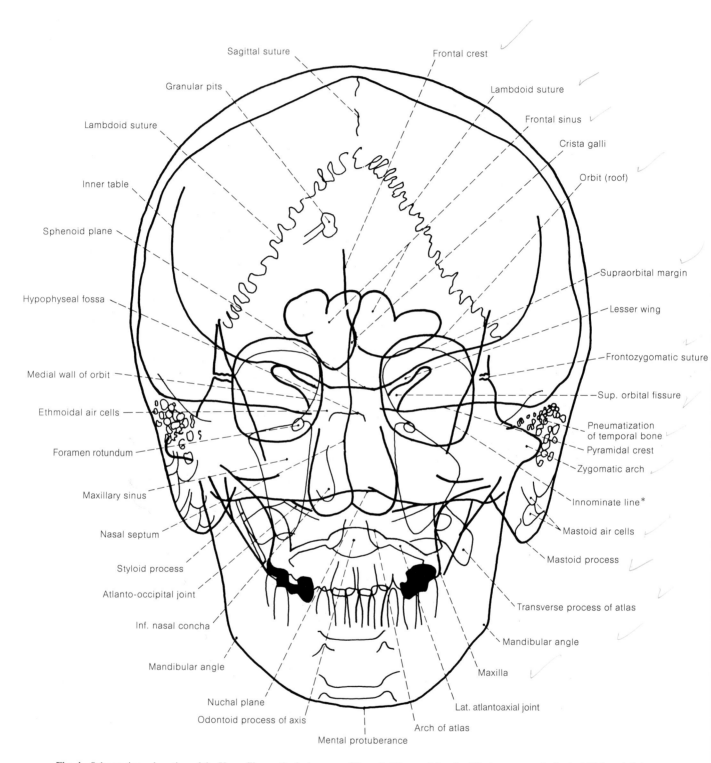

Sagittal suture

Granular pits

Lambdoid suture

Inner table

Sphenoid plane

Hypophyseal fossa

Medial wall of orbit

Ethmoidal air cells

Foramen rotundum

Maxillary sinus

Nasal septum

Styloid process

Atlanto-occipital joint

Inf. nasal concha

Mandibular angle

Nuchal plane

Odontoid process of axis

Mental protuberance

Frontal crest

Lambdoid suture

Frontal sinus

Crista galli

Orbit (roof)

Supraorbital margin

Lesser wing

Frontozygomatic suture

Sup. orbital fissure

Pneumatization of temporal bone

Pyramidal crest

Zygomatic arch

Innominate line*

Mastoid air cells

Mastoid process

Transverse process of atlas

Mandibular angle

Maxilla

Lat. atlantoaxial joint

Arch of atlas

**Fig. 4.** Schematic explanation of the X-ray film on the facing page. (From L. WICKE: Atlas der Röntgenanatomie, 2nd ed. Urban & Schwarzenberg, Munich–Vienna–Baltimore 1980.) * roentgenologic terminology (super positions).

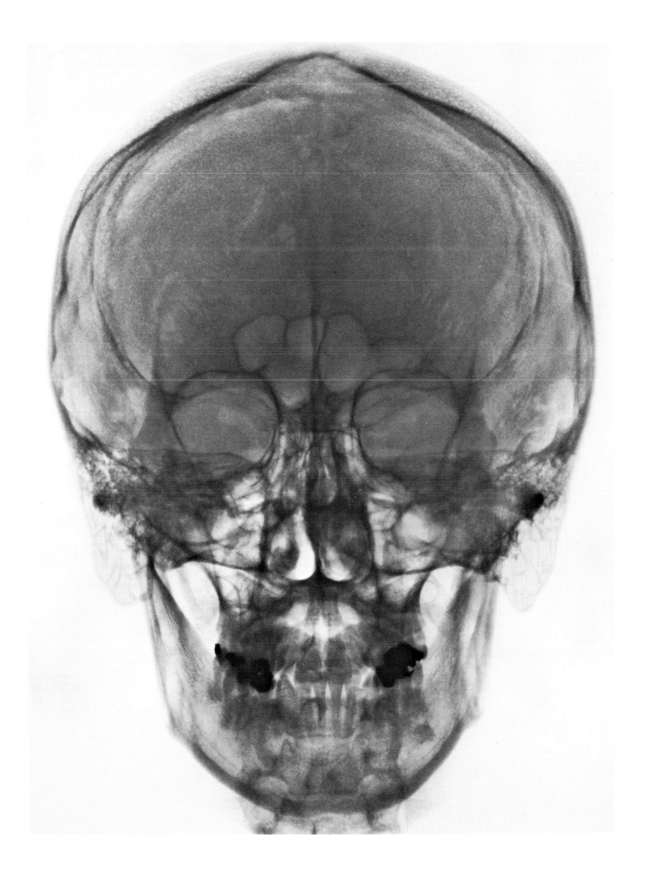

**Fig. 5.** X-ray film of the skull, sagittal projection. (From L. WICKE: Atlas der Röntgenanatomie, 2nd ed. Urban & Schwarzenberg, Munich–Vienna–Baltimore 1980.)

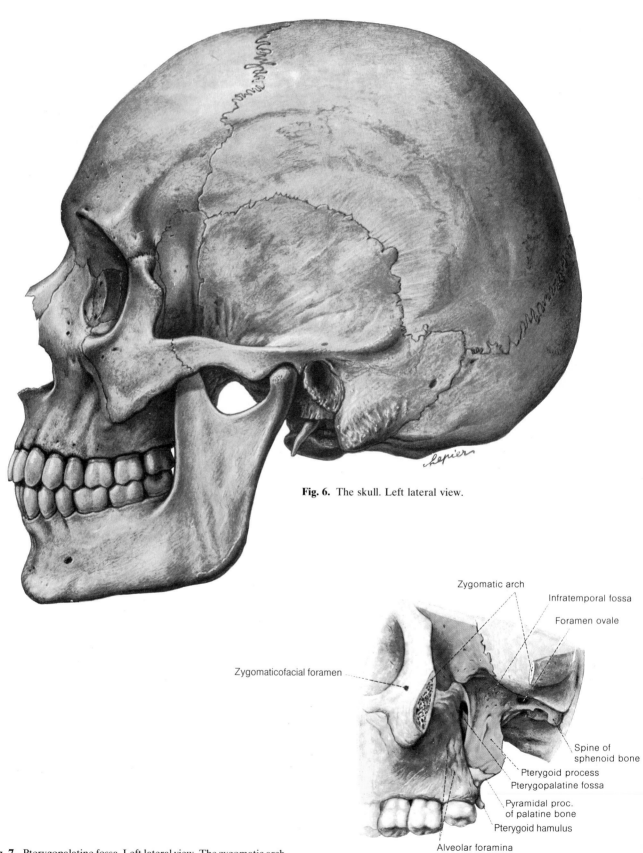

**Fig. 6.** The skull. Left lateral view.

Zygomatic arch

Infratemporal fossa

Foramen ovale

Zygomaticofacial foramen

Spine of
sphenoid bone

Pterygoid process

Pterygopalatine fossa

Pyramidal proc.
of palatine bone

Pterygoid hamulus

Alveolar foramina

**Fig. 7.** Pterygopalatine fossa. Left lateral view. The zygomatic arch
was removed.

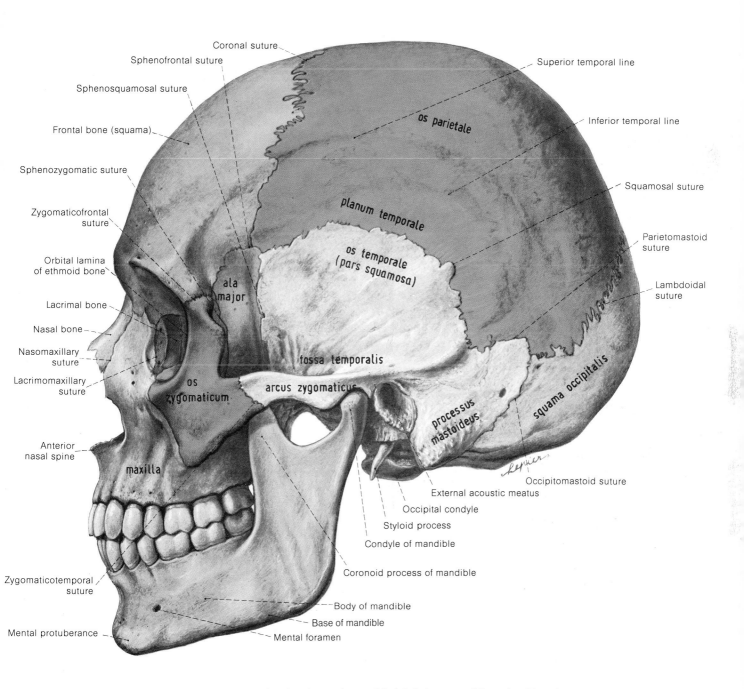

Coronal suture
Sphenofrontal suture
Sphenosquamosal suture
Frontal bone (squama)
Sphenozygomatic suture
Zygomaticofrontal suture
Orbital lamina of ethmoid bone
Lacrimal bone
Nasal bone
Nasomaxillary suture
Lacrimomaxillary suture
Anterior nasal spine
Zygomaticotemporal suture
Mental protuberance

Superior temporal line
os parietale
Inferior temporal line
Squamosal suture
Parietomastoid suture
Lambdoidal suture

planum temporale
os temporale (pars squamosa)
ala major
fossa temporalis
os zygomaticum
arcus zygomaticus
processus mastoideus
squama occipitalis
maxilla

Occipitomastoid suture
External acoustic meatus
Occipital condyle
Styloid process
Condyle of mandible
Coronoid process of mandible
Body of mandible
Base of mandible
Mental foramen

**Fig. 8.** The skull. Left lateral view. The bones forming the cranium and facial skeleton are differentiated by color.

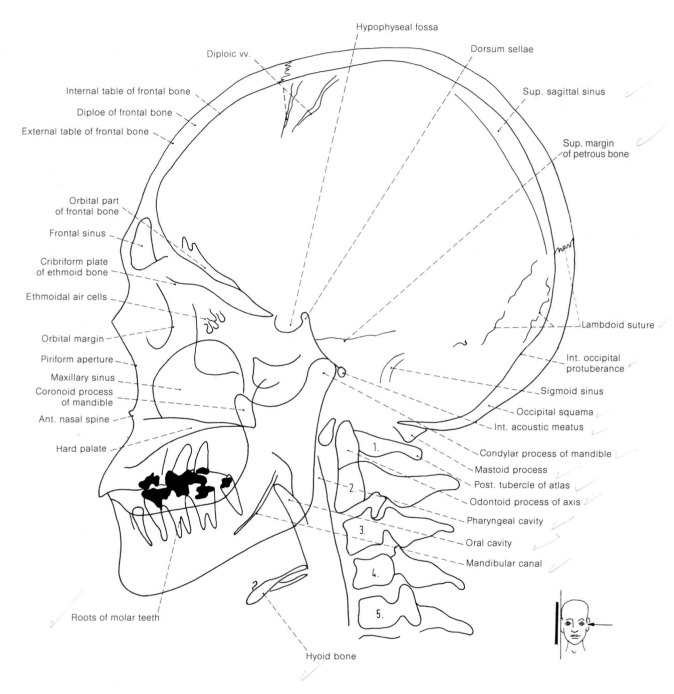

**Fig. 9.** Schematic explanation of the X-ray film on the facing page. (From L. WICKE: Atlas der Röntgenanatomie, 2nd ed. Urban & Schwarzenberg, Munich–Vienna–Baltimore 1980.) 1–5 = Cervical vertebrae

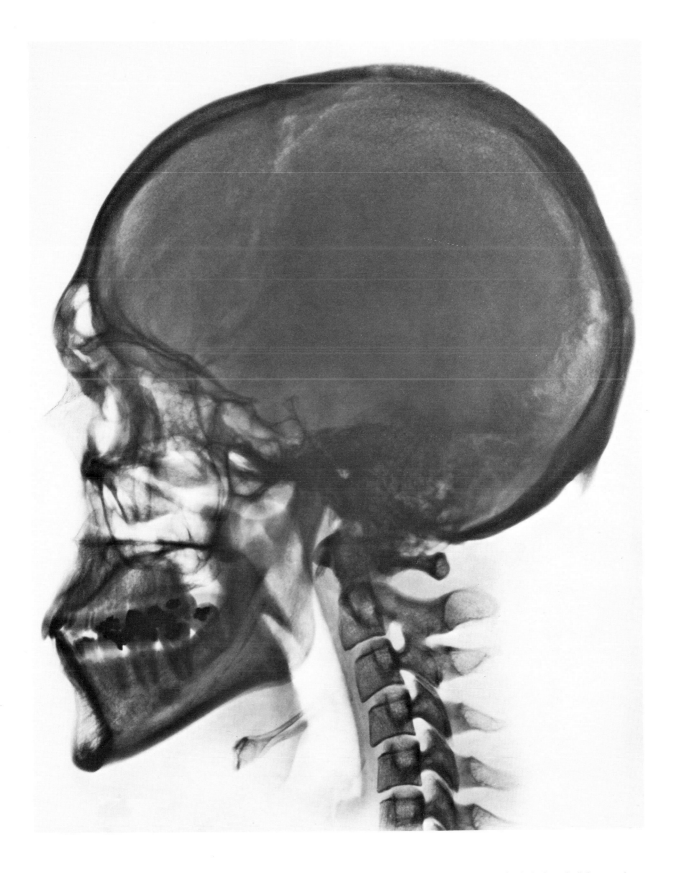

**Fig. 10.** X-ray film of the skull, lateral projection. (From L. WICKE: Atlas der Röntgenanatomie, 2nd ed. Urban & Schwarzenberg, Munich–Vienna–Baltimore 1980.)

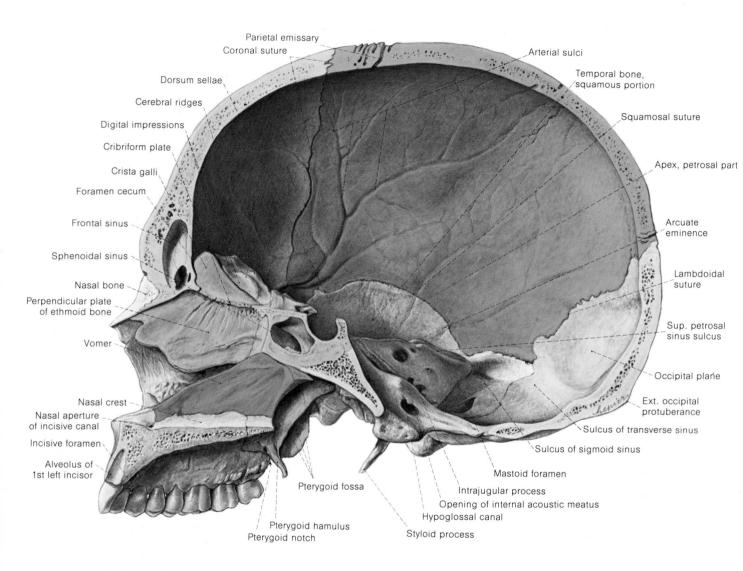

**Fig. 11.** Paramedian sagittal section through the human skull. The bones are differentiated by color.

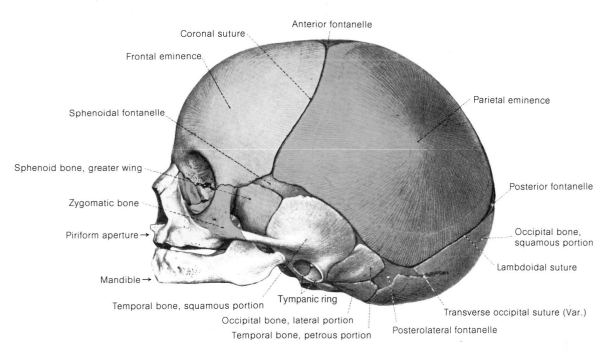

**Fig. 12.** Skull of a new-born, lateral view.

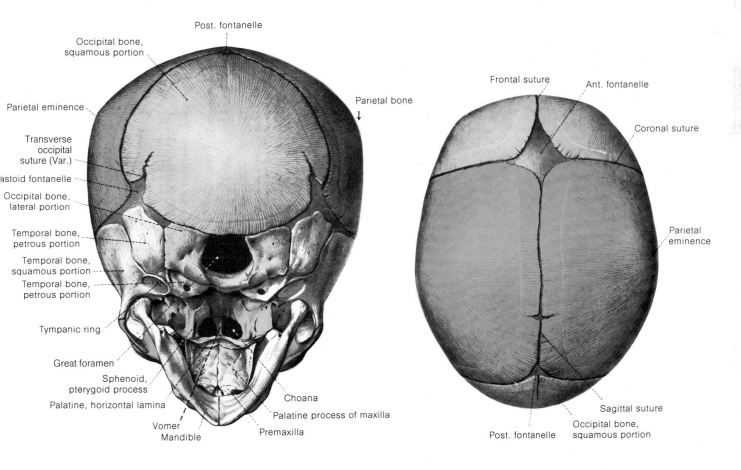

**Fig. 13.** Skull of a new-born. View from below. Base of the skull. **Fig. 14.** Skull of a new-born. View from above.

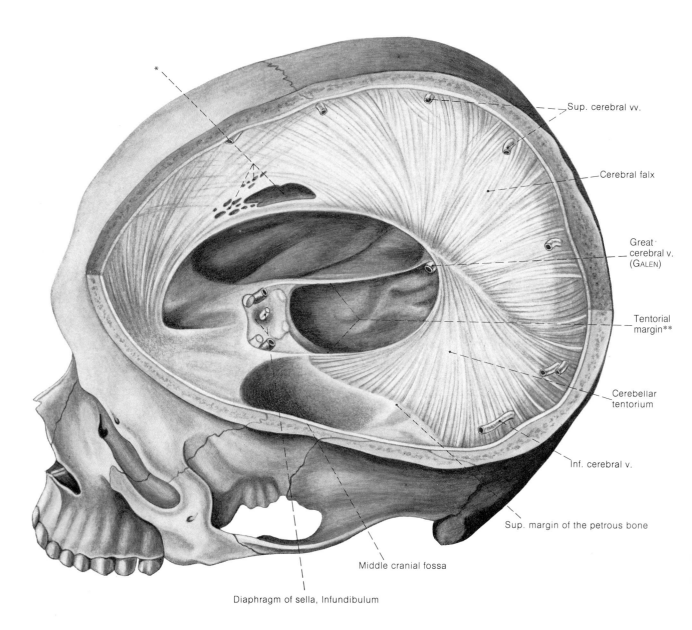

*

Sup. cerebral vv.

Cerebral falx

Great cerebral v. (GALEN)

Tentorial margin**

Cerebellar tentorium

Inf. cerebral v.

Sup. margin of the petrous bone

Middle cranial fossa

Diaphragm of sella, Infundibulum

**Fig. 15.** The major subdivisions of the neurocranial cavity by means of dural septa. Falx, tentorium. After removal of the brain the partition of the cranial cavity into three chambers is evident. Supratentorial space for the right and left cerebral hemispheres and infratentorial space for brain stem and cerebellum. The tentorial notch accommodates the midbrain and the cisterna ambiens. View from left and above (after FERNER/KAUTZKY: Angewandte Anatomie des Gehirns und seiner Hüllen. In Handbuch der Neurochirurgie I/1. Springer, Berlin–Göttingen–Heidelberg 1959). * = voids in the substance of the falx. ** = boundary of the tentorial notch.

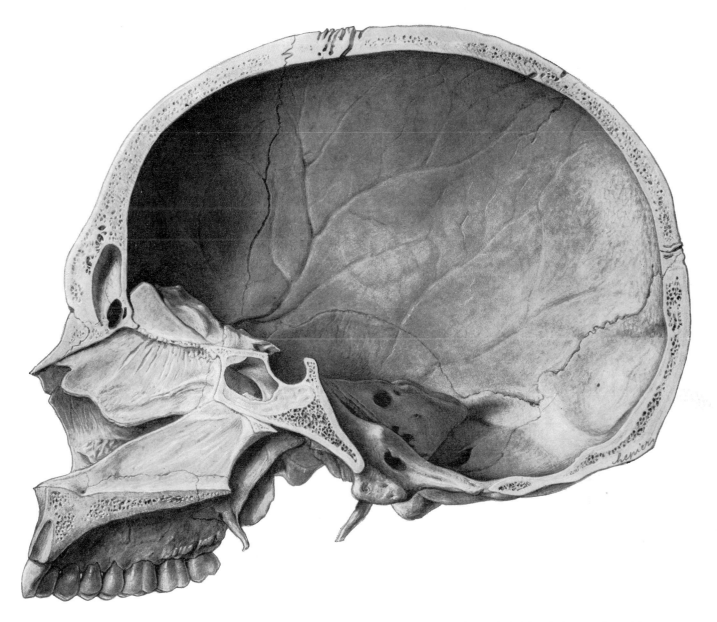

**Fig. 16.** The skull without the mandible. Right sagittal section with bony nasal septum. Note the arterial sulci at the inner surface of the bones in which the branches of the middle meningeal artery ascend between dura mater and bone. (Their injury leads to hemorrhage into the epidural space: epidural hematoma.)

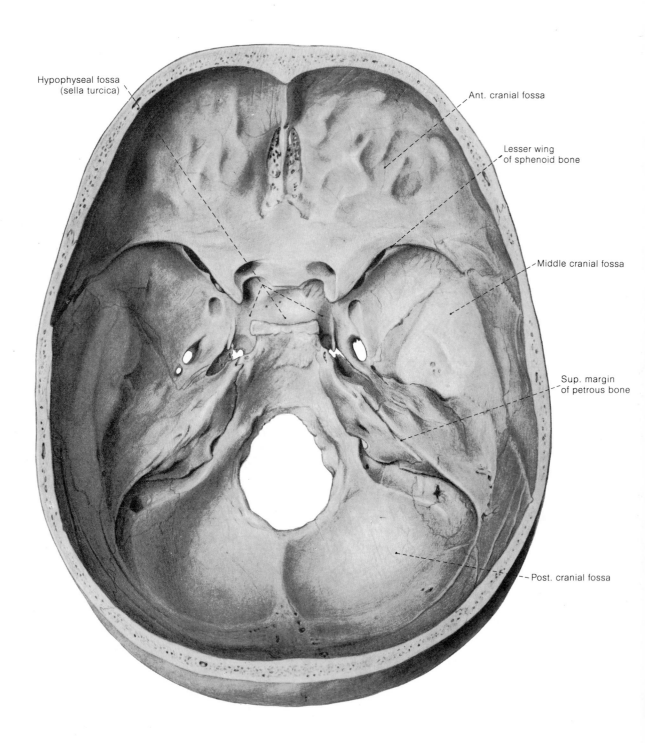

Hypophyseal fossa
(sella turcica)

Ant. cranial fossa

Lesser wing
of sphenoid bone

Middle cranial fossa

Sup. margin
of petrous bone

Post. cranial fossa

**Fig. 17.** The base of the skull. Inner (cerebral) surface.

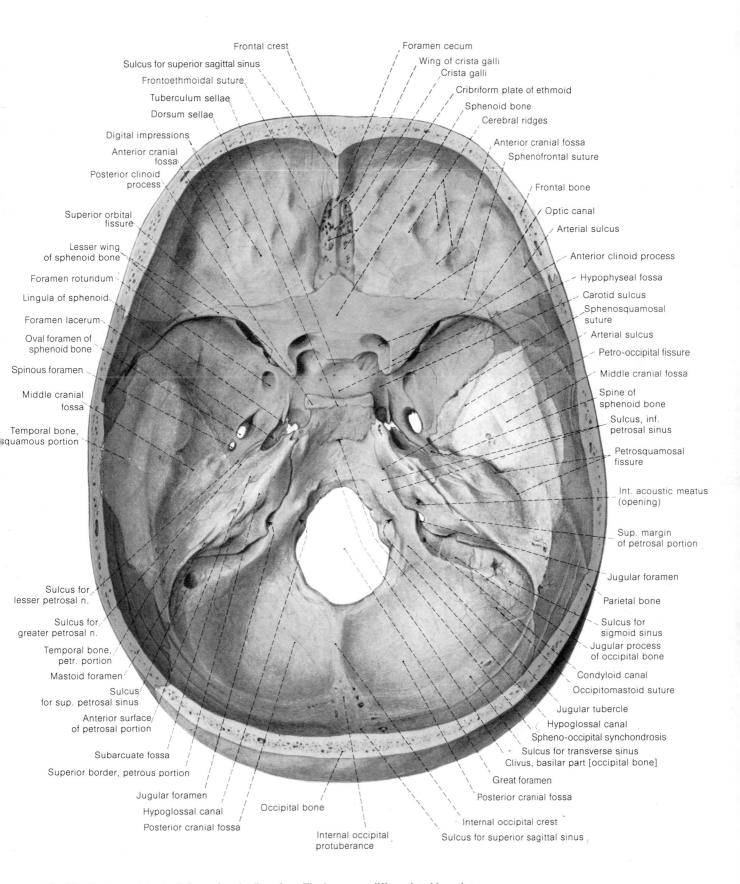

Frontal crest

Foramen cecum

Sulcus for superior sagittal sinus

Wing of crista galli

Crista galli

Frontoethmoidal suture

Cribriform plate of ethmoid

Tuberculum sellae

Sphenoid bone

Dorsum sellae

Cerebral ridges

Digital impressions

Anterior cranial fossa

Anterior cranial fossa

Sphenofrontal suture

Posterior clinoid process

Frontal bone

Optic canal

Superior orbital fissure

Arterial sulcus

Lesser wing of sphenoid bone

Anterior clinoid process

Foramen rotundum

Hypophyseal fossa

Lingula of sphenoid

Carotid sulcus

Foramen lacerum

Sphenosquamosal suture

Oval foramen of sphenoid bone

Arterial sulcus

Spinous foramen

Petro-occipital fissure

Middle cranial fossa

Temporal bone, squamous portion

Middle cranial fossa

Spine of sphenoid bone

Sulcus, inf. petrosal sinus

Petrosquamosal fissure

Int. acoustic meatus (opening)

Sulcus for lesser petrosal n.

Sup. margin of petrosal portion

Sulcus for greater petrosal n.

Jugular foramen

Temporal bone, petr. portion

Parietal bone

Mastoid foramen

Sulcus for sigmoid sinus

Sulcus for sup. petrosal sinus

Jugular process of occipital bone

Anterior surface of petrosal portion

Condyloid canal

Occipitomastoid suture

Subarcuate fossa

Jugular tubercle

Superior border, petrous portion

Hypoglossal canal

Spheno-occipital synchondrosis

Jugular foramen

Sulcus for transverse sinus

Hypoglossal canal

Clivus, basilar part [occipital bone]

Posterior cranial fossa

Great foramen

Occipital bone

Posterior cranial fossa

Internal occipital protuberance

Internal occipital crest

Sulcus for superior sagittal sinus

**Fig. 18.** The base of the skull. Inner (cerebral) surface. The bones are differentiated by color.

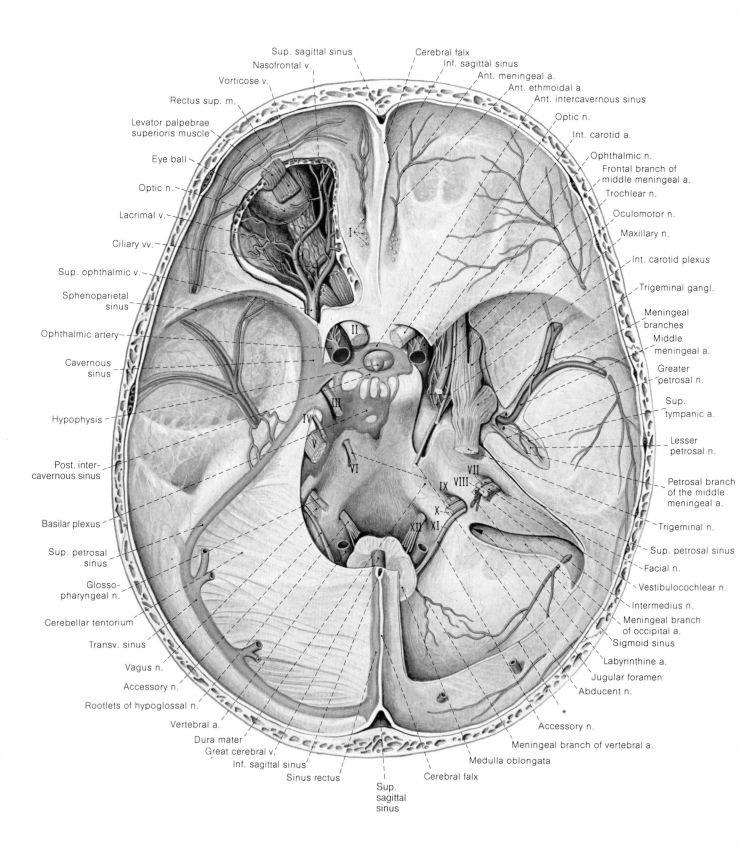

**Fig. 19.** Dura mater with its arteries and sinuses; arteries and veins of the orbit; cranial nerves (I–XII) in the floor of the cranial cavity existing through the dura mater. The roof of the left orbit is removed, sigmoid and cavernous sinus on the right side are opened, the right trigeminal ganglion and middle meningeal artery are exposed. Concerning the position of the internal carotid artery within the cavernous sinus compare Fig. 131. * cut edge of tentorium.

16

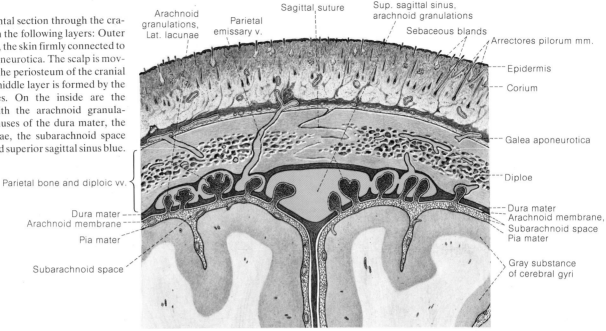

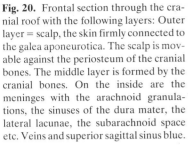

**Fig. 20.** Frontal section through the cranial roof with the following layers: Outer layer = scalp, the skin firmly connected to the galea aponeurotica. The scalp is movable against the periosteum of the cranial bones. The middle layer is formed by the cranial bones. On the inside are the meninges with the arachnoid granulations, the sinuses of the dura mater, the lateral lacunae, the subarachnoid space etc. Veins and superior sagittal sinus blue.

Arachnoid granulations, Lat. lacunae

Parietal emissary v.

Sagittal suture

Sup. sagittal sinus, arachnoid granulations

Sebaceous blands

Arrectores pilorum mm.

Epidermis

Corium

Galea aponeurotica

Diploe

Dura mater
Arachnoid membrane,
Subarachnoid space
Pia mater

Gray substance of cerebral gyri

Parietal bone and diploic vv.

Dura mater
Arachnoid membrane
Pia mater

Subarachnoid space

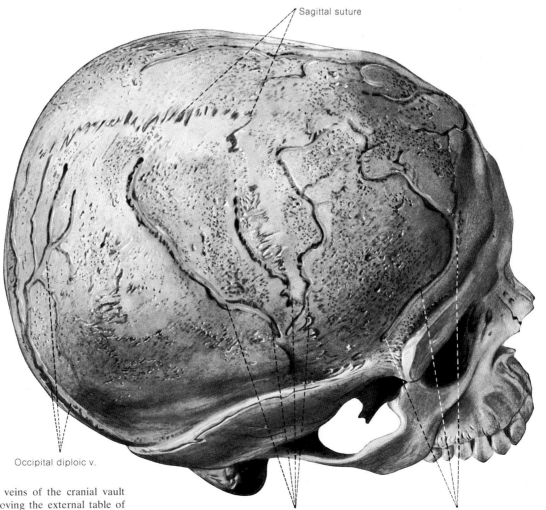

Sagittal suture

Occipital diploic v.

**Fig. 21.** Diploic veins of the cranial vault exposed by removing the external table of the flat cranial bones.

Ant. and post. temporal deploic vv.

Frontal diploic v.

17

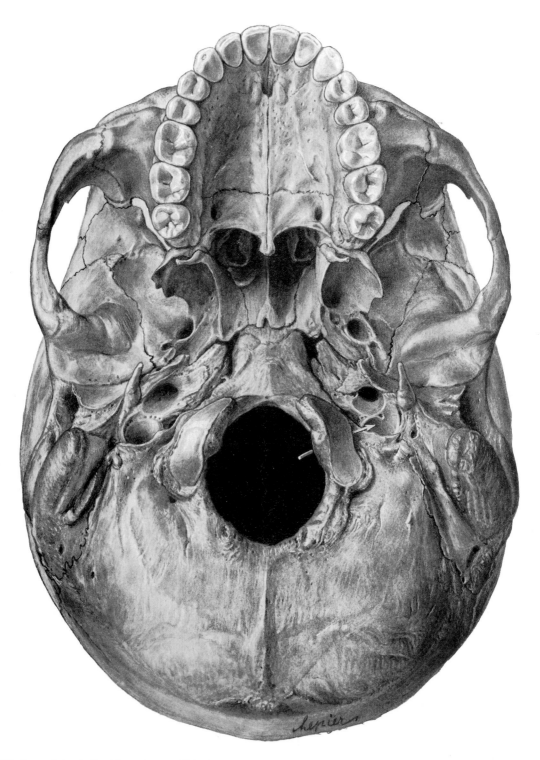

**Fig. 22.** The base of the skull, without the mandible, from below. Arrow in the hypoglossal canal.

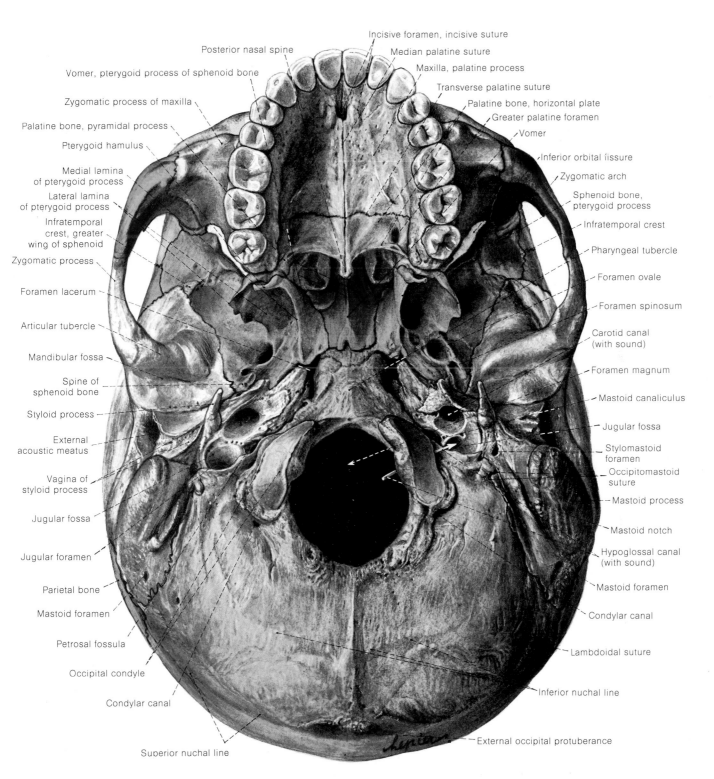

**Fig. 23.** The base of the skull, without the mandible. The visible bones of the neurocranium and the viscerocranium are differentiated by color.

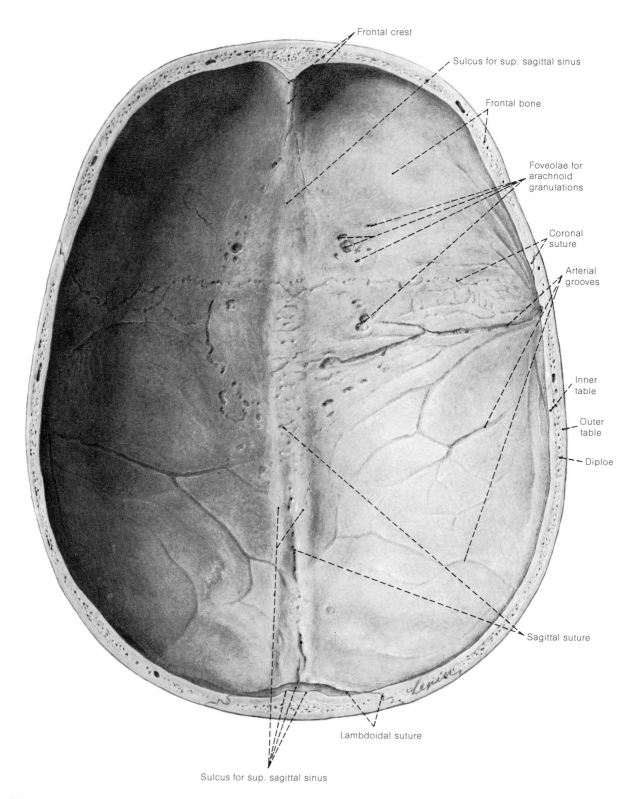

Frontal crest

Sulcus for sup. sagittal sinus

Frontal bone

Foveolae for arachnoid granulations

Coronal suture

Arterial grooves

Inner table

Outer table

Diploe

Sagittal suture

Lambdoidal suture

Sulcus for sup. sagittal sinus

**Fig. 24.** Interior view of the calvarium. Note the bony sulci for the branches of the middle meningeal artery, the foveae for the arachnoid granulations, the laminated construction of the cranial bones, and the ossification of the sutures.

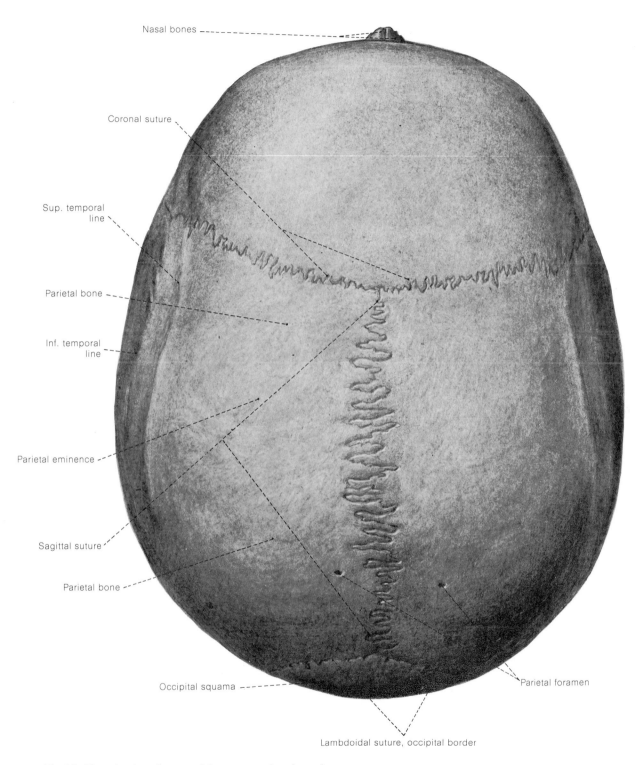

Nasal bones

Coronal suture

Sup. temporal line

Parietal bone

Inf. temporal line

Parietal eminence

Sagittal suture

Parietal bone

Occipital squama

Parietal foramen

Lambdoidal suture, occipital border

**Fig. 25.** The calvarium. Sutures of the neurocranium from above.

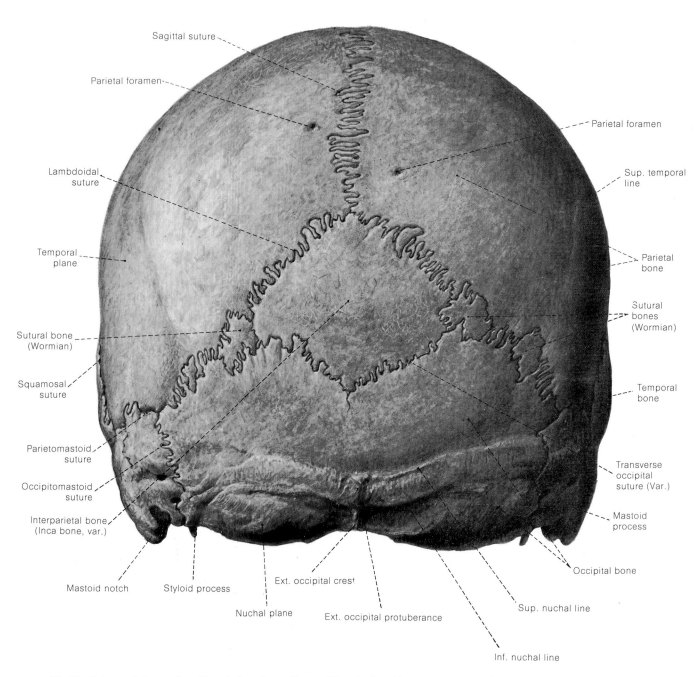

**Fig. 26.** Sutures of the cranium. Dorsal view. Sutural bones (Wormian) and interparietal bones (so-called Inca bone).

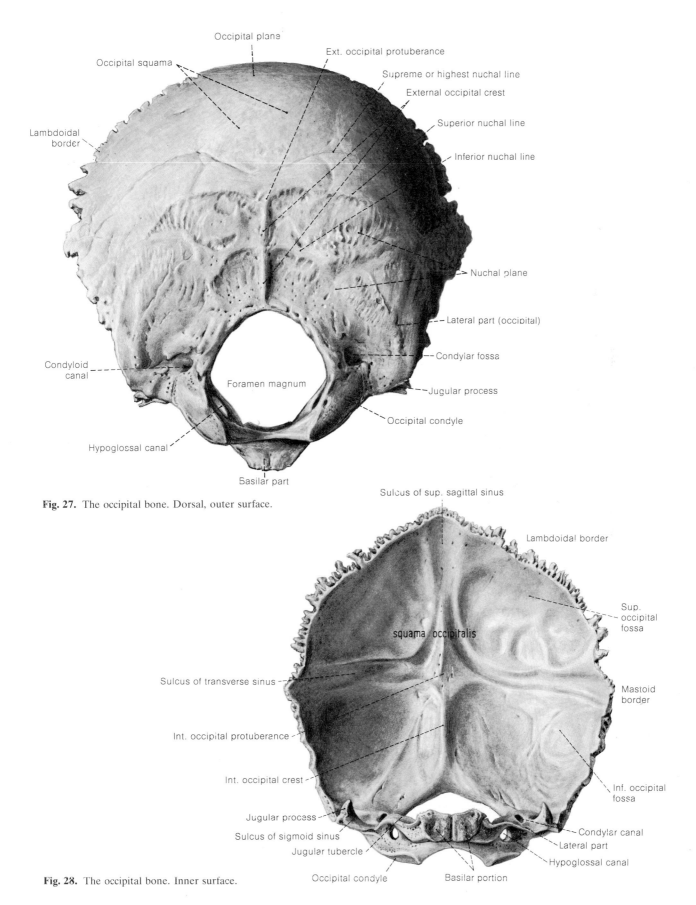

**Fig. 27.** The occipital bone. Dorsal, outer surface.

**Fig. 28.** The occipital bone. Inner surface.

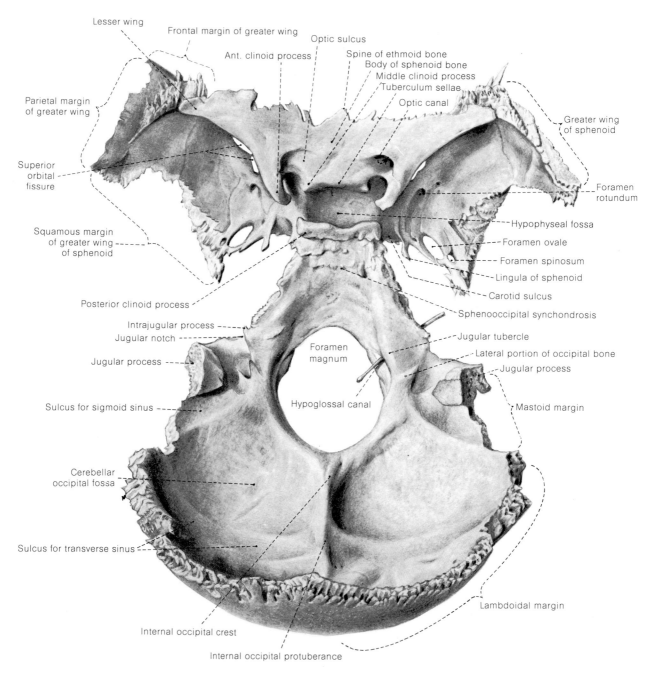

**Fig. 29.** Occipital and sphenoid bones. Seen from inside the skull. These are the bones of a growing youth, so the sphenooccipital synchondrosis is still present. The petrous part of the temporal bone in the space between the occipital and sphenoid bones is not shown.

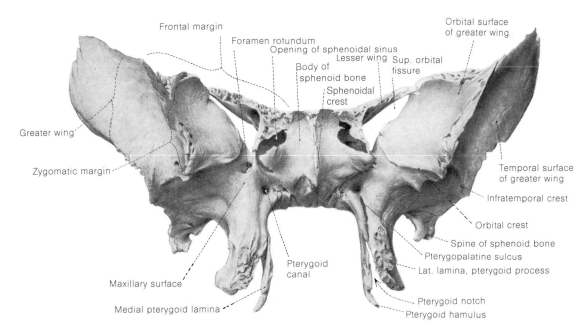

Frontal margin
Foramen rotundum
Opening of sphenoidal sinus
Lesser wing
Body of
sphenoid bone
Sphenoidal
crest
Sup. orbital
fissure
Orbital surface
of greater wing

Greater wing

Zygomatic margin

Temporal surface
of greater wing

Infratemporal crest

Orbital crest

Spine of sphenoid bone

Pterygopalatine sulcus

Lat. lamina, pterygoid process

Maxillary surface

Pterygoid
canal

Medial pterygoid lamina

Pterygoid notch
Pterygoid hamulus

**Fig. 30.** Sphenoid bone. Ventral view.

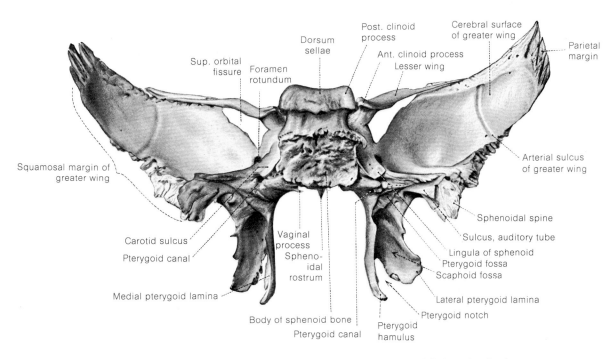

Dorsum
sellae
Post. clinoid
process
Cerebral surface
of greater wing
Parietal
margin

Sup. orbital
fissure
Foramen
rotundum
Ant. clinoid process
Lesser wing

Squamosal margin of
greater wing

Arterial sulcus
of greater wing

Sphenoidal spine

Carotid sulcus
Pterygoid canal

Vaginal
process
Spheno-
idal
rostrum

Sulcus, auditory tube

Lingula of sphenoid
Pterygoid fossa
Scaphoid fossa

Medial pterygoid lamina

Lateral pterygoid lamina
Pterygoid notch

Body of sphenoid bone

Pterygoid
hamulus

Pterygoid canal

**Fig. 31.** Sphenoid bone. Dorsal view. From a young person with an unossified sphenooccipital synchondrosis.

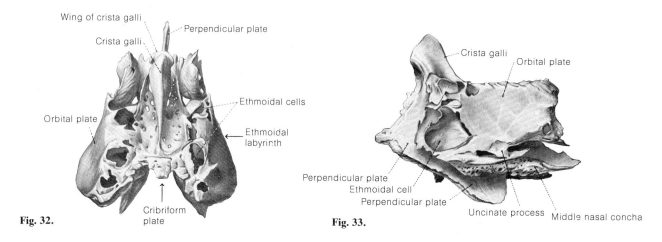

Wing of crista galli

Perpendicular plate

Crista galli

Orbital plate

Ethmoidal cells

Ethmoidal labyrinth

Cribriform plate

**Fig. 32.**

Crista galli

Orbital plate

Perpendicular plate

Ethmoidal cell

Perpendicular plate

Uncinate process

Middle nasal concha

**Fig. 33.**

**Figs. 32 and 33.** Ethmoid bone. Fig. 32 Cranial view; Fig. 33 Lateral view.

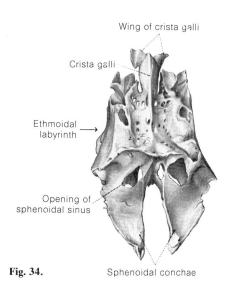

Wing of crista galli

Crista galli

Ethmoidal labyrinth

Opening of sphenoidal sinus

**Fig. 34.** Sphenoidal conchae

◁ **Fig. 34.** Ethmoid bone and sphenoidal conchae. From above and dorsal.

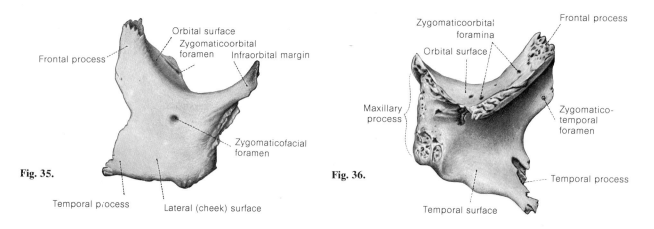

Orbital surface

Zygomaticoorbital foramen

Frontal process

Infraorbital margin

Frontal process

Zygomaticofacial foramen

**Fig. 35.**

Temporal process

Lateral (cheek) surface

Zygomaticoorbital foramina

Frontal process

Orbital surface

Maxillary process

Zygomatico-temporal foramen

**Fig. 36.**

Temporal process

Temporal surface

**Figs. 35 and 36.** Right zygomatic bone. Fig. 35 Lateral, external surface; Fig. 36 Medial, temporal surface.

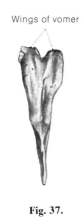

Wings of vomer

**Fig. 37.**

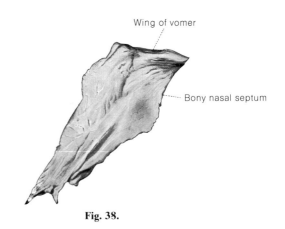

Wing of vomer

Bony nasal septum

**Fig. 38.**

**Figs. 37 and 38.** Vomer. Fig. 37 Dorsal view. Fig. 38 Lateral view.

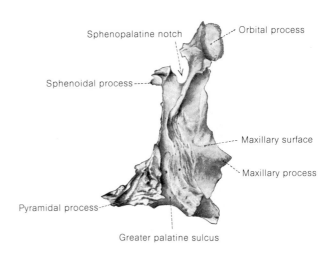

Sphenopalatine notch

Orbital process

Sphenoidal process

Maxillary surface

Maxillary process

Pyramidal process

Greater palatine sulcus

**Fig. 39.**

**Figs. 39–41.** Right palatine bone. Fig. 39 Lateral view. Fig. 40 Dorsal View. Fig. 41 Medial view.

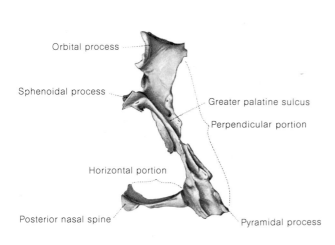

Orbital process

Sphenoidal process

Greater palatine sulcus

Perpendicular portion

Horizontal portion

Posterior nasal spine

Pyramidal process

**Fig. 40.**

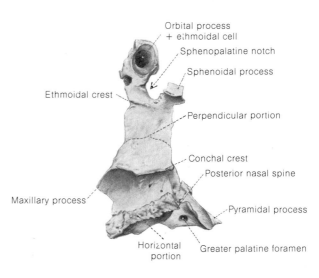

Orbital process + ethmoidal cell

Sphenopalatine notch

Sphenoidal process

Ethmoidal crest

Perpendicular portion

Conchal crest

Posterior nasal spine

Maxillary process

Pyramidal process

Greater palatine foramen

Horizontal portion

**Fig. 41.**

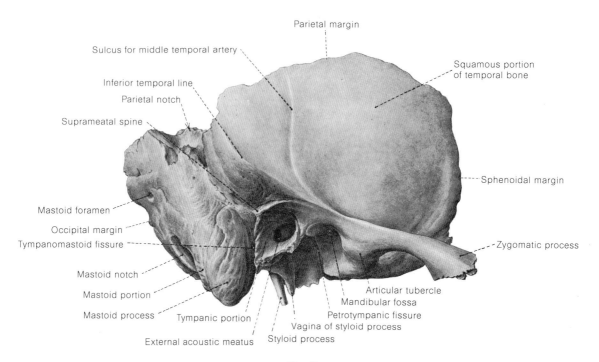

Parietal margin

Sulcus for middle temporal artery

Squamous portion of temporal bone

Inferior temporal line

Parietal notch

Suprameatal spine

Sphenoidal margin

Mastoid foramen

Occipital margin

Tympanomastoid fissure

Zygomatic process

Mastoid notch

Mastoid portion

Articular tubercle

Mandibular fossa

Mastoid process

Tympanic portion

Petrotympanic fissure

Vagina of styloid process

External acoustic meatus

Styloid process

**Fig. 42.**

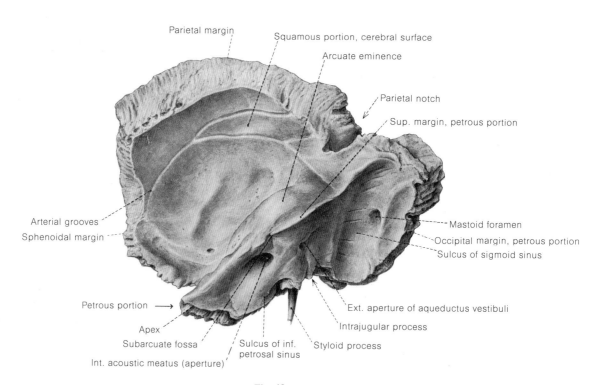

Parietal margin

Squamous portion, cerebral surface

Arcuate eminence

Parietal notch

Sup. margin, petrous portion

Arterial grooves

Sphenoidal margin

Mastoid foramen

Occipital margin, petrous portion

Sulcus of sigmoid sinus

Petrous portion →

Ext. aperture of aqueductus vestibuli

Apex

Intrajugular process

Subarcuate fossa

Sulcus of inf. petrosal sinus

Styloid process

Int. acoustic meatus (aperture)

**Fig. 43.**

**Figs. 42 and 43.** Right temporal bone. Fig. 42 Lateral view. Fig. 43 Medial view.

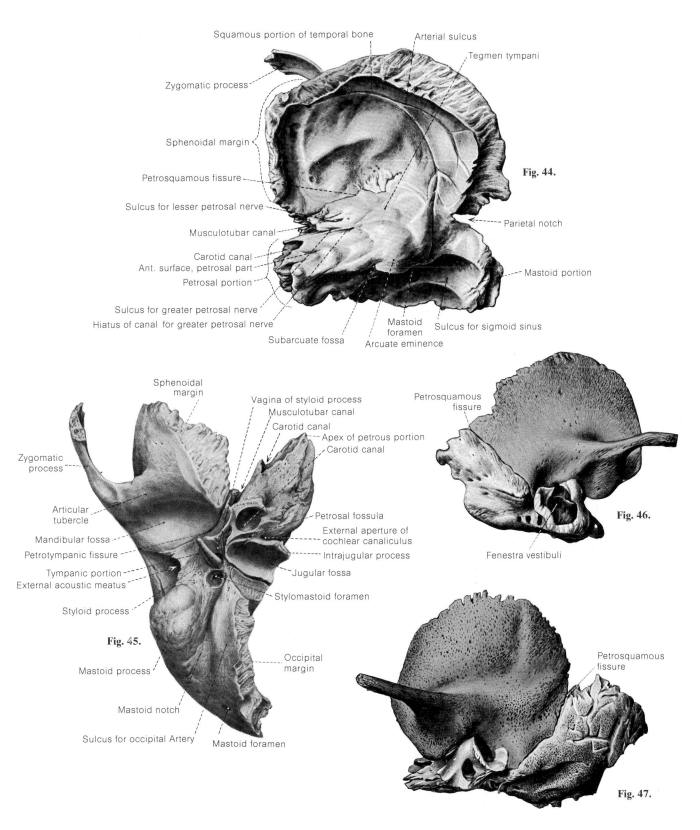

Squamous portion of temporal bone

Arterial sulcus

Tegmen tympani

Zygomatic process

Sphenoidal margin

Fig. 44.

Petrosquamous fissure

Sulcus for lesser petrosal nerve

Parietal notch

Musculotubar canal

Carotid canal
Ant. surface, petrosal part

Petrosal portion

Mastoid portion

Sulcus for greater petrosal nerve

Hiatus of canal for greater petrosal nerve

Mastoid
foramen

Sulcus for sigmoid sinus

Subarcuate fossa

Arcuate eminence

Sphenoidal
margin

Vagina of styloid process

Musculotubar canal

Carotid canal

Apex of petrous portion

Carotid canal

Petrosquamous
fissure

Zygomatic
process

Articular
tubercle

Mandibular fossa

Petrotympanic fissure

Tympanic portion

External acoustic meatus

Styloid process

Fig. 45.

Mastoid process

Occipital
margin

Mastoid notch

Sulcus for occipital Artery

Mastoid foramen

Petrosal fossula

External aperture of
cochlear canaliculus

Intrajugular process

Jugular fossa

Stylomastoid foramen

Petrosquamous
fissure

Fig. 46.

Fenestra vestibuli

Petrosquamous
fissure

Fig. 47.

**Fig. 44.** Right temporal bone. Inner surface. Head-on view of apex of petrous portion.
**Fig. 45.** Right temporal bone, seen from below.
**Figs. 46 and 47.** Right and left temporal bones of a new-born. Squamous portion, green; petrosal portion, yellow; tympanic portion, not colored.

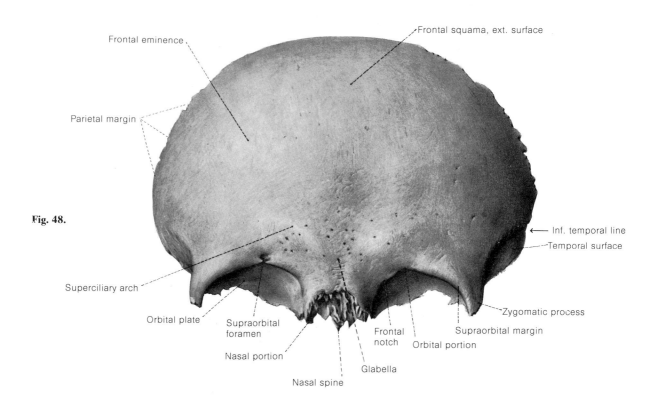

Frontal eminence

Frontal squama, ext. surface

Parietal margin

**Fig. 48.**

Inf. temporal line

Temporal surface

Superciliary arch

Orbital plate

Supraorbital foramen

Nasal portion

Frontal notch

Orbital portion

Zygomatic process

Supraorbital margin

Glabella

Nasal spine

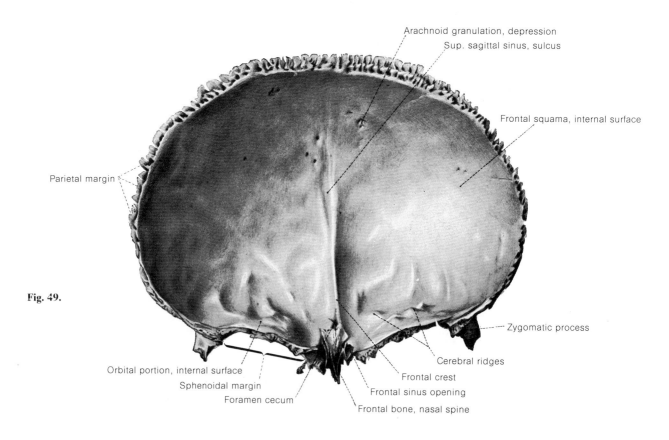

Arachnoid granulation, depression

Sup. sagittal sinus, sulcus

Frontal squama, internal surface

Parietal margin

**Fig. 49.**

Zygomatic process

Orbital portion, internal surface

Sphenoidal margin

Foramen cecum

Cerebral ridges

Frontal crest

Frontal sinus opening

Frontal bone, nasal spine

**Figs. 48 and 49.** Frontal bone. Fig. 48 Ventral or external view. Fig. 49 Dorsal or internal view.

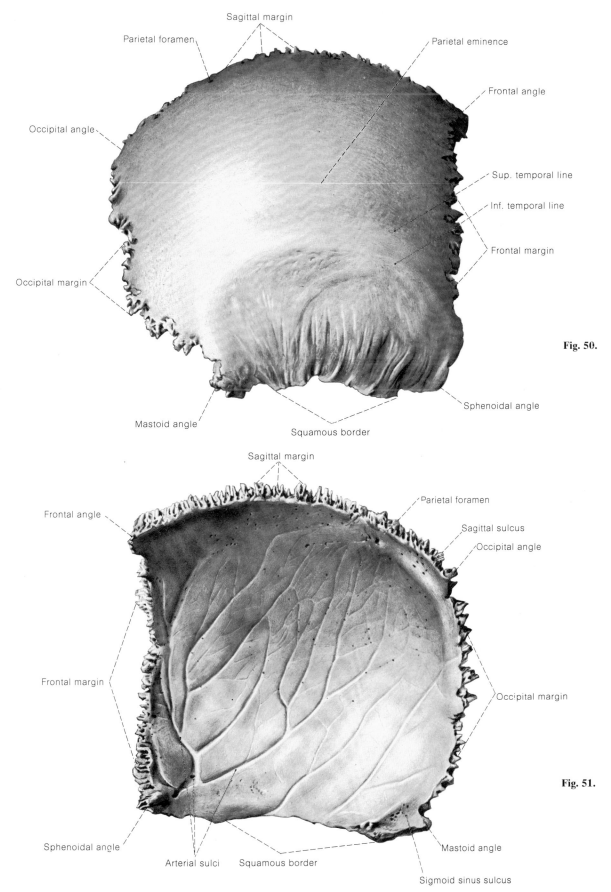

Figs. 50 and 51. Right parietal bone. Fig. 50 External view. Fig. 51 Internal view.

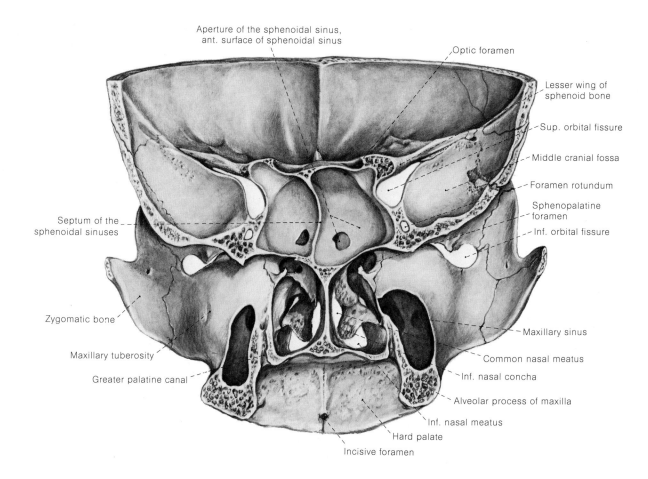

**Fig. 52.** Frontal section through the skull in the area of the sella turcica. Dorsal view.

# Brain, Meninges, Blood Vessels

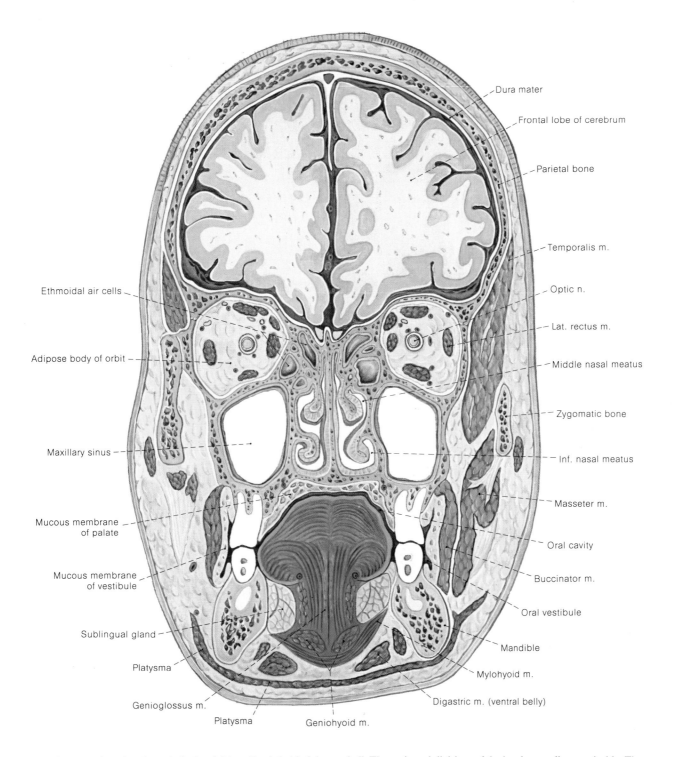

Dura mater

Frontal lobe of cerebrum

Parietal bone

Temporalis m.

Optic n.

Lat. rectus m.

Middle nasal meatus

Zygomatic bone

Inf. nasal meatus

Masseter m.

Oral cavity

Buccinator m.

Oral vestibule

Mandible

Mylohyoid m.

Digastric m. (ventral belly)

Ethmoidal air cells

Adipose body of orbit

Maxillary sinus

Mucous membrane of palate

Mucous membrane of vestibule

Sublingual gland

Platysma

Genioglossus m.

Platysma

Geniohyoid m.

**Fig. 53.** Frontal section through the head, immediately behind the eye ball. The major subdivisions of the head are well recognizable. The upper third represents the neurocranium containing the brain. The middle third contains the paired nasal cavity with the ethmoidal cells, the orbits and the maxillary sinuses. The lower third, separated by the palate from the nasal cavity, contains the oral cavity with the tongue and the sublingual region with the sublingual gland. The border toward the neck is formed by the plate-like mylohyoid muscle (oral diaphragm).

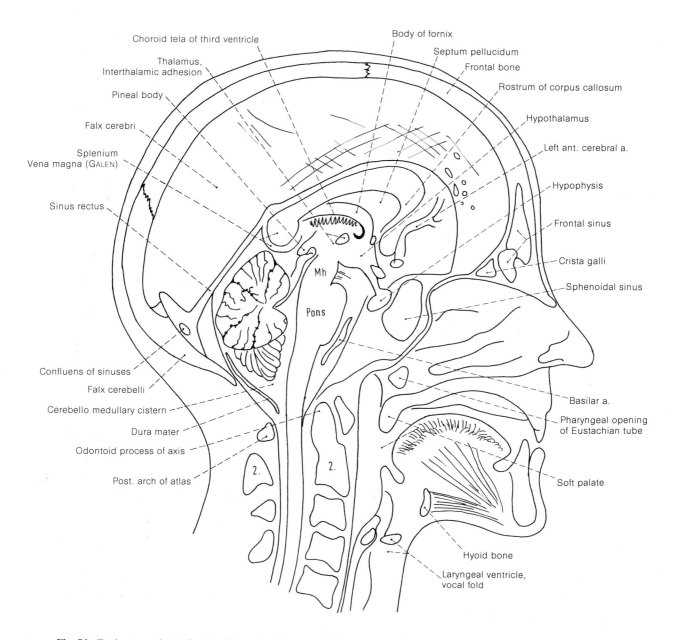

Choroid tela of third ventricle

Thalamus,
Interthalamic adhesion

Pineal body

Falx cerebri

Splenium
Vena magna (GALEN)

Sinus rectus

Body of fornix

Septum pellucidum

Frontal bone

Rostrum of corpus callosum

Hypothalamus

Left ant. cerebral a.

Hypophysis

Frontal sinus

Crista galli

Sphenoidal sinus

Mh

Pons

Confluens of sinuses

Falx cerebelli

Cerebello medullary cistern

Dura mater

Odontoid process of axis

Post. arch of atlas

2.

2.

Basilar a.

Pharyngeal opening
of Eustachian tube

Soft palate

Hyoid bone

Laryngeal ventricle,
vocal fold

**Fig. 54.** Explanatory sketch for Fig. 55 on the facing page. Mh = mesencephalon.

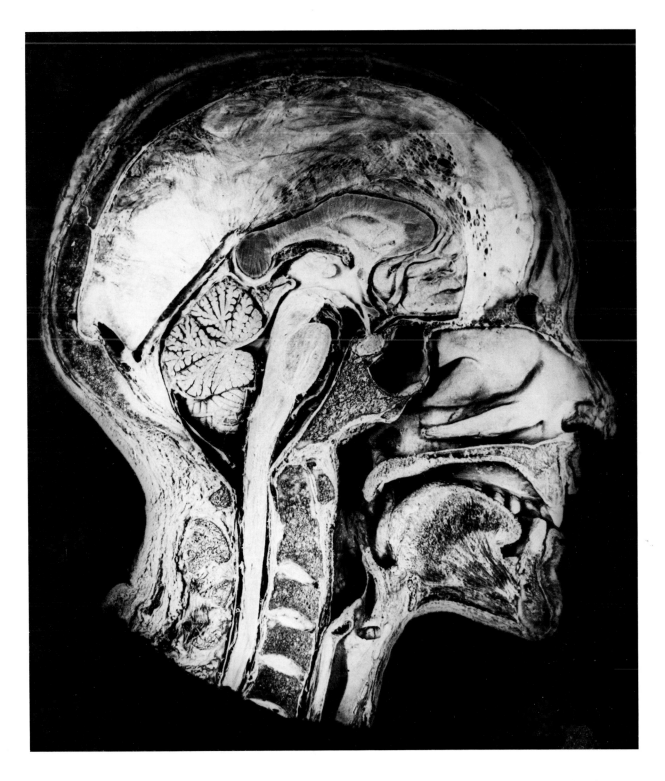

**Fig. 55.** Median sagittal section through the head of a 50-year-old woman (reduced to ⁴/₅). Neurocranium and viscerocranium. (Specimen from the collection of the Anatomical Institute Vienna, Prof. HOCHSTETTER.)

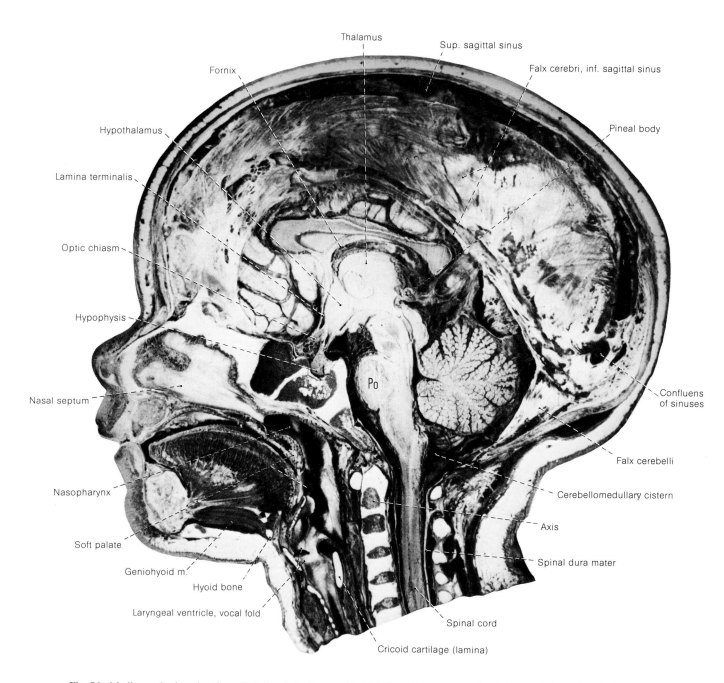

**Fig. 56.** Median sagittal section through the head of a 3-year-old child. Note: the upper margin of the pons is located at the level of the dorsum sellae; the corpus callosum, especially the body, is still small. Infundibulum and hypophyseal stalk are positioned almost vertically downward, without pronounced bend. In many bones, only larger or smaller ossification centers are developed, otherwise they are still cartilaginous. The pneumatization of the sphenoid bone is still in an initial stage, the cartilaginous sphenooccipital synchondrosis is still broad (specimen by Prof. HOCHSTETTER, Vienna). Po = pons.

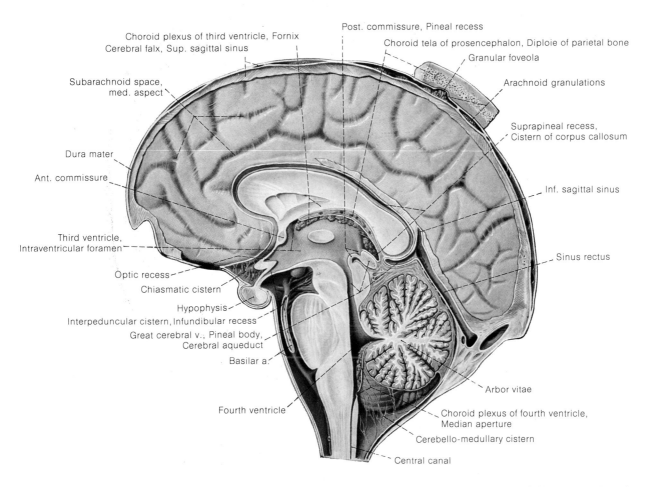

Choroid plexus of third ventricle, Fornix
Cerebral falx, Sup. sagittal sinus
Post. commissure, Pineal recess
Choroid tela of prosencephalon, Diploie of parietal bone
Granular foveola
Arachnoid granulations
Subarachnoid space, med. aspect
Suprapineal recess, Cistern of corpus callosum
Dura mater
Inf. sagittal sinus
Ant. commissure
Third ventricle, Intraventricular foramen
Sinus rectus
Optic recess
Chiasmatic cistern
Hypophysis
Interpeduncular cistern, Infundibular recess
Great cerebral v., Pineal body, Cerebral aqueduct
Basilar a.
Arbor vitae
Fourth ventricle
Choroid plexus of fourth ventricle, Median aperture
Cerebello-medullary cistern
Central canal

**Fig. 57.** Paramedian section through the neurocranium. Situs of the brain in the cranial cavity. The cerebrospinal fluid spaces are shown in blue. (From PERNKOPF: Atlas der topographischen und angewandten Anatomie des Menschen, Vol. 1, 2nd ed. [Ed. H. FERNER]. Urban & Schwarzenberg, Munich–Vienna–Baltimore 1980.)

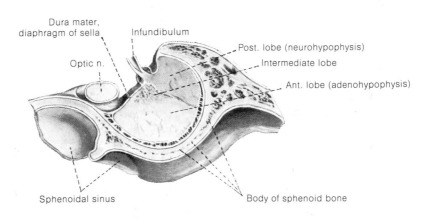

Dura mater, diaphragm of sella
Infundibulum
Post. lobe (neurohypophysis)
Intermediate lobe
Optic n.
Ant. lobe (adenohypophysis)
Sphenoidal sinus
Body of sphenoid bone

**Fig. 58.** Median section through the hypophysis. Situs of the hypophysis in the sella turcica.

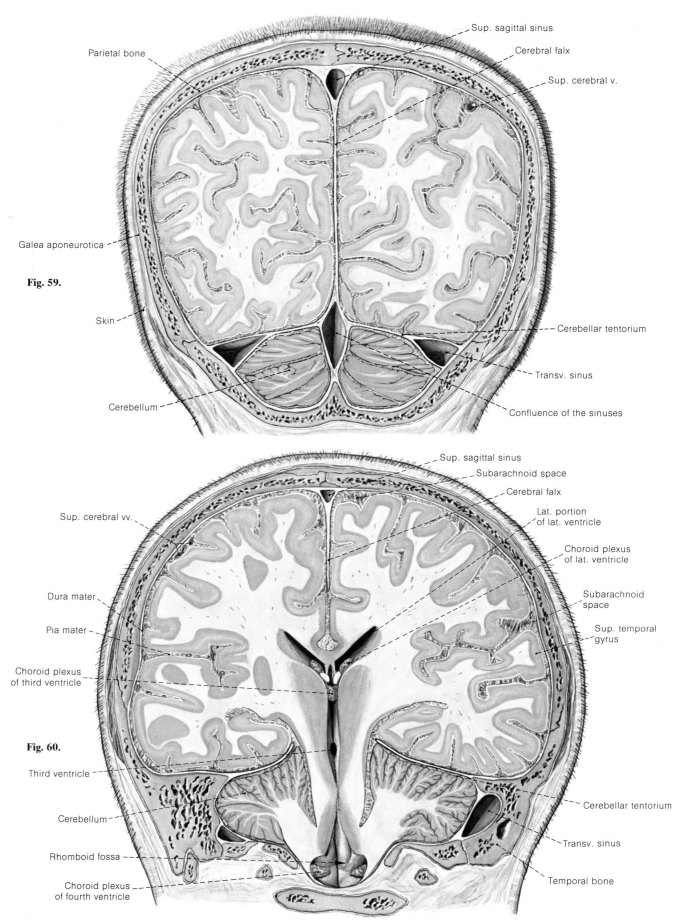

Parietal bone

Sup. sagittal sinus

Cerebral falx

Sup. cerebral v.

Galea aponeurotica

**Fig. 59.**

Skin

Cerebellar tentorium

Transv. sinus

Cerebellum

Confluence of the sinuses

Sup. sagittal sinus

Subarachnoid space

Cerebral falx

Sup. cerebral vv.

Lat. portion of lat. ventricle

Choroid plexus of lat. ventricle

Dura mater

Subarachnoid space

Pia mater

Sup. temporal gyrus

Choroid plexus of third ventricle

**Fig. 60.**

Third ventricle

Cerebellum

Cerebellar tentorium

Rhomboid fossa

Transv. sinus

Choroid plexus of fourth ventricle

Temporal bone

◁ **Fig. 59.** Frontal section through the neurocranium at the plane of the confluens of the sinuses. Color key as in Fig. 60.

**Fig. 60.** Frontal section through the neurocranium at the plane of the third ventricle. Dura mater white, arachnoid membrane and pia mater red, contents of sinuses and veins blue.

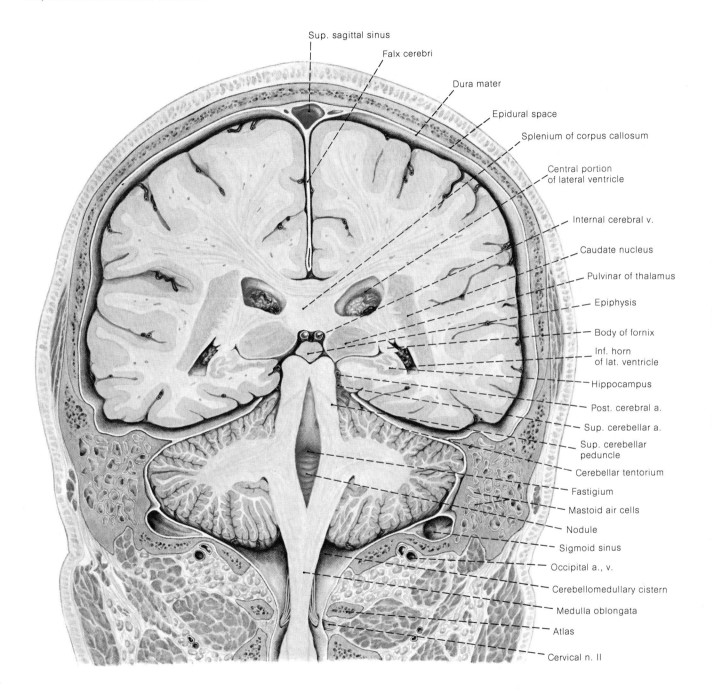

Sup. sagittal sinus

Falx cerebri

Dura mater

Epidural space

Splenium of corpus callosum

Central portion of lateral ventricle

Internal cerebral v.

Caudate nucleus

Pulvinar of thalamus

Epiphysis

Body of fornix

Inf. horn of lat. ventricle

Hippocampus

Post. cerebral a.

Sup. cerebellar a.

Sup. cerebellar peduncle

Cerebellar tentorium

Fastigium

Mastoid air cells

Nodule

Sigmoid sinus

Occipital a., v.

Cerebellomedullary cistern

Medulla oblongata

Atlas

Cervical n. II

**Fig. 61.** Frontal section through the neurocranium, Dural septa. Cerebrum above the cerebellar tentorium within the supratentorial space. Rhombencephalon (cerebellum, pons and medulla oblongata) in the infratentorial space. The dural septa (falx cerebri and cerebellar tentorium) prevent coarse mass movements of the soft central nervous substance in transverse and vertical directions. Pressure differences may cause herniations of parts of the cerebrum into the tentorial notch, e.g., parahippocampal gyrus, splenium of corpus callosum etc. The cerebellar tonsils may be forced into the foramen magnum. Note the triangular contour of the superior sagittal sinus and its relation to the inner periosteum and dura mater proper. The dural sinuses are incompressible and non-contractible because they possess no muscular tissue in their walls. The sigmoid sinus is protected from compression by its position well within the bony substance of the petrous portion of the temporal bone. (From PERNKOPF: Atlas der topographischen und angewandten Anatomie des Menschen, Vol. 1, 2nd ed. [Ed. H. FERNER]. Urban & Schwarzenberg, Munich–Vienna–Baltimore 1980.)

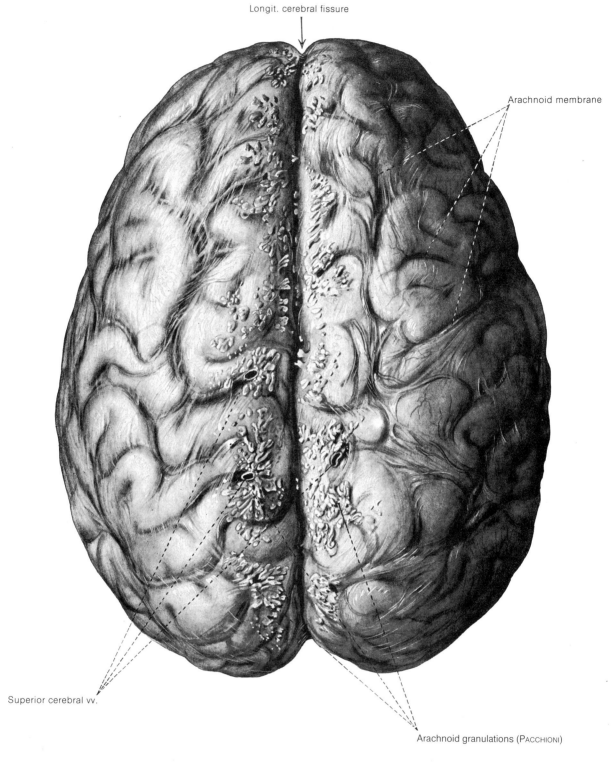

Longit. cerebral fissure

Arachnoid membrane

Superior cerebral vv.

Arachnoid granulations (PACCHIONI)

**Fig. 62.** Telencephalon with leptomeninges seen from above. The large superior cerebral veins are located within the subarachnoid space.

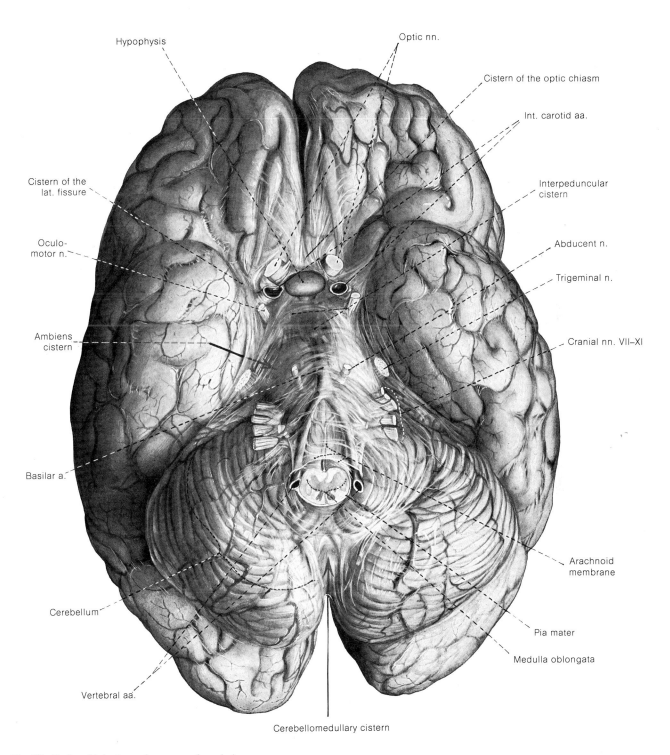

Hypophysis

Optic nn.

Cistern of the optic chiasm

Int. carotid aa.

Cistern of the lat. fissure

Interpeduncular cistern

Oculo-motor n.

Abducent n.

Trigeminal n.

Ambiens cistern

Cranial nn. VII–XI

Basilar a.

Arachnoid membrane

Cerebellum

Pia mater

Vertebral aa.

Medulla oblongata

Cerebellomedullary cistern

**Fig. 63.** Brain with leptomeninges seen from below.

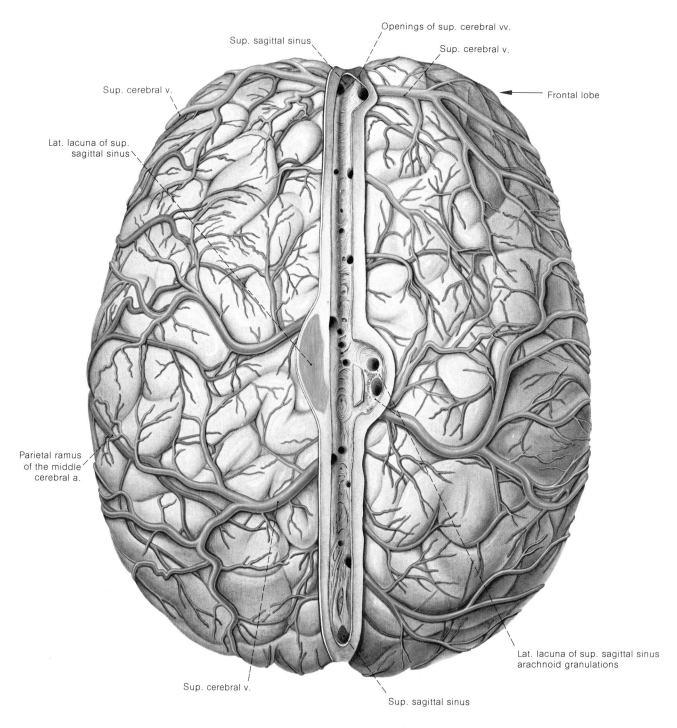

Openings of sup. cerebral vv.

Sup. sagittal sinus

Sup. cerebral v.

Sup. cerebral v.

Frontal lobe

Lat. lacuna of sup.
sagittal sinus

Parietal ramus
of the middle
cerebral a.

Lat. lacuna of sup. sagittal sinus
arachnoid granulations

Sup. cerebral v.

Sup. sagittal sinus

**Fig. 64.** Superior sagittal sinus, lateral lacunae, veins and arteries of the brain seen from above. A strip of dura mater has been maintained alongside the superior sagittal sinus, the sinus itself as well as a lateral lacuna on the right side have been opened. The branches of the middle cerebral artery ascend along the convexity of the brain but do not reach the crest of the pallium. Here, the terminal branches of the anterior cerebral artery extend beyond the pallial crest to the convexity. The superior cerebral veins empty into the superior sagittal sinus and its lateral lacunae.

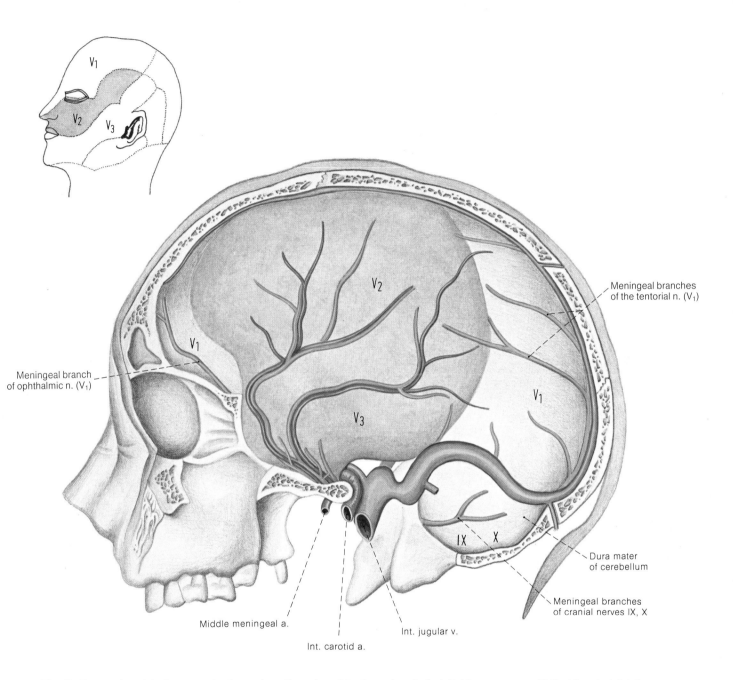

**Fig. 65.** Innervation of the dura mater by the meningeal branches of the three trigeminal subdivisions; compare with the trigeminal distribution to the cutaneous areas of the face. The meningeal branches of $V_2$ and $V_3$ accompany the branches of the middle meningeal artery. Nevi vasculosi of the face are associated by analogous vascular anomalies in corresponding areas of the meninges (STURGE-WEBER syndrome). (After Prof. KAUTZKY, Hamburg.)

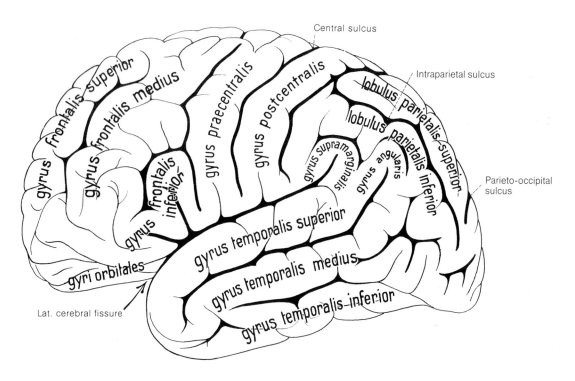

**Fig. 66.** Sulci and gyri of the pallium. Lateral view.

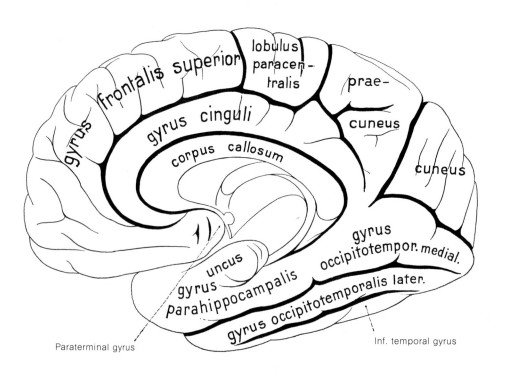

**Fig. 67.** Sulci and gyri of the pallium. Medial view. The brain is halved in the median plane. The brain stem together with the cerebellum has been removed by an oblique section through the thalamus.

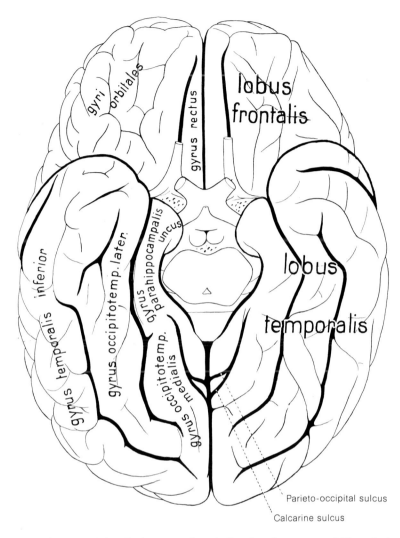

**Fig. 68.** Sulci and gyri of the pallium. Basal view. Brain stem and cerebellum have been removed. Hypophysis, olfactory tracts and optic nerves have been sectioned.

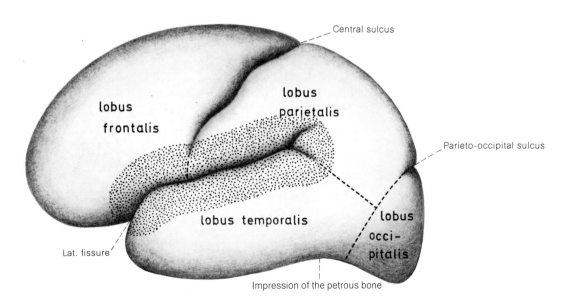

**Fig. 69.** The lobes of the telencephalon. The region of the frontal, frontoparietal and temporal opercula is shown by stippling.

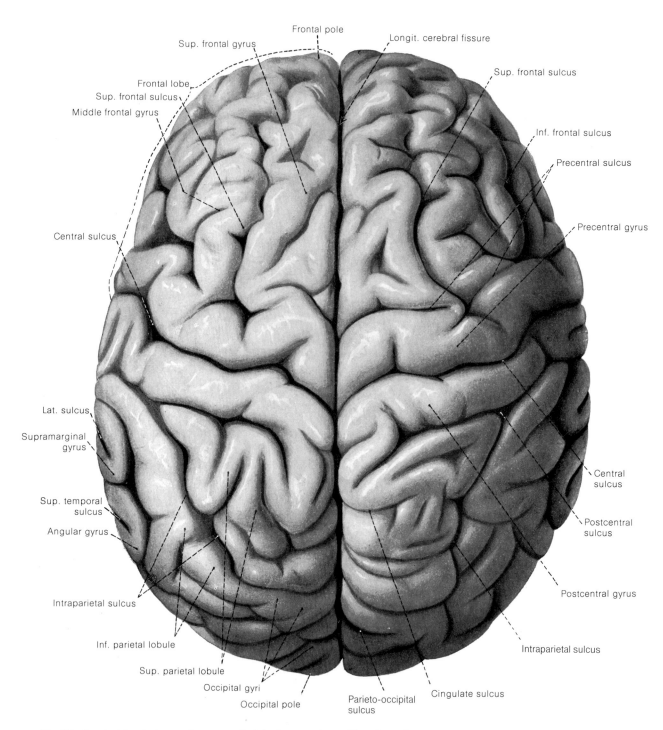

**Fig. 70.** Cerebral hemispheres after removal of the leptomeninges. View from above.

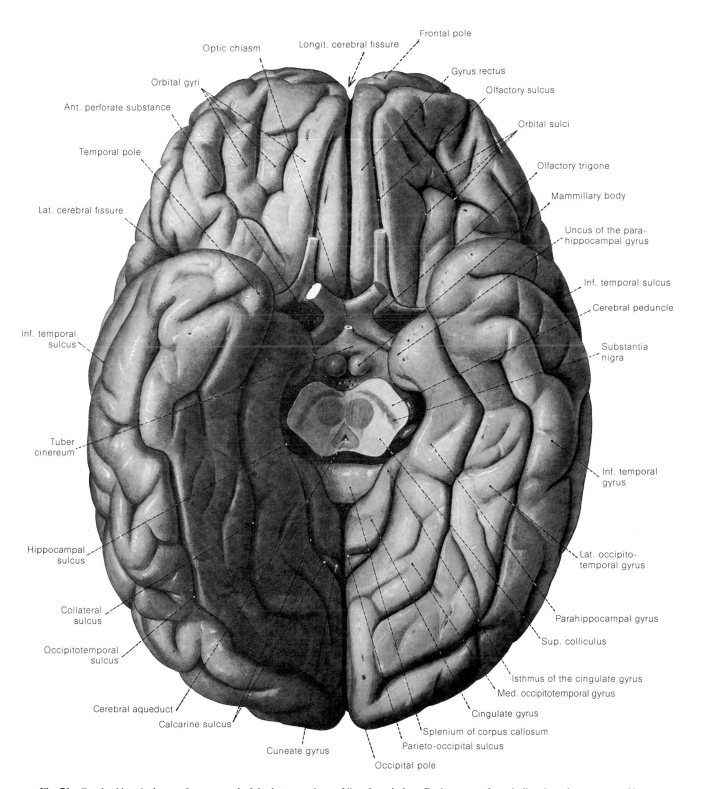

Optic chiasm

Longit. cerebral fissure

Frontal pole

Gyrus rectus

Orbital gyri

Olfactory sulcus

Ant. perforate substance

Orbital sulci

Temporal pole

Olfactory trigone

Mammillary body

Lat. cerebral fissure

Uncus of the para-hippocampal gyrus

Inf. temporal sulcus

Cerebral peduncle

Inf. temporal sulcus

Substantia nigra

Tuber cinereum

Inf. temporal gyrus

Hippocampal sulcus

Lat. occipito-temporal gyrus

Collateral sulcus

Parahippocampal gyrus

Occipitotemporal sulcus

Sup. colliculus

Isthmus of the cingulate gyrus

Cerebral aqueduct

Med. occipitotemporal gyrus

Calcarine sulcus

Cingulate gyrus

Splenium of corpus callosum

Cuneate gyrus

Parieto-occipital sulcus

Occipital pole

**Fig. 71.** Cerebral hemispheres after removal of the leptomeninges. View from below. Brain stem and cerebellum have been removed by a cross section through the midbrain. The section through the midbrain reveals the red nucleus on both sides under the substantia nigra.

47

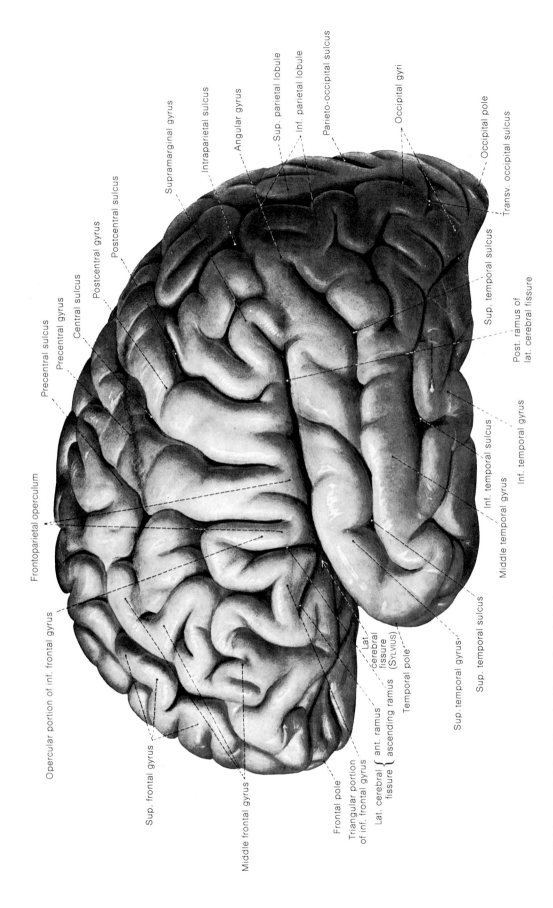

**Fig. 72.** Sulci and gyri of the left cerebral hemisphere. Lateral view.

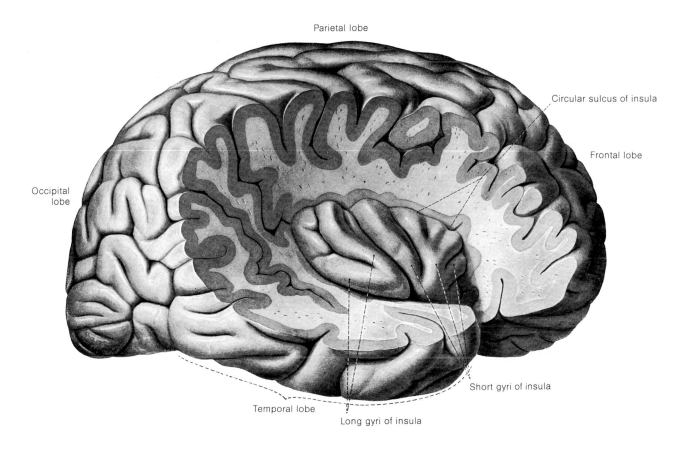

Parietal lobe

Circular sulcus of insula

Frontal lobe

Occipital lobe

Short gyri of insula

Temporal lobe

Long gyri of insula

**Fig. 73.** Right hemisphere. Lateral view. The insula is brought into view by removing the frontal, frontoparietal and temporal opercular portions.

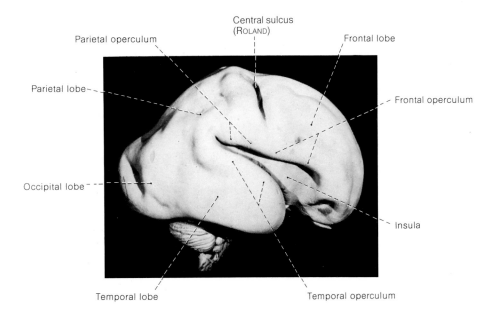

Parietal operculum

Central sulcus (ROLAND)

Frontal lobe

Parietal lobe

Frontal operculum

Occipital lobe

Insula

Temporal lobe

Temporal operculum

**Fig. 74.** Brain of a human fetus of 20 cm Crown-Rump-Length (CRL), natural size (Collection HOCHSTETTER); fronto-occipital diameter = 7 cm. Gyri have not yet developed, only the primary sulci are formed: central sulcus and lateral fissure. The opercula do not yet cover the insular cortex. In the depth of the lateral fissure one observes the as yet smooth insular cortex without gyri and sulci.

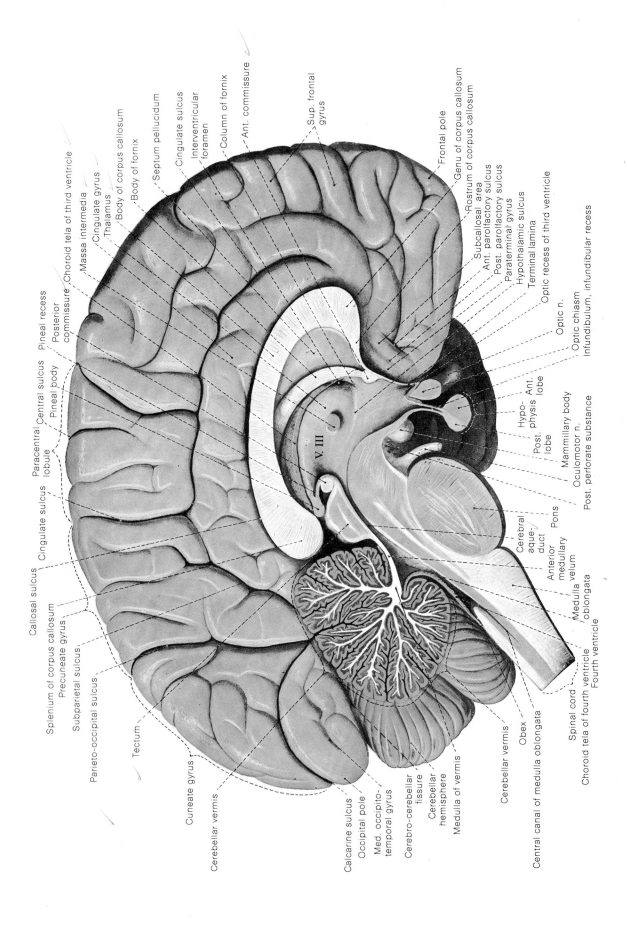

**Fig. 75.** Sagittal section through the brain. Medial aspect of the left half of the brain. V. III = third ventricle.

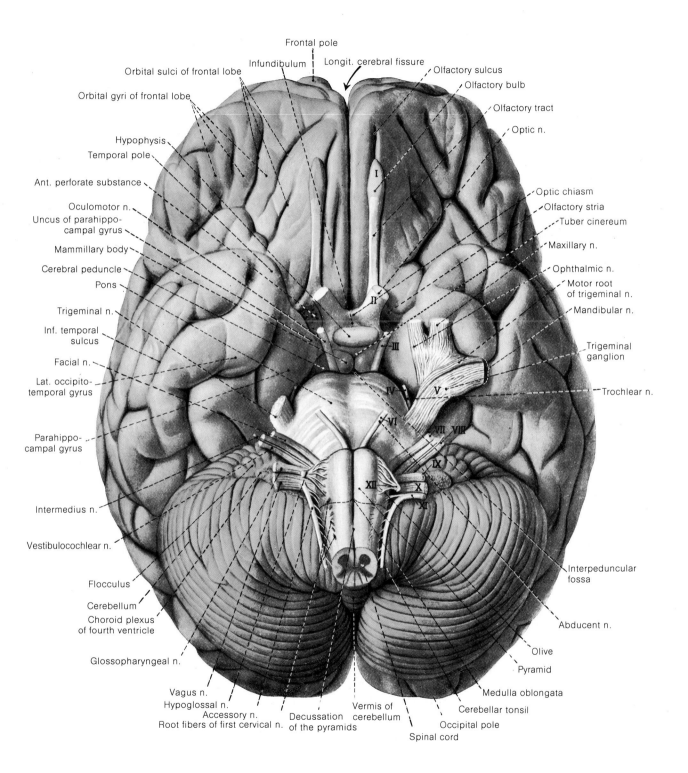

Frontal pole

Infundibulum

Longit. cerebral fissure

Orbital sulci of frontal lobe

Orbital gyri of frontal lobe

Olfactory sulcus

Olfactory bulb

Olfactory tract

Optic n.

Hypophysis

Temporal pole

Ant. perforate substance

Oculomotor n.

Uncus of parahippo-
campal gyrus

Mammillary body

Cerebral peduncle

Pons

Trigeminal n.

Inf. temporal
sulcus

Facial n.

Lat. occipito-
temporal gyrus

Parahippo-
campal gyrus

Intermedius n.

Vestibulocochlear n.

Flocculus

Cerebellum

Choroid plexus
of fourth ventricle

Glossopharyngeal n.

Vagus n.

Hypoglossal n.

Accessory n.

Root fibers of first cervical n.

Decussation
of the pyramids

Vermis of
cerebellum

Optic chiasm

Olfactory stria

Tuber cinereum

Maxillary n.

Ophthalmic n.

Motor root
of trigeminal n.

Mandibular n.

Trigeminal
ganglion

Trochlear n.

Interpeduncular
fossa

Abducent n.

Olive

Pyramid

Medulla oblongata

Cerebellar tonsil

Occipital pole

Spinal cord

**Fig. 76.** Basal view of the brain revealing the sites of origin of the cranial nerves (I–XII). Telencephalon yellow, cerebellum orange, brain stem and cranial nerves white. The left trigeminal ganglion is preserved. The hypophysis is slightly deflected posteriorly in order to reveal the infundibulum.

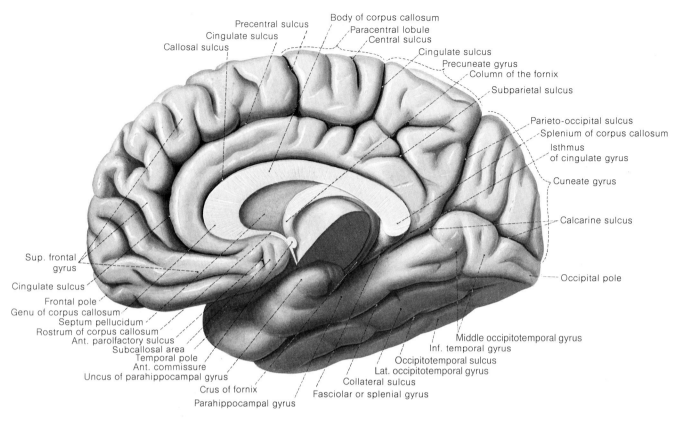

Precentral sulcus
Cingulate sulcus
Callosal sulcus
Body of corpus callosum
Paracentral lobule
Central sulcus
Cingulate sulcus
Precuneate gyrus
Column of the fornix
Subparietal sulcus
Parieto-occipital sulcus
Splenium of corpus callosum
Isthmus of cingulate gyrus
Cuneate gyrus
Calcarine sulcus
Occipital pole
Sup. frontal gyrus
Cingulate sulcus
Frontal pole
Genu of corpus callosum
Septum pellucidum
Rostrum of corpus callosum
Ant. parolfactory sulcus
Subcallosal area
Temporal pole
Ant. commissure
Uncus of parahippocampal gyrus
Crus of fornix
Parahippocampal gyrus
Middle occipitotemporal gyrus
Inf. temporal gyrus
Occipitotemporal sulcus
Lat. occipitotemporal gyrus
Collateral sulcus
Fasciolar or splenial gyrus

**Fig. 77.** Right cerebral hemisphere. The brain has been halved in the midline, the brain stem together with the cerebellum have been removed by an oblique section through the thalamus. View onto the medial and inferior surface of the hemisphere.

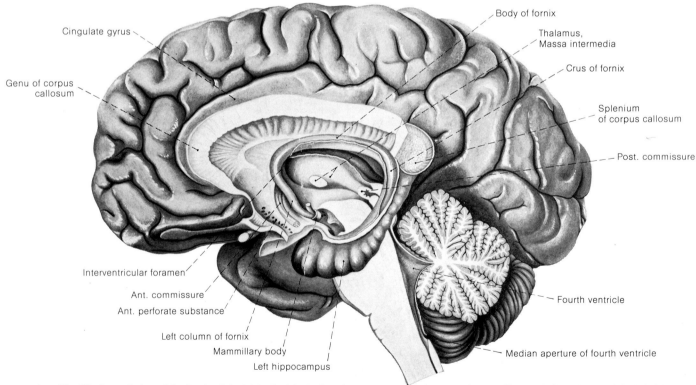

Cingulate gyrus
Genu of corpus callosum
Body of fornix
Thalamus, Massa intermedia
Crus of fornix
Splenium of corpus callosum
Post. commissure
Interventricular foramen
Ant. commissure
Ant. perforate substance
Left column of fornix
Mammillary body
Left hippocampus
Fourth ventricle
Median aperture of fourth ventricle

**Fig. 78.** Lateral view of the fornix of the left half of the brain. Hippocampus, anterior commissure, olfactory bulb and tract of the left side are also shown. The corpus callosum has been sectioned in a left parasagittal plane, the brain stem in the sagittal plane. (After PERNKOPF: Atlas der topographischen und angewandten Anatomie des Menschen, Vol. 1, 2nd ed. [Ed. H. FERNER]. Urban & Schwarzenberg, Munich–Vienna–Baltimore 1980.)

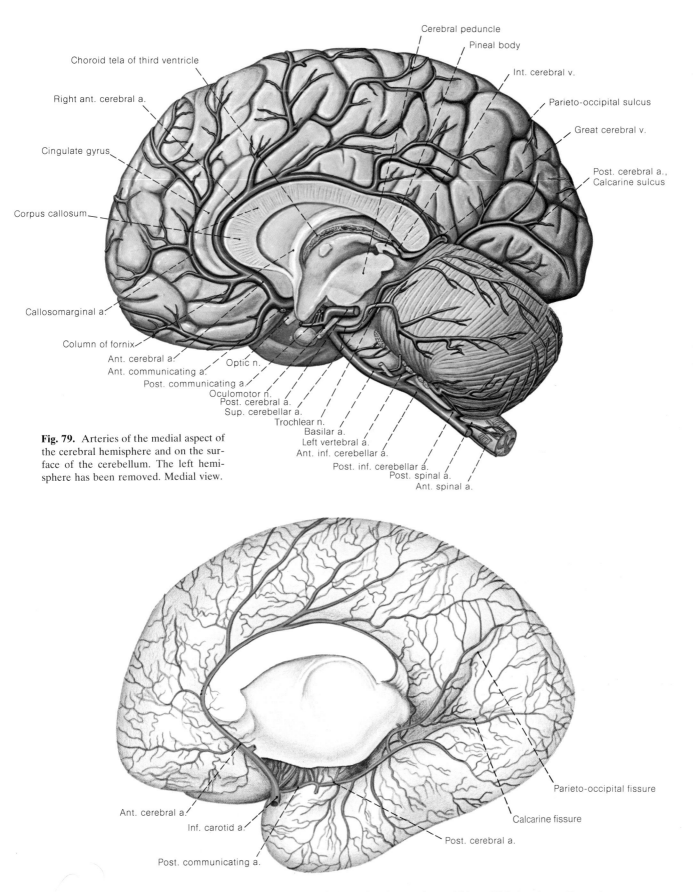

**Fig. 79.** Arteries of the medial aspect of the cerebral hemisphere and on the surface of the cerebellum. The left hemisphere has been removed. Medial view.

Labels (Fig. 79):
Choroid tela of third ventricle
Right ant. cerebral a.
Cingulate gyrus
Corpus callosum
Callosomarginal a.
Column of fornix
Ant. cerebral a.
Ant. communicating a.
Post. communicating a.
Optic n.
Oculomotor n.
Post. cerebral a.
Sup. cerebellar a.
Trochlear n.
Basilar a.
Left vertebral a.
Ant. inf. cerebellar a.
Post. inf. cerebellar a.
Post. spinal a.
Ant. spinal a.
Cerebral peduncle
Pineal body
Int. cerebral v.
Parieto-occipital sulcus
Great cerebral v.
Post. cerebral a., Calcarine sulcus

Labels (Fig. 80):
Ant. cerebral a.
Inf. carotid a.
Post. communicating a.
Post. cerebral a.
Calcarine fissure
Parieto-occipital fissure

**Fig. 80.** Arteries on the medial and basal surfaces of the hemispheres in a human fetus of 28 cm CRL (specimen: FERNER).

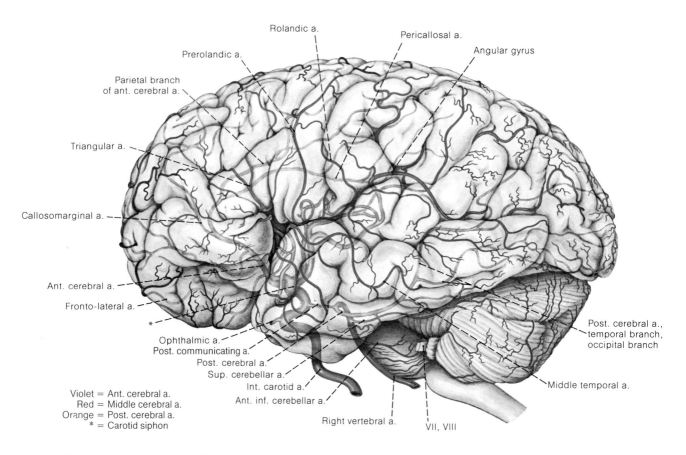

Rolandic a.

Pericallosal a.

Prerolandic a.

Angular gyrus

Parietal branch
of ant. cerebral a.

Triangular a.

Callosomarginal a.

Ant. cerebral a.

Fronto-lateral a.

*

Ophthalmic a.
Post. communicating a.
Post. cerebral a.
Sup. cerebellar a.
Int. carotid a.
Ant. inf. cerebellar a.

Post. cerebral a.,
temporal branch,
occipital branch

Middle temporal a.

Right vertebral a.

VII, VIII

Violet = Ant. cerebral a.
Red = Middle cerebral a.
Orange = Post. cerebral a.
* = Carotid siphon

**Fig. 81.** Arteries of the left hemisphere. Lateral view. Injected specimen. The cerebral matter is rendered transparent, so that the representation is directly comparable to an arteriogram. The terminal branches of the anterior and posterior cerebral arteries extend beyond the pallial crest onto the convexity. (From PERNKOPF: Atlas der topographischen und angewandten Anatomie des Menschen, Vol. 1, 2nd ed. [Ed. H. FERNER]. Urban & Schwarzenberg, Munich–Vienna–Baltimore 1980.)

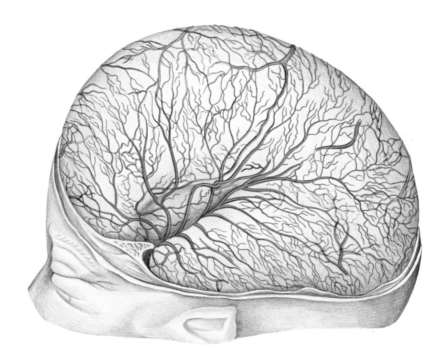

**Fig. 82.** Arteries on the convex surfaces of the hemispheres in a human fetus of 28 cm CRL. The branches of the middle cerebral artery ascend over the opercula in a fan-shaped manner (specimen: FERNER).

54

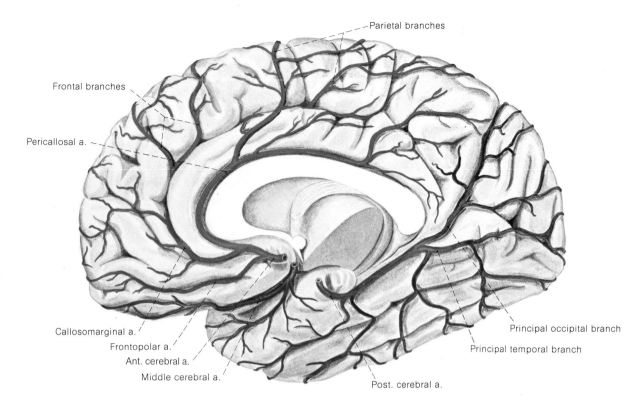

Parietal branches

Frontal branches

Pericallosal a.

Callosomarginal a.

Frontopolar a.

Ant. cerebral a.

Middle cerebral a.

Post. cerebral a.

Principal occipital branch

Principal temporal branch

**Fig. 83.** The arteries of the medial and basal hemispheric surfaces. Note: The branches of the anterior and posterior cerebral arteries extend over the pallial crest to the convexity of the hemisphere where they supply a region of about one fingers width. The anterior cerebral artery supplies the medial surface up to the parieto-occipital sulcus, the posterior cerebral artery supplies the basal surface of the hemisphere and the cuneus with the exception of the upper surface of the base of the frontal brain.

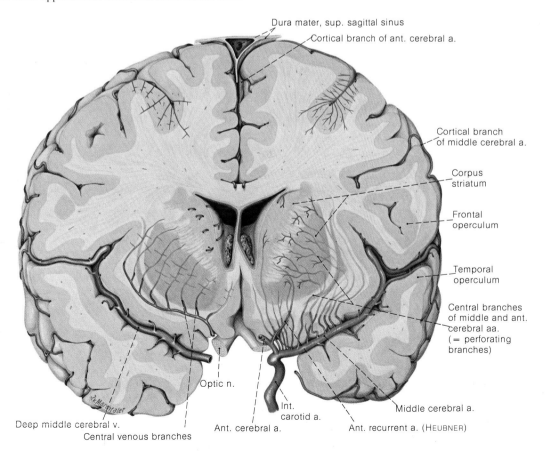

Dura mater, sup. sagittal sinus

Cortical branch of ant. cerebral a.

Cortical branch of middle cerebral a.

Corpus striatum

Frontal operculum

Temporal operculum

Central branches of middle and ant. cerebral aa. (= perforating branches)

Middle cerebral a.

Ant. recurrent a. (HEUBNER)

Ant. cerebral a.

Int. carotid a.

Optic n.

Central venous branches

Deep middle cerebral v.

**Fig. 84.** Vascularization of the telencephalon as seen in a semidiagrammatic frontal section. On the right side of the illustration, arteries; on the left side, veins (after corrosion preparations by H. FERNER). Note the central branches (striate branches) from the middle and anterior cerebral arteries for the basal ganglia and the internal capsule. The anterior recurrent artery (of HEUBNER) springs from the anterior cerebral artery. (Original: FERNER.)

55

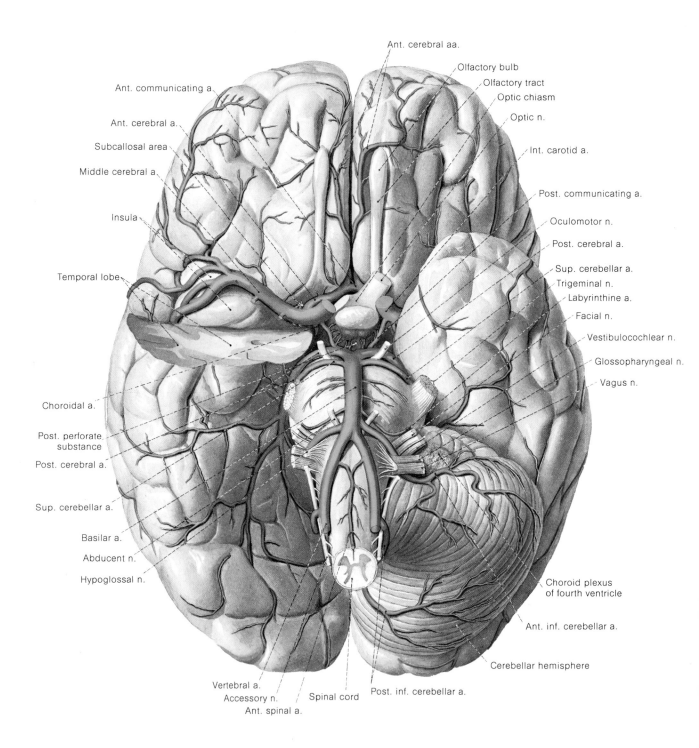

Ant. cerebral aa.

Olfactory bulb

Olfactory tract

Optic chiasm

Optic n.

Ant. communicating a.

Ant. cerebral a.

Subcallosal area

Middle cerebral a.

Insula

Temporal lobe

Int. carotid a.

Post. communicating a.

Oculomotor n.

Post. cerebral a.

Sup. cerebellar a.

Trigeminal n.

Labyrinthine a.

Facial n.

Vestibulocochlear n.

Glossopharyngeal n.

Vagus n.

Choroidal a.

Post. perforate substance

Post. cerebral a.

Sup. cerebellar a.

Basilar a.

Abducent n.

Hypoglossal n.

Choroid plexus of fourth ventricle

Ant. inf. cerebellar a.

Cerebellar hemisphere

Vertebral a.

Accessory n.

Ant. spinal a.

Spinal cord

Post. inf. cerebellar a.

**Fig. 85.** Arteries at the base of the brain, arterial circle of WILLIS. The optic nerve, the anterior portion of the temporal lobe and the cerebellar hemisphere of the right side have been removed.

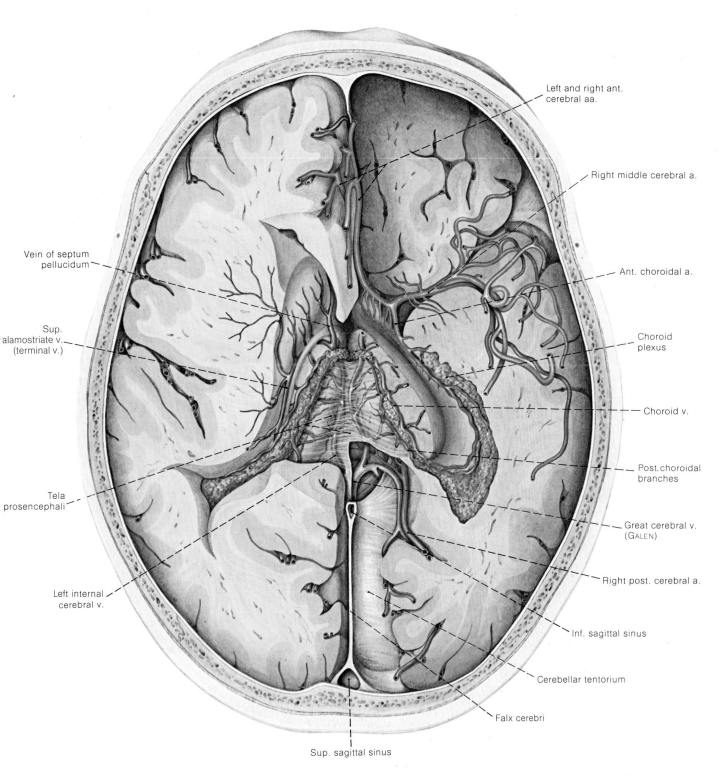

Left and right ant. cerebral aa.

Right middle cerebral a.

Ant. choroidal a.

Vein of septum pellucidum

Choroid plexus

Sup. alamostriate v. (terminal v.)

Choroid v.

Post. choroidal branches

Tela prosencephali

Great cerebral v. (GALEN)

Left internal cerebral v.

Right post. cerebral a.

Inf. sagittal sinus

Cerebellar tentorium

Falx cerebri

Sup. sagittal sinus

**Fig. 86.** Horizontal section through the brain showing the branches of the anterior, middle, and posterior arteries as well as the internal cerebral veins. (From PERNKOPF: Atlas der topographischen und angewandten Anatomie des Menschen, Vol. 1, 2nd ed. [Ed. H. FERNER]. Urban & Schwarzenberg, Munich–Vienna–Baltimore 1980.)

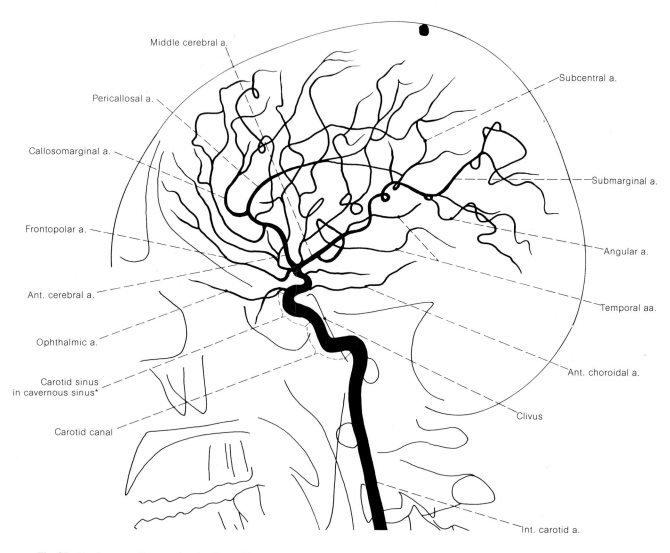

Middle cerebral a.

Pericallosal a.

Callosomarginal a.

Frontopolar a.

Ant. cerebral a.

Ophthalmic a.

Carotid sinus in cavernous sinus*

Carotid canal

Subcentral a.

Submarginal a.

Angular a.

Temporal aa.

Ant. choroidal a.

Clivus

Int. carotid a.

**Fig. 87.** Explanatory diagram for the X-ray film on the facing page. (From L. WICKE: Atlas der Röntgenanatomie, 2nd ed. Urban & Schwarzenberg, Munich–Vienna–Baltimore 1980.) * Carotid siphon.

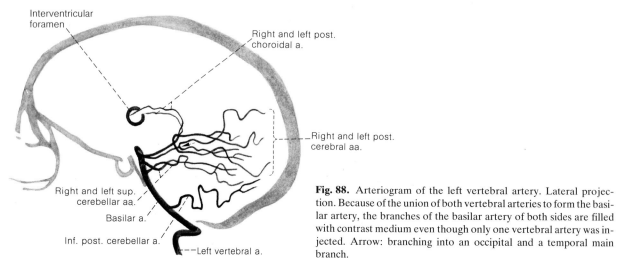

Interventricular foramen

Right and left post. choroidal a.

Right and left post. cerebral aa.

Right and left sup. cerebellar aa.

Basilar a.

Inf. post. cerebellar a.

Left vertebral a.

**Fig. 88.** Arteriogram of the left vertebral artery. Lateral projection. Because of the union of both vertebral arteries to form the basilar artery, the branches of the basilar artery of both sides are filled with contrast medium even though only one vertebral artery was injected. Arrow: branching into an occipital and a temporal main branch.

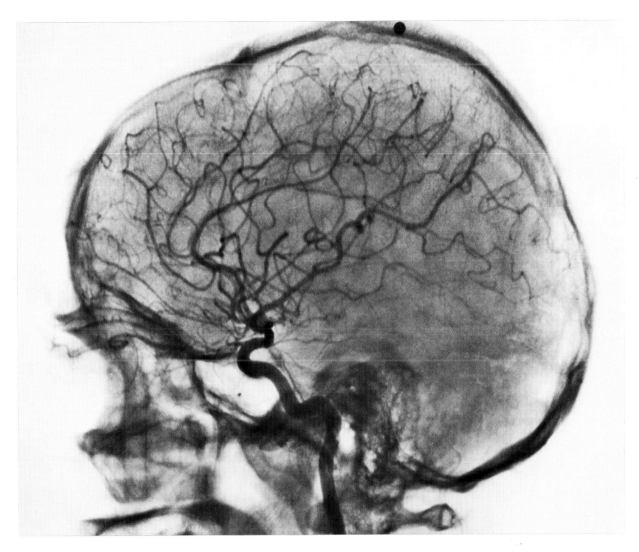

**Fig. 89.** Carotid arteriogram (lateral projection). Original (from L. WICKE: Atlas der Röntgenanatomie, 2nd ed. Urban & Schwarzenberg, Munich–Vienna–Baltimore 1980). Filled are the two terminal branches of the internal carotid artery, i.e., the middle cerebral artery with the Sylvian vascular system in the center of the film; and the anterior cerebral artery with its characteristic course, anteriorly convex and delineating the outer contour of the corpus callosum.

The internal carotid artery penetrates the bony base of the skull through the carotid canal in the area of the apex of the petrous bone. After leaving the bony canal near the apex of the petrous bone it is separated from the trigeminal ganglion by a thin bony or connective tissue septum. It ascends in a sulcus at the lateral surface of the body of the sphenoid bone, and here it is in close vicinity with the frontal pole of the trigeminal ganglion (ganglionic segment). The artery then bends rostral and, in the sagittal plane, slightly ascends forward toward the base of the anterior clinoid process. This is the "cavernous sinus-segment" which extends from the tip of the pyramid to the base of the anterior clinoid process. It lies in a shallow sulcus in the lateral wall of the body of the sphenoid bone. Below the base of the anterior clinoid process, the artery bends sharply backward ("carotid knee"), perforates the dura mater and arachnoid membrane and, running posteriorly, comes to lie below the optic nerve entering through the optic foramen (Fig. 94). From here it courses within the subarachnoid space ("cisternal segment"), and finally divides into its terminal branches ("carotid fork").

In roentgenological terminology, these tortuous segments from the ganglionic segment to the carotid fork are called "carotid siphon".

# Brain, Meninges, Cerebral Vessels

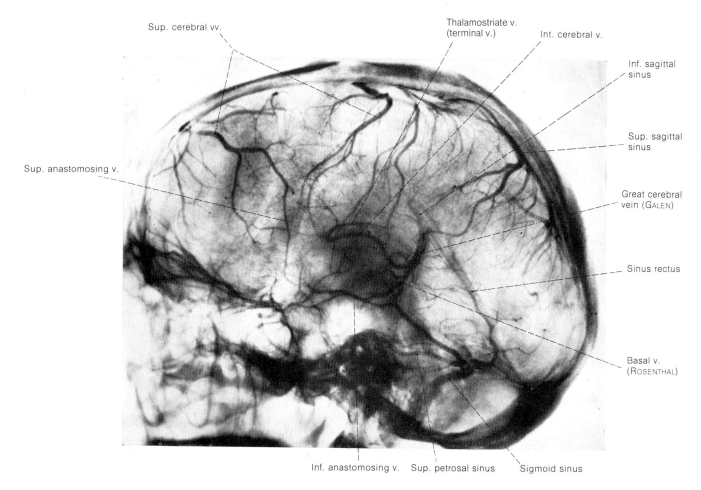

Sup. cerebral vv.

Thalamostriate v. (terminal v.)

Int. cerebral v.

Inf. sagittal sinus

Sup. sagittal sinus

Great cerebral vein (GALEN)

Sinus rectus

Basal v. (ROSENTHAL)

Sup. anastomosing v.

Inf. anastomosing v.    Sup. petrosal sinus    Sigmoid sinus

**Fig. 90.** Phlebo-sinogram, lateral projection. Recognizable are the superior cerebral veins ascending toward the superior sagittal sinus, the centrally located internal cerebral vein, and the arch of the great cerebral vein of GALEN. (From PERNKOPF: Atlas der topographischen und angewandten Anatomie des Menschen, Vol. 1, 2nd ed. [Ed. H. FERNER]. Urban & Schwarzenberg, Munich–Vienna–Baltimore 1980.)

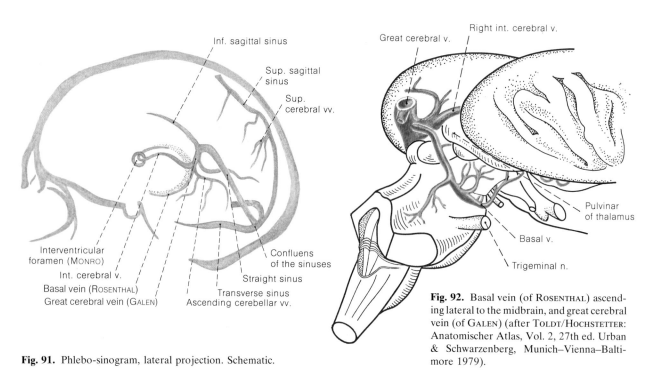

Inf. sagittal sinus

Sup. sagittal sinus

Sup. cerebral vv.

Interventricular foramen (MONRO)

Int. cerebral v.

Basal vein (ROSENTHAL)

Great cerebral vein (GALEN)

Confluens of the sinuses

Straight sinus

Transverse sinus
Ascending cerebellar vv.

**Fig. 91.** Phlebo-sinogram, lateral projection. Schematic.

Great cerebral v.

Right int. cerebral v.

Pulvinar of thalamus

Basal v.

Trigeminal n.

**Fig. 92.** Basal vein (of ROSENTHAL) ascending lateral to the midbrain, and great cerebral vein (of GALEN) (after TOLDT/HOCHSTETTER: Anatomischer Atlas, Vol. 2, 27th ed. Urban & Schwarzenberg, Munich–Vienna–Baltimore 1979).

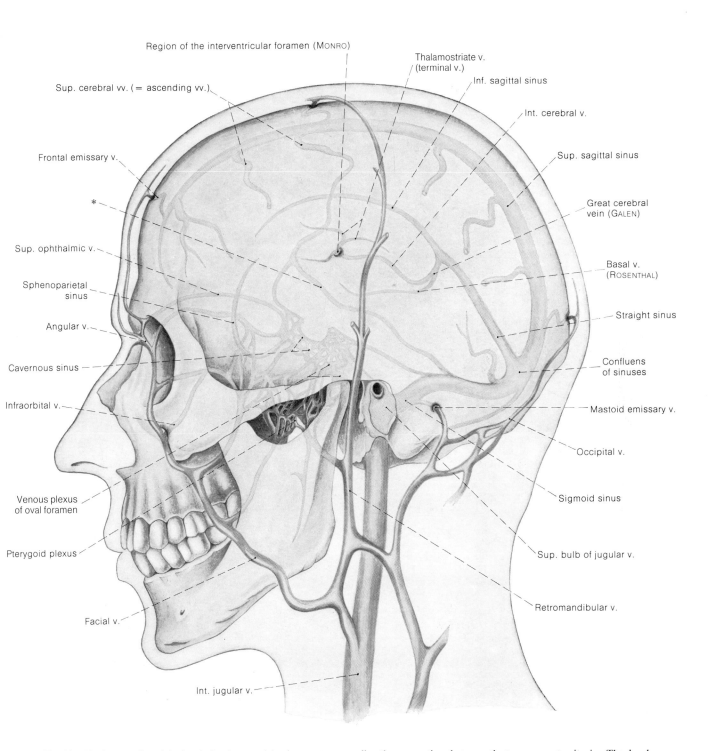

Region of the interventricular foramen (MONRO)

Thalamostriate v. (terminal v.)

Sup. cerebral vv. (= ascending vv.)

Inf. sagittal sinus

Int. cerebral v.

Frontal emissary v.

Sup. sagittal sinus

*

Great cerebral vein (GALEN)

Sup. ophthalmic v.

Basal v. (ROSENTHAL)

Sphenoparietal sinus

Straight sinus

Angular v.

Confluens of sinuses

Cavernous sinus

Infraorbital v.

Mastoid emissary v.

Occipital v.

Venous plexus of oval foramen

Sigmoid sinus

Pterygoid plexus

Sup. bulb of jugular v.

Retromandibular v.

Facial v.

Int. jugular v.

**Fig. 93.** The larger veins of the head, the sinuses of the dura mater, as well as the connections between the two venous territories. The dural sinuses and the veins covered by bones are drawn transparently. (After FERNER/KAUTZKY: Handbuch der Neurochirurgie, Vol. 1. Springer 1959.) * So-called anastomosis of LABBÉ.

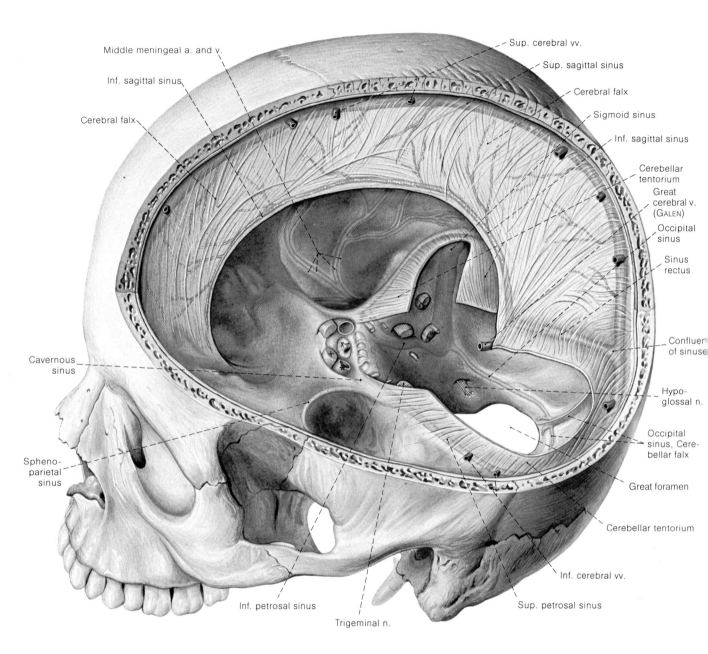

Middle meningeal a. and v.

Inf. sagittal sinus

Cerebral falx

Cavernous sinus

Spheno-parietal sinus

Inf. petrosal sinus

Trigeminal n.

Sup. cerebral vv.

Sup. sagittal sinus

Cerebral falx

Sigmoid sinus

Inf. sagittal sinus

Cerebellar tentorium

Great cerebral v. (GALEN)

Occipital sinus

Sinus rectus

Confluen of sinuse

Hypo-glossal n.

Occipital sinus, Cerebellar falx

Great foramen

Cerebellar tentorium

Inf. cerebral vv.

Sup. petrosal sinus

**Fig. 94.** Dura mater and its sinuses seen from above and left. A large portion has been removed from the left side of the tentorium and a narrow strip from the right side. * Int. carotid a.; × = hypophysis; + = optic n.

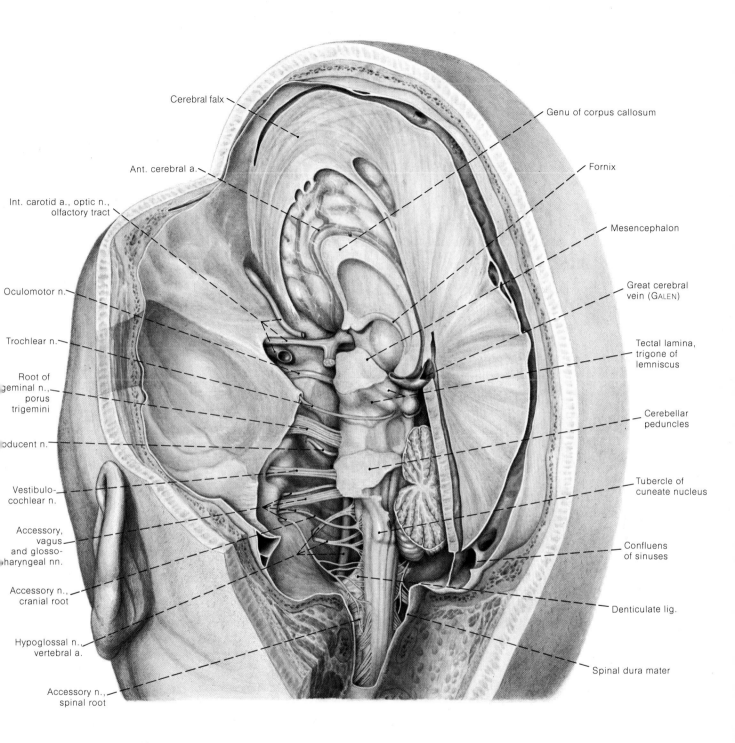

Cerebral falx

Ant. cerebral a.

Int. carotid a., optic n.,
olfactory tract

Oculomotor n.

Trochlear n.

Root of
geminal n.,
porus
trigemini

oducent n.

Vestibulo-
cochlear n.

Accessory,
vagus
and glosso-
pharyngeal nn.

Accessory n.,
cranial root

Hypoglossal n.,
vertebral a.

Accessory n.,
spinal root

Genu of corpus callosum

Fornix

Mesencephalon

Great cerebral
vein (GALEN)

Tectal lamina,
trigone of
lemniscus

Cerebellar
peduncles

Tubercle of
cuneate nucleus

Confluens
of sinuses

Denticulate lig.

Spinal dura mater

**Fig. 95.** The brain in situ. The left hemispheres of both the cerebrum and cerebellum were removed. Brain stem in situ. Intracranial (lep-tomeningeal) portion of all twelve cranial nerves. (From PERNKOPF: Atlas der topographischen und angewandten Anatomie des Menschen, Vol. 1, 2nd ed. [Ed. H. FERNER]. Urban & Schwarzenberg, Munich–Vienna–Baltimore 1980.)

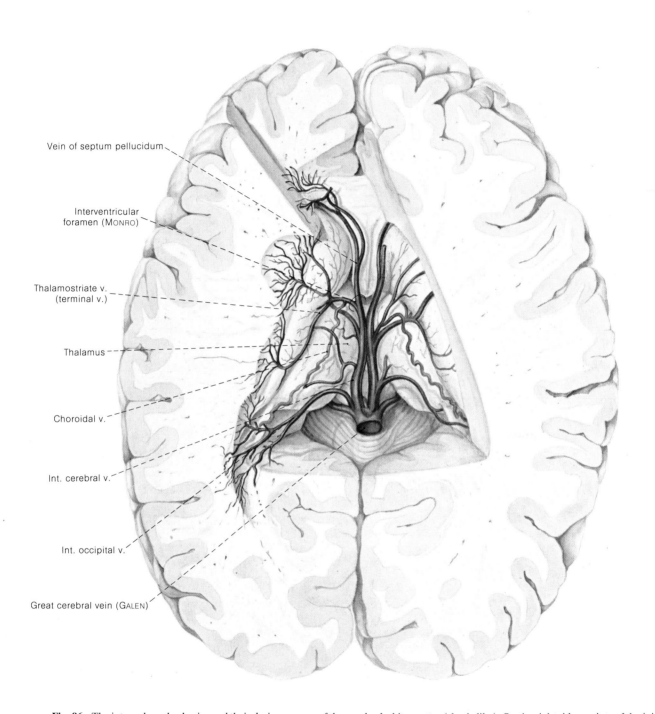

Vein of septum pellucidum

Interventricular
foramen (MONRO)

Thalamostriate v.
(terminal v.)

Thalamus

Choroidal v.

Int. cerebral v.

Int. occipital v.

Great cerebral vein (GALEN)

**Fig. 96.** The internal cerebral veins and their drainage areas of the cerebral white matter (shrub-like). On the right side: variety of the joining pattern (from H. FERNER, Z. Anat. 120, 1958).

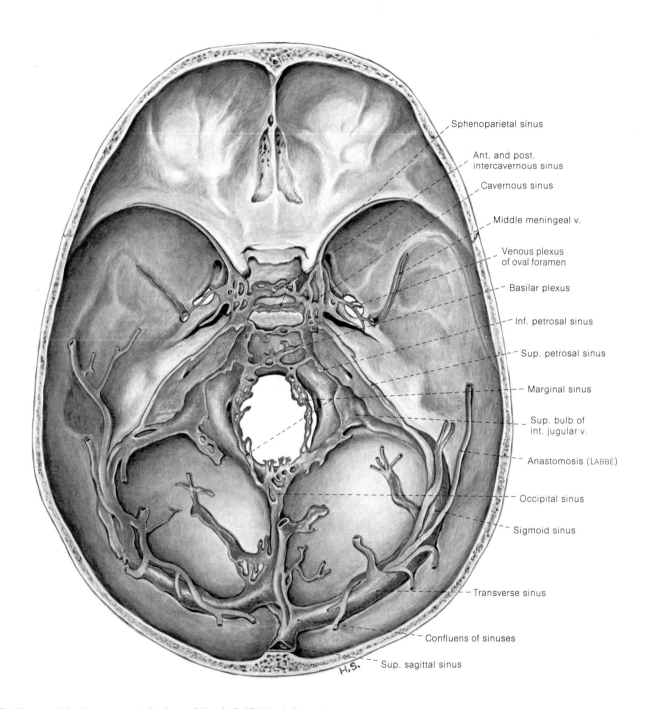

Sphenoparietal sinus

Ant. and post.
intercavernous sinus

Cavernous sinus

Middle meningeal v.

Venous plexus
of oval foramen

Basilar plexus

Inf. petrosal sinus

Sup. petrosal sinus

Marginal sinus

Sup. bulb of
int. jugular v.

Anastomosis (LABBÉ)

Occipital sinus

Sigmoid sinus

Transverse sinus

Confluens of sinuses

Sup. sagittal sinus

**Fig. 97.** Sinuses of the dura mater at the base of the skull (Original: FERNER).

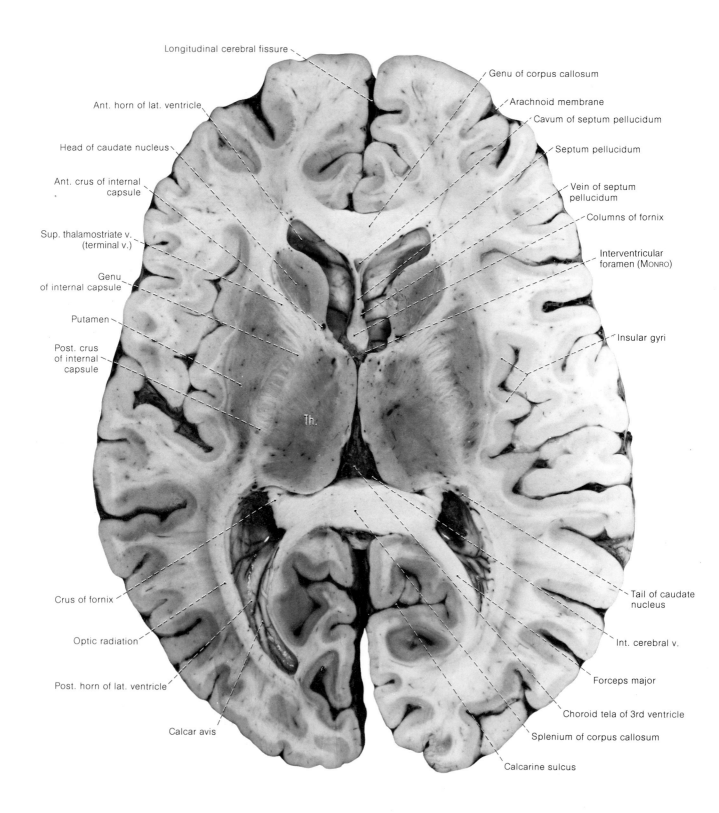

Longitudinal cerebral fissure

Ant. horn of lat. ventricle

Head of caudate nucleus

Ant. crus of internal capsule

Sup. thalamostriate v. (terminal v.)

Genu of internal capsule

Putamen

Post. crus of internal capsule

Th.

Crus of fornix

Optic radiation

Post. horn of lat. ventricle

Calcar avis

Genu of corpus callosum

Arachnoid membrane

Cavum of septum pellucidum

Septum pellucidum

Vein of septum pellucidum

Columns of fornix

Interventricular foramen (MONRO)

Insular gyri

Tail of caudate nucleus

Int. cerebral v.

Forceps major

Choroid tela of 3rd ventricle

Splenium of corpus callosum

Calcarine sulcus

**Fig. 98.** Horizontal section through the telencephalon at the level of the basal ganglia and the interventricular foramina of MONRO (compare illustration on facing page). Th = Thalamus.

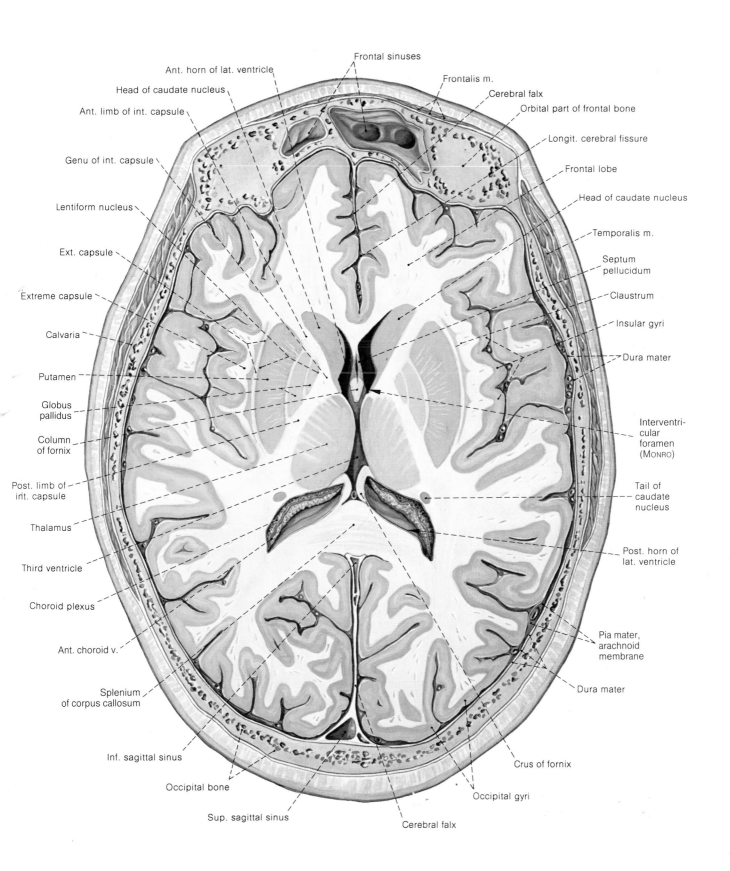

Ant. horn of lat. ventricle

Frontal sinuses

Head of caudate nucleus

Frontalis m.

Cerebral falx

Ant. limb of int. capsule

Orbital part of frontal bone

Longit. cerebral fissure

Genu of int. capsule

Frontal lobe

Head of caudate nucleus

Lentiform nucleus

Temporalis m.

Ext. capsule

Septum pellucidum

Extreme capsule

Claustrum

Calvaria

Insular gyri

Putamen

Dura mater

Globus pallidus

Interventricular foramen (MONRO)

Column of fornix

Post. limb of int. capsule

Tail of caudate nucleus

Thalamus

Third ventricle

Post. horn of lat. ventricle

Choroid plexus

Ant. choroid v.

Pia mater, arachnoid membrane

Splenium of corpus callosum

Dura mater

Inf. sagittal sinus

Crus of fornix

Occipital bone

Occipital gyri

Sup. sagittal sinus

Cerebral falx

**Fig. 99.** Horizontal section through the neurocranium at the level of the basal ganglia and the internal capsule.

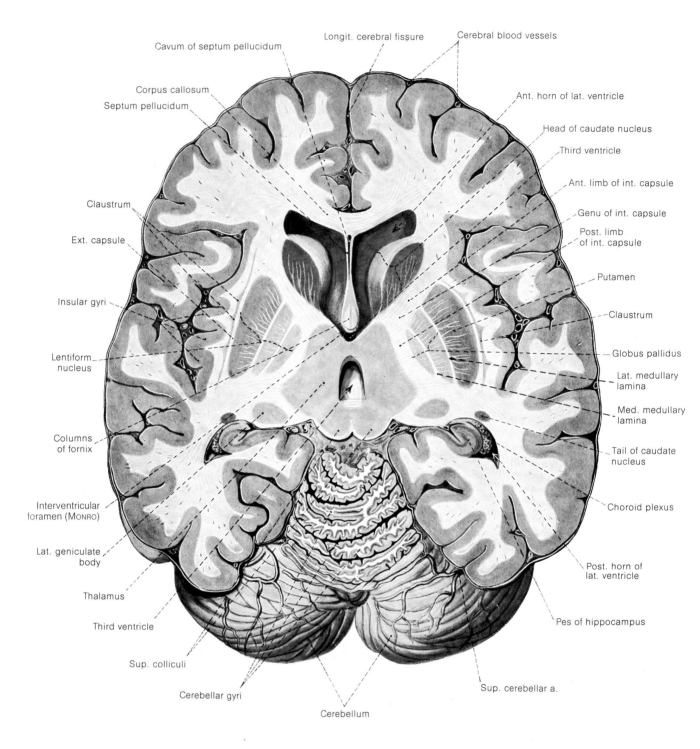

Cavum of septum pellucidum

Longit. cerebral fissure

Cerebral blood vessels

Corpus callosum

Septum pellucidum

Ant. horn of lat. ventricle

Head of caudate nucleus

Third ventricle

Claustrum

Ant. limb of int. capsule

Genu of int. capsule

Ext. capsule

Post. limb of int. capsule

Putamen

Insular gyri

Claustrum

Lentiform nucleus

Globus pallidus

Lat. medullary lamina

Med. medullary lamina

Columns of fornix

Tail of caudate nucleus

Choroid plexus

Interventricular foramen (Monro)

Lat. geniculate body

Post. horn of lat. ventricle

Thalamus

Pes of hippocampus

Third ventricle

Sup. colliculi

Cerebellar gyri

Sup. cerebellar a.

Cerebellum

**Fig. 100.** Horizontal section through the telencephalon at the level of the basal ganglia and the internal capsule. The plane of section is somewhat lower than that in Fig. 99, so that the mesencephalon and the vermis of the cerebellum are included in the section.

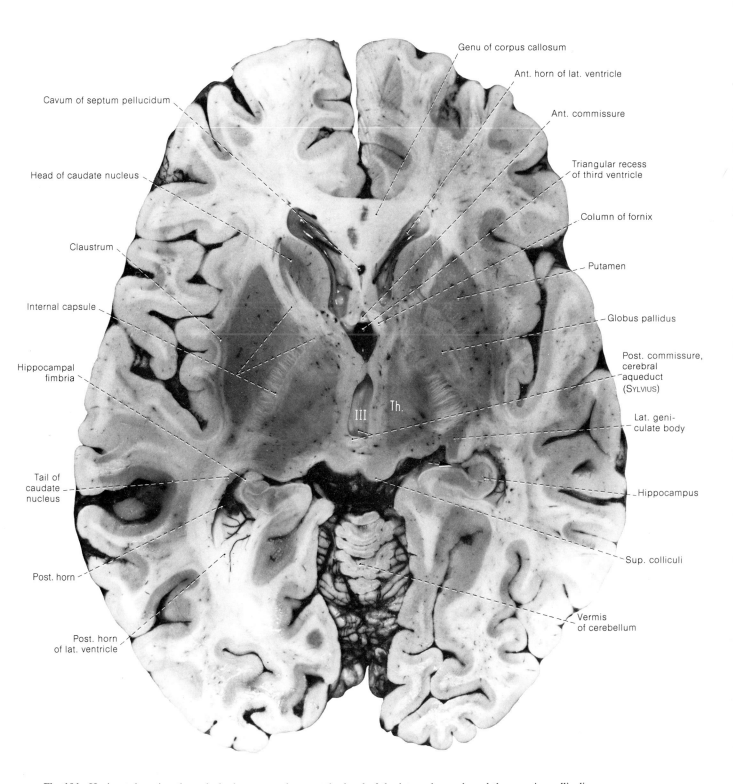

Genu of corpus callosum

Ant. horn of lat. ventricle

Cavum of septum pellucidum

Ant. commissure

Head of caudate nucleus

Triangular recess of third ventricle

Column of fornix

Claustrum

Putamen

Internal capsule

Globus pallidus

Hippocampal fimbria

Post. commissure, cerebral aqueduct (SYLVIUS)

Lat. geniculate body

III    Th.

Tail of caudate nucleus

Hippocampus

Post. horn

Sup. colliculi

Vermis of cerebellum

Post. horn of lat. ventricle

**Fig. 101.** Horizontal section through the human cerebrum at the level of the internal capsule and the superior colliculi. Arrow = Hippocampal fissure, III = third ventricle, Th = Thalamus.

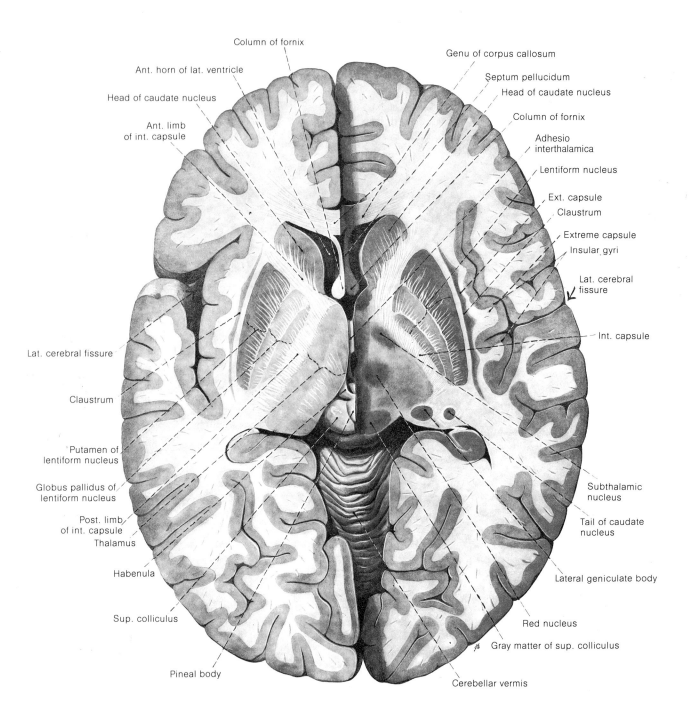

Column of fornix

Ant. horn of lat. ventricle

Head of caudate nucleus

Ant. limb
of int. capsule

Genu of corpus callosum

Septum pellucidum

Head of caudate nucleus

Column of fornix

Adhesio
interthalamica

Lentiform nucleus

Ext. capsule

Claustrum

Extreme capsule

Insular gyri

Lat. cerebral
fissure

Int. capsule

Lat. cerebral fissure

Claustrum

Putamen of
lentiform nucleus

Globus pallidus of
lentiform nucleus

Post. limb
of int. capsule

Thalamus

Habenula

Sup. colliculus

Pineal body

Subthalamic
nucleus

Tail of caudate
nucleus

Lateral geniculate body

Red nucleus

Gray matter of sup. colliculus

Cerebellar vermis

**Fig. 102.** Horizontal section through the telencephalon to show the basal ganglia (thalamus, lentiform nucleus, caudate nucleus) and the internal capsule. The plane of section on the left side is at the level of the thalamus; on the right side it is about 1 cm lower going through the lamina quadrigemina and the subthalamic nucleus.

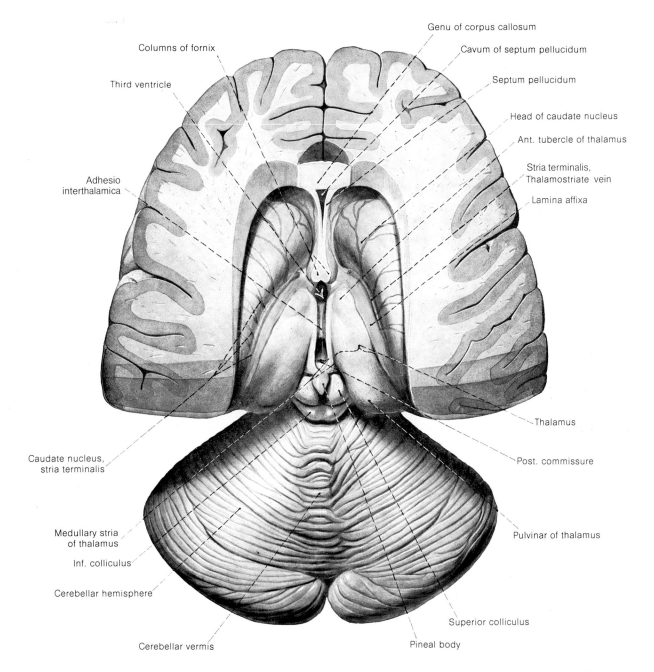

Columns of fornix

Third ventricle

Adhesio
interthalamica

Genu of corpus callosum

Cavum of septum pellucidum

Septum pellucidum

Head of caudate nucleus

Ant. tubercle of thalamus

Stria terminalis,
Thalamostriate vein

Lamina affixa

Thalamus

Post. commissure

Caudate nucleus,
stria terminalis

Medullary stria
of thalamus

Inf. colliculus

Cerebellar hemisphere

Pulvinar of thalamus

Superior colliculus

Cerebellar vermis

Pineal body

**Fig. 103.** Basal ganglia of the forebrain (thalamus and caudate nucleus), third ventricle, lamina quadrigemina and cerebellum seen from above. The columns of the fornix, choroid plexus of the third ventricle as well as temporal and occipital lobes of the telencephalic hemispheres have been removed. The lamina affixa, that is the extremely thin portion of the telencephalic wall that abuts the thalamus, is shown in yellow.

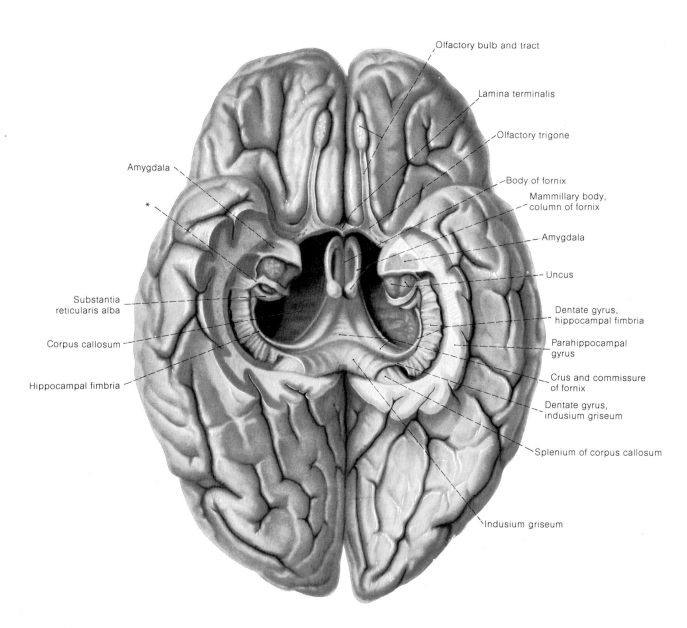

**Fig. 104.** Basal surface of the telencephalon. Dissection of the two fornices. (From PERNKOPF: Atlas der topographischen und angewandten Anatomie des Menschen, Vol. 1, 2nd ed. [Ed. H. FERNER]. Urban & Schwarzenberg, Munich–Vienna–Baltimore 1980.) * = ribbon of uncus.

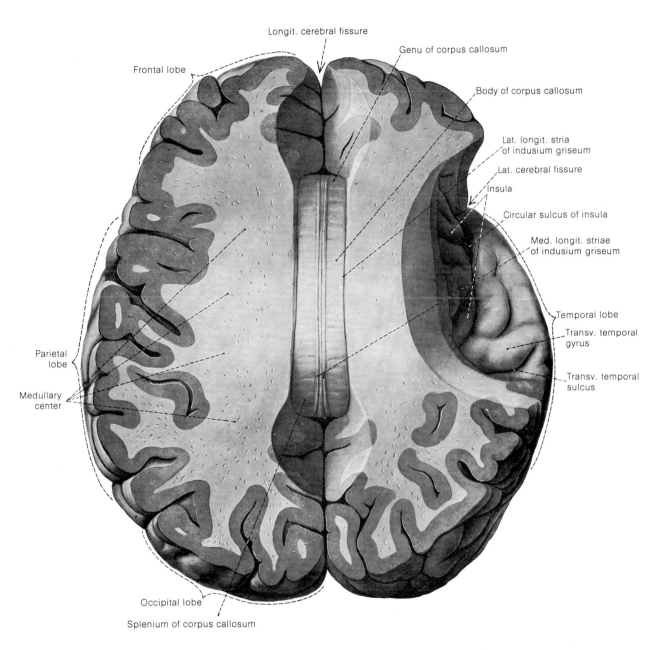

Longit. cerebral fissure

Genu of corpus callosum

Frontal lobe

Body of corpus callosum

Lat. longit. stria of indusium griseum

Lat. cerebral fissure

Insula

Circular sulcus of insula

Med. longit. striae of indusium griseum

Temporal lobe

Transv. temporal gyrus

Transv. temporal sulcus

Parietal lobe

Medullary center

Occipital lobe

Splenium of corpus callosum

**Fig. 105.** Horizontal section through both hemispheres. The corpus callosum is exposed. View from above. The insula is dissected free on the right side; anteriorly the genu and posteriorly the splenium of the corpus callosum have been exposed.

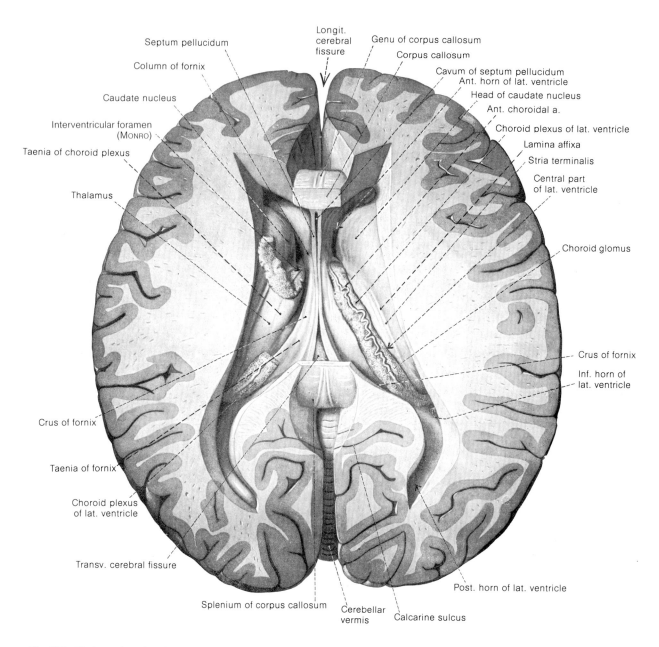

Septum pellucidum

Longit. cerebral fissure

Genu of corpus callosum

Column of fornix

Corpus callosum

Caudate nucleus

Cavum of septum pellucidum
Ant. horn of lat. ventricle

Interventricular foramen (MONRO)

Head of caudate nucleus

Ant. choroidal a.

Taenia of choroid plexus

Choroid plexus of lat. ventricle

Lamina affixa

Stria terminalis

Thalamus

Central part of lat. ventricle

Choroid glomus

Crus of fornix

Inf. horn of lat. ventricle

Crus of fornix

Taenia of fornix

Choroid plexus of lat. ventricle

Transv. cerebral fissure

Post. horn of lat. ventricle

Splenium of corpus callosum

Cerebellar vermis

Calcarine sulcus

**Fig. 106.** Horizontal section through both hemispheres. The lateral ventricles are opened and seen from above. Fornix and septum pellucidum are visible following partial removal of the corpus callosum. On the left side the choroid plexus has been sectioned and reflected.

**Fig. 107.** Frontal section through the telencephalon rostral to the thalamus. The anterior horns of the lateral ventricles do not possess a ▷ choroid plexus.

**Fig. 108.** The fornix exposed in its entire extent and in its natural position. The brain has been halved in the midline, the brain stem together with the cerebellum has been removed by an oblique section through the thalamus. The parahippocampal gyrus has been removed to such an extent as to reveal the hippocampal fimbria and the dentate gyrus. After removal of the lateral wall of the third ventricle (hypothalamic area) the column of the fornix and mammillothalamic tract have been dissected free down to the mammillary body. View from medial and below.

74

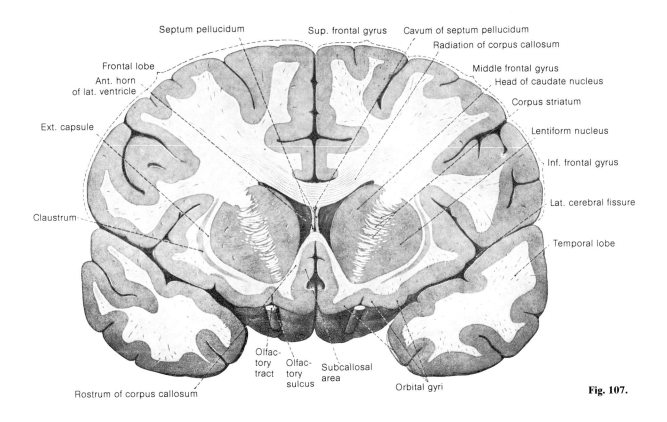

Septum pellucidum — Sup. frontal gyrus — Cavum of septum pellucidum

Radiation of corpus callosum

Frontal lobe

Middle frontal gyrus

Ant. horn of lat. ventricle

Head of caudate nucleus

Corpus striatum

Ext. capsule

Lentiform nucleus

Inf. frontal gyrus

Lat. cerebral fissure

Claustrum

Temporal lobe

Olfactory tract

Olfactory sulcus

Subcallosal area

Orbital gyri

Rostrum of corpus callosum

**Fig. 107.**

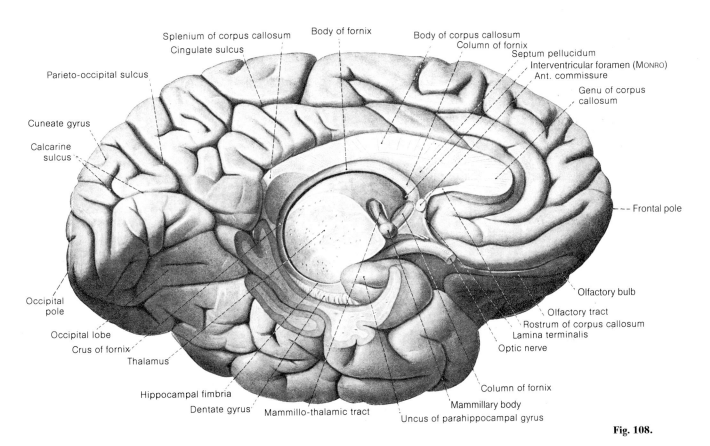

Splenium of corpus callosum — Body of fornix — Body of corpus callosum

Cingulate sulcus

Column of fornix

Septum pellucidum

Parieto-occipital sulcus

Interventricular foramen (Monro)

Ant. commissure

Genu of corpus callosum

Cuneate gyrus

Calcarine sulcus

Frontal pole

Occipital pole

Olfactory bulb

Olfactory tract

Rostrum of corpus callosum

Lamina terminalis

Occipital lobe

Optic nerve

Crus of fornix

Thalamus

Column of fornix

Hippocampal fimbria

Mammillary body

Dentate gyrus

Mammillo-thalamic tract

Uncus of parahippocampal gyrus

**Fig. 108.**

75

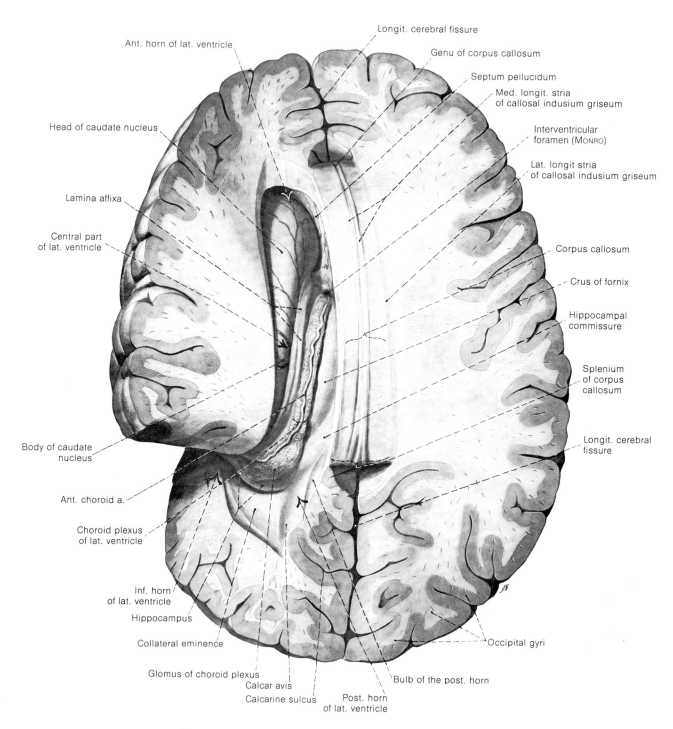

Ant. horn of lat. ventricle

Longit. cerebral fissure

Genu of corpus callosum

Septum pellucidum

Med. longit. stria
of callosal indusium griseum

Head of caudate nucleus

Interventricular
foramen (MONRO)

Lat. longit stria
of callosal indusium griseum

Lamina affixa

Central part
of lat. ventricle

Corpus callosum

Crus of fornix

Hippocampal
commissure

Splenium
of corpus
callosum

Body of caudate
nucleus

Longit. cerebral
fissure

Ant. choroid a.

Choroid plexus
of lat. ventricle

Inf. horn
of lat. ventricle

Hippocampus

Collateral eminence

Occipital gyri

Glomus of choroid plexus

Calcar avis

Calcarine sulcus

Post. horn
of lat. ventricle

Bulb of the post. horn

**Fig. 109.** Horizontal section through both hemispheres. The corpus callosum and the left lateral ventricle are seen from above and left. Preparation similar to the one in Fig. 105, but the roof of the left lateral ventricle has also been removed.

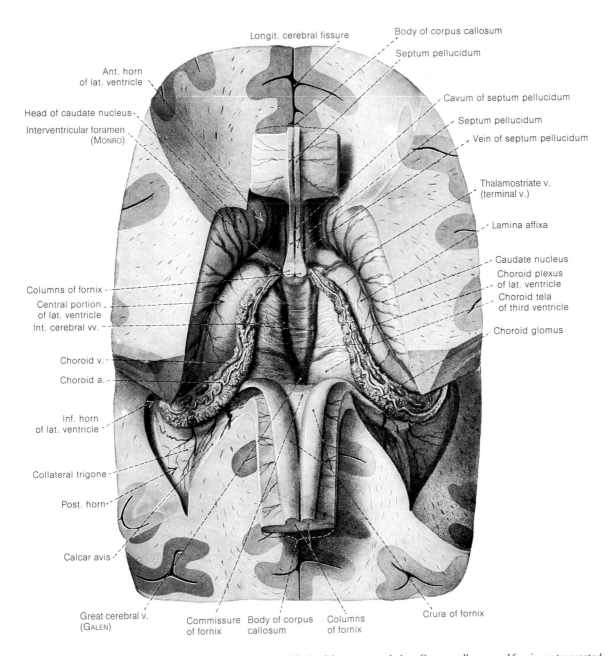

Longit. cerebral fissure

Body of corpus callosum

Septum pellucidum

Ant. horn
of lat. ventricle

Head of caudate nucleus

Interventricular foramen
(MONRO)

Cavum of septum pellucidum

Septum pellucidum

Vein of septum pellucidum

Thalamostriate v.
(terminal v.)

Lamina affixa

Caudate nucleus

Choroid plexus
of lat. ventricle

Choroid tela
of third ventricle

Columns of fornix

Central portion
of lat. ventricle

Int. cerebral vv.

Choroid v.

Choroid a.

Choroid glomus

Inf. horn
of lat. ventricle

Collateral trigone

Post. horn

Calcar avis

Great cerebral v.
(GALEN)

Commissure
of fornix

Body of corpus
callosum

Columns
of fornix

Crura of fornix

**Fig. 110.** Lateral ventricles opened from above to expose the choroid tela of the prosencephalon. Corpus callosum and fornix are transected and deflected forward and backward.

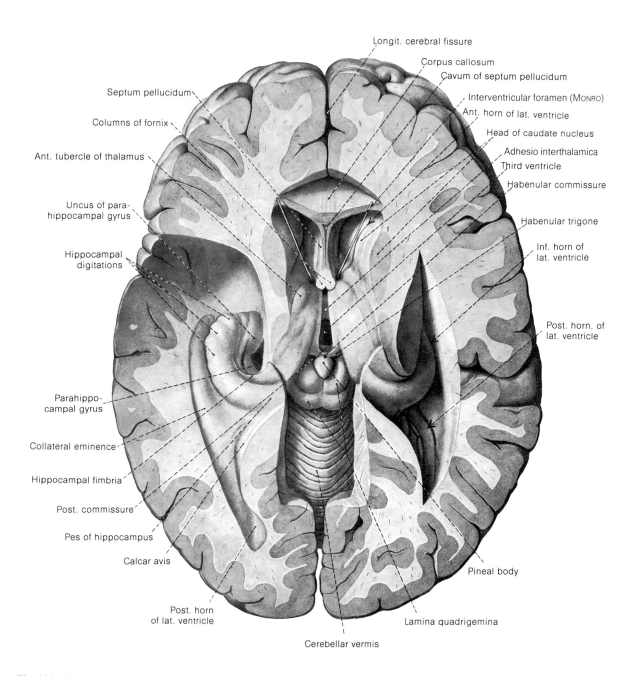

Longit. cerebral fissure

Corpus callosum

Cavum of septum pellucidum

Interventricular foramen (MONRO)

Ant. horn of lat. ventricle

Head of caudate nucleus

Adhesio interthalamica

Third ventricle

Habenular commissure

Habenular trigone

Inf. horn of lat. ventricle

Post. horn. of lat. ventricle

Pineal body

Lamina quadrigemina

Septum pellucidum

Columns of fornix

Ant. tubercle of thalamus

Uncus of para-hippocampal gyrus

Hippocampal digitations

Parahippo-campal gyrus

Collateral eminence

Hippocampal fimbria

Post. commissure

Pes of hippocampus

Calcar avis

Post. horn of lat. ventricle

Cerebellar vermis

**Fig. 111.** Horizontal section through both hemispheres. Lateral ventricles and third ventricle are seen from above. The body and splenium of the corpus callosum as well as the columns of the fornix and the choroid tela of the third ventricle have been removed. The left temporal lobe has been excavated down to the inferior horn of the lateral ventricle. Probe in the interventricular foramen.

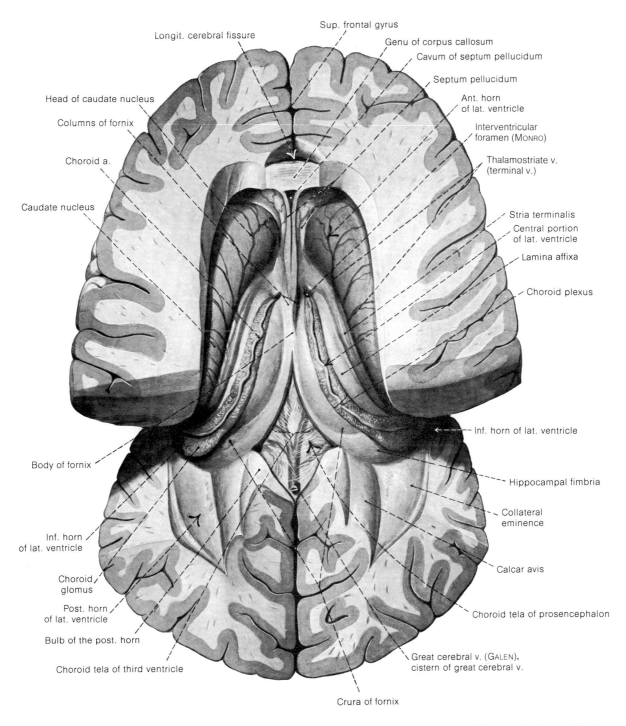

Longit. cerebral fissure

Sup. frontal gyrus

Genu of corpus callosum

Cavum of septum pellucidum

Septum pellucidum

Head of caudate nucleus

Ant. horn
of lat. ventricle

Columns of fornix

Interventricular
foramen (MONRO)

Choroid a.

Thalamostriate v.
(terminal v.)

Caudate nucleus

Stria terminalis

Central portion
of lat. ventricle

Lamina affixa

Choroid plexus

Inf. horn of lat. ventricle

Body of fornix

Hippocampal fimbria

Collateral
eminence

Inf. horn
of lat. ventricle

Calcar avis

Choroid
glomus

Post. horn
of lat. ventricle

Choroid tela of prosencephalon

Bulb of the post. horn

Great cerebral v. (GALEN),
cistern of great cerebral v.

Choroid tela of third ventricle

Crura of fornix

**Fig. 112.** Lateral ventricles opened from above. The major portion of the corpus callosum has been removed. The posterior horns of both lateral ventricles have been exposed.

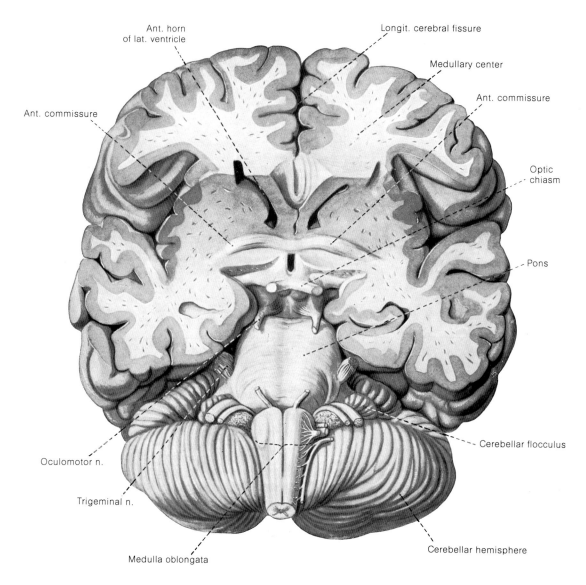

Ant. horn
of lat. ventricle

Longit. cerebral fissure

Medullary center

Ant. commissure

Ant. commissure

Optic chiasm

Pons

Cerebellar flocculus

Oculomotor n.

Trigeminal n.

Cerebellar hemisphere

Medulla oblongata

**Fig. 113.** Anterior commissure exposed by a curved section from the base of the brain. The section shows only the middle portion of the commissure; its anterior and posterior radiations are not seen.

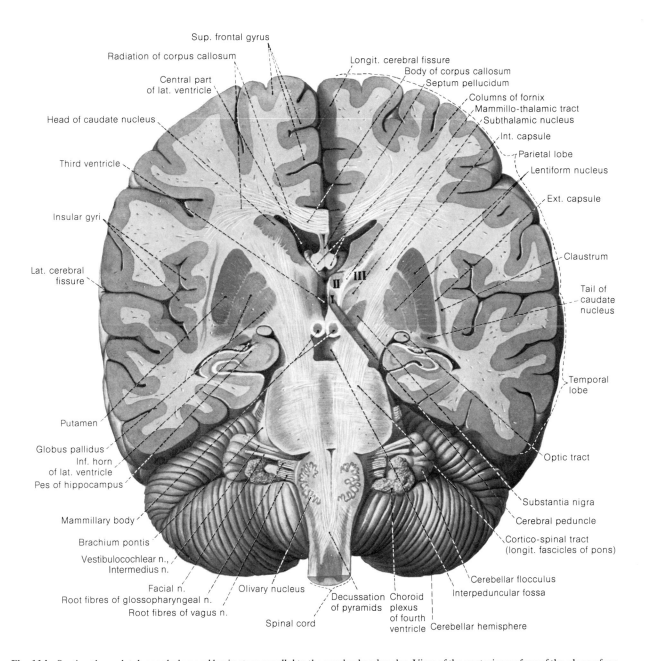

Sup. frontal gyrus
Radiation of corpus callosum
Central part of lat. ventricle
Head of caudate nucleus
Third ventricle
Insular gyri
Lat. cerebral fissure
Putamen
Globus pallidus
Inf. horn of lat. ventricle
Pes of hippocampus
Mammillary body
Brachium pontis
Vestibulocochlear n., Intermedius n.
Facial n.
Root fibres of glossopharyngeal n.
Root fibres of vagus n.
Olivary nucleus
Spinal cord
Decussation of pyramids
Choroid plexus of fourth ventricle
Cerebellar hemisphere

Longit. cerebral fissure
Body of corpus callosum
Septum pellucidum
Columns of fornix
Mammillo-thalamic tract
Subthalamic nucleus
Int. capsule
Parietal lobe
Lentiform nucleus
Ext. capsule
Claustrum
Tail of caudate nucleus
Temporal lobe
Optic tract
Substantia nigra
Cerebral peduncle
Cortico-spinal tract (longit. fascicles of pons)
Cerebellar flocculus
Interpeduncular fossa

II  III
I

**Fig. 114.** Section through telencephalon and brain stem parallel to the cerebral peduncles. View of the posterior surface of the plane of sectioning. On the right side of the figure the section reaches back to about the middle of the cerebral peduncle (oblique section). I–III thalamic nuclei. I = medial nucleus, II = anterior nucleus, III = lateral nucleus.

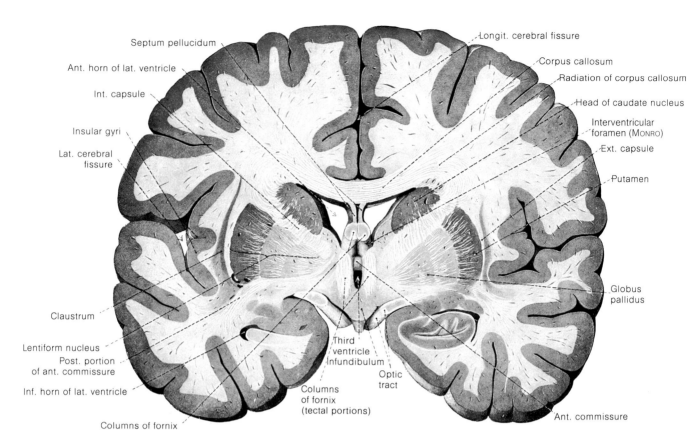

Septum pellucidum

Ant. horn of lat. ventricle

Int. capsule

Insular gyri

Lat. cerebral fissure

Claustrum

Lentiform nucleus

Post. portion of ant. commissure

Inf. horn of lat. ventricle

Columns of fornix

Longit. cerebral fissure

Corpus callosum

Radiation of corpus callosum

Head of caudate nucleus

Interventricular foramen (MONRO)

Ext. capsule

Putamen

Globus pallidus

Third ventricle

Infundibulum

Optic tract

Columns of fornix (tectal portions)

Ant. commissure

**Fig. 115.** Frontal section through the telencephalon immediately behind the anterior commissure.

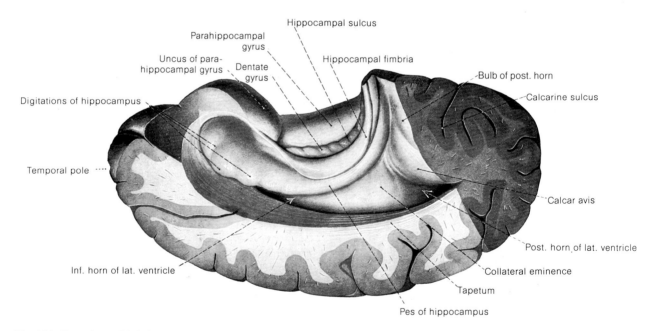

Hippocampal sulcus

Parahippocampal gyrus

Uncus of para-hippocampal gyrus

Dentate gyrus

Hippocampal fimbria

Digitations of hippocampus

Temporal pole

Inf. horn of lat. ventricle

Bulb of post. horn

Calcarine sulcus

Calcar avis

Post. horn of lat. ventricle

Collateral eminence

Tapetum

Pes of hippocampus

**Fig. 116.** Posterior and inferior horns of the lateral ventricle, opened from lateral. View of the hippocampus.

**Fig. 117.** Frontal section through the telencephalon at the plane of the mammillary bodies and the thalamus. In Figs. 115 and 117 the ▷ observer views the anterior cut surface.

**Fig. 118.** Frontal section through the human telencephalon. View from posterior.

82

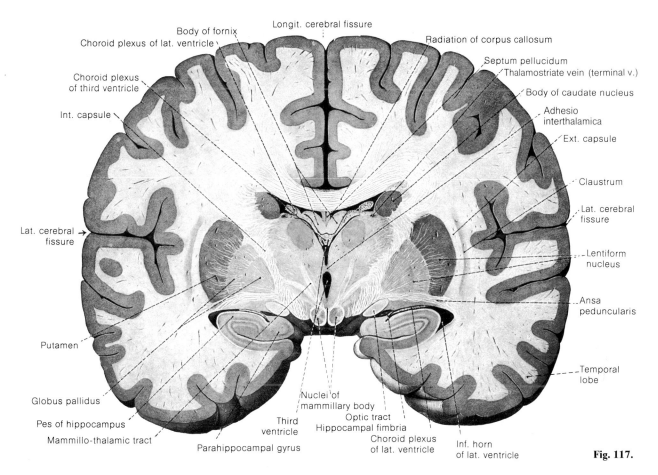

Longit. cerebral fissure

Body of fornix

Choroid plexus of lat. ventricle

Radiation of corpus callosum

Septum pellucidum

Thalamostriate vein (terminal v.)

Choroid plexus of third ventricle

Body of caudate nucleus

Adhesio interthalamica

Int. capsule

Ext. capsule

Claustrum

Lat. cerebral fissure

Lat. cerebral fissure

Lentiform nucleus

Ansa peduncularis

Putamen

Temporal lobe

Globus pallidus

Pes of hippocampus

Nuclei of mammillary body

Optic tract

Mammillo-thalamic tract

Third ventricle

Hippocampal fimbria

Choroid plexus of lat. ventricle

Inf. horn of lat. ventricle

Parahippocampal gyrus

**Fig. 117.**

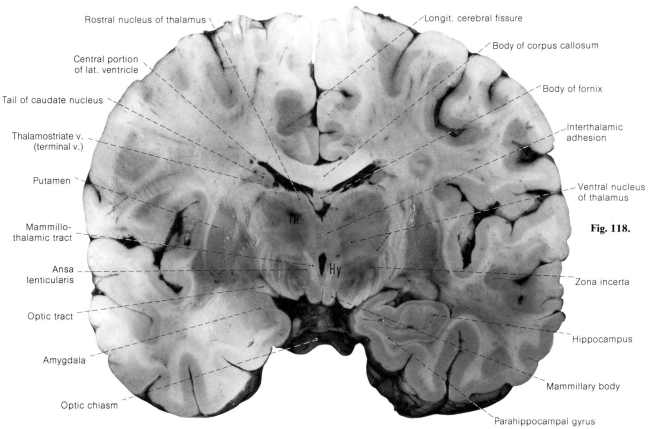

Rostral nucleus of thalamus

Longit. cerebral fissure

Body of corpus callosum

Central portion of lat. ventricle

Body of fornix

Tail of caudate nucleus

Interthalamic adhesion

Thalamostriate v. (terminal v.)

Putamen

Ventral nucleus of thalamus

**Fig. 118.**

Mammillo-thalamic tract

Ansa lenticularis

Zona incerta

Optic tract

Hippocampus

Amygdala

Mammillary body

Optic chiasm

Parahippocampal gyrus

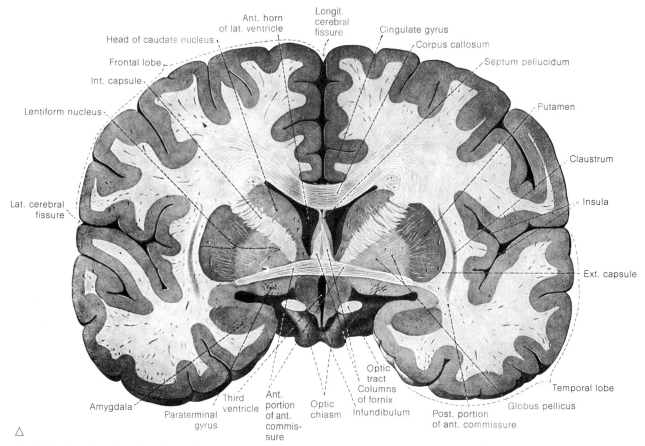

**Fig. 119.** Frontal section through the telencephalon in the plane of the anterior commissure. Sectioned surface seen from behind.

**Fig. 120.** Frontal section through the cerebrum in front of thalamus, optic chiasm, and foramen of MONRO. Anterior horn of lateral ventricle without choroid plexus. (From PERNKOPF: Atlas der topographischen und angewandten Anatomie des Menschen, Vol. 1, 2nd ed. [Ed. H. FERNER]. Urban & Schwarzenberg, Munich–Vienna–Baltimore 1980.)

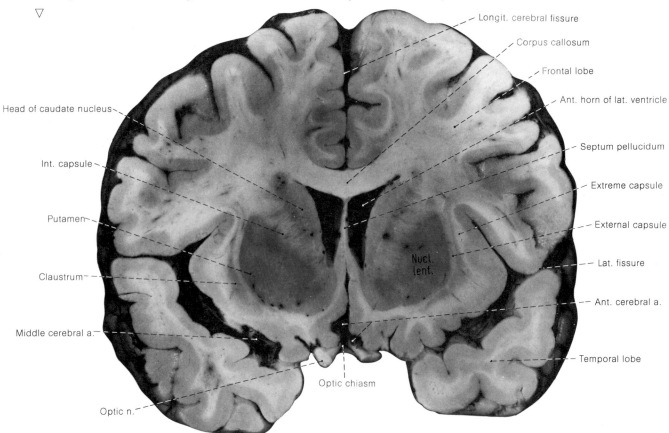

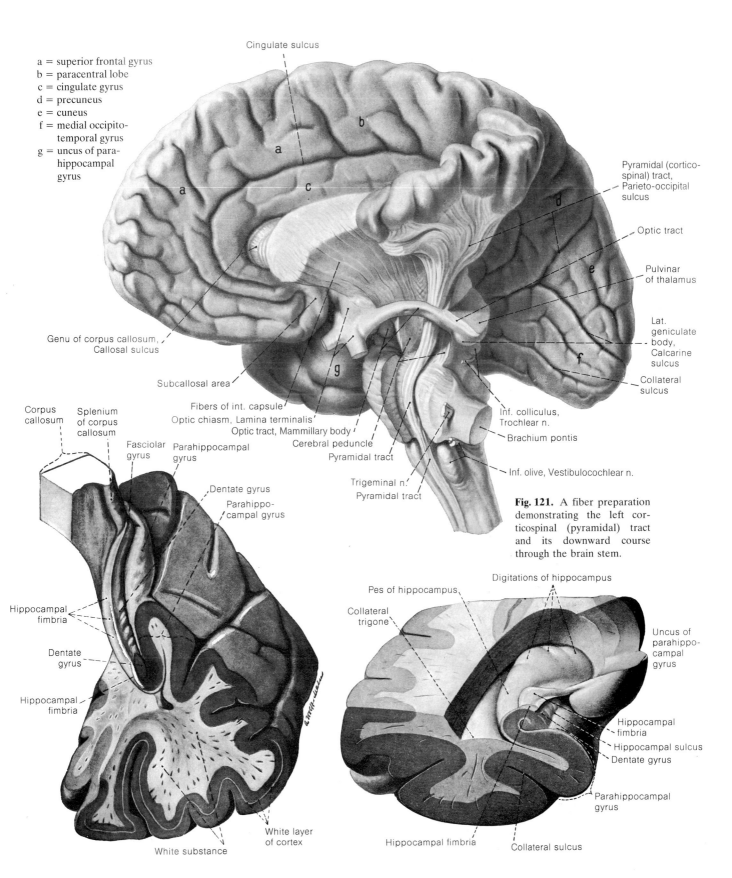

a = superior frontal gyrus
b = paracentral lobe
c = cingulate gyrus
d = precuneus
e = cuneus
f = medial occipito-
    temporal gyrus
g = uncus of para-
    hippocampal
    gyrus

Cingulate sulcus

Pyramidal (cortico-
spinal) tract,
Parieto-occipital
sulcus

Optic tract

Pulvinar
of thalamus

Lat.
geniculate
body,
Calcarine
sulcus

Collateral
sulcus

Genu of corpus callosum,
Callosal sulcus

Subcallosal area

Fibers of int. capsule
Optic chiasm, Lamina terminalis
Optic tract, Mammillary body
Cerebral peduncle
Pyramidal tract

Trigeminal n.
Pyramidal tract

Inf. colliculus,
Trochlear n.

Brachium pontis

Inf. olive, Vestibulocochlear n.

**Fig. 121.** A fiber preparation demonstrating the left corticospinal (pyramidal) tract and its downward course through the brain stem.

Corpus
callosum

Splenium
of corpus
callosum

Fasciolar
gyrus

Parahippocampal
gyrus

Dentate gyrus

Parahippo-
campal gyrus

Hippocampal
fimbria

Dentate
gyrus

Hippocampal
fimbria

White layer
of cortex

White substance

Pes of hippocampus

Digitations of hippocampus

Collateral
trigone

Uncus of
parahippo-
campal
gyrus

Hippocampal
fimbria

Hippocampal sulcus

Dentate gyrus

Parahippocampal
gyrus

Hippocampal fimbria

Collateral sulcus

**Fig. 122.** Anterior end of the temporal lobe with the splenium of the corpus callosum. View from behind and below. The transition of the dentate gyrus into the fasciolar gyrus is visible.

**Fig. 123.** Anterior end of the temporal lobe after opening the inferior horn of the lateral ventricle by frontal section. View from behind and above.

85

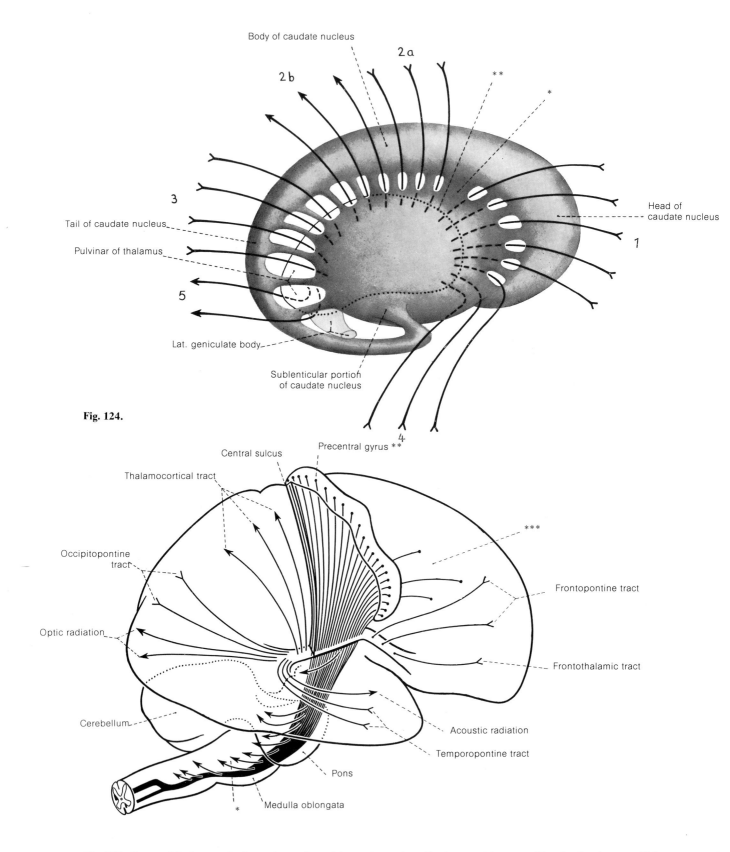

Body of caudate nucleus

2 a

2 b

**

*

3

Tail of caudate nucleus

Pulvinar of thalamus

Head of caudate nucleus

1

5

Lat. geniculate body

Sublenticular portion of caudate nucleus

**Fig. 124.**

Central sulcus

Precentral gyrus **

4

Thalamocortical tract

***

Occipitopontine tract

Frontopontine tract

Optic radiation

Frontothalamic tract

Cerebellum

Acoustic radiation

Temporopontine tract

Pons

*

Medulla oblongata

**Fig. 125.** Course of the long projection pathways through internal capsule and brain stem. * Arrows = fibers leaving the pyramidal tract toward the lamina quadrigemina (corticotectal tract), toward the pontine nuclei (corticopontine tract), toward the cerebellum (corticocerebellar tract) and toward the nuclei of the medulla oblongata (corticobulbar tract). The pyramidal tract continues as crossed lateral corticospinal tract and as uncrossed ventral corticospinal tract. ** First neurons of the pyramidal tract; their fibers converge and occupy the anterior two thirds of the posterior limb of the internal capsule (compare Fig. 126). *** Motor pathways from the medial frontal gyrus.

◁ **Fig. 124.** Thalamic radiation, caudate nucleus and putamen in lateral view. The outline of the medially located thalamus is indicated anteriorly by a dotted line, posteriorly by a solid line. 1 = anterior limb; 2 a b and 3 = posterior limb; 4 = inf. thalamic peduncle (not part of internal capsule); 5 = ventrolenticular and sublentiform portions including optic radiation. * Bridges of gray substance between caudate nucleus and putamen. ** This dotted and solid line indicates the position of the thalamus located medial to the lentiform nucleus. Between the two is the internal capsule through which the fibers of the thalamic radiation take their course (arrows).

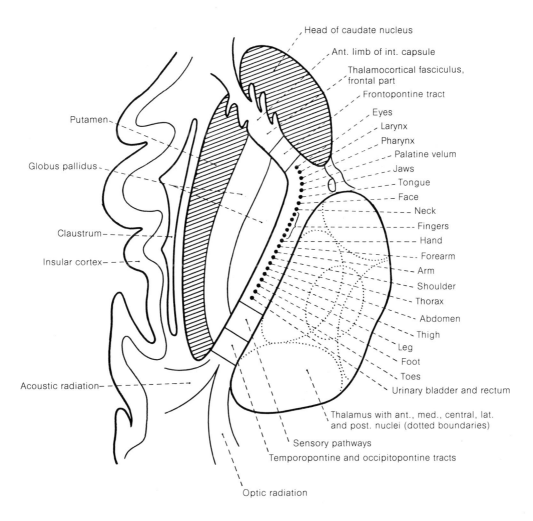

Head of caudate nucleus
Ant. limb of int. capsule
Thalamocortical fasciculus, frontal part
Frontopontine tract
Eyes
Larynx
Pharynx
Palatine velum
Jaws
Tongue
Face
Neck
Fingers
Hand
Forearm
Arm
Shoulder
Thorax
Abdomen
Thigh
Leg
Foot
Toes
Urinary bladder and rectum
Thalamus with ant., med., central, lat. and post. nuclei (dotted boundaries)
Sensory pathways
Temporopontine and occipitopontine tracts
Optic radiation

Putamen
Globus pallidus
Claustrum
Insular cortex
Acoustic radiation

**Fig. 126.** Disposition of the fiber systems within the internal capsule with special emphasis on the somatotopic arrangement of the motor pathways (pyramidal tract).

NOTE: Most of the long pathways between cerebral cortex and lower centers of brain stem and spinal cord (ascending and descending pathways) take their course through an L-shaped area located between the lentiform nucleus on the lateral side and the thalamus and caudate nucleus on the medial side. The entirety of these fibers forms the internal capsule in which can be distinguished an anterior limb, a genu, and a posterior limb. These designations are based upon the appearance of the internal capsule in a horizontally sectioned cerebral hemisphere. In three dimensional view, additionally a sublentiform and a retrolentiform portion of the internal capsule may be distinguished. The anterior limb of the internal capsule contains the thalamocortical and frontopontine pathways, the genu contains the corticobulbar pathways, and in the posterior limb – arranged from rostral to caudal – are located the corticospinal tract, thalamocortical tract, temporo-occipital pontine pathways as well as the acoustic and optic radiations.

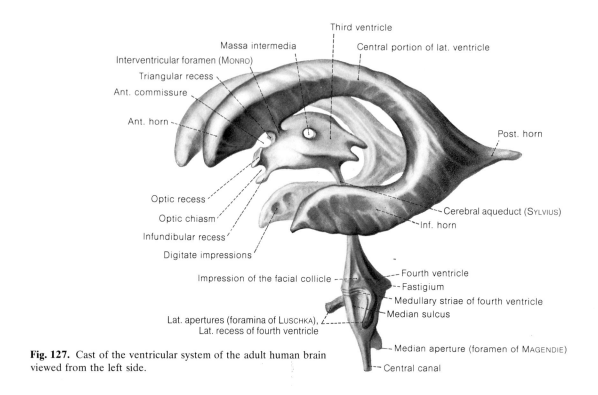

Third ventricle

Massa intermedia

Central portion of lat. ventricle

Interventricular foramen (MONRO)

Triangular recess

Ant. commissure

Ant. horn

Post. horn

Optic recess

Optic chiasm

Infundibular recess

Digitate impressions

Cerebral aqueduct (SYLVIUS)

Inf. horn

Impression of the facial collicle

Fourth ventricle

Fastigium

Medullary striae of fourth ventricle

Median sulcus

Lat. apertures (foramina of LUSCHKA),
Lat. recess of fourth ventricle

Median aperture (foramen of MAGENDIE)

Central canal

**Fig. 127.** Cast of the ventricular system of the adult human brain viewed from the left side.

NOTE: Obstruction of the narrow passages of the ventricular system, i.e., cerebral aqueduct and median and lateral apertures of the fourth ventricle may lead to the condition called internal obstructive hydrocephalus.

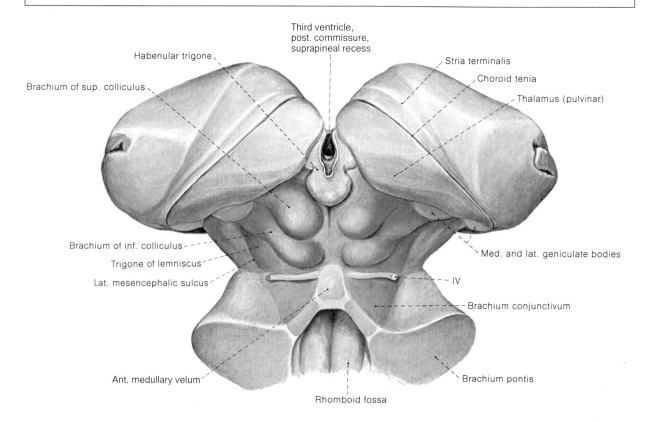

Habenular trigone

Third ventricle,
post. commissure,
suprapineal recess

Stria terminalis

Choroid tenia

Brachium of sup. colliculus

Thalamus (pulvinar)

Brachium of inf. colliculus

Trigone of lemniscus

Lat. mesencephalic sulcus

Med. and lat. geniculate bodies

IV

Brachium conjunctivum

Ant. medullary velum

Brachium pontis

Rhomboid fossa

**Fig. 128.** Mesencephalon (red), seen from above. View of the lamina quadrigemina; medial and lateral geniculate bodies green.

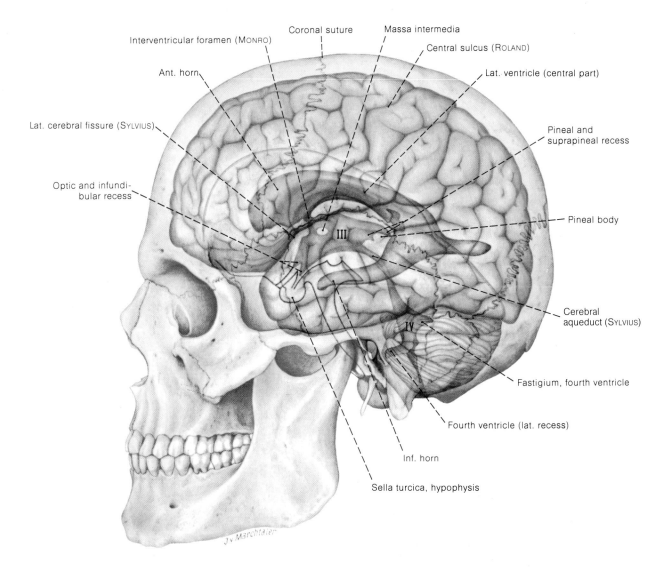

**Fig. 129.** Lateral view of the ventricles of the brain in their topographical position within the brain and the bony skull. Normally, the anterior horn does not extend forward beyond the coronal suture. The basal contour of the brain stem and the median contour of the inside of the base of the skull are indicated by a simple line (Preparation by FERNER and KAUTZKY). (From PERNKOPF: Atlas der topographischen und angewandten Anatomie des Menschen, Vol. 1, 2nd ed. [Ed. H. FERNER]. Urban & Schwarzenberg, Munich–Vienna–Baltimore 1980.)

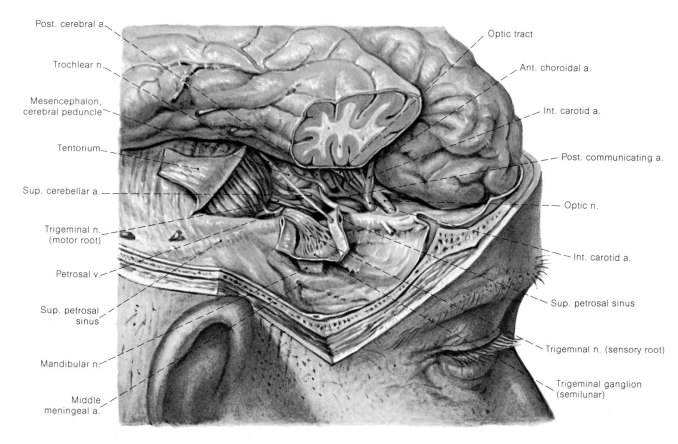

Post. cerebral a.

Trochlear n.

Mesencephalon, cerebral peduncle

Tentorium

Sup. cerebellar a.

Trigeminal n. (motor root)

Petrosal v.

Sup. petrosal sinus

Mandibular n.

Middle meningeal a.

Optic tract

Ant. choroidal a.

Int. carotid a.

Post. communicating a.

Optic n.

Int. carotid a.

Sup. petrosal sinus

Trigeminal n. (sensory root)

Trigeminal ganglion (semilunar)

**Fig. 130.** The middle cranial fossa and the intracranial portion of the trigeminal nerve. The dural pouch (= cavum MECKELI) containing the trigeminal ganglion and the distal part of the root of the trigeminal nerve, surrounded by arachnoid membrane and cerebrospinal fluid (trigeminal cistern), has been opened. The superior petrosal sinus has been cut at the trigeminal porus, the temporal lobe has been elevated. (From FERNER and KAUTZKY: Handbuch der Neurochirurgie. Springer, Heidelberg 1959.)

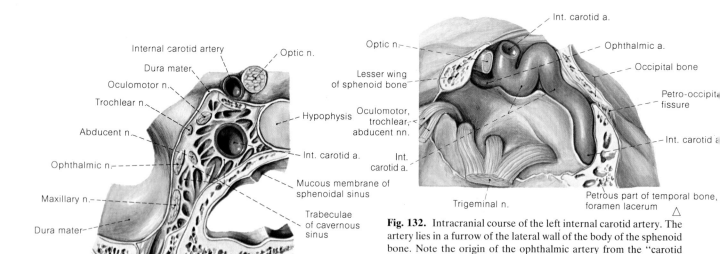

Internal carotid artery

Dura mater

Oculomotor n.

Trochlear n.

Abducent n.

Ophthalmic n.

Maxillary n.

Dura mater

Optic n.

Hypophysis

Int. carotid a.

Mucous membrane of sphenoidal sinus

Trabeculae of cavernous sinus

Body of sphenoid bone

Optic n.

Lesser wing of sphenoid bone

Oculomotor, trochlear, abducent nn.

Int. carotid a.

Trigeminal n.

Int. carotid a.

Ophthalmic a.

Occipital bone

Petro-occipital fissure

Int. carotid a.

Petrous part of temporal bone, foramen lacerum

**Fig. 132.** Intracranial course of the left internal carotid artery. The artery lies in a furrow of the lateral wall of the body of the sphenoid bone. Note the origin of the ophthalmic artery from the "carotid knee" and the S-shaped curve ("carotid siphon") of the carotid artery within the carotid sulcus next to the sella turcica. Trigeminal, oculomotor, trochlear and abducent nerves have been deflected laterally.

**Fig. 131.** Frontal section through the left cavernous sinus at the plane of the hypophysis. The internal carotid artery (lower cross section) is surrounded by the venous chambers of the sinus. After forming the "carotid knee", from which the ophthalmic artery arises, the carotid artery penetrates the dura mater and appears below the optic nerve where it enters the optic canal (upper cross section). This segment of the artery is surrounded by cerebrospinal fluid ("cisternal segment"). The carotid cross sections have different diameters because of the origin of the ophthalmic artery.

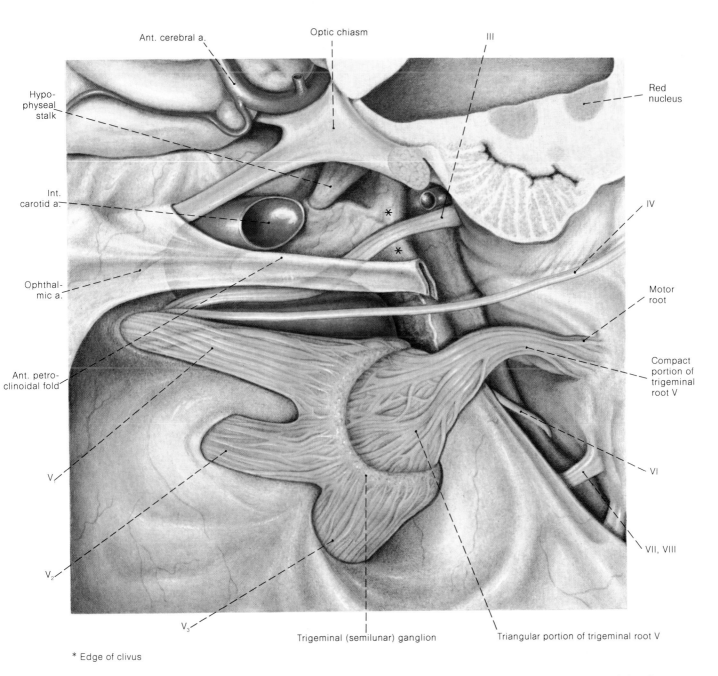

Ant. cerebral a.

Optic chiasm

III

Red nucleus

Hypo-physeal stalk

Int. carotid a.

*

*

IV

Ophthal-mic a.

Motor root

Compact portion of trigeminal root V

Ant. petro-clinoidal fold

V₁

VI

V₂

VII, VIII

V₃

Trigeminal (semilunar) ganglion

Triangular portion of trigeminal root V

\* Edge of clivus

**Fig. 133.** Topography of the region of the sella and the intracranial portions of the left trigeminal nerve (viewed from lateral and above). The lateral dural wall of the cavernous sinus below the anterior petroclinoidal fold, the dura mater above the trigeminal ganglion and its branches as well as the tentorium have been removed. One recognizes the ganglionic segment, the cavernous-sinus-segment and the cisternal segment of the internal carotid artery. The oculomotor nerve courses over the edge of the clivus. Note the position of the infundibulum, the inclination of the hypophyseal stalk and its relationship to the optic chiasm. The third ventricle is opened, the midbrain is cross-sectioned behind the optic tract. (From FERNER and KAUTZKY: Handbuch der Neurochirurgie. Springer, Heidelberg 1959.)

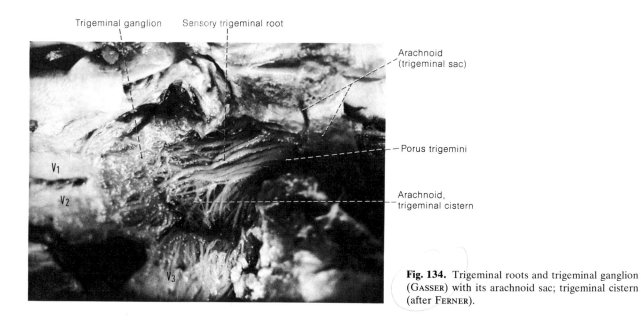

Trigeminal ganglion    Sensory trigeminal root

Arachnoid
(trigeminal sac)

Porus trigemini

Arachnoid,
trigeminal cistern

V₁

V₂

V₃

**Fig. 134.** Trigeminal roots and trigeminal ganglion (Gasser) with its arachnoid sac; trigeminal cistern (after Ferner).

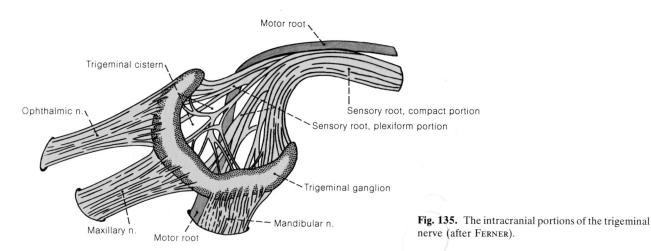

Motor root

Trigeminal cistern

Ophthalmic n.

Sensory root, compact portion

Sensory root, plexiform portion

Trigeminal ganglion

Maxillary n.    Motor root    Mandibular n.

**Fig. 135.** The intracranial portions of the trigeminal nerve (after Ferner).

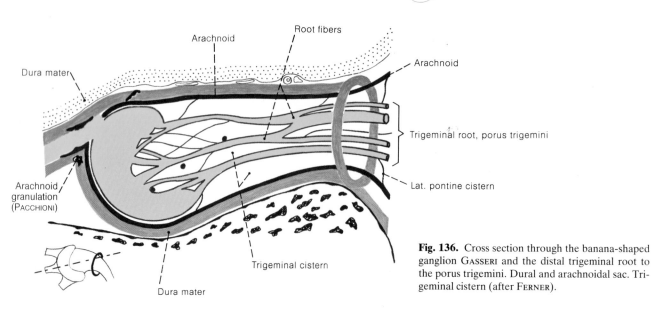

Root fibers

Arachnoid

Dura mater

Arachnoid

Trigeminal root, porus trigemini

Arachnoid
granulation
(Pacchioni)

Lat. pontine cistern

Trigeminal cistern

Dura mater

**Fig. 136.** Cross section through the banana-shaped ganglion Gasseri and the distal trigeminal root to the porus trigemini. Dural and arachnoidal sac. Trigeminal cistern (after Ferner).

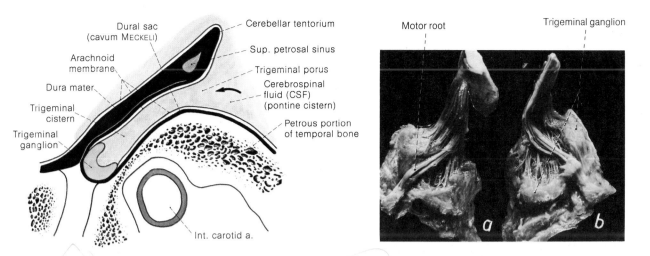

**Fig. 136a.** Frontal section through the trigeminal cistern and the CSF-communication through the trigeminal porus between pontine cistern and trigeminal cistern. CSF green (after FERNER).

**Fig. 137.** The left and right trigeminal ganglion with the sensory and the compact motor roots, medial view (after FERNER).

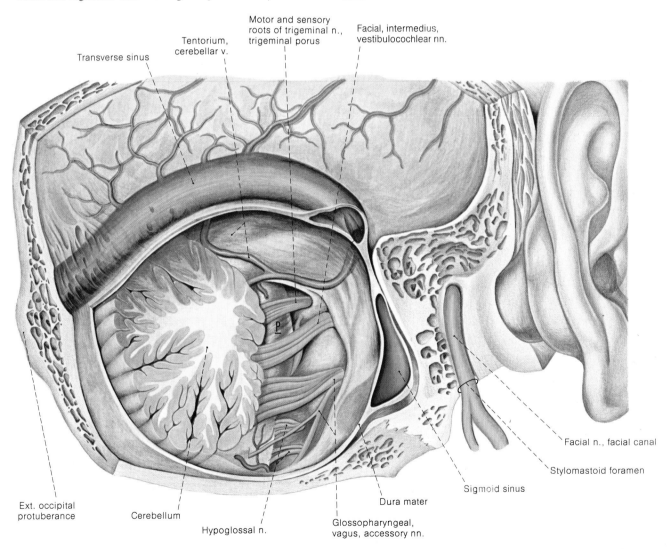

**Fig. 138.** View into the subtentorial space after partial removal of the right cerebellar hemisphere. P = pons.

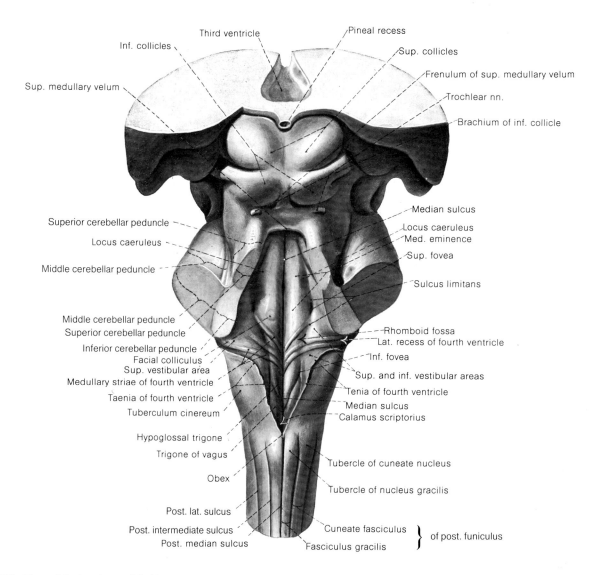

Third ventricle

Inf. collicles

Pineal recess

Sup. collicles

Sup. medullary velum

Frenulum of sup. medullary velum

Trochlear nn.

Brachium of inf. collicle

Superior cerebellar peduncle

Locus caeruleus

Middle cerebellar peduncle

Median sulcus

Locus caeruleus

Med. eminence

Sup. fovea

Sulcus limitans

Middle cerebellar peduncle

Superior cerebellar peduncle

Inferior cerebellar peduncle

Facial colliculus

Sup. vestibular area

Medullary striae of fourth ventricle

Taenia of fourth ventricle

Tuberculum cinereum

Hypoglossal trigone

Trigone of vagus

Obex

Post. lat. sulcus

Post. intermediate sulcus

Post. median sulcus

Rhomboid fossa

Lat. recess of fourth ventricle

Inf. fovea

Sup. and inf. vestibular areas

Tenia of fourth ventricle

Median sulcus

Calamus scriptorius

Tubercle of cuneate nucleus

Tubercle of nucleus gracilis

Cuneate fasciculus

Fasciculus gracilis

} of post. funiculus

**Fig. 139.** Floor of the fourth ventricle (rhomboid fossa). Dorsal view of the lamina tecti (quadrigemina). Cerebellum and pineal body have been removed.

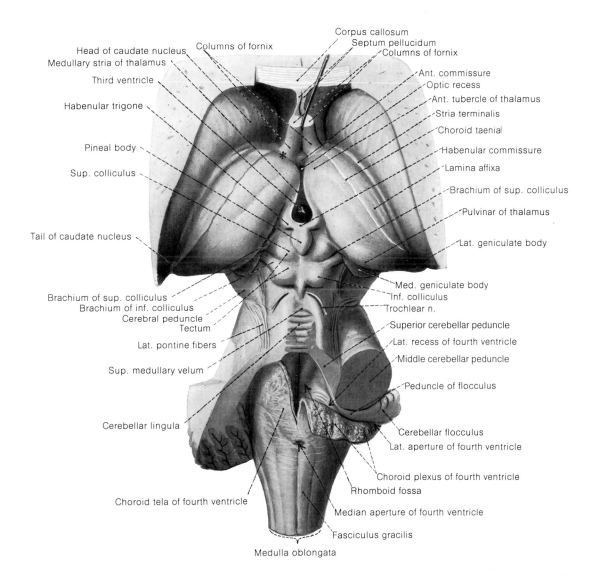

Head of caudate nucleus
Medullary stria of thalamus
Columns of fornix
Corpus callosum
Septum pellucidum
Columns of fornix
Third ventricle
Ant. commissure
Optic recess
Ant. tubercle of thalamus
Habenular trigone
Stria terminalis
Choroid taenia
Pineal body
Habenular commissure
Lamina affixa
Sup. colliculus
Brachium of sup. colliculus
Pulvinar of thalamus
Tail of caudate nucleus
Lat. geniculate body
Brachium of sup. colliculus
Med. geniculate body
Brachium of inf. colliculus
Inf. colliculus
Cerebral peduncle
Trochlear n.
Tectum
Superior cerebellar peduncle
Lat. pontine fibers
Lat. recess of fourth ventricle
Middle cerebellar peduncle
Sup. medullary velum
Peduncle of flocculus
Cerebellar lingula
Cerebellar flocculus
Lat. aperture of fourth ventricle
Choroid plexus of fourth ventricle
Rhomboid fossa
Choroid tela of fourth ventricle
Median aperture of fourth ventricle
Fasciculus gracilis
Medulla oblongata

**Fig. 140.** Brain stem seen from dorsal and above. The caudate nuclei, thalami and third ventricle have been made visible by removing the corpus callosum, the fornix and the choroid tela of the third ventricle. The cerebellum has been removed except the flocculus on the right side and a part of the hemisphere on the left side. The choroid tela of the fourth ventricle has been split in the midline and is reflected on the right side. * = interventricular foramen.

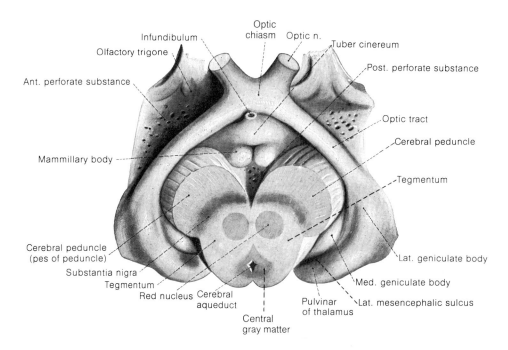

**Fig. 141.**

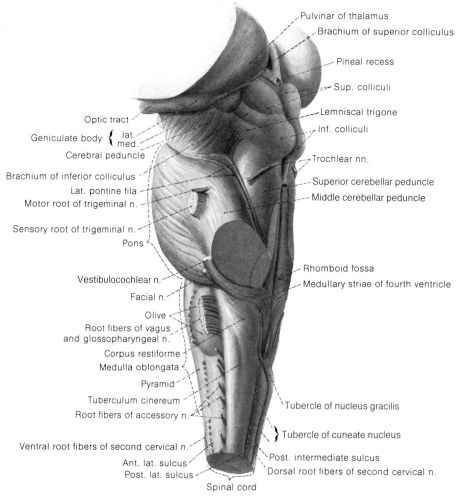

**Fig. 142.** Brain stem seen from left and somewhat dorsal.

**Fig. 141.** Section through the midbrain. View from behind. Optic tract, geniculate bodies, hypothalamus. Compare with Fig. 143.

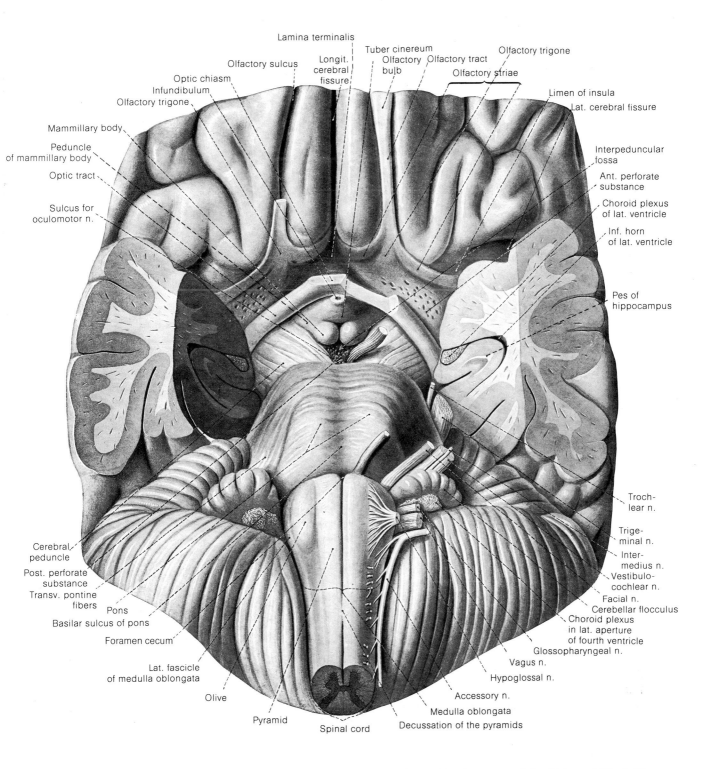

Lamina terminalis
Olfactory sulcus
Optic chiasm
Infundibulum
Olfactory trigone
Mammillary body
Peduncle of mammillary body
Optic tract
Sulcus for oculomotor n.
Longit. cerebral fissure
Tuber cinereum
Olfactory bulb
Olfactory tract
Olfactory striae
Olfactory trigone
Limen of insula
Lat. cerebral fissure
Interpeduncular fossa
Ant. perforate substance
Choroid plexus of lat. ventricle
Inf. horn of lat. ventricle
Pes of hippocampus
Cerebral peduncle
Post. perforate substance
Transv. pontine fibers
Pons
Basilar sulcus of pons
Foramen cecum
Lat. fascicle of medulla oblongata
Olive
Pyramid
Spinal cord
Decussation of the pyramids
Medulla oblongata
Accessory n.
Hypoglossal n.
Vagus n.
Glossopharyngeal n.
Choroid plexus in lat. aperture of fourth ventricle
Cerebellar flocculus
Facial n.
Vestibulocochlear n.
Intermedius n.
Trigeminal n.
Trochlear n.

**Fig. 143.** Basal view of the brain stem with adjacent parts of the brain: diencephalon, midbrain, pons, medulla oblongata (bulbus). The temporal poles have been removed. The origins of the cranial nerves are preserved on the left side, on the right side they have been removed. Somewhat enlarged over natural size.

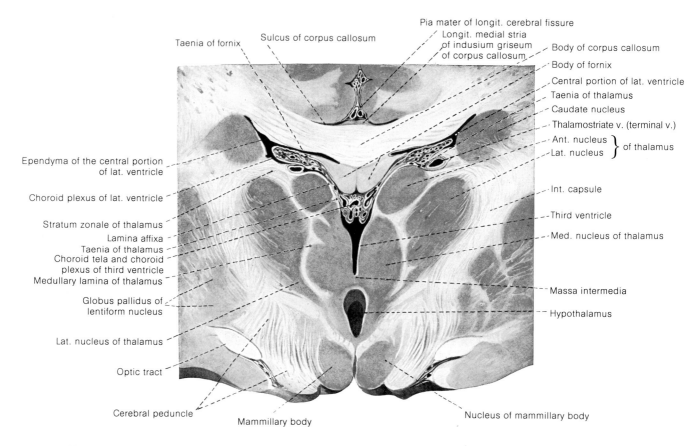

**Fig. 144.** Frontal section through lateral ventricles, third ventricle, corpus callosum, fornix and hypothalamus at the plane of the mammillary bodies.

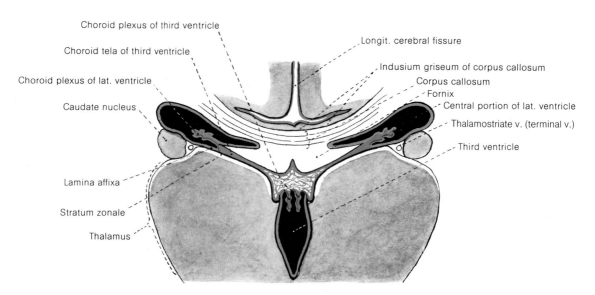

**Fig. 145.** Schematic representation of a transverse section through the central portion of the lateral ventricle. Roof of the third ventricle, choroid tela of the third ventricle. Pia mater and arachnoid membrane are shown in red, the ependyma and the epithelium of the choroid plexus in blue. Compare with Fig. 144.

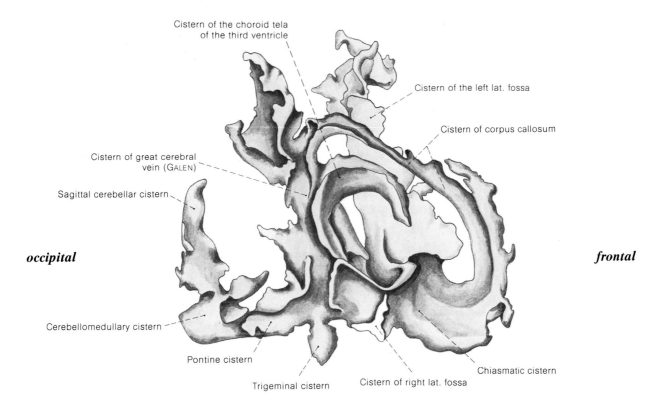

Cistern of the choroid tela
of the third ventricle

Cistern of the left lat. fossa

Cistern of corpus callosum

Cistern of great cerebral
vein (GALEN)

Sagittal cerebellar cistern

*occipital*

*frontal*

Cerebellomedullary cistern

Pontine cistern

Chiasmatic cistern

Trigeminal cistern

Cistern of right lat. fossa

**Fig. 146.** Cast of the cisternal spaces around the human brain, after NAFFZIGER. Extracerebral CSF-spaces.

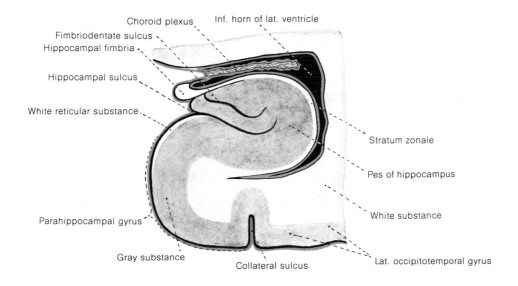

Choroid plexus

Inf. horn of lat. ventricle

Fimbriodentate sulcus

Hippocampal fimbria

Hippocampal sulcus

White reticular substance

Stratum zonale

Pes of hippocampus

White substance

Parahippocampal gyrus

Gray substance

Collateral sulcus

Lat. occipitotemporal gyrus

**Fig. 147.** Schematic representation of a frontal section through the inferior horn of the lateral ventricle. The pia mater is shown in red, the ependyma and epithelium of the choroid plexus in blue. Compare with Fig. 102.

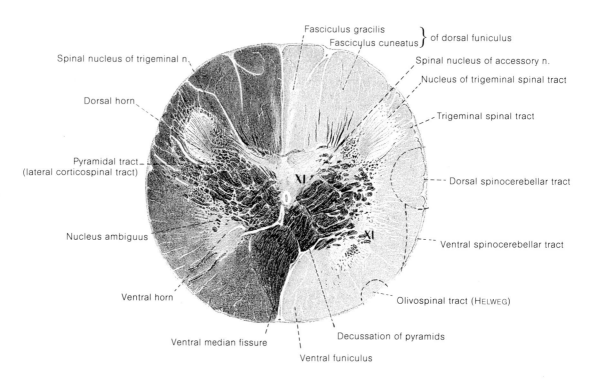

Fasciculus gracilis
Fasciculus cuneatus } of dorsal funiculus

Spinal nucleus of trigeminal n.

Spinal nucleus of accessory n.

Nucleus of trigeminal spinal tract

Dorsal horn

Trigeminal spinal tract

Pyramidal tract
(lateral corticospinal tract)

Dorsal spinocerebellar tract

Nucleus ambiguus

Ventral spinocerebellar tract

Ventral horn

Olivospinal tract (HELWEG)

Ventral median fissure

Decussation of pyramids

Ventral funiculus

**Fig. 148.** Cross section through the medulla oblongata at the level of the lower pole of the decussation of the pyramids.

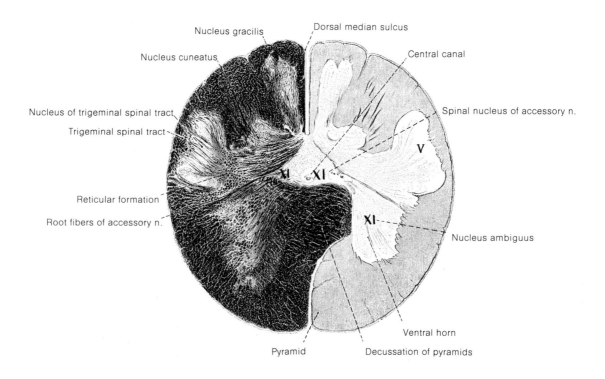

Nucleus gracilis

Dorsal median sulcus

Nucleus cuneatus

Central canal

Nucleus of trigeminal spinal tract

Spinal nucleus of accessory n.

Trigeminal spinal tract

Reticular formation

Root fibers of accessory n.

Nucleus ambiguus

Ventral horn

Pyramid

Decussation of pyramids

**Fig. 149.** Cross section through the medulla oblongata at the level of the upper pole of the decussation of the pyramids. The Roman numerals indicate the position of the corresponding cranial nerve nuclei.

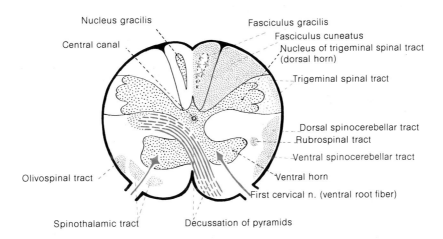

Nucleus gracilis

Central canal

Fasciculus gracilis

Fasciculus cuneatus

Nucleus of trigeminal spinal tract (dorsal horn)

Trigeminal spinal tract

Dorsal spinocerebellar tract

Rubrospinal tract

Ventral spinocerebellar tract

Ventral horn

First cervical n. (ventral root fiber)

Olivospinal tract

Spinothalamic tract

Decussation of pyramids

**Fig. 150.** Architecture of the medulla oblongata at the level of the decussation of the pyramids. Schematic cross section.

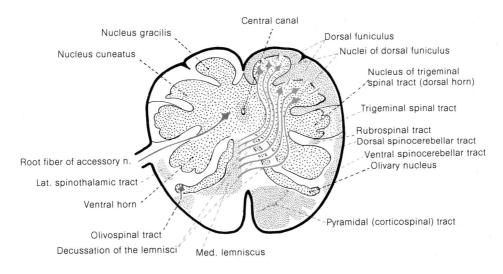

Nucleus gracilis

Nucleus cuneatus

Central canal

Dorsal funiculus

Nuclei of dorsal funiculus

Nucleus of trigeminal spinal tract (dorsal horn)

Trigeminal spinal tract

Rubrospinal tract

Dorsal spinocerebellar tract

Ventral spinocerebellar tract

Olivary nucleus

Root fiber of accessory n.

Lat. spinothalamic tract

Ventral horn

Olivospinal tract

Pyramidal (corticospinal) tract

Decussation of the lemnisci

Med. lemniscus

**Fig. 151.** Architecture of the medulla oblongata at the level of the decussation of the lemnisci. Schematic cross section.

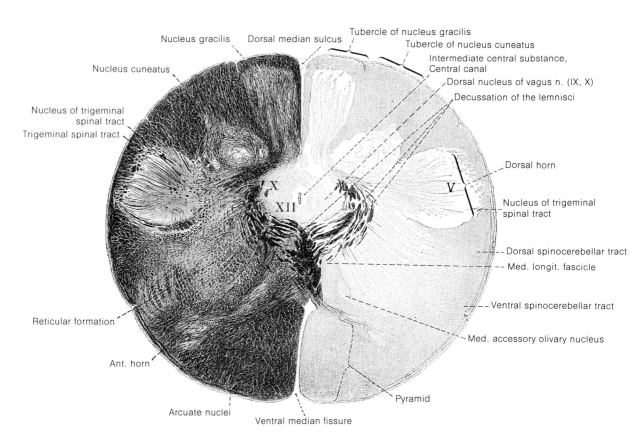

**Fig. 152.** Cross section through the medulla oblongata at the level of the decussation of the lemnisci.

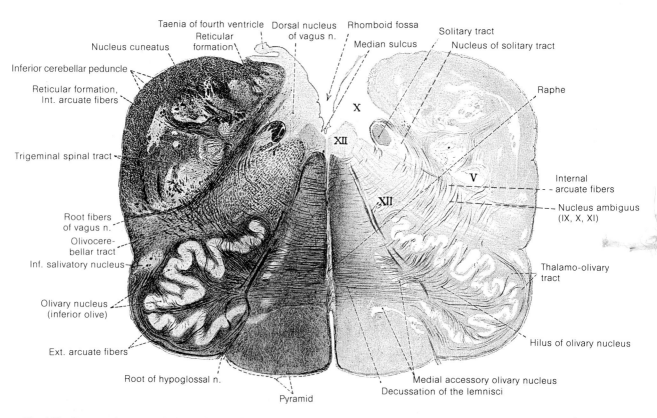

**Fig. 153.** Cross section through the medulla oblongata at the level of the obex.

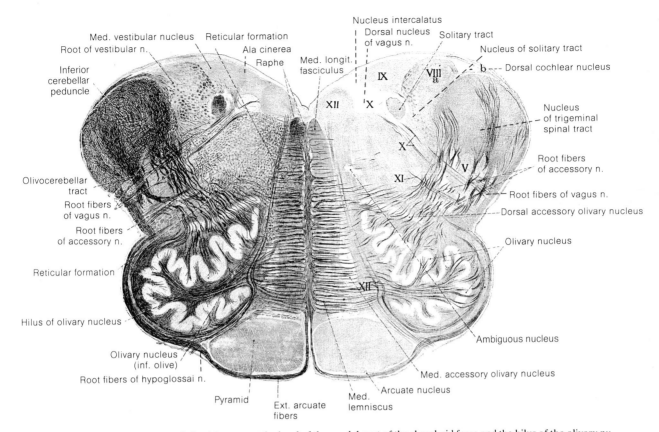

**Fig. 154.** Cross section through the medulla oblongata at the level of the caudal part of the rhomboid fossa and the hilus of the olivary nucleus. The Roman numerals indicate the location of the nuclei of the corresponding cranial nerves. VIII a = vestibular nucleus, b = cochlear nucleus.

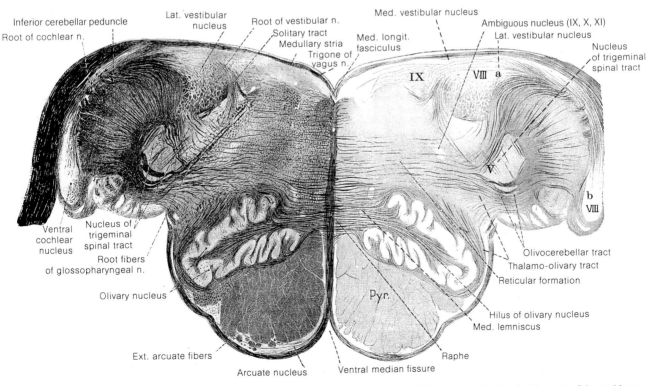

**Fig. 155.** Cross section through the medulla oblongata in the middle area of the rhomboid fossa and at the level of the root of the cochlear nerve. The Roman numerals indicate the nuclei of the corresponding cranial nerves. VIII a = vestibular nucleus, VIII b = cochlear nucleus.

103

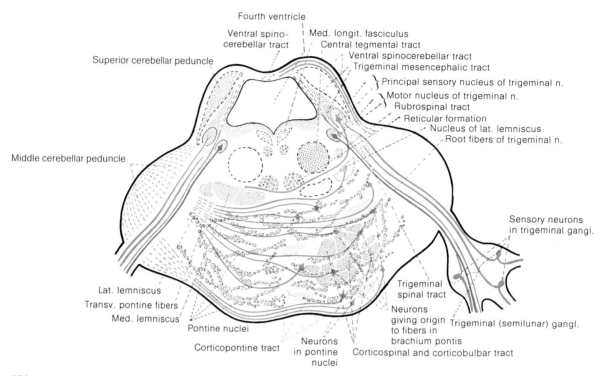

Fourth ventricle
Ventral spino-
cerebellar tract
Superior cerebellar peduncle
Med. longit. fasciculus
Central tegmental tract
Ventral spinocerebellar tract
Trigeminal mesencephalic tract
Principal sensory nucleus of trigeminal n.
Motor nucleus of trigeminal n.
Rubrospinal tract
Reticular formation
Nucleus of lat. lemniscus
Root fibers of trigeminal n.
Middle cerebellar peduncle
Sensory neurons
in trigeminal gangl.
Lat. lemniscus
Transv. pontine fibers
Med. lemniscus
Pontine nuclei
Corticopontine tract
Neurons
in pontine
nuclei
Trigeminal
spinal tract
Neurons
giving origin
to fibers in
brachium pontis
Corticospinal and corticobulbar tract
Trigeminal (semilunar) gangl.

**Fig. 156.** Architecture of the pons at the level of the trigeminal nuclei. Schematic cross section.

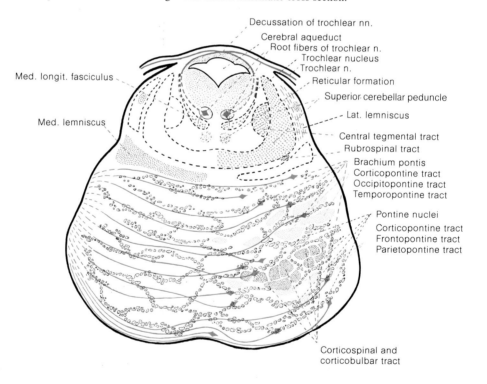

Decussation of trochlear nn.
Cerebral aqueduct
Root fibers of trochlear n.
Trochlear nucleus
Trochlear n.
Reticular formation
Superior cerebellar peduncle
Lat. lemniscus
Med. longit. fasciculus
Med. lemniscus
Central tegmental tract
Rubrospinal tract
Brachium pontis
Corticopontine tract
Occipitopontine tract
Temporopontine tract
Pontine nuclei
Corticopontine tract
Frontopontine tract
Parietopontine tract
Corticospinal and
corticobulbar tract

**Fig. 157.** Architecture of the pons at the level of the trochlear nuclei. Schematic cross section.
Red and yellow: descending pathways; blue: ascending pathways.

**Fig. 158.** Position and extent of motor and parasympathetic cranial nuclei in the tegmentum (after M. CLARA, 1942). ▷

**Fig. 159.** The position and extent of the sensory cranial nuclei in the tegmentum.

**Fig. 160.** Position and extent of cranial nerve nuclei of the brain stem. On the left side the motor (red) and parasympathetic (yellow) nuclei; on the right side the sensory nuclei (blue).

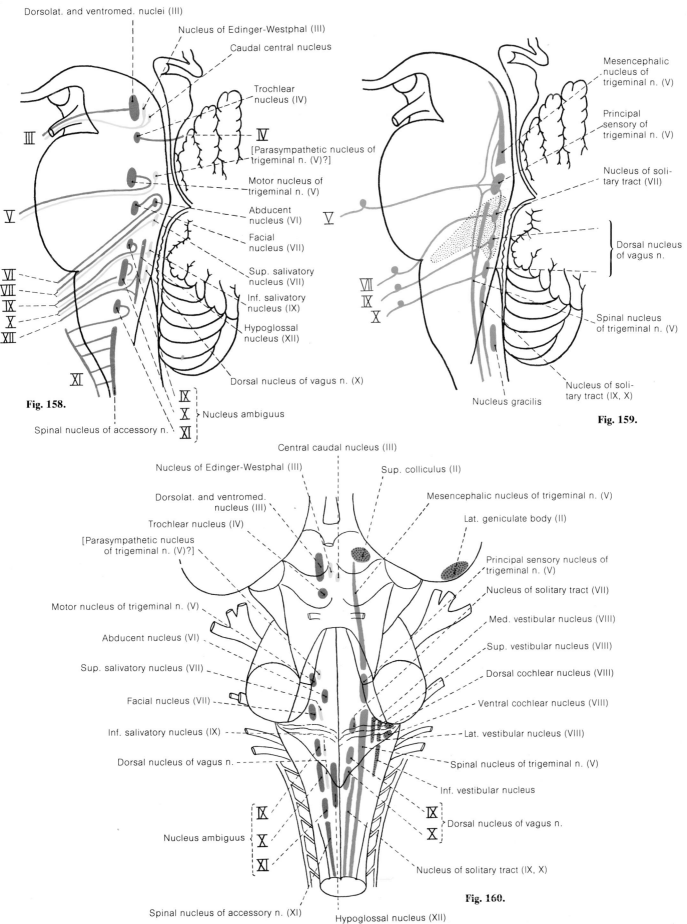

Dorsolat. and ventromed. nuclei (III)

Nucleus of Edinger-Westphal (III)

Caudal central nucleus

Trochlear nucleus (IV)

[Parasympathetic nucleus of trigeminal n. (V)?]

Motor nucleus of trigeminal n. (V)

Abducent nucleus (VI)

Facial nucleus (VII)

Sup. salivatory nucleus (VII)

Inf. salivatory nucleus (IX)

Hypoglossal nucleus (XII)

Dorsal nucleus of vagus n. (X)

III

IV

V

VI
VII
IX
X
XII

XI

**Fig. 158.**

Spinal nucleus of accessory n.

IX
X
XI } Nucleus ambiguus

Mesencephalic nucleus of trigeminal n. (V)

Principal sensory of trigeminal n. (V)

Nucleus of solitary tract (VII)

Dorsal nucleus of vagus n.

Spinal nucleus of trigeminal n. (V)

Nucleus of solitary tract (IX, X)

Nucleus gracilis

V

VII
IX
X

**Fig. 159.**

Central caudal nucleus (III)

Nucleus of Edinger-Westphal (III)

Sup. colliculus (II)

Dorsolat. and ventromed. nucleus (III)

Mesencephalic nucleus of trigeminal n. (V)

Trochlear nucleus (IV)

Lat. geniculate body (II)

[Parasympathetic nucleus of trigeminal n. (V)?]

Principal sensory nucleus of trigeminal n. (V)

Motor nucleus of trigeminal n. (V)

Nucleus of solitary tract (VII)

Abducent nucleus (VI)

Med. vestibular nucleus (VIII)

Sup. salivatory nucleus (VII)

Sup. vestibular nucleus (VIII)

Facial nucleus (VII)

Dorsal cochlear nucleus (VIII)

Ventral cochlear nucleus (VIII)

Inf. salivatory nucleus (IX)

Lat. vestibular nucleus (VIII)

Dorsal nucleus of vagus n.

Spinal nucleus of trigeminal n. (V)

Inf. vestibular nucleus

IX
X
XI

IX
X } Dorsal nucleus of vagus n.

Nucleus ambiguus

Nucleus of solitary tract (IX, X)

Spinal nucleus of accessory n. (XI)

Hypoglossal nucleus (XII)

**Fig. 160.**

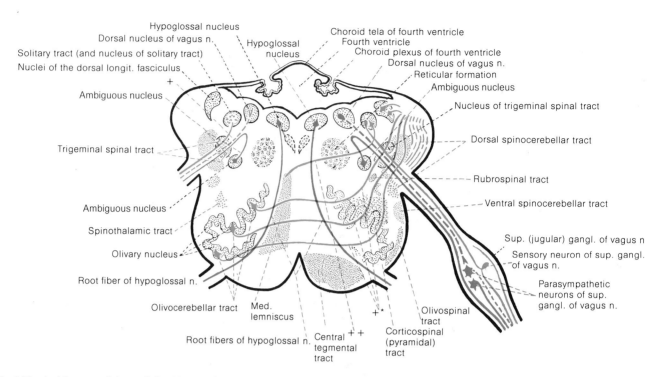

Hypoglossal nucleus
Dorsal nucleus of vagus n.
Solitary tract (and nucleus of solitary tract)
Nuclei of the dorsal longit. fasciculus
Ambiguous nucleus
Trigeminal spinal tract
Ambiguous nucleus
Spinothalamic tract
Olivary nucleus
Root fiber of hypoglossal n.
Olivocerebellar tract
Med. lemniscus
Root fibers of hypoglossal n.
Central tegmental tract

Hypoglossal nucleus
Choroid tela of fourth ventricle
Fourth ventricle
Choroid plexus of fourth ventricle
Dorsal nucleus of vagus n.
Reticular formation
Ambiguous nucleus
Nucleus of trigeminal spinal tract
Dorsal spinocerebellar tract
Rubrospinal tract
Ventral spinocerebellar tract
Sup. (jugular) gangl. of vagus n.
Sensory neuron of sup. gangl. of vagus n.
Parasympathetic neurons of sup. gangl. of vagus n.
Olivospinal tract
Corticospinal (pyramidal) tract

**Fig. 161.** Architecture of the medulla oblongata in the region of the caudal part of the rhomboid fossa. Schematic cross section; compare with Fig. 154. Red: descending pathways; blue: ascending pathways.

+ * = *olivocerebellar fibers;*      + = *afferent fibers to dorsal nucleus of vagus;*      + + = *fibers from solitary tract to med. lemniscus*

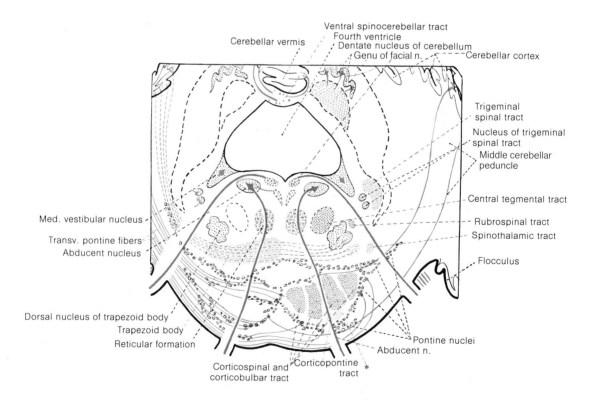

Cerebellar vermis
Ventral spinocerebellar tract
Fourth ventricle
Dentate nucleus of cerebellum
Genu of facial n.
Cerebellar cortex
Trigeminal spinal tract
Nucleus of trigeminal spinal tract
Middle cerebellar peduncle
Central tegmental tract
Rubrospinal tract
Spinothalamic tract
Flocculus
Med. vestibular nucleus
Transv. pontine fibers
Abducent nucleus
Dorsal nucleus of trapezoid body
Trapezoid body
Reticular formation
Pontine nuclei
Abducent n.
Corticospinal and corticobulbar tract
Corticopontine tract

**Fig. 162.** Architecture of the caudal portion of the pons. Schematic cross section. Red and yellow: descending pathways; blue: ascending pathways. * Fibers from the cerebellar cortex to the pontine nuclei.

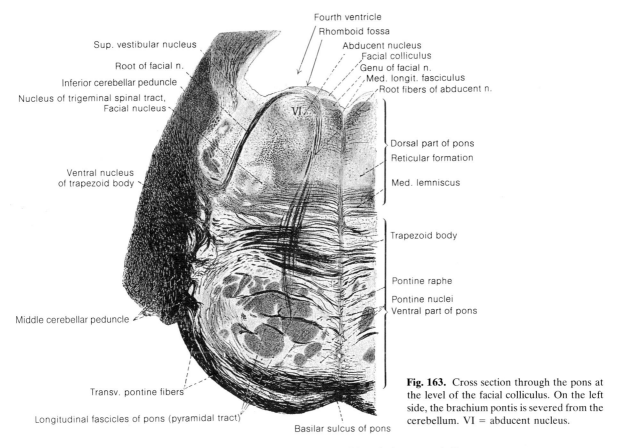

Sup. vestibular nucleus

Root of facial n.

Inferior cerebellar peduncle

Nucleus of trigeminal spinal tract,
Facial nucleus

Ventral nucleus
of trapezoid body

Middle cerebellar peduncle

Transv. pontine fibers

Longitudinal fascicles of pons (pyramidal tract)

Fourth ventricle
Rhomboid fossa
Abducent nucleus
Facial colliculus
Genu of facial n.
Med. longit. fasciculus
Root fibers of abducent n.

Dorsal part of pons
Reticular formation

Med. lemniscus

Trapezoid body

Pontine raphe
Pontine nuclei
Ventral part of pons

Basilar sulcus of pons

**Fig. 163.** Cross section through the pons at the level of the facial colliculus. On the left side, the brachium pontis is severed from the cerebellum. VI = abducent nucleus.

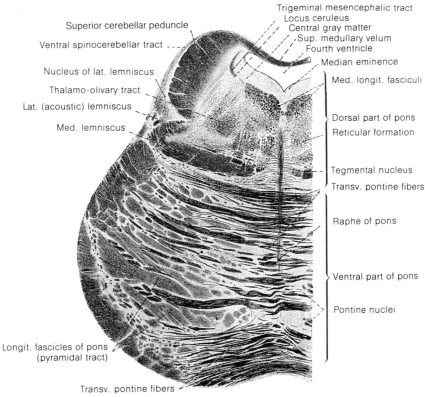

Superior cerebellar peduncle

Ventral spinocerebellar tract

Nucleus of lat. lemniscus

Thalamo-olivary tract

Lat. (acoustic) lemniscus

Med. lemniscus

Trigeminal mesencephalic tract
Locus ceruleus
Central gray matter
Sup. medullary velum
Fourth ventricle
Median eminence

Med. longit. fasciculi

Dorsal part of pons
Reticular formation

Tegmental nucleus
Transv. pontine fibers

Raphe of pons

Ventral part of pons

Pontine nuclei

Longit. fascicles of pons
(pyramidal tract)

Transv. pontine fibers

**Fig. 164.** Cross section through the middle portion of the pons.

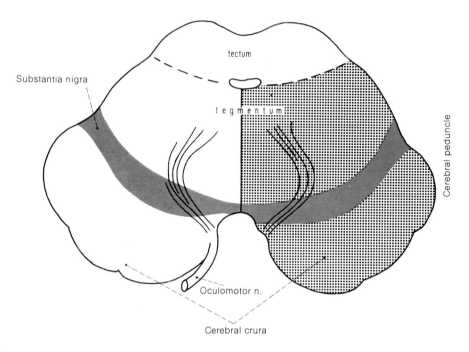

**Fig. 165.** Subdivisions of the midbrain: tectum, tegmentum, crura cerebri. Screened: cerebral peduncle.

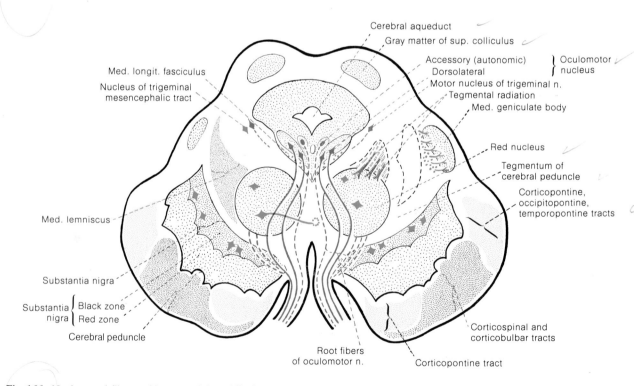

**Fig. 166.** Nuclear and fiber architecture of the midbrain.

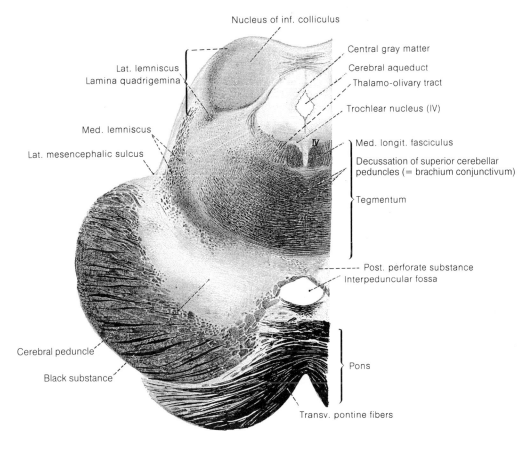

Nucleus of inf. colliculus

Central gray matter

Cerebral aqueduct

Thalamo-olivary tract

Lat. lemniscus
Lamina quadrigemina

Trochlear nucleus (IV)

Med. lemniscus

Lat. mesencephalic sulcus

Med. longit. fasciculus

Decussation of superior cerebellar peduncles (= brachium conjunctivum)

Tegmentum

Post. perforate substance
Interpeduncular fossa

Cerebral peduncle

Black substance

Pons

Transv. pontine fibers

**Fig. 167.** Cross section through the midbrain at the level of the inferior colliculi.

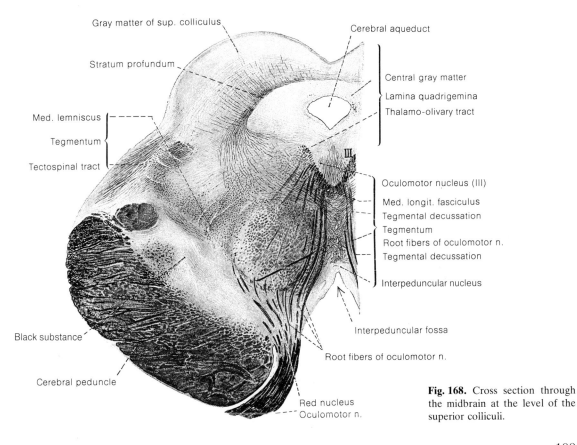

Gray matter of sup. colliculus

Cerebral aqueduct

Stratum profundum

Central gray matter

Lamina quadrigemina

Thalamo-olivary tract

Med. lemniscus

Tegmentum

Tectospinal tract

Oculomotor nucleus (III)

Med. longit. fasciculus
Tegmental decussation
Tegmentum
Root fibers of oculomotor n.
Tegmental decussation

Interpeduncular nucleus

Black substance

Interpeduncular fossa

Cerebral peduncle

Root fibers of oculomotor n.

Red nucleus
Oculomotor n.

**Fig. 168.** Cross section through the midbrain at the level of the superior colliculi.

109

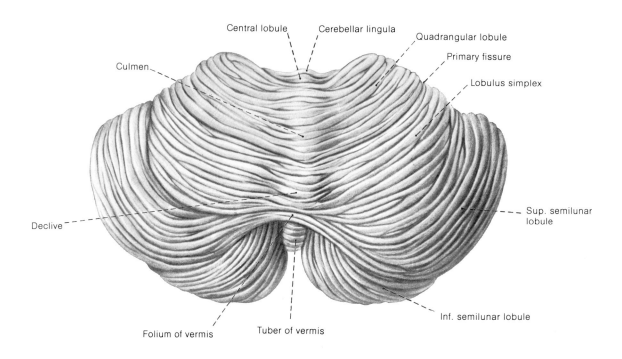

Central lobule
Cerebellar lingula
Quadrangular lobule
Primary fissure
Lobulus simplex
Culmen
Sup. semilunar lobule
Declive
Inf. semilunar lobule
Folium of vermis
Tuber of vermis

**Fig. 169.** Cerebellum viewed from above and behind. Portions of the paleocerebellum are shown in yellow.

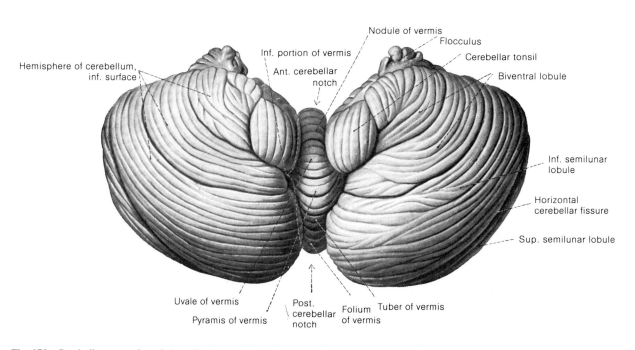

Nodule of vermis
Flocculus
Inf. portion of vermis
Cerebellar tonsil
Hemisphere of cerebellum, inf. surface
Ant. cerebellar notch
Biventral lobule
Inf. semilunar lobule
Horizontal cerebellar fissure
Sup. semilunar lobule
Uvale of vermis
Post. cerebellar notch
Folium of vermis
Tuber of vermis
Pyramis of vermis

**Fig. 170.** Cerebellum seen from below. Portions of the paleocerebellum are shown in yellow.

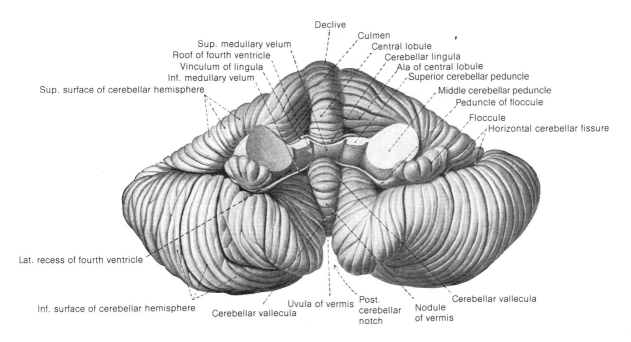

**Fig. 171.** Anterior view of cerebellum. Cerebral peduncles cut transversely.

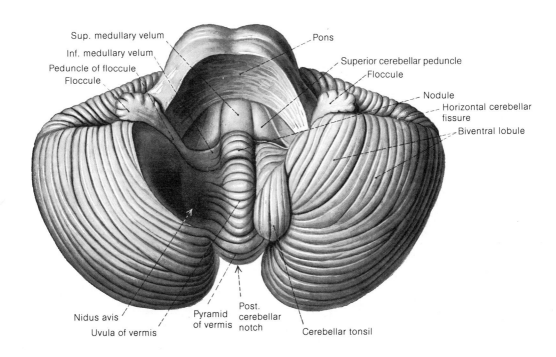

**Fig. 172.** Inferior cerebellar surface after removal of the right tonsil and a part of the biventral lobule. Pons sectioned transversely. View from below onto the roof of the fourth ventricle.

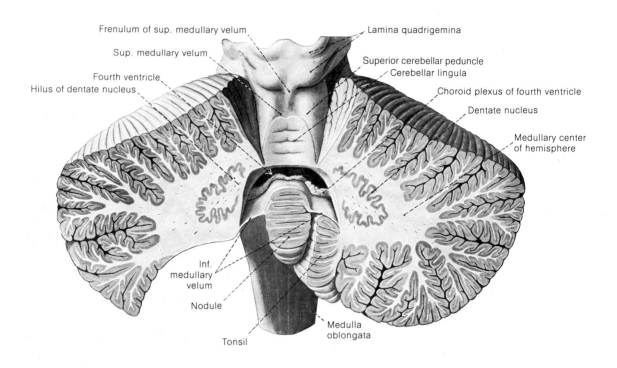

**Fig. 173.** Transverse section through the cerebellum exposing the fourth ventricle.

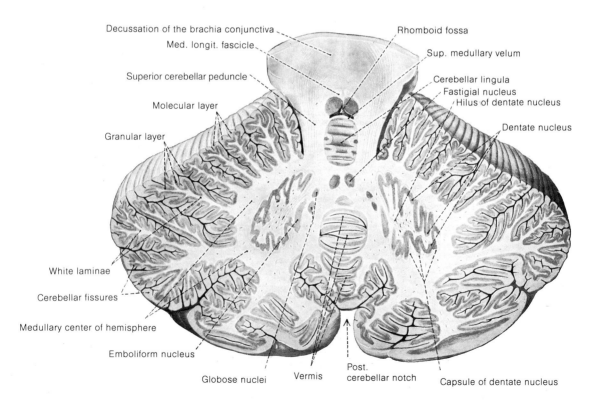

**Fig. 174.** Section through the cerebellum parallel to the brachium conjunctivum. Cerebellar nuclei.

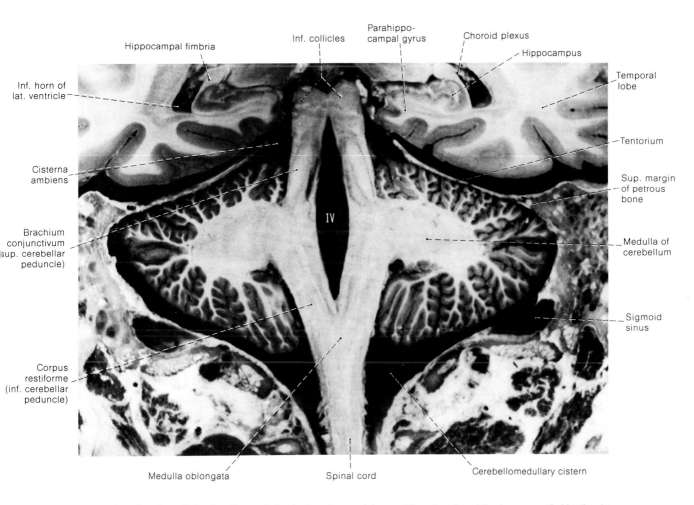

Hippocampal fimbria

Inf. collicles

Parahippo-campal gyrus

Choroid plexus

Hippocampus

Inf. horn of lat. ventricle

Temporal lobe

Tentorium

Cisterna ambiens

Sup. margin of petrous bone

IV

Brachium conjunctivum (sup. cerebellar peduncle)

Medulla of cerebellum

Sigmoid sinus

Corpus restiforme (inf. cerebellar peduncle)

Medulla oblongata

Spinal cord

Cerebellomedullary cistern

**Fig. 175.** Frontal section through the rhombencephalon in the subtentorial space. Note that the midbrain, surrounded by the cisterna ambiens, is located in the area of the tentorial notch. Isthmus of the rhombencephalon (from KAUTZKY-FERNER, Springer, Heidelberg 1959).

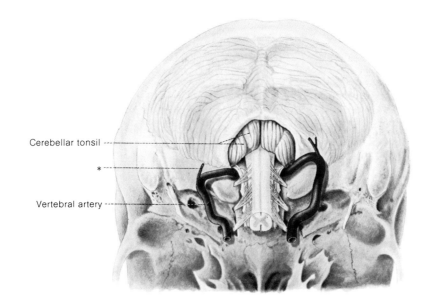

Cerebellar tonsil

*

Vertebral artery

**Fig. 176.** The parts of the brain in the area of the foramen magnum, viewed from below. The spinal cord is deflected forward (from KAUTZ-KY-FERNER, Springer, Heidelberg 1959). * Muscular branch (collateral).

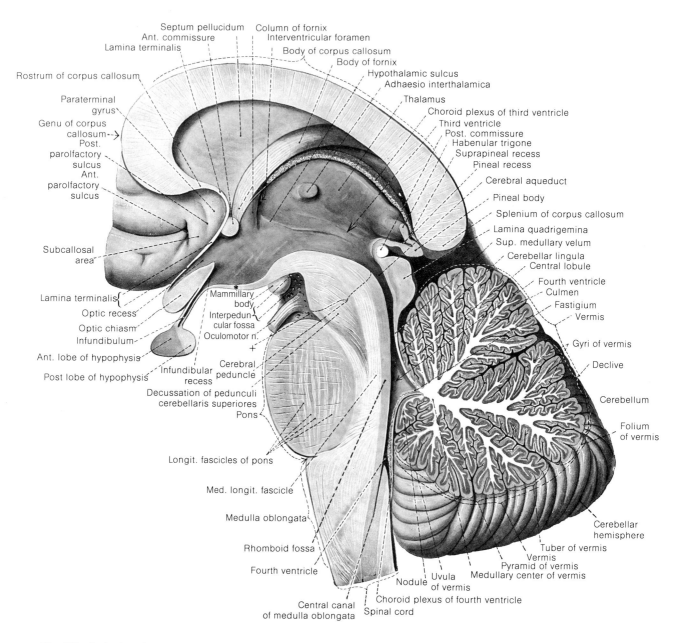

**Fig. 177.** Sagittal section through the brain stem. Cut surface of the right half. Walls of the third and fourth ventricle as well as of the cerebral aqueduct are shown in yellow. * = Tuber cinereum; + = Interpeduncular fossa.

**Fig. 178.** Paramedian sagittal section through the human brain. WEIGERT's myelin stain (myelinated tracts black, nuclear areas gray). Compare with figure on facing page. The myelinated fiber tracts are easily recognized as black regions, e.g., corpus callosum medulla of cerebellum, pyramidal tract, medial lemniscus, optic chiasm and others. The cortical regions and the subcortical nuclei are lightly stained (cortex around the corpus callosum (because of the paramedian section, thalamus, hypothalamus). Nuclear areas with significant fiber = admixtures are stained with intermediate intensity, e.g., pons with pontine nuclei as well as corticopontine and pontocerebellar tracts. Of intermediate staining intensity are also thalamus and other nuclear areas (from KAUTZKY-FERNER, Springer, Heidelberg 1959).  ▷

**Fig. 179.** Suboccipital tap, anatomical situation. (From PERNKOPF: Atlas der topographischen und angewandten Anatomie des Menschen,  ▷ Vol. 1, 2nd ed. [Ed. H. FERNER]. Urban & Schwarzenberg, Munich–Vienna–Baltimore 1980.)

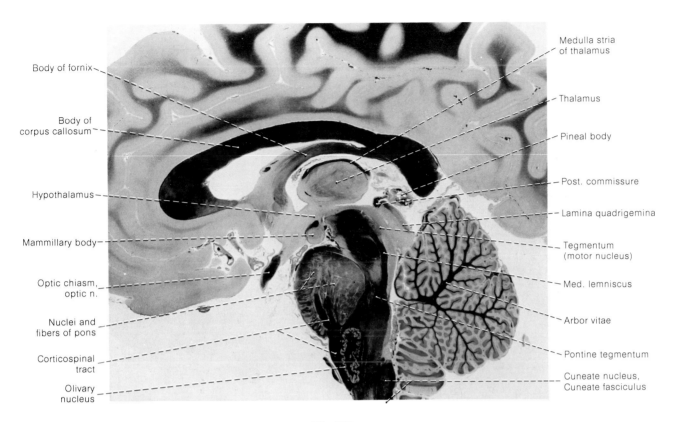

Body of fornix

Body of
corpus callosum

Hypothalamus

Mammillary body

Optic chiasm,
optic n.

Nuclei and
fibers of pons

Corticospinal
tract

Olivary
nucleus

Medulla stria
of thalamus

Thalamus

Pineal body

Post. commissure

Lamina quadrigemina

Tegmentum
(motor nucleus)

Med. lemniscus

Arbor vitae

Pontine tegmentum

Cuneate nucleus,
Cuneate fasciculus

**Fig. 178.**

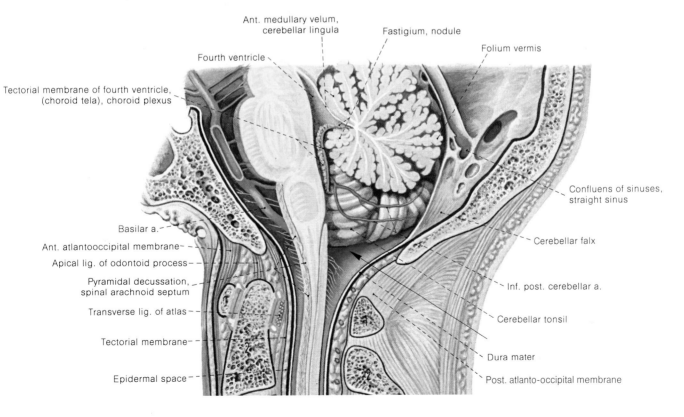

Ant. medullary velum,
cerebellar lingula

Fastigium, nodule

Folium vermis

Fourth ventricle

Tectorial membrane of fourth ventricle,
(choroid tela), choroid plexus

Confluens of sinuses,
straight sinus

Basilar a.

Ant. atlantooccipital membrane

Apical lig. of odontoid process

Pyramidal decussation,
spinal arachnoid septum

Transverse lig. of atlas

Tectorial membrane

Epidermal space

Cerebellar falx

Inf. post. cerebellar a.

Cerebellar tonsil

Dura mater

Post. atlanto-occipital membrane

**Fig. 179.**

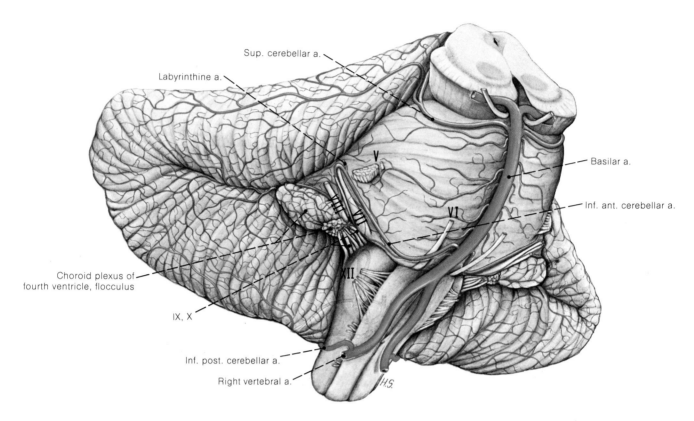

**Fig. 180.** Arteries of the rhombencephalon (Original: Dozent Dr. Tschabitscher, Vienna).

### Arteries of the Cerebellum

The cerebellum is supplied by three paired arteries:
1. Inferior posterior cerebellar artery from the vertebral a.
2. Inferior anterior cerebellar a.
3. Superior cerebellar a., the latter two from the basilar a. They are interconnected by anastomoses. Characteristic for the cerebellar arteries is their arched course from ventral around the brain stem toward dorsal. The branches course along the folia in order to penetrate into the fissures. The arteries underlie the larger veins.

1. **Inferior posterior cerebellar a.** It originates 1–3 cm caudal to the union of the two vertebral arteries and lies between the root fibers of the vagus group, bends around the medulla oblongata and comes to lie upon the choroid tela of the fourth ventricle (branches supply the choroid plexus), it passes to the inferior surface of the cerebellum and loops around the tonsil. Its supply territory is the inferior cerebellar surface.

2. **Inferior anterior cerebellar a.** Originating from the basilar artery, it crosses the abducent n., and then forms a loop whose cortex may read into the internal acoustic meatus. The distal limb of the loop parallels the facial and vestibulocochlear nerves. In most cases, it gives off the labyrinthine a. Its end branches reach the floccule and the lateral positions of the choroid plexus of the fourth ventricle.

3. **Superior cerebellar a.** It originates from the anterior part of the basilar a. shortly before its division, courses within the cisterna ambiens along the anterior margin of the pons around the cerebral peduncle toward dorsal and is, in its initial portion, separated from the posterior cerebral a. by the oculomotor n. The superior cerebellar a. divides into two main branches which both parallel the trochlear nerve and reach the lamina quadrigemina. The artery supplies the superior surface of the cerebellum, the cerebellar nuclei (dentate nucleus etc.).

# Spinal Cord, Spinal Nerves, Sympathetic Trunk

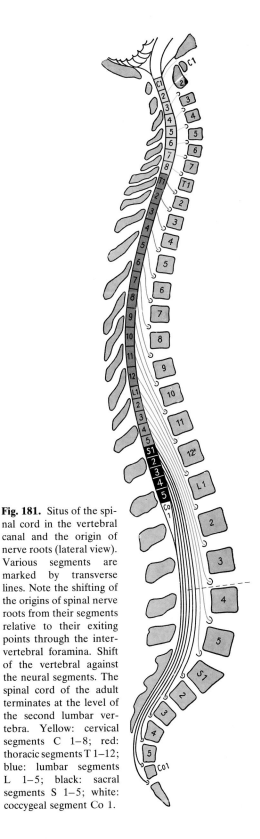

**Fig. 181.** Situs of the spinal cord in the vertebral canal and the origin of nerve roots (lateral view). Various segments are marked by transverse lines. Note the shifting of the origins of spinal nerve roots from their segments relative to their exiting points through the intervertebral foramina. Shift of the vertebral against the neural segments. The spinal cord of the adult terminates at the level of the second lumbar vertebra. Yellow: cervical segments C 1–8; red: thoracic segments T 1–12; blue: lumbar segments L 1–5; black: sacral segments S 1–5; white: coccygeal segment Co 1.

Inf. ganglion of vagus n.
Sup. cervical ganglion
Sup. cardiac n.
Sup. cardiac branch (X)
Cervical sympathetic trunk
Middle cervical ganglion
Middle cardiac n.
Stellate ganglion
Recurrent laryngeal n.
Inf. cardiac n.
Lowest cardiac n.
Thoracic spinal ganglion 3
Cardiac plexus
Left recurrent n.
Roots of greater splanchnic n.
Thoracic symp. ganglion 7
Ant. and post. vagal trunk
Greater splanchnic n.
Lesser splanchnic n.
Celiac plexus
Lumbar spinal ganglion 1
Sup. mesenteric plexus
Lumbar symp. ganglion 1
Lumbar splanchnic nn.
Inf. mesenteric ganglion
Interganglionic branch
Sacral symp. ganglion 1
Sup. hypogastric plexus
Inf. hypogastric plexus
Pelvic plexus
Coccygeal ganglion impar

Renal plexus

**Fig. 182.** The sympathetic trunk, its relationships to the spinal nerves and its branches, e.g., splanchnic nerves.

# Spinal Cord, Spinal Nerves, Sympathetic Trunk

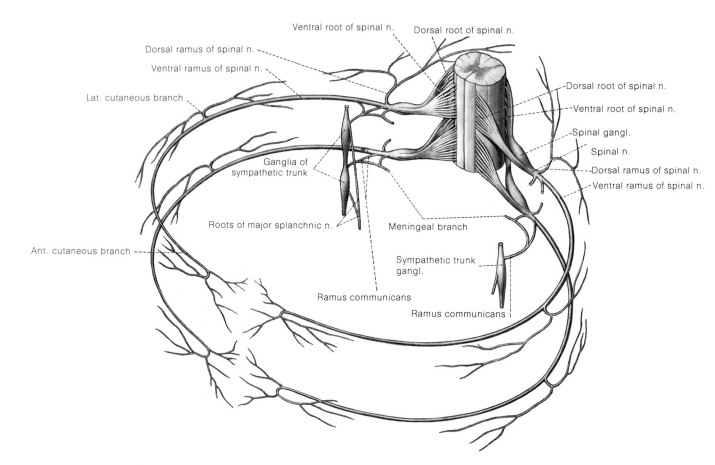

**Fig. 183.** Representation of two thoracic spinal cord segments with corresponding segmental spinal nerves and their branches. Also depicted are the connections with the sympathetic trunk.

## Explanation

A **"spinal cord segment"** (neural segment) is that conceptual disk of spinal cord that is defined by the extent of the exiting radicular fibers for one spinal nerve. The spinal cord segments are designated by the letters $C_1$–$C_8$, $Th_1$–$Th_{12}$, $L_1$–$L_5$, $S_1$–$S_5$, and $Co_1$. Thus there are 8 cervical, 12 thoracic, 5 lumbar, 5 sacral, and 1 coccygeal segments. The latter is located at the level of the second lumbar vertebra.

In contrast, the **"vertebral segments"** correspond to the vertebral bodies. Since the spinal cord reaches only to the second lumbar vertebra, the spinal cord segments do not topically correspond to the vertebral segments. The positional difference increases downward. Thus, the 10th thoracic spinal cord segment is located approximately at the level of the 8th thoracic vertebra, and the 5th neural sacral segment is at the level of the first lumbar vertebra. Therefore, the root fibers of spinal cord segments must, in order to reach their intervertebral foramina, descend steeper the more caudal they are.

The **cauda equina.** Since the dural and arachnoid sacs do not terminate at the same level as the spinal cord but extend downward to the second sacral vertebra, the descending anterior and posterior root fibers that originate from the lumbar and sacral segments are located within this sac surrounding the filum terminale. Their entirety represents the cauda equina.

The **lumbar tap** is performed by inserting a canula into the CSF sac of the cauda equina between the third and fourth lumbar vertebra. CSF can thus be obtained for diagnostic purposes. Also, local anesthetics can be administered here in order to achieve anesthesia in areas below the umbilicus.

A **"peripheral segment"** is that area of the body the various tissues of which are supplied by a single spinal nerve, namely:

1. the cutaneous area (cutis, subcutis, epidermis) of a spinal nerve is the **dermatome.** The dermatomes are belt or ribbon-shaped cutaneous areas that are especially evident on the trunk. Here, the course of the intercostal nerves corresponds to the dermatomes because in the thoracic area the ventral rami of the spinal nerves do not form plexuses.

2. the influence area of one spinal nerve upon skeletal muscles is a **myotome.**

3. the influence area of spinal nerve upon viscera is an **enterotome.**

The majority of skeletal muscles is innervated by more than one root; only those muscles located centrally within a myotome, for all practical purposes, are dependent on this particular root of a spinal nerve. Such muscles may serve to recognize the primary source of innervation for that particular myotome, e.g., the diaphragm for $C_3$, $C_4$, the deltoid muscle for $C_5$, the extensor hallucis longus muscle for $L_5$.

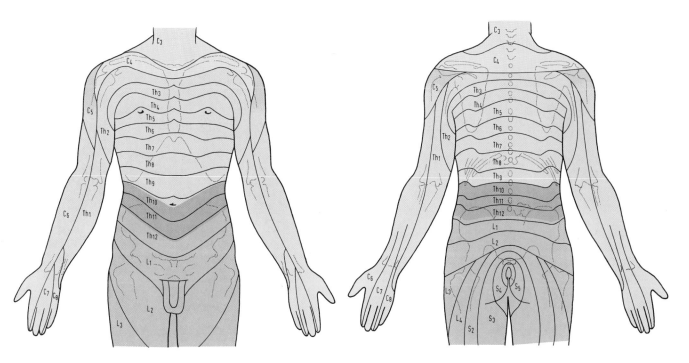

**Fig. 184.** Segmental distribution of dermatomes on the ventral and dorsal aspect of the body. The letters and numerals refer to the corresponding spinal cord segments. (Improved schema of Hansen and Schliack.)

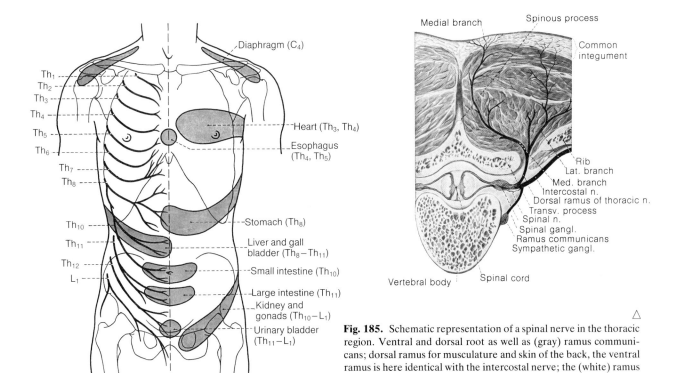

**Fig. 185.** Schematic representation of a spinal nerve in the thoracic region. Ventral and dorsal root as well as (gray) ramus communicans; dorsal ramus for musculature and skin of the back, the ventral ramus is here identical with the intercostal nerve; the (white) ramus communicans contains the preganglionic sympathetic fibers.

**Fig. 184 a.** Segmental survey innervation of the viscera. Frequently, the pain associated with certain irritative visceral diseases is referred to the corresponding skin segment or dermatome (hyperesthesia and hyperalgesia). Explanation: The afferent dorsal roots of spinal nerves contain not only fibers from dermatomes but also afferent, vegetative fibers from corresponding viscera. The hyperesthetic and hyperalgesic skin areas are called HEAD's zones (HEAD, English neurologist, 1861–1940). These are of practical importance for the diagnosis of visceral diseases. Reflex pain may be treated by anesthesia or transection of dorsal roots.

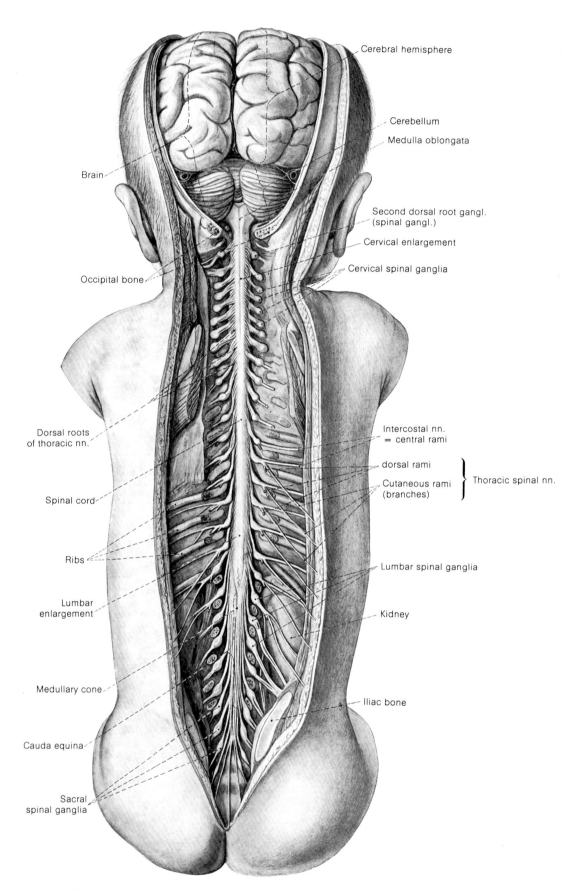

Cerebral hemisphere

Cerebellum

Medulla oblongata

Brain

Second dorsal root gangl. (spinal gangl.)

Cervical enlargement

Cervical spinal ganglia

Occipital bone

Dorsal roots of thoracic nn.

Intercostal nn. = central rami

dorsal rami

Cutaneous rami (branches)

Thoracic spinal nn.

Spinal cord

Ribs

Lumbar spinal ganglia

Lumbar enlargement

Kidney

Medullary cone

Iliac bone

Cauda equina

Sacral spinal ganglia

**Fig. 186.** Central nervous system (brain and spinal cord) of a newborn exposed from dorsal. The spinal dura mater is completely removed. Dissection of dorsal root ganglia and spinal nerves.

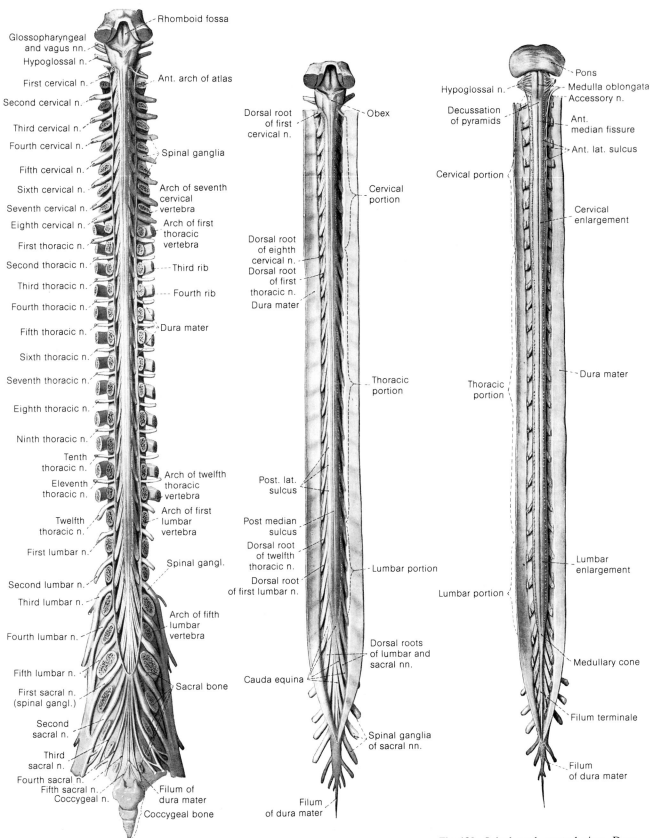

Fig. 187 labels (left figure):
Rhomboid fossa
Glossopharyngeal and vagus nn.
Hypoglossal n.
First cervical n.
Second cervical n.
Ant. arch of atlas
Third cervical n.
Fourth cervical n.
Spinal ganglia
Fifth cervical n.
Sixth cervical n.
Arch of seventh cervical vertebra
Seventh cervical n.
Eighth cervical n.
Arch of first thoracic vertebra
First thoracic n.
Second thoracic n.
Third rib
Third thoracic n.
Fourth rib
Fourth thoracic n.
Fifth thoracic n.
Dura mater
Sixth thoracic n.
Seventh thoracic n.
Eighth thoracic n.
Ninth thoracic n.
Tenth thoracic n.
Eleventh thoracic n.
Arch of twelfth thoracic vertebra
Twelfth thoracic n.
Arch of first lumbar vertebra
First lumbar n.
Spinal gangl.
Second lumbar n.
Third lumbar n.
Arch of fifth lumbar vertebra
Fourth lumbar n.
Fifth lumbar n.
Sacral bone
First sacral n. (spinal gangl.)
Second sacral n.
Third sacral n.
Fourth sacral n.
Fifth sacral n.
Coccygeal n.
Filum of dura mater
Coccygeal bone

Fig. 188 labels (middle figure):
Dorsal root of first cervical n.
Obex
Cervical portion
Dorsal root of eighth cervical n.
Dorsal root of first thoracic n.
Dura mater
Thoracic portion
Post. lat. sulcus
Post median sulcus
Dorsal root of twelfth thoracic n.
Dorsal root of first lumbar n.
Lumbar portion
Dorsal roots of lumbar and sacral nn.
Cauda equina
Spinal ganglia of sacral nn.
Filum of dura mater

Fig. 189 labels (right figure):
Hypoglossal n.
Pons
Medulla oblongata
Accessory n.
Decussation of pyramids
Ant. median fissure
Ant. lat. sulcus
Cervical portion
Cervical enlargement
Thoracic portion
Dura mater
Lumbar enlargement
Lumbar portion
Medullary cone
Filum terminale
Filum of dura mater

**Fig. 187.** Spinal cord within the vertebral canal, dorsal view. Neural arches and dura mater have been partially removed. Bones shown in yellow.

**Fig. 188.** Spinal cord and roots of spinal nerves, dorsal view. Dura mater split longitudinally and reflected.

**Fig. 189.** Spinal cord, ventral view. Dura mater split longitudinally. The anterior roots of spinal nerves are severed at their origin from the spinal cord; the dorsal roots are seen from ventral.

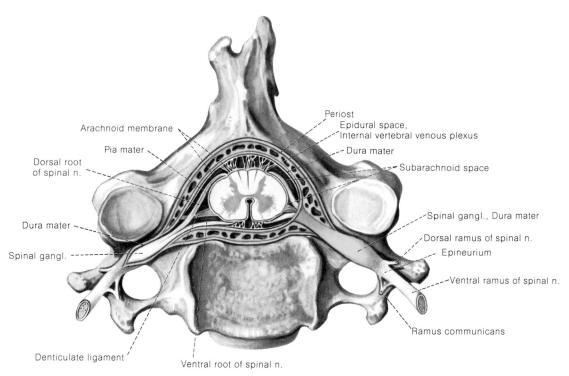

Arachnoid membrane

Pia mater

Dorsal root
of spinal n.

Dura mater

Spinal gangl.

Denticulate ligament

Ventral root of spinal n.

Periost

Epidural space,
Internal vertebral venous plexus

Dura mater

Subarachnoid space

Spinal gangl., Dura mater

Dorsal ramus of spinal n.

Epineurium

Ventral ramus of spinal n.

Ramus communicans

**Fig. 190.** Spinal cord with meninges within the vertebral canal. Cervical level. On the left side of the figure the dura mater has been split to expose the spinal ganglion. Dura and periosteum of the vertebral canal yellow.

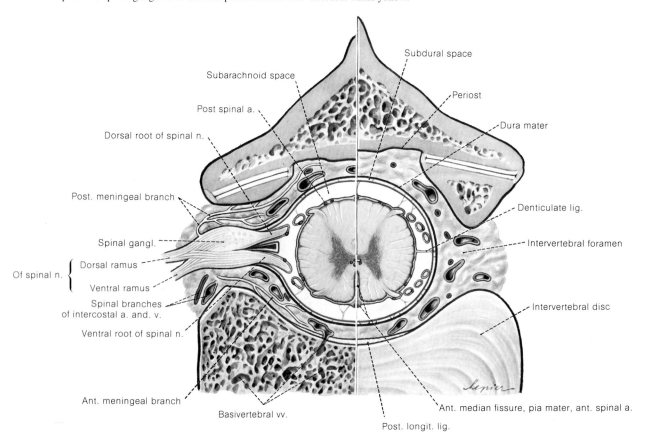

Subarachnoid space

Post spinal a.

Dorsal root of spinal n.

Post. meningeal branch

Spinal gangl.

Of spinal n. { Dorsal ramus

Ventral ramus

Spinal branches
of intercostal a. and. v.

Ventral root of spinal n.

Ant. meningeal branch

Basivertebral vv.

Subdural space

Periost

Dura mater

Denticulate lig.

Intervertebral foramen

Intervertebral disc

Ant. median fissure, pia mater, ant. spinal a.

Post. longit. lig.

**Fig. 191.** Contents of the vertebral canal at a thoracic level. On the right side the cross section passes through an intervertebral disc, on the left through a vertebral body. Dura mater black, arachnoid membrane red, pia mater light blue, arteries red, veins blue. (After PERN-KOPF/FERNER: Atlas der topographischen und syngewandten Anatomie des Menschen, Vol. 2. Urban & Schwarzenberg, Munich–Berlin 1964.)

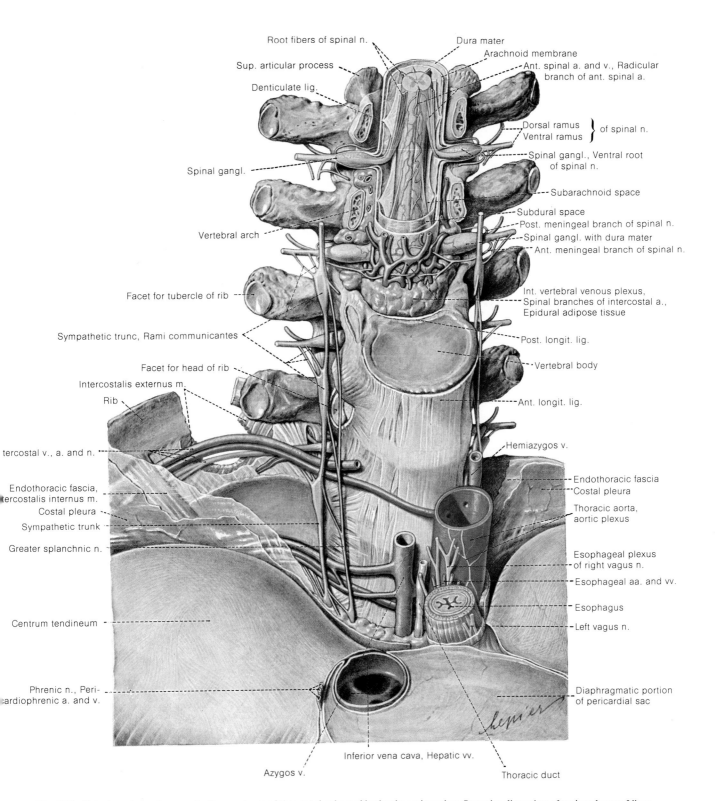

Root fibers of spinal n.

Sup. articular process

Denticulate lig.

Spinal gangl.

Vertebral arch

Facet for tubercle of rib

Sympathetic trunc, Rami communicantes

Facet for head of rib

Intercostalis externus m.

Rib

tercostal v., a. and n.

Endothoracic fascia, tercostalis internus m.

Costal pleura

Sympathetic trunk

Greater splanchnic n.

Centrum tendineum

Phrenic n., Peri-cardiophrenic a. and v.

Azygos v.

Inferior vena cava, Hepatic vv.

Dura mater

Arachnoid membrane

Ant. spinal a. and v., Radicular branch of ant. spinal a.

Dorsal ramus } of spinal n.
Ventral ramus }

Spinal gangl., Ventral root of spinal n.

Subarachnoid space

Subdural space

Post. meningeal branch of spinal n.

Spinal gangl. with dura mater

Ant. meningeal branch of spinal n.

Int. vertebral venous plexus, Spinal branches of intercostal a., Epidural adipose tissue

Post. longit. lig.

Vertebral body

Ant. longit. lig.

Hemiazygos v.

Endothoracic fascia

Costal pleura

Thoracic aorta, aortic plexus

Esophageal plexus of right vagus n.

Esophageal aa. and vv.

Esophagus

Left vagus n.

Diaphragmatic portion of pericardial sac

Thoracic duct

**Fig. 192.** Spinal cord, meninges and other contents of the vertebral canal in the thoracic region. Stepwise dissection of various layers. View from ventral and above.

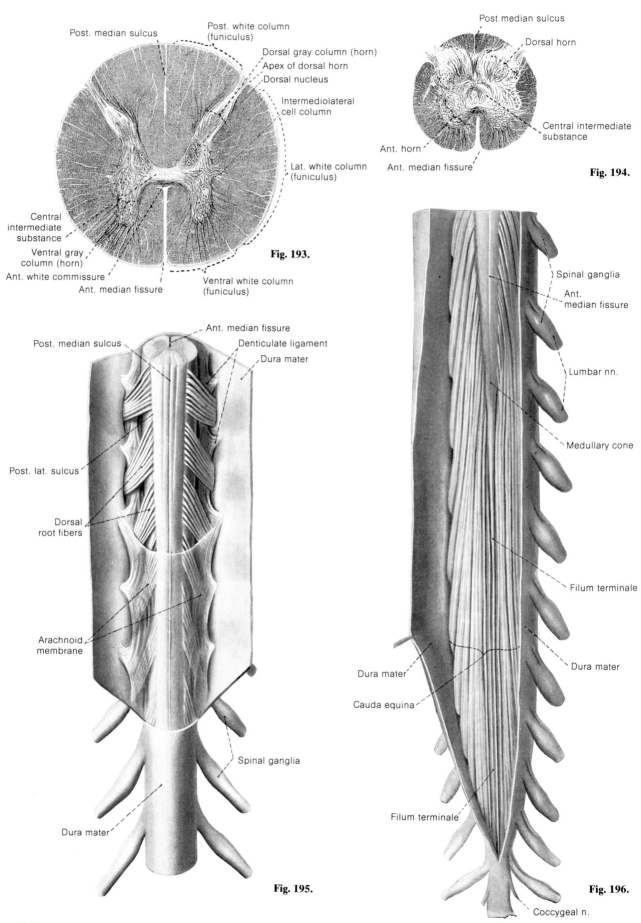

Post. median sulcus

Post. white column (funiculus)

Dorsal gray column (horn)

Apex of dorsal horn

Dorsal nucleus

Intermediolateral cell column

Lat. white column (funiculus)

Central intermediate substance

Ventral gray column (horn)

Ant. white commissure

Ant. median fissure

Ventral white column (funiculus)

**Fig. 193.**

Post median sulcus

Dorsal horn

Central intermediate substance

Ant. horn

Ant. median fissure

**Fig. 194.**

Post. median sulcus

Ant. median fissure

Denticulate ligament

Dura mater

Post. lat. sulcus

Dorsal root fibers

Arachnoid membrane

Spinal ganglia

Dura mater

**Fig. 195.**

Spinal ganglia

Ant. median fissure

Lumbar nn.

Medullary cone

Filum terminale

Dura mater

Dura mater

Cauda equina

Filum terminale

**Fig. 196.**

Coccygeal n.

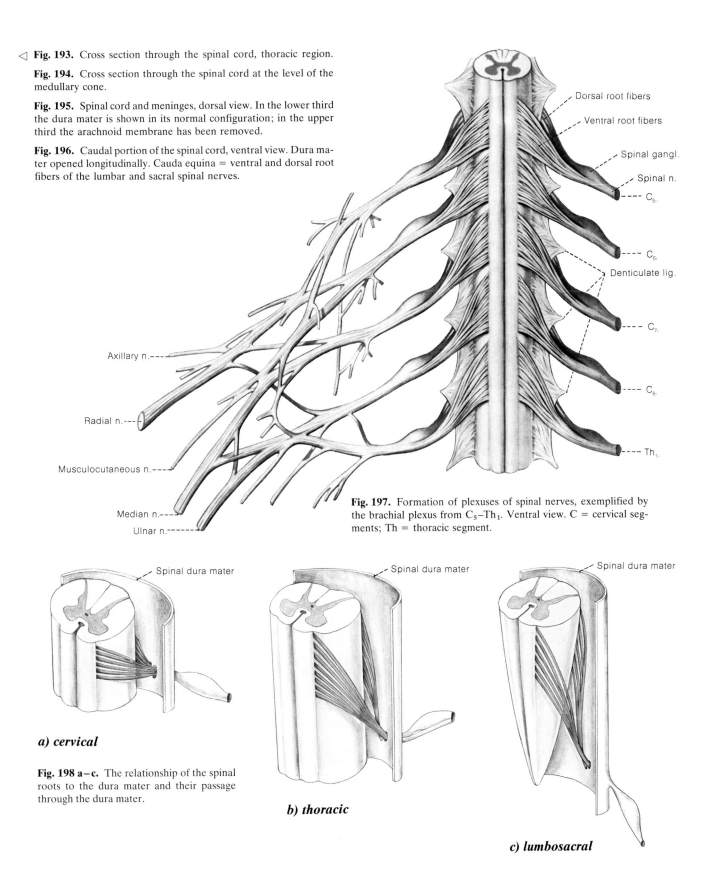

**Fig. 193.** Cross section through the spinal cord, thoracic region.

**Fig. 194.** Cross section through the spinal cord at the level of the medullary cone.

**Fig. 195.** Spinal cord and meninges, dorsal view. In the lower third the dura mater is shown in its normal configuration; in the upper third the arachnoid membrane has been removed.

**Fig. 196.** Caudal portion of the spinal cord, ventral view. Dura mater opened longitudinally. Cauda equina = ventral and dorsal root fibers of the lumbar and sacral spinal nerves.

Dorsal root fibers

Ventral root fibers

Spinal gangl.

Spinal n.

C₅,

C₆,

Denticulate lig.

C₇,

C₈,

Th₁,

Axillary n.

Radial n.

Musculocutaneous n.

Median n.

Ulnar n.

**Fig. 197.** Formation of plexuses of spinal nerves, exemplified by the brachial plexus from $C_5$–$Th_1$. Ventral view. C = cervical segments; Th = thoracic segment.

Spinal dura mater

Spinal dura mater

Spinal dura mater

*a) cervical*

**Fig. 198 a–c.** The relationship of the spinal roots to the dura mater and their passage through the dura mater.

*b) thoracic*

*c) lumbosacral*

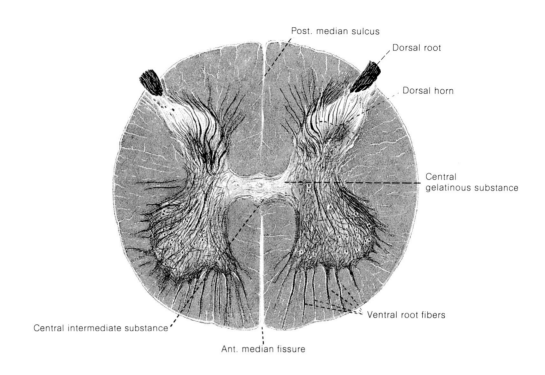

**Fig. 199.** Cross section through the spinal cord at the level of the lumbar enlargement.

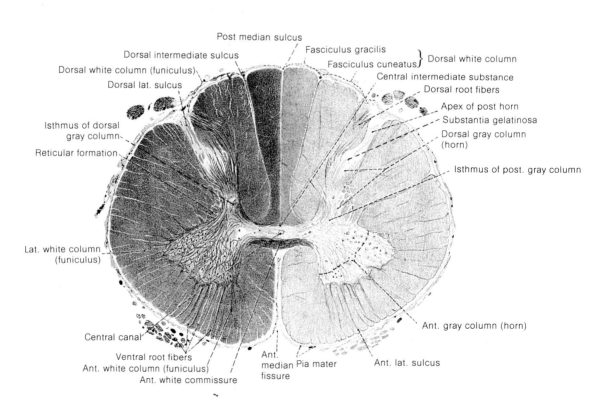

**Fig. 200.** Cross section through the spinal cord at the level of the cervical enlargement (silver technique).

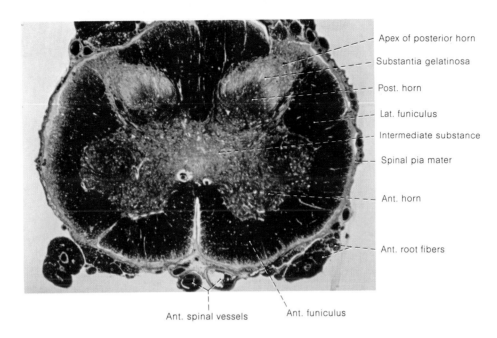

Apex of posterior horn
Substantia gelatinosa
Post. horn
Lat. funiculus
Intermediate substance
Spinal pia mater
Ant. horn
Ant. root fibers
Ant. spinal vessels
Ant. funiculus

**Fig. 201.** Cross section through the spinal cord of an adult human at the level of the lumbar enlargement, WEIGERT's myelin stain (preparation FERNER).

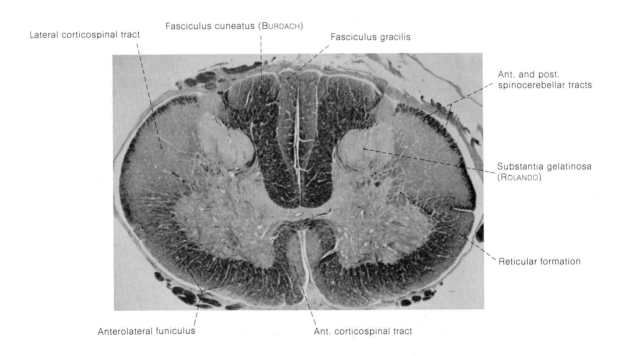

Lateral corticospinal tract
Fasciculus cuneatus (BURDACH)
Fasciculus gracilis
Ant. and post. spinocerebellar tracts
Substantia gelatinosa (ROLANDO)
Reticular formation
Anterolateral funiculus
Ant. corticospinal tract

**Fig. 202.** Cervical spinal cord of a newborn, histological section, 12 ×, WEIGERT's myelin stain (nuclear areas yellowish, tracts brownblack). Lateral and ventral pyramidal tracts are not yet myelinated sind therefore appear as lighter areas. Example for myelogenesis. (Preparation FERNER.)

127

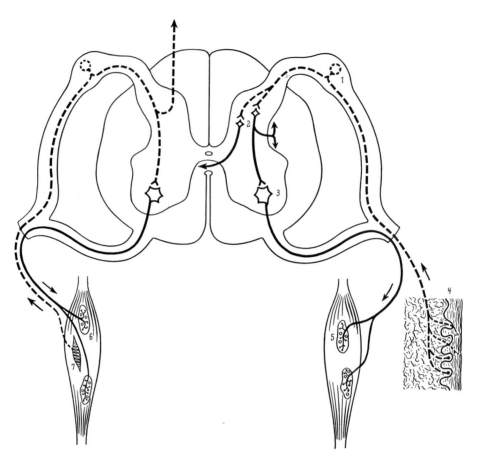

**Fig. 203.** Diagram of a monosynaptic (left) and a polysynaptic (right) reflex arc of the spinal cord. Afferent limb = broken line, efferent limb = solid line. 1 Dorsal root ganglion, 2 Interneurons, 3 Alpha motor neuron, 4 Sensory endings in skin, 5, 6 Motor end plates, 7 Neuromuscular spindle. Included among the basic mechanisms of the spinal cord are the following: 1. The direct bineuronal monosynaptic proprioceptive reflex arc (e.g., knee jerk reflex). 2. The indirect plurineuronal polysynaptic reflex arc in which several neurons of the ipsilateral or contralateral side are involved (e.g., plantar reflex, cremasteric reflex, abdominal reflex, mucous membrane (reflex). 3. The medial longitudinal fasciculus, descending branches of dorsal funicular fibers and others.

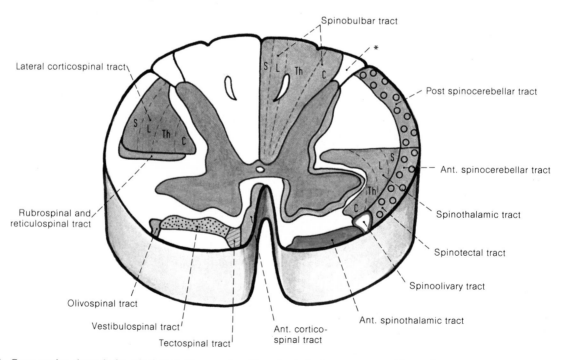

**Fig. 204.** Cross section through the spinal cord. Topography of long tracts (red: motor tracts; blue and green: sensory afferent tracts). * Entry zone of post. root.

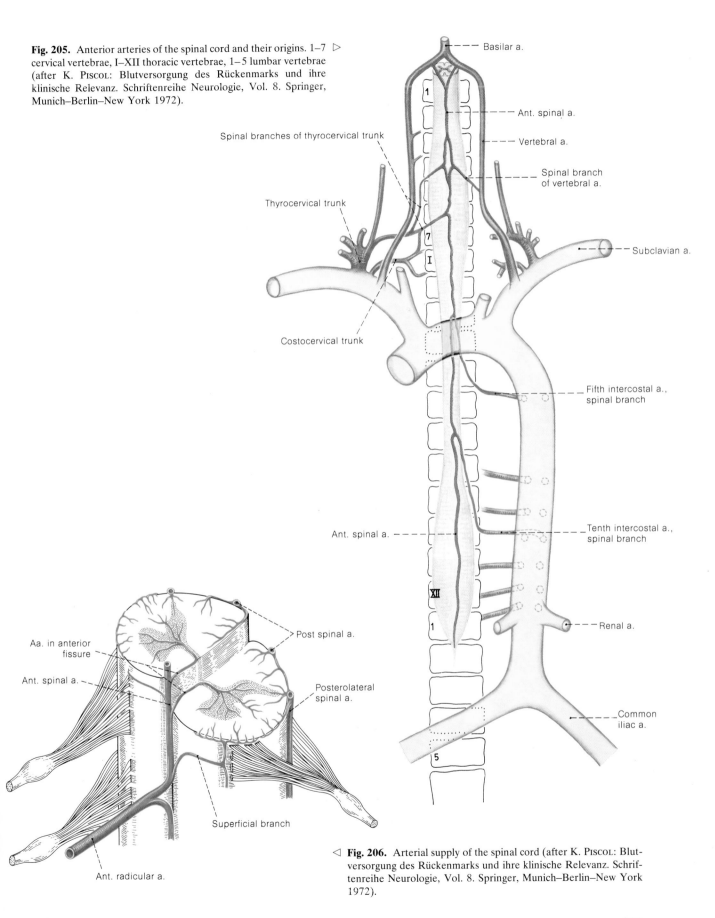

**Fig. 205.** Anterior arteries of the spinal cord and their origins. 1–7 ▷ cervical vertebrae, I–XII thoracic vertebrae, 1–5 lumbar vertebrae (after K. PISCOL: Blutversorgung des Rückenmarks und ihre klinische Relevanz. Schriftenreihe Neurologie, Vol. 8. Springer, Munich–Berlin–New York 1972).

Basilar a.

Ant. spinal a.

Vertebral a.

Spinal branch of vertebral a.

Spinal branches of thyrocervical trunk

Thyrocervical trunk

Subclavian a.

Costocervical trunk

Fifth intercostal a., spinal branch

Ant. spinal a.

Tenth intercostal a., spinal branch

Renal a.

Aa. in anterior fissure

Ant. spinal a.

Post spinal a.

Posterolateral spinal a.

Common iliac a.

Superficial branch

Ant. radicular a.

◁ **Fig. 206.** Arterial supply of the spinal cord (after K. PISCOL: Blutversorgung des Rückenmarks und ihre klinische Relevanz. Schriftenreihe Neurologie, Vol. 8. Springer, Munich–Berlin–New York 1972).

129

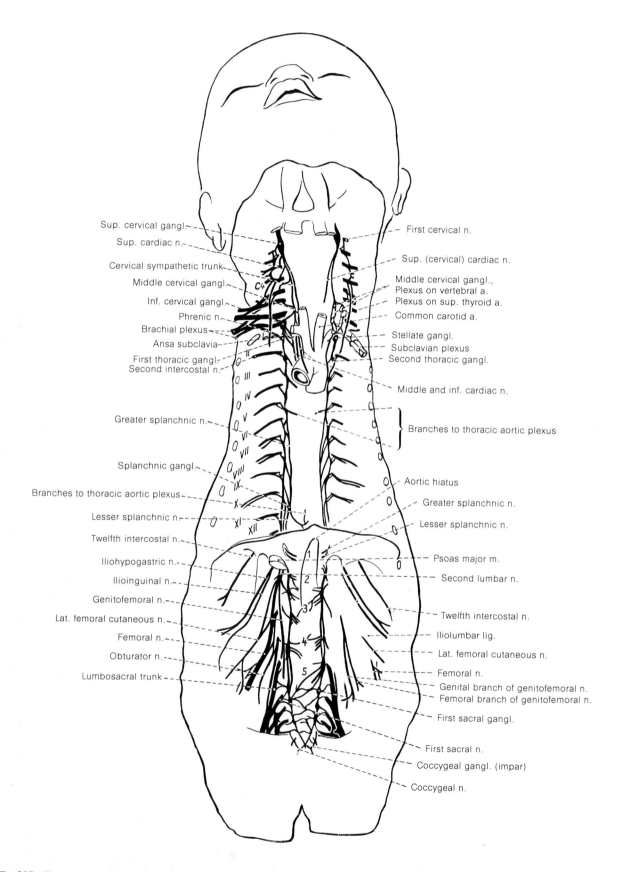

Sup. cervical gangl.

Sup. cardiac n.

Cervical sympathetic trunk

Middle cervical gangl.

Inf. cervical gangl.

Phrenic n.

Brachial plexus

Ansa subclavia

First thoracic gangl.
Second intercostal n.

Greater splanchnic n.

Splanchnic gangl.

Branches to thoracic aortic plexus

Lesser splanchnic n.

Twelfth intercostal n.

Iliohypogastric n.

Ilioinguinal n.

Genitofemoral n.

Lat. femoral cutaneous n.

Femoral n.

Obturator n.

Lumbosacral trunk

First cervical n.

Sup. (cervical) cardiac n.

Middle cervical gangl.,
Plexus on vertebral a.
Plexus on sup. thyroid a.

Common carotid a.

Stellate gangl.
Subclavian plexus
Second thoracic gangl.

Middle and inf. cardiac n.

Branches to thoracic aortic plexus

Aortic hiatus

Greater splanchnic n.

Lesser splanchnic n.

Psoas major m.

Second lumbar n.

Twelfth intercostal n.

Iliolumbar lig.

Lat. femoral cutaneous n.

Femoral n.

Genital branch of genitofemoral n.
Femoral branch of genitofemoral n.

First sacral gangl.

First sacral n.

Coccygeal gangl. (impar)

Coccygeal n.

**Fig. 207.** The sympathetic trunk and its connections to the spinal nerves in a newborn; explanatory diagram for Fig. 208 on facing page.

The **sympathetic trunk** is a paired nervous chain extending on both sides of the spinal column from the base of the skull to the tip of the coccyx. It is characterized by knot-like enlargements, the **paravertebral ganglia.** At the base of the skull it continues cephalad as a sympathetic fiber network around the internal carotid artery and its branches, and also establishes other connections with cranial nerves (internal carotid plexus, caroticotympanic nerve, deep petrosal nerve). Via carotid and ophthalmic arteries, sympathetic nerve fibers reach the orbit and the eye ball (dilatator pupillae muscle, etc.). Sometimes, this is referred to as the "cranial portion" of the sympathicus.

Topographically, the sympathetic trunk is composed of a cervical, thoracic, abdominal, and pelvic segment. In the neck, it is located behind the prevertebral fascia on the anterior face of the longus colli muscle. In the thoracic area it is covered by the costovertebral pleura and in the abdomen and pelvis by the peritoneum.

The **cervical portion** of the sympathetic trunk has three ganglia (superior, middle and inferior cervical ganglion). The superior ganglion measures about 2 cm in length and lies at the level of atlas and axis. From its inferior pole originates the superior cervical cardiac nerve which courses along the common carotid artery to the heart. The middle cervical ganglion lies in the area of the transverse portion of the inferior thyroid artery; it is inconstant. It gives rise to the middle cervical cardiac nerve. The inferior cervical ganglion lies at the level of the superior thoracic aperture behind the origin of the vertebral artery; it gives off the inferior cervical cardiac nerve. (The branches of the vagus nerve for the heart are named **rami** cardiaci [cardiac **branches**].) Between the middle and inferior cervical ganglion, the sympathetic trunk forms a loop around the subclavian artery, the ansa subclavia. In most cases, the inferior cervical ganglion is united with the first thoracic ganglion to form a large common ganglion, the stellate ganglion on the anterior surface of the capitulum of the first rib. The **12 thoracic sympathetic ganglia** lie near the heads of the ribs and are interconnected by interganglionic branches. They are connected to the segmental spinal nerves by one or more rami communicantes. Additionally, from the 5th to the 10th thoracic ganglia originate medial branches that unite to form the **greater splanchnic nerve,** from the 10th to the 12th originate branches to form the **lesser splanchnic nerve.** These pass through gaps in the lumbar portion of the diaphragm into the abdominal area where they enter the **celiac ganglion.** Direct branches reach the aorta and the bronchial tree.

From the second to the fourth thoracic ganglion originate the **thoracic cardiac nerves** which also carry pain fibers. In the abdominal and pelvic areas, the sympathetic trunk lies in the groove between vertebral bodies and psoas major muscle. The lumbar and sacral ganglia are not precisely segmental any more. The lumbar and sacral splanchnic branches reach to the prevertebral ganglia associated with the aorta and its branches. At the level of the coccyx the two sympathetic truncs unite in a common ganglion impar.

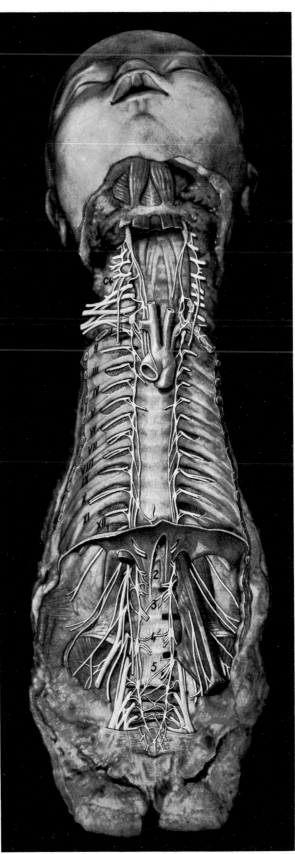

**Fig. 208.** The sympathetic trunk of the newborn. The brachial plexus and the lumbosacral plexus are depicted on the right side of the preparation. The sympathetic trunk and its ganglia in lumbar and sacral levels are emphasized by underlying markers (preparation in the Anatomical Institute Münster).

# Spinal Cord, Spinal Nerves, Sympathetic Trunk

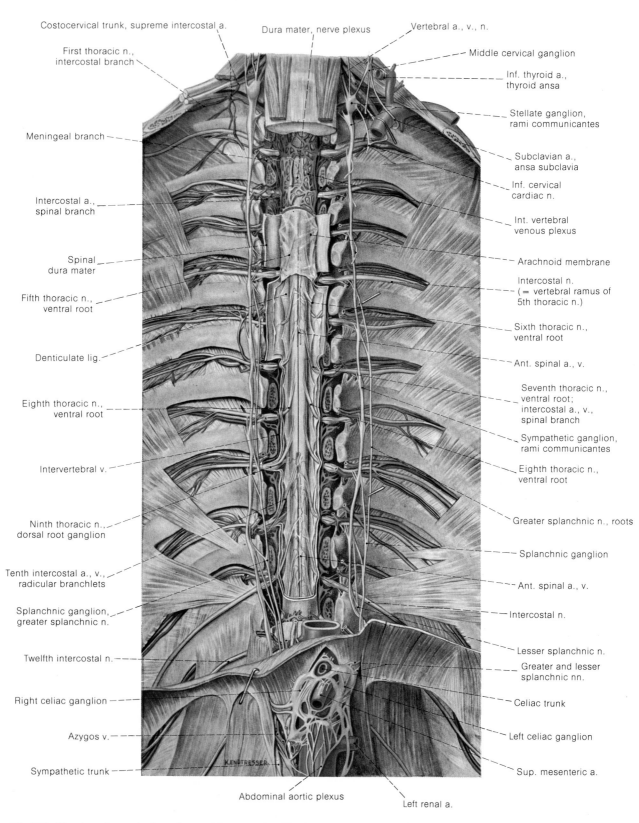

**Fig. 209.** The thoracic vertebral canal opened from anterior. The dura mater has been opened so as to visualize the spinal nerves, their root fibers, their anterior and posterior rami, the dorsal root ganglia and the connections of the spinal nerves with the sympathetic trunk. (From Pernkopf: Atlas der topographischen und angewandten Anatomie des Menschen, Vol. 2, 2nd ed. [Ed. H. Ferner]. Urban & Schwarzenberg, Munich–Vienna–Baltimore 1980.)

# Superficial and Deep Facial Region

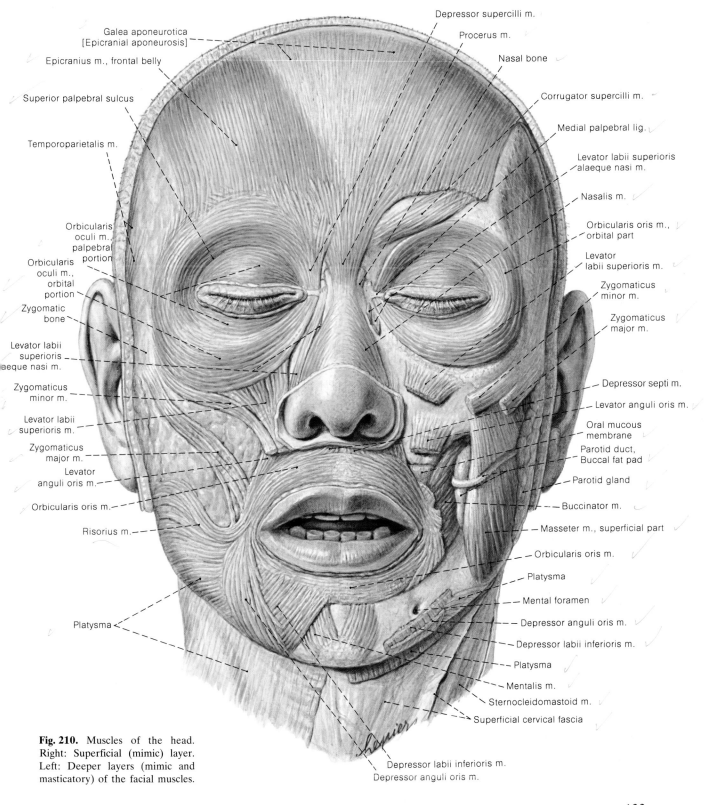

Depressor supercilli m.

Procerus m.

Nasal bone

Galea aponeurotica
[Epicranial aponeurosis]

Epicranius m., frontal belly

Superior palpebral sulcus

Corrugator supercilli m.

Medial palpebral lig.

Temporoparietalis m.

Levator labii superioris
alaeque nasi m.

Nasalis m.

Orbicularis
oculi m.,
palpebral
portion

Orbicularis oris m.,
orbital part

Levator
labii superioris m.

Orbicularis
oculi m.,
orbital
portion

Zygomaticus
minor m.

Zygomatic
bone

Zygomaticus
major m.

Levator labii
superioris
aeque nasi m.

Zygomaticus
minor m.

Depressor septi m.

Levator anguli oris m.

Levator labii
superioris m.

Oral mucous
membrane

Zygomaticus
major m.

Parotid duct,
Buccal fat pad

Levator
anguli oris m.

Parotid gland

Orbicularis oris m.

Buccinator m.

Risorius m.

Masseter m., superficial part

Orbicularis oris m.

Platysma

Mental foramen

Platysma

Depressor anguli oris m.

Depressor labii inferioris m.

Platysma

Mentalis m.

Sternocleidomastoid m.

Superficial cervical fascia

**Fig. 210.** Muscles of the head.
Right: Superficial (mimic) layer.
Left: Deeper layers (mimic and
masticatory) of the facial muscles.

Depressor labii inferioris m.
Depressor anguli oris m.

**Facial Muscles**

| Name | Origin | Insertion |
|---|---|---|
| 1. **Levator labii superioris alaeque nasi muscle** | Frontal process of maxilla | Ala of nose and upper lip |
| 2. **Levator labii superioris muscle** | Infraorbital margin | Ala of nose and upper lip |
| 3. **Zygomaticus minor muscle** | Malar surface of zygomatic bone | Near angle of mouth |
| 4. **Zygomaticus major muscle** | Lateral surface of zygomatic bone | Angle of mouth |
| 5. **Risorius muscle** (a part of the Platysma) | Masseteric fascia | Angle of mouth |
| 6. **Depressor anguli oris muscle** | Oblique line of mandible | Angle of mouth; lower lip |
| 7. **Levator anguli oris muscle** | Canine fossa of maxilla | Musculature of upper lip; angle of mouth |
| 8. **Depressor labii inferioris muscle** | Mandible between symphysis and mental foramen | Lower lip |
| 9. **Orbicularis oris muscle** | The following specifications: Marginal part: fibers blended with adjacent muscles Labial part: fibers restricted to lips | Protrudes and shapes lips |
| 10. **Buccinator muscle** | Outer surface of mandible; alveolar process of maxilla; pterygomandibular raphe | Angle of mouth and lips; its interlacing fibers contribute to Orbicularis oris m. |
| 11. **Mentalis muscle** | Incisive fossa of mandible | Skin of chin |

*Nerve:*   Facial nerve (Fig. 218)

*Function:*   Moves lips, ala of nose, cheeks, skin of chin. Risorius: draws angle of mouth laterally (smiling)

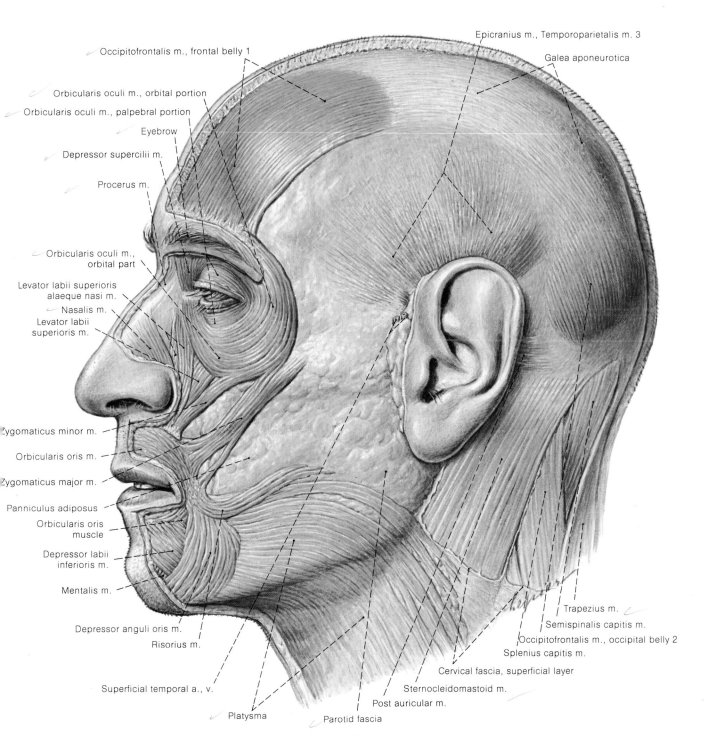

Occipitofrontalis m., frontal belly 1

Orbicularis oculi m., orbital portion

Orbicularis oculi m., palpebral portion

Eyebrow

Depressor supercilii m.

Procerus m.

Orbicularis oculi m., orbital part

Levator labii superioris alaeque nasi m.

Nasalis m.

Levator labii superioris m.

Zygomaticus minor m.

Orbicularis oris m.

Zygomaticus major m.

Panniculus adiposus

Orbicularis oris muscle

Depressor labii inferioris m.

Mentalis m.

Depressor anguli oris m.

Risorius m.

Superficial temporal a., v.

Platysma

Parotid fascia

Epicranius m., Temporoparietalis m. 3

Galea aponeurotica

Trapezius m.

Semispinalis capitis m.

Occipitofrontalis m., occipital belly 2

Splenius capitis m.

Cervical fascia, superficial layer

Sternocleidomastoid m.

Post auricular m.

**Fig. 211.** Lateral aspect of the head with mimic musculature and superficial layers of the cervical musculature. The three parts of the Epicranial muscles are designated 1, 2, 3.

135

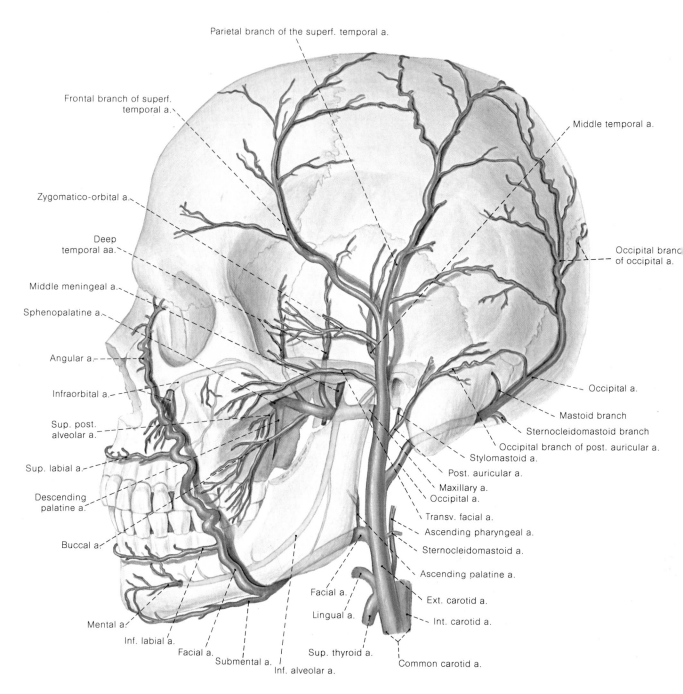

Parietal branch of the superf. temporal a.

Frontal branch of superf. temporal a.

Middle temporal a.

Zygomatico-orbital a.

Deep temporal aa.

Occipital branch of occipital a.

Middle meningeal a.

Sphenopalatine a.

Angular a.

Infraorbital a.

Occipital a.

Mastoid branch

Sup. post. alveolar a.

Sternocleidomastoid branch

Occipital branch of post. auricular a.

Stylomastoid a.

Sup. labial a.

Post. auricular a.

Descending palatine a.

Maxillary a.

Occipital a.

Transv. facial a.

Buccal a.

Ascending pharyngeal a.

Sternocleidomastoid a.

Ascending palatine a.

Mental a.

Facial a.

Lingual a.

Ext. carotid a.

Int. carotid a.

Inf. labial a.

Facial a.

Submental a.

Sup. thyroid a.

Inf. alveolar a.

Common carotid a.

**Fig. 212.** Diagram of the external carotid artery and its branches.

136

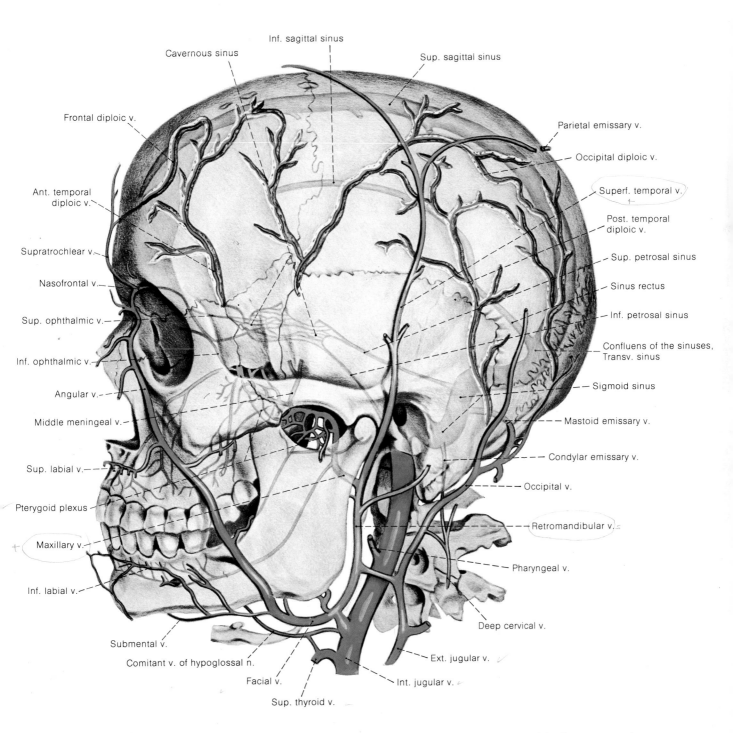

**Fig. 213.** Diploic veins and large veins of the head. Veins seen through bony structures and the venous sinuses of the dura mater are shown in lighter blue. (After PERNKOPF: Atlas der topographischen und angewandten Anatomie des Menschen, Vol. 1, 2nd. [Ed. H. FERNER]. Urban & Schwarzenberg, Munich–Vienna–Baltimore 1980.)

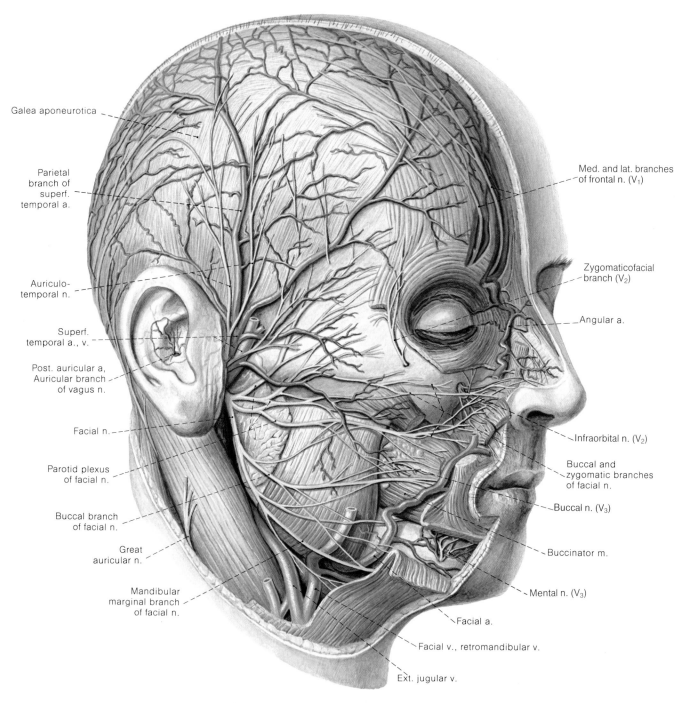

**Fig. 214.** Nerves and arteries of the head, intermediate layer. Superficial portions of the parotid gland have been removed in order to expose the stem and the parotid plexus of the facial nerve.

Galea aponeurotica

Parietal branch of superf. temporal a.

Auriculo-temporal n.

Superf. temporal a., v.

Post. auricular a, Auricular branch of vagus n.

Facial n.

Parotid plexus of facial n.

Buccal branch of facial n.

Great auricular n.

Mandibular marginal branch of facial n.

Med. and lat. branches of frontal n. (V₁)

Zygomaticofacial branch (V₂)

Angular a.

Infraorbital n. (V₂)

Buccal and zygomatic branches of facial n.

Buccal n. (V₃)

Buccinator m.

Mental n. (V₃)

Facial a.

Facial v., retromandibular v.

Ext. jugular v.

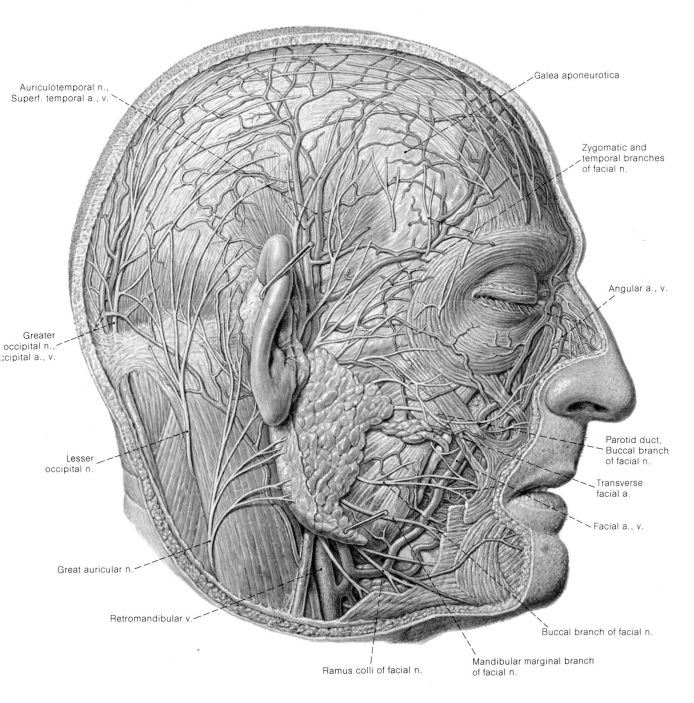

Auriculotemporal n.,
Superf. temporal a., v.

Galea aponeurotica

Zygomatic and
temporal branches
of facial n.

Angular a., v.

Greater
occipital n.,
occipital a., v.

Lesser
occipital n.

Parotid duct,
Buccal branch
of facial n.

Transverse
facial a.

Facial a., v.

Great auricular n.

Retromandibular v.

Buccal branch of facial n.

Ramus colli of facial n.

Mandibular marginal branch
of facial n.

**Fig. 215.** Superficial nerves and vessels of head.

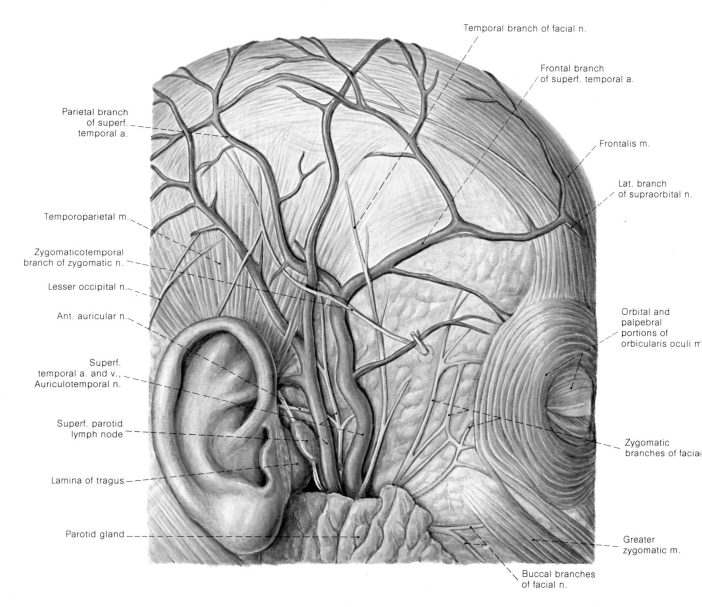

Temporal branch of facial n.

Frontal branch
of superf. temporal a.

Parietal branch
of superf.
temporal a.

Frontalis m.

Lat. branch
of supraorbital n.

Temporoparietal m.

Zygomaticotemporal
branch of zygomatic n.

Lesser occipital n.

Ant. auricular n.

Orbital and
palpebral
portions of
orbicularis oculi m

Superf.
temporal a. and v.,
Auriculotemporal n.

Superf. parotid
lymph node

Zygomatic
branches of facia

Lamina of tragus

Parotid gland

Greater
zygomatic m.

Buccal branches
of facial n.

**Fig. 216.** Superficial layer of the temporal region with superficial temporal artery, auriculotemporal nerve, branches of facial nerve, and zygomaticotemporal branch of zygomatic nerve.

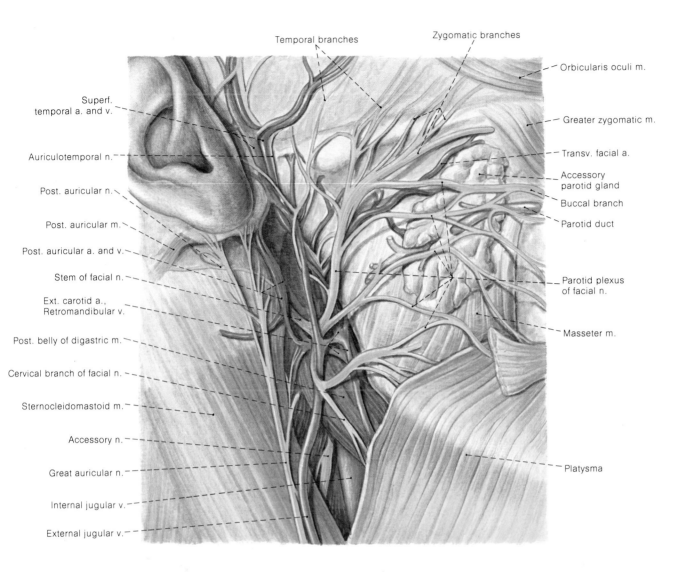

Temporal branches — Zygomatic branches

Orbicularis oculi m.

Superf. temporal a. and v.

Greater zygomatic m.

Auriculotemporal n.

Transv. facial a.

Accessory parotid gland

Post. auricular n.

Buccal branch

Post. auricular m.

Parotid duct

Post. auricular a. and v.

Stem of facial n.

Parotid plexus of facial n.

Ext. carotid a., Retromandibular v.

Post. belly of digastric m.

Masseter m.

Cervical branch of facial n.

Sternocleidomastoid m.

Accessory n.

Great auricular n.

Internal jugular v.

Platysma

External jugular v.

**Fig. 217.** Blood vessels and nerves in the area of the retromandibular fossa and the parotideomasseteric region. The major portion of the parotid gland has been removed. Note the ramification of the stem of the facial nerve to form the parotid plexus and the radially arranged branches for the facial muscles.

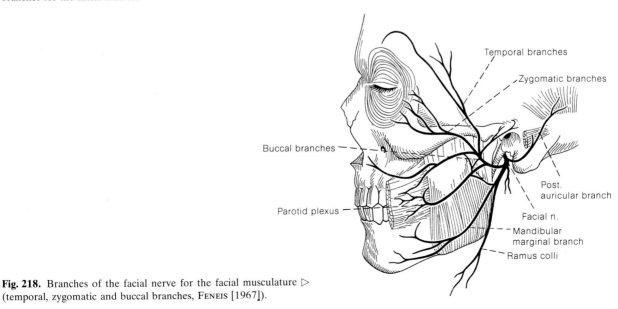

Temporal branches

Zygomatic branches

Buccal branches

Parotid plexus

Post. auricular branch

Facial n.

Mandibular marginal branch

Ramus colli

**Fig. 218.** Branches of the facial nerve for the facial musculature ▷ (temporal, zygomatic and buccal branches, FENEIS [1967]).

141

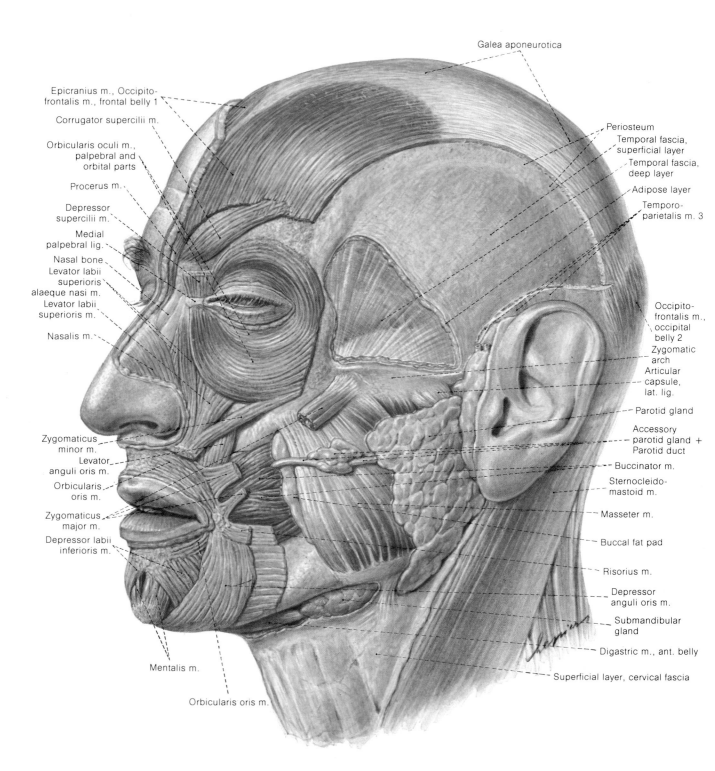

Galea aponeurotica

Epicranius m., Occipito-
frontalis m., frontal belly 1

Corrugator supercilii m.

Orbicularis oculi m.,
palpebral and
orbital parts

Procerus m.

Depressor
supercilii m.

Medial
palpebral lig.

Nasal bone
Levator labii
superioris
alaeque nasi m.
Levator labii
superioris m.

Nasalis m.

Zygomaticus
minor m.

Levator
anguli oris m.

Orbicularis
oris m.

Zygomaticus
major m.

Depressor labii
inferioris m.

Mentalis m.

Orbicularis oris m.

Periosteum
Temporal fascia,
superficial layer
Temporal fascia,
deep layer
Adipose layer
Temporo-
parietalis m. 3

Occipito-
frontalis m.,
occipital
belly 2
Zygomatic
arch
Articular
capsule,
lat. lig.

Parotid gland

Accessory
parotid gland +
Parotid duct

Buccinator m.

Sternocleido-
mastoid m.

Masseter m.

Buccal fat pad

Risorius m.

Depressor
anguli oris m.

Submandibular
gland

Digastric m., ant. belly

Superficial layer, cervical fascia

**Fig. 219.** The head and upper cervical region from the left side. Mimic musculature, part of the Masseter muscles, salivary glands, the Sternocleidomastoid muscle and some of the upper cervical muscles. The three parts of the Epicranius muscle designated 1, 2, 3.

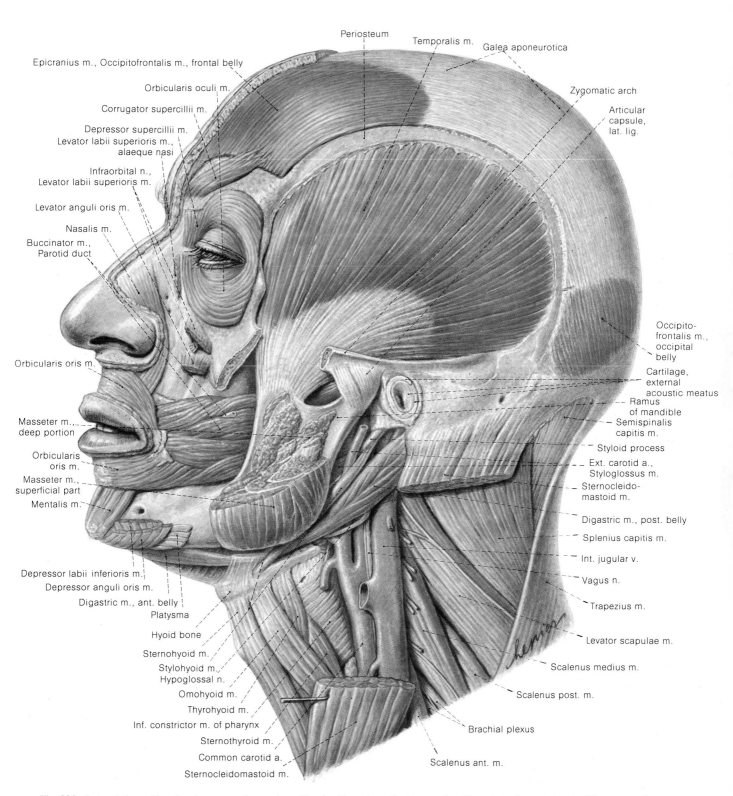

Periosteum

Temporalis m.

Galea aponeurotica

Epicranius m., Occipitofrontalis m., frontal belly

Zygomatic arch

Orbicularis oculi m.

Articular capsule, lat. lig.

Corrugator supercillii m.

Depressor supercillii m.

Levator labii superioris m., alaeque nasi

Infraorbital n., Levator labii superioris m.

Levator anguli oris m.

Nasalis m.

Buccinator m., Parotid duct

Occipito-frontalis m., occipital belly

Orbicularis oris m.

Cartilage, external acoustic meatus

Ramus of mandible

Masseter m., deep portion

Semispinalis capitis m.

Styloid process

Orbicularis oris m.

Ext. carotid a., Styloglossus m.

Masseter m., superficial part

Sternocleido-mastoid m.

Mentalis m.

Digastric m., post. belly

Splenius capitis m.

Int. jugular v.

Vagus n.

Depressor labii inferioris m.

Trapezius m.

Depressor anguli oris m.

Digastric m., ant. belly

Levator scapulae m.

Platysma

Hyoid bone

Scalenus medius m.

Sternohyoid m.

Stylohyoid m.

Hypoglossal n.

Scalenus post. m.

Omohyoid m.

Thyrohyoid m.

Inf. constrictor m. of pharynx

Brachial plexus

Sternothyroid m.

Common carotid a.

Scalenus ant. m.

Sternocleidomastoid m.

**Fig. 220.** Lateral view of head and upper neck muscles with mimetic and masticator muscles. The external ear and part of the zygomatic arch were removed. A wide piece of the upper half of the Sternocleidomastoid was removed to display the large vessels. The Masseter muscle was partly removed to display its tendinous insertions between the muscle bundles. A few mimic muscles were cut off near their origins.

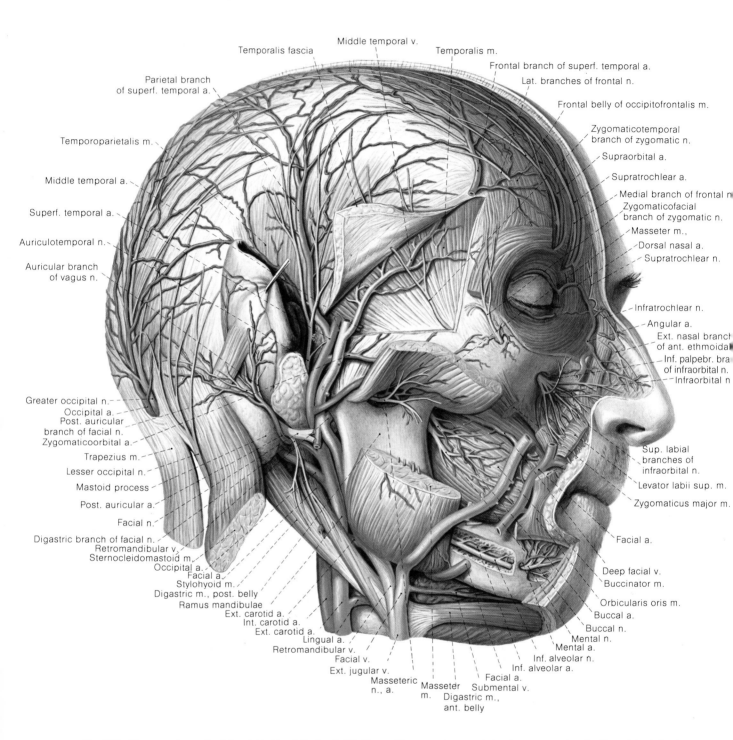

**Fig. 221.** Nerves and vessels of the right side of the head, third layer. The masseter muscle has been severed and reflected, both laminae of the temporal fascia have been reflected from the upper margin of the zygomatic arch, parotid gland and facial nerve have been removed, several facial muscles have been partially removed, the mandibular canal has been opened.

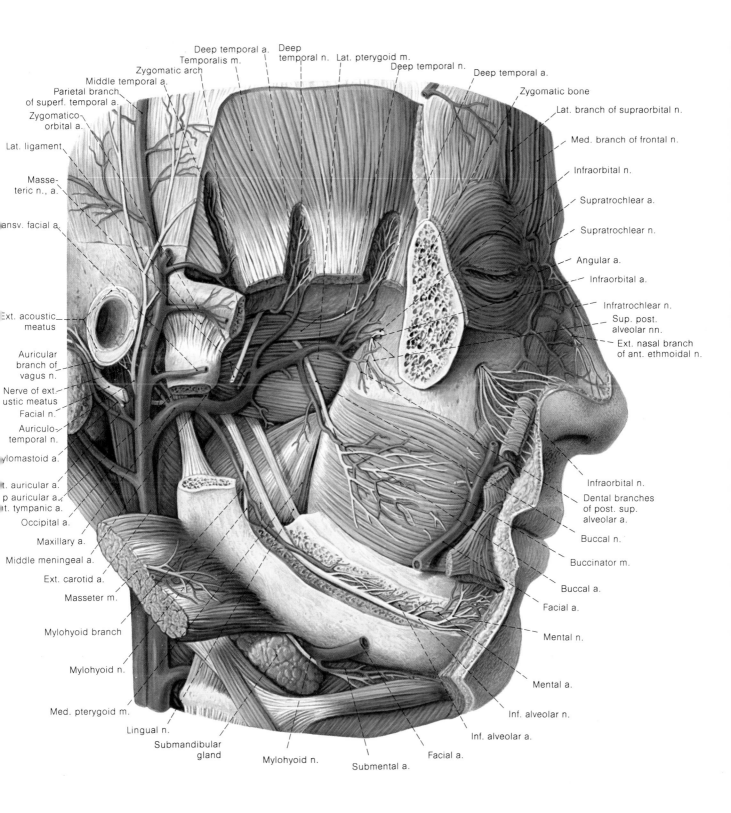

**Fig. 222.** Nerves and vessels of the right side of the face, deep layer: maxillary artery and its branches. Preparation similar to the one in Fig. 224, but the insertion of the temporalis muscle together with the coronoid process of the mandible have been removed and the deep temporal arteries have been exposed.

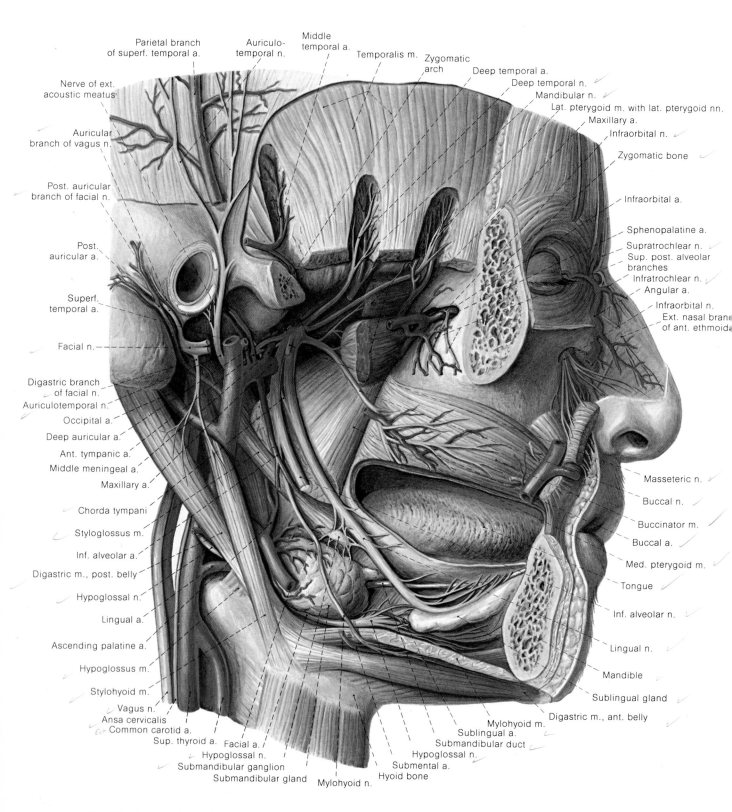

**Fig. 223.** Nerves and vessels of the right side of the face, deep layer: mandibular nerve and its branches. Preparation similar to the one in Fig. 222, but the condylar process of the mandible has been disjointed and removed together with the rest of the right lower jaw. The lower half of the buccinator muscle and the underlying oral mucosa have been removed.

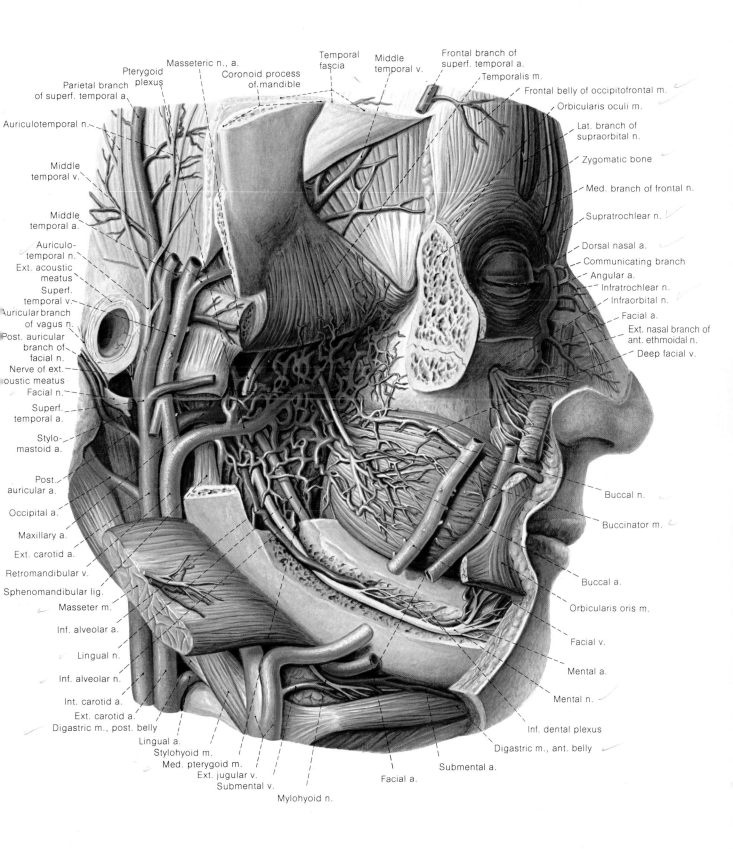

Temporal fascia
Middle temporal v.
Frontal branch of superf. temporal a.
Masseteric n., a.
Coronoid process of mandible
Temporalis m.
Pterygoid plexus
Frontal belly of occipitofrontal m.
Parietal branch of superf. temporal a
Orbicularis oculi m.
Auriculotemporal n.
Lat. branch of supraorbital n.
Middle temporal v.
Zygomatic bone
Med. branch of frontal n.
Middle temporal a.
Supratrochlear n.
Auriculo-temporal n.
Dorsal nasal a.
Ext. acoustic meatus
Communicating branch
Superf. temporal v.
Angular a.
Auricular branch of vagus n.
Infratrochlear n.
Post. auricular branch of facial n.
Infraorbital n.
Nerve of ext. acoustic meatus
Facial a.
Ext. nasal branch of ant. ethmoidal n.
Facial n.
Deep facial v.
Superf. temporal a.
Stylo-mastoid a.
Post. auricular a.
Buccal n.
Occipital a.
Buccinator m.
Maxillary a.
Ext. carotid a.
Retromandibular v.
Buccal a.
Sphenomandibular lig.
Orbicularis oris m.
Masseter m.
Inf. alveolar a.
Facial v.
Lingual n.
Mental a.
Inf. alveolar n.
Mental n.
Int. carotid a.
Ext. carotid a.
Inf. dental plexus
Digastric m., post. belly
Digastric m., ant. belly
Lingual a.
Stylohyoid m.
Med. pterygoid m.
Ext. jugular v.
Submental v.
Facial a.
Submental a.
Mylohyoid n.

**Fig. 224.** Nerves and vessels of the right side of the face, fourth layer. Zygomatic arch and neck of mandible have been removed, the mandibular canal has been opened, the temporalis muscle together with the coronoid process of the mandible have been reflected upward. Note the venous plexus between the pterygoid muscles.

147

## Epicranius Muscles

| Name | Origin | Insertion |
|---|---|---|
| **Occipitofrontalis muscle, Frontal belly:** | Supraorbital margin, skin of forehead and eyebrows | Galea aponeurotica |
| **Occipitofrontalis muscle, Occipital belly:** | Supreme nuchal line | Galea aponeurotica |
| **Temporoparietalis muscle** | Superficial lamina, temporal fascia near ear | On skin and temporal fascia above and in front of ear |

*Nerve:*    Facial nerve

*Function:*    Moves scalp, wrinkles forehead

## Muscles of the Nose

**Nasalis muscle**

| | Origin | Insertion |
|---|---|---|
| Transverse part: | Area over canine teeth (the maxilla) | Aponeurosis over bridge of nose |
| Alar part: | Area over the lateral incisors (alar cartilage) | Skin at tip of nose |
| **Depressor septi muscle** | Incisive fossa of maxilla | Alar cartilage and septum of nose |

*Nerve:*    Facial nerve

*Function:*    Slightly moves nose, namely, ala of the nose (dilates and contracts nostrils)

## Muscles of the Eyelids

| Name | Origin | Insertion |
|---|---|---|
| **Orbicularis oculi muscle** | | |
| Orbital portion | Frontal process of maxilla; medial angle of eye; medial palpebral lig. | Surrounds orbital opening as a sphincter, some fibers go to eyebrow |
| Palpebral portion | Medial palpebral ligament | Lateral palpebral raphe |
| Lacrimal portion | Posterior lacrimal crest | Tarsus of each eyelid |
| **Depressor supercilii muscles** | Nasal process of frontal bone | Skin of eyebrow |

*Nerve:*    Facial nerve, temporal and zygomatic branches

*Function:*    Closes lids, compresses lacrimal sac, moves eyebrows

| | | |
|---|---|---|
| **Corrugator supercili muscle** | Nasal process of frontal bone | Skin of eyebrow |
| **Procerus muscle** | Bridge of nose and lateral nasal cartilage | Skin of forehead between eyebrows |

*Nerve:*    Facial nerve, temporal branch

*Function:*    Acts upon skin of forehead (glabella) and eyebrows

# Nose, Nasal Cavity, Paranasal Sinuses

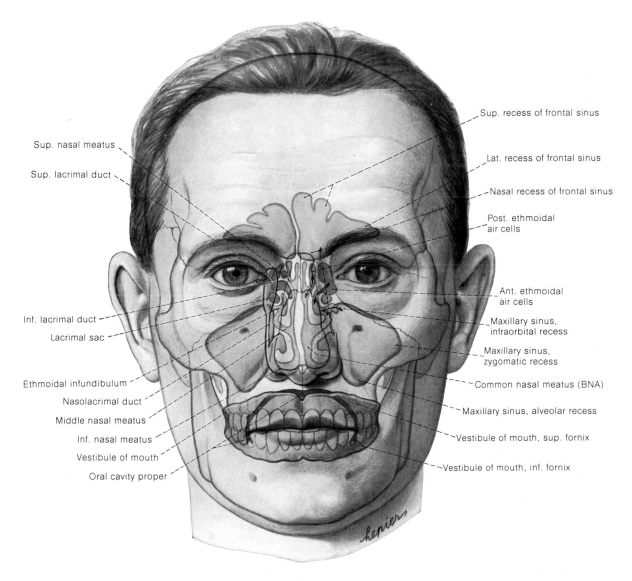

Sup. nasal meatus

Sup. lacrimal duct

Inf. lacrimal duct

Lacrimal sac

Ethmoidal infundibulum

Nasolacrimal duct

Middle nasal meatus

Inf. nasal meatus

Vestibule of mouth

Oral cavity proper

Sup. recess of frontal sinus

Lat. recess of frontal sinus

Nasal recess of frontal sinus

Post. ethmoidal air cells

Ant. ethmoidal air cells

Maxillary sinus, infraorbital recess

Maxillary sinus, zygomatic recess

Common nasal meatus (BNA)

Maxillary sinus, alveolar recess

Vestibule of mouth, sup. fornix

Vestibule of mouth, inf. fornix

**Fig. 225.** Phantom projection of mucous membranes of the facial part of the skull. Ventral view. Contour of the mouth and nasal cavities as well as the paranasal sinuses shown in different colors. (From PERNKOPF: Atlas der topographischen und angewandten Anatomie des Menschen, Vol. 1, 2nd ed. [Ed. H. FERNER]. Urban & Schwarzenberg, Munich–Vienna–Baltimore 1980.)

**Nasal cavity,** Survey: The nasal cavity is a paired narrow space in the middle of the viscerocranium extending in sagittal direction from the piriform aperture to the choanae. The right and left nasal cavities are separated from each other by the nasal septum. The lateral wall of the nasal cavity is subdivided by the three nasal conchae. The space next to the septum is the common nasal meatus. Beneath each concha are the superior, middle and inferior nasal meatus. The floor of the nasal cavity is formed by the superior side of the palate; its roof is connected to the neurocranium through the cribriform plate. From each nasal cavity originate several paired paranasal sinuses that are lined with mucous membrane and are filled with air. These are the maxillary sinus, frontal sinus, sphenoidal sinus, and the ethmoidal air cells.

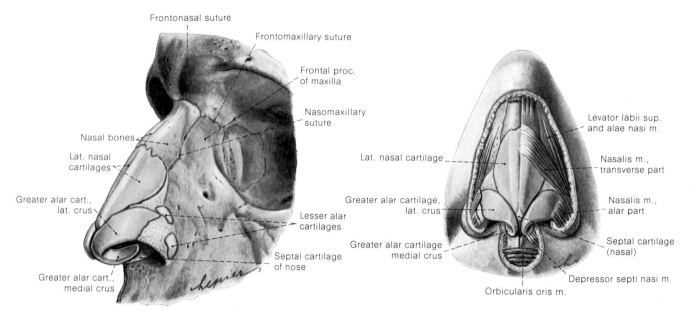

**Fig. 226.** Skeleton and cartilages of external nose. Left view. Nasal cartilages, blue.

**Fig. 227.** Nasal cartilages and muscles. Front view. Cartilages, blue.

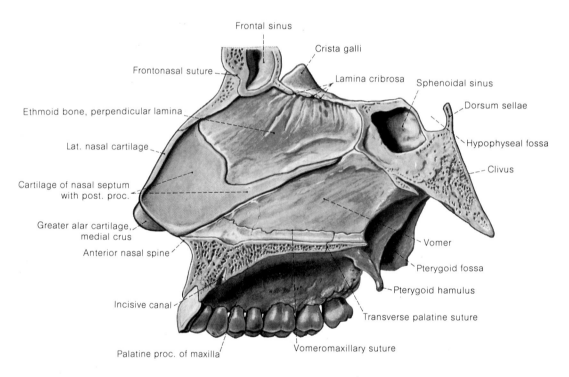

**Fig. 228.** Osseous and cartilaginous nasal septum. Cartilages, blue.

**Nasal nerves:** for motor functions fibers from the facial nerve; for sensory functions fibers from the trigeminal nerve: ant. ethmoidal nerve with branches for nasal septum, lateral nasal wall, tip and wings of nose (ext. nasal branch); post. ethmoidal nerve for sphenoidal sinus and posterior ethmoidal cells; supraorbital nerve for frontal sinus; posterior superior lateral nasal branches for the two upper conchae and posterior ethmoidal cells; posterior inferior lateral nasal branches for the inferior concha and the two inferior nasal meatus; posterior superior medial branches for the upper part of the septum; superior posterior alveolar branches for the maxillary sinus; external nasal branches for the outside of the nasal wings. Olfactory fibers for sense of smell (comp. Fig. 229, 232).

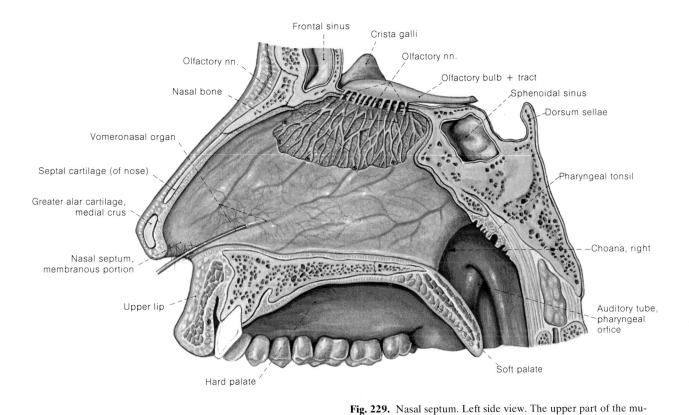

Frontal sinus
Crista galli
Olfactory nn.
Olfactory nn.
Nasal bone
Olfactory bulb + tract
Sphenoidal sinus
Vomeronasal organ
Dorsum sellae
Septal cartilage (of nose)
Greater alar cartilage, medial crus
Pharyngeal tonsil
Nasal septum, membranous portion
Choana, right
Upper lip
Auditory tube, pharyngeal orfice
Hard palate
Soft palate

**Fig. 229.** Nasal septum. Left side view. The upper part of the mucous membrane of the nasal septum is removed to display the medial olfactory nerves. The lateral olfactory nerves were severed at the cribriform openings. Sound inserted in short blind duct of the rudimentary human vomeronasal organ (JACOBSON's) which occurs occasionally. The arteries and veins of the nasal septum show through the mucous membrane.

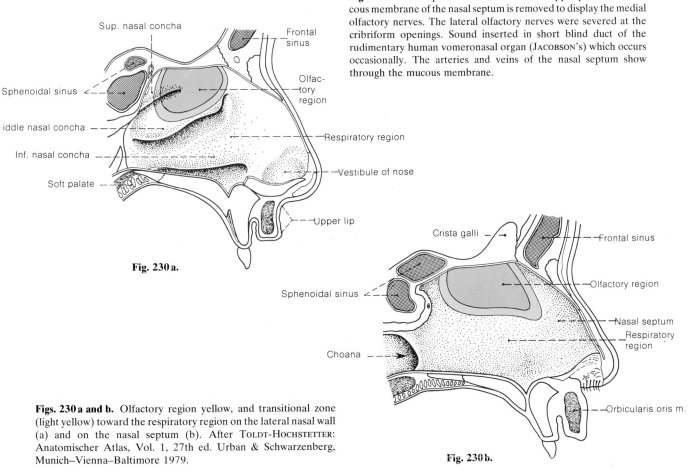

Sup. nasal concha
Frontal sinus
Sphenoidal sinus
Olfactory region
Middle nasal concha
Respiratory region
Inf. nasal concha
Vestibule of nose
Soft palate
Upper lip

**Fig. 230 a.**

Crista galli
Frontal sinus
Sphenoidal sinus
Olfactory region
Nasal septum
Respiratory region
Choana
Orbicularis oris m.

**Fig. 230 b.**

**Figs. 230 a and b.** Olfactory region yellow, and transitional zone (light yellow) toward the respiratory region on the lateral nasal wall (a) and on the nasal septum (b). After TOLDT-HOCHSTETTER: Anatomischer Atlas, Vol. 1, 27th ed. Urban & Schwarzenberg, Munich–Vienna–Baltimore 1979.

# Nose, Nasal Cavity, Paranasal Sinuses

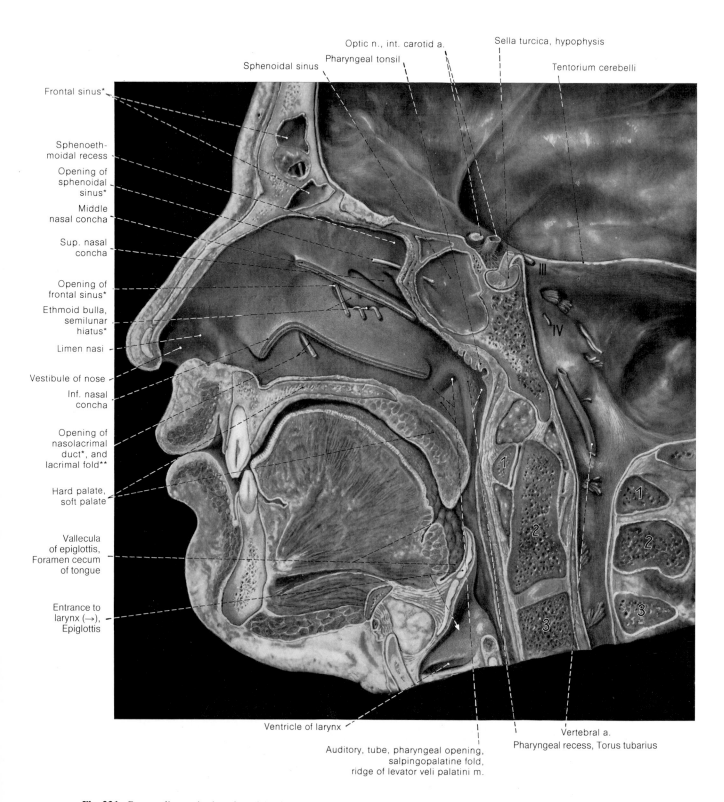

Optic n., int. carotid a.

Pharyngeal tonsil

Sella turcica, hypophysis

Sphenoidal sinus

Tentorium cerebelli

Frontal sinus*

Sphenoeth-moidal recess

Opening of sphenoidal sinus*

Middle nasal concha

Sup. nasal concha

Opening of frontal sinus*

Ethmoid bulla, semilunar hiatus*

Limen nasi

Vestibule of nose

Inf. nasal concha

Opening of nasolacrimal duct*, and lacrimal fold**

Hard palate, soft palate

Vallecula of epiglottis, Foramen cecum of tongue

Entrance to larynx (→), Epiglottis

Ventricle of larynx

Auditory, tube, pharyngeal opening, salpingopalatine fold, ridge of levator veli palatini m.

Vertebral a.
Pharyngeal recess, Torus tubarius

**Fig. 231.** Paramedian sagittal section of the right half of the head. Lateral wall of nasal cavity. Middle and inferior nasal conchae cut off near their base. Openings of paranasal sinus with probes. * Probe, ** HASNER'S valve.
1 Atlas, 2 Axis, 3 Third cervical vertebra. III Oculomotor nerve. IV Trochlear nerves. The other cranial and superior spinal nerves are not specifically indicated. Probes in apertures of sphenoidal and frontal sinuses, the nasolacrimal duct, and two probes in the maxillary sinus.

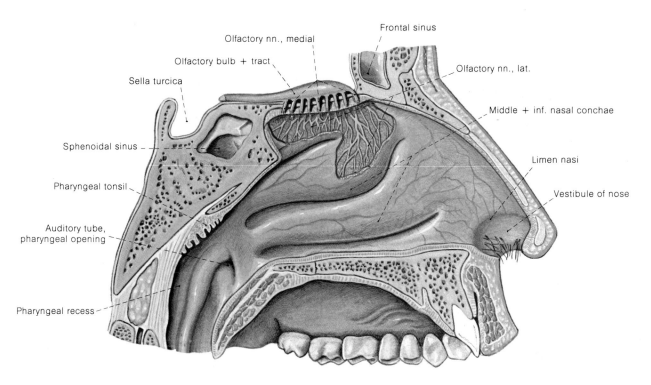

**Fig. 232.** Lateral wall of the left nasal cavity. The medial olfactory nerves from the olfactory bulb were cut; the mucous membrane in the region of the superior and middle conchae was removed to show the lateral row of olfactory nerves.

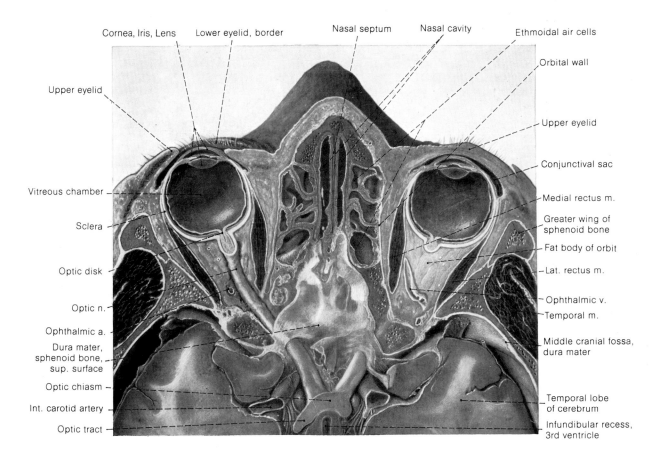

**Fig. 233.** Horizontal section through the head in the region of the eyes, the ethmoidal labyrinth, and optic chiasma. Seen from above.

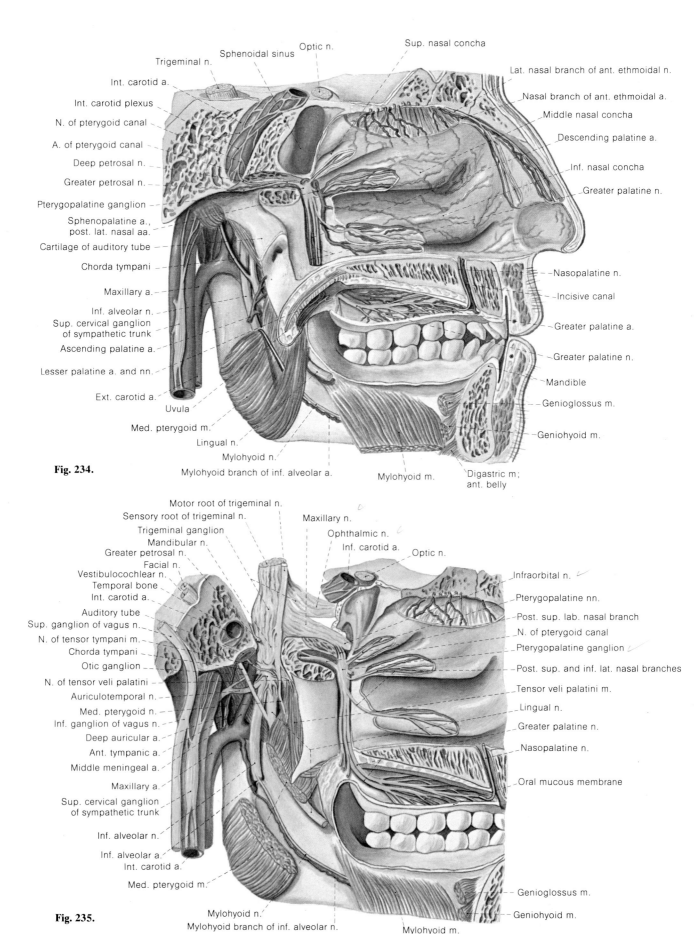

Fig. 234.

Fig. 235.

**Fig. 234.** Nerves and arteries of the lateral nasal wall and the palate with the pterygopalatine ganglion. The carotid, pterygopalatine and pterygoid canals have been opened. The tongue has been removed.

**Fig. 235.** The ramification of the trigeminal nerve, seen from medial. Maxillary nerve with pterygopalatine ganglion and mandibular nerve which otic ganglion. The body of the sphenoid bone has mostly been removed.

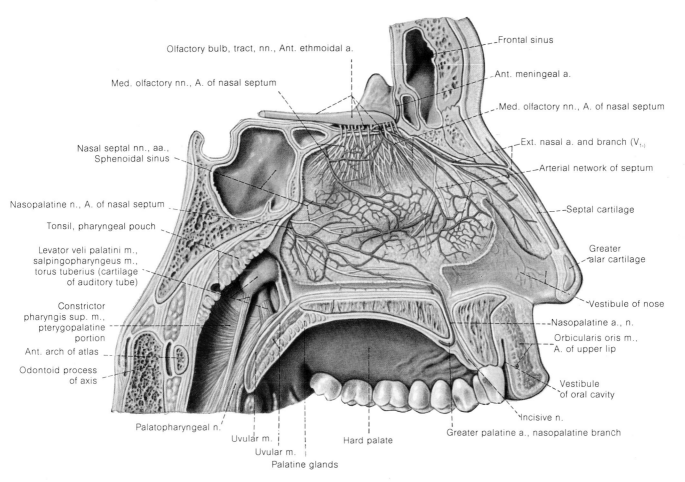

**Fig. 236.** Arteries and nerves in the area of the nasal septum. The mucous membrane has been removed. Musculature of the nasopharynx. (From PERNKOPF: Atlas der topographischen und angewandten Anatomie des Menschen, Vol. 1, 2nd ed. [Ed. H. FERNER]. Urban & Schwarzenberg, Munich–Vienna–Baltimore 1980.)

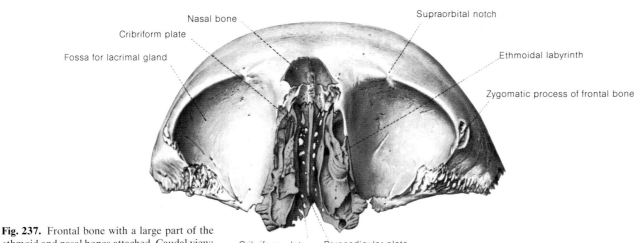

**Fig. 237.** Frontal bone with a large part of the ethmoid and nasal bones attached. Caudal view: Frontal bone, not colored; ethmoid, orange.

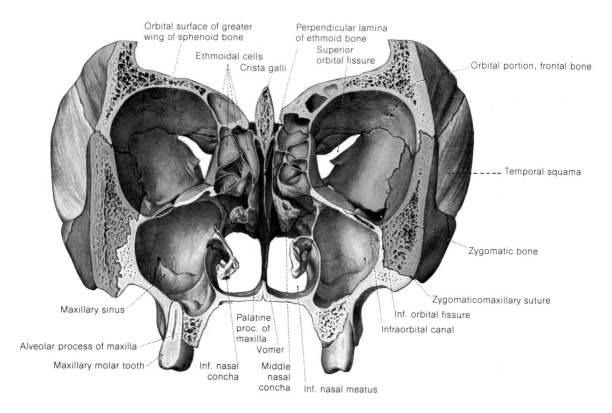

Orbital surface of greater wing of sphenoid bone
Ethmoidal cells
Crista galli
Perpendicular lamina of ethmoid bone
Superior orbital fissure
Orbital portion, frontal bone
Temporal squama
Zygomatic bone
Zygomaticomaxillary suture
Inf. orbital fissure
Infraorbital canal
Maxillary sinus
Alveolar process of maxilla
Maxillary molar tooth
Inf. nasal concha
Palatine proc. of maxilla
Vomer
Middle nasal concha
Inf. nasal meatus

**Fig. 238.** Frontal section through the anterior part of the skull. Orbit, Nasal cavity, Maxillary sinus, Ethmoidal air cells.

**Fig. 239.** Bony portion of the nasal septum. Seen from the left side. Ethmoid, orange; vomer, reddish.

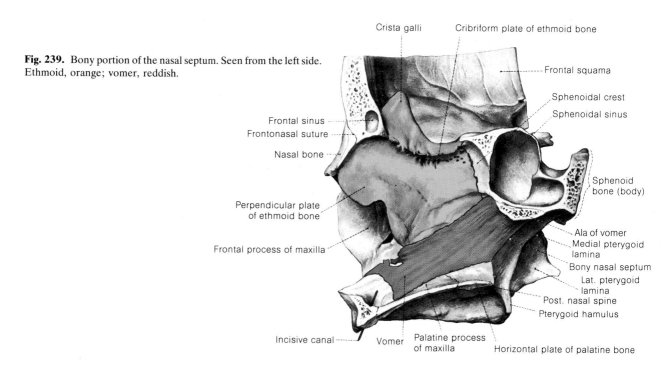

Crista galli
Cribriform plate of ethmoid bone
Frontal squama
Sphenoidal crest
Sphenoidal sinus
Frontal sinus
Frontonasal suture
Nasal bone
Sphenoid bone (body)
Perpendicular plate of ethmoid bone
Ala of vomer
Medial pterygoid lamina
Bony nasal septum
Lat. pterygoid lamina
Post. nasal spine
Pterygoid hamulus
Frontal process of maxilla
Incisive canal
Vomer
Palatine process of maxilla
Horizontal plate of palatine bone

The paranasal sinuses are extensions of the nasal cavity that are lined with a mucous membrane and filled with air: Maxillary sinus, Frontal sinus, Sphenoidal sinus, Ethmoidal air cells, Ethmoidal bulla.

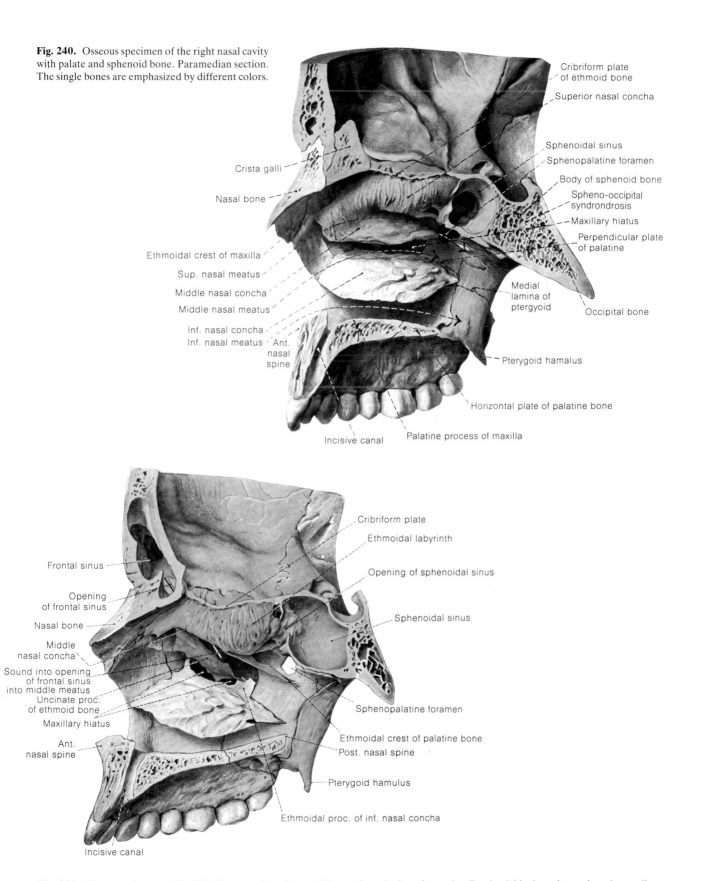

**Fig. 240.** Osseous specimen of the right nasal cavity with palate and sphenoid bone. Paramedian section. The single bones are emphasized by different colors.

Cribriform plate of ethmoid bone

Superior nasal concha

Sphenoidal sinus

Sphenopalatine foramen

Body of sphenoid bone

Spheno-occipital syndrondrosis

Maxillary hiatus

Perpendicular plate of palatine

Crista galli

Nasal bone

Occipital bone

Ethmoidal crest of maxilla

Sup. nasal meatus

Middle nasal concha

Middle nasal meatus

Inf. nasal concha

Inf. nasal meatus

Ant. nasal spine

Medial lamina of ptergyoid

Pterygoid hamalus

Horizontal plate of palatine bone

Incisive canal

Palatine process of maxilla

Cribriform plate

Ethmoidal labyrinth

Opening of sphenoidal sinus

Frontal sinus

Opening of frontal sinus

Nasal bone

Middle nasal concha

Sound into opening of frontal sinus into middle meatus

Uncinate proc. of ethmoid bone

Maxillary hiatus

Ant. nasal spine

Sphenoidal sinus

Sphenopalatine foramen

Ethmoidal crest of palatine bone

Post. nasal spine

Pterygoid hamulus

Ethmoidal proc. of inf. nasal concha

Incisive canal

**Fig. 241.** The same view as in Fig. 240 after resection of the middle nasal concha in order to visualize the sickle shaped entry into the maxillary sinus.

157

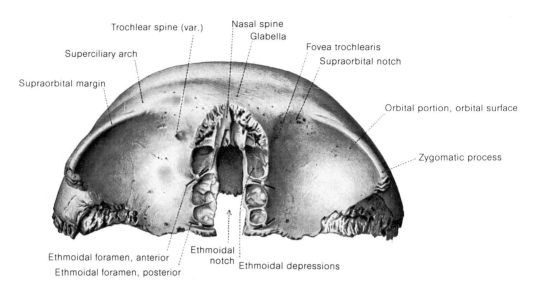

Trochlear spine (var.)
Nasal spine
Glabella
Superciliary arch
Fovea trochlearis
Supraorbital notch
Supraorbital margin

Orbital portion, orbital surface

Zygomatic process

Ethmoidal foramen, anterior
Ethmoidal notch
Ethmoidal foramen, posterior
Ethmoidal depressions

**Fig. 242.** Frontal bone. Seen from below.

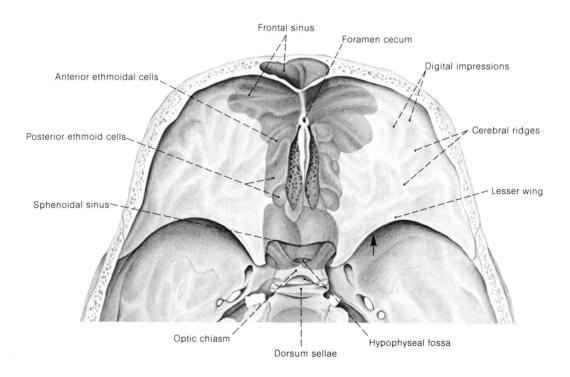

Frontal sinus
Foramen cecum
Digital impressions
Anterior ethmoidal cells
Posterior ethmoid cells
Cerebral ridges
Lesser wing
Sphenoidal sinus

Optic chiasm
Hypophyseal fossa
Dorsum sellae

**Fig. 243.** Paranasal air sinuses and their projection on the anterior cranial fossa from which they are separated by only thin bony plates. The arrow points to the entrance of the superior orbital fissure.

**Fig. 245.** Inferior nasal concha with bony core and very thick mucous membrane with arteries, venous plexuses and pseudoerectile tissues. ▷

158

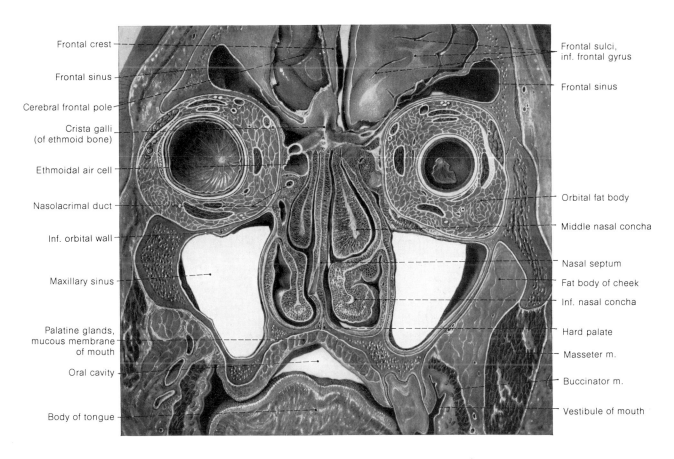

Frontal crest

Frontal sinus

Cerebral frontal pole

Crista galli
(of ethmoid bone)

Ethmoidal air cell

Nasolacrimal duct

Inf. orbital wall

Maxillary sinus

Palatine glands,
mucous membrane
of mouth

Oral cavity

Body of tongue

Frontal sulci,
inf. frontal gyrus

Frontal sinus

Orbital fat body

Middle nasal concha

Nasal septum

Fat body of cheek

Inf. nasal concha

Hard palate

Masseter m.

Buccinator m.

Vestibule of mouth

**Fig. 244.** Frontal section through the head showing orbits, nasal cavity, maxillary sinuses and roof of oral cavity.

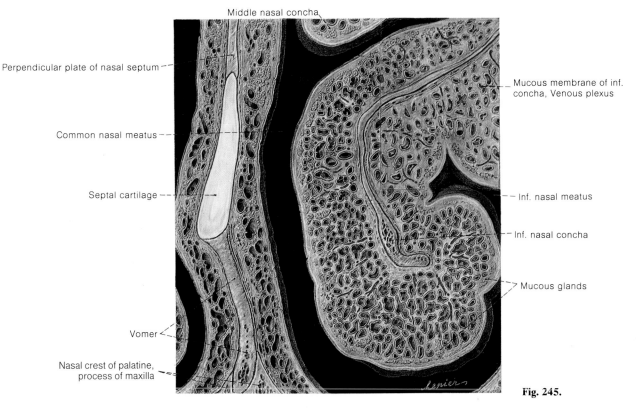

Middle nasal concha

Perpendicular plate of nasal septum

Common nasal meatus

Septal cartilage

Vomer

Nasal crest of palatine,
process of maxilla

Mucous membrane of inf.
concha, Venous plexus

Inf. nasal meatus

Inf. nasal concha

Mucous glands

**Fig. 245.**

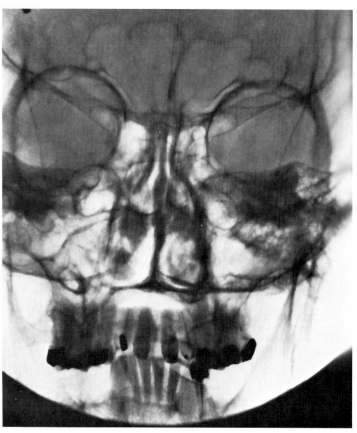

**Fig. 246.** X-ray film of the paranasal sinuses; sagittal projection. Original film. (From L. WICKE: Atlas der Röntgenanatomie, 2nd ed. Urban & Schwarzenberg, Munich–Vienna–Baltimore 1980.)

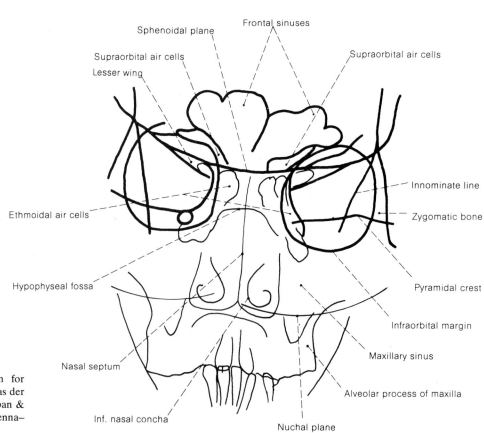

**Fig. 247.** Explanatory diagram for Fig. 246. (From L. WICKE: Atlas der Röntgenanatomie, 2nd ed. Urban & Schwarzenberg, Munich–Vienna–Baltimore 1980.)

Sphenoidal plane

Frontal sinuses

Supraorbital air cells

Supraorbital air cells

Lesser wing

Innominate line

Ethmoidal air cells

Zygomatic bone

Hypophyseal fossa

Pyramidal crest

Infraorbital margin

Maxillary sinus

Nasal septum

Alveolar process of maxilla

Inf. nasal concha

Nuchal plane

# Oral Cavity, Teeth, Masticatory System

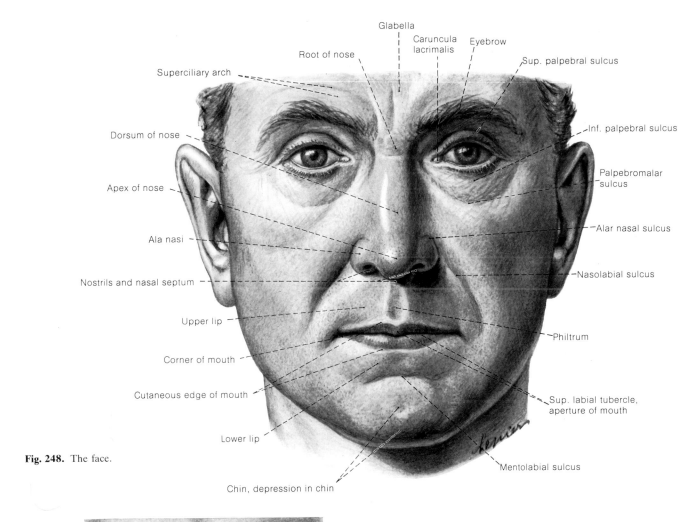

Glabella

Root of nose

Caruncula lacrimalis

Eyebrow

Sup. palpebral sulcus

Superciliary arch

Inf. palpebral sulcus

Dorsum of nose

Palpebromalar sulcus

Apex of nose

Alar nasal sulcus

Ala nasi

Nasolabial sulcus

Nostrils and nasal septum

Upper lip

Philtrum

Corner of mouth

Cutaneous edge of mouth

Sup. labial tubercle, aperture of mouth

Lower lip

Mentolabial sulcus

Chin, depression in chin

**Fig. 248.** The face.

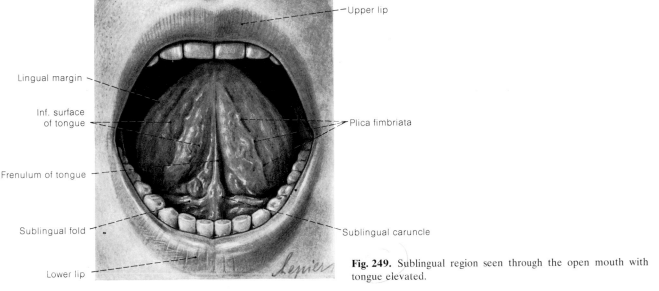

Upper lip

Lingual margin

Inf. surface of tongue

Plica fimbriata

Frenulum of tongue

Sublingual fold

Sublingual caruncle

Lower lip

**Fig. 249.** Sublingual region seen through the open mouth with tongue elevated.

161

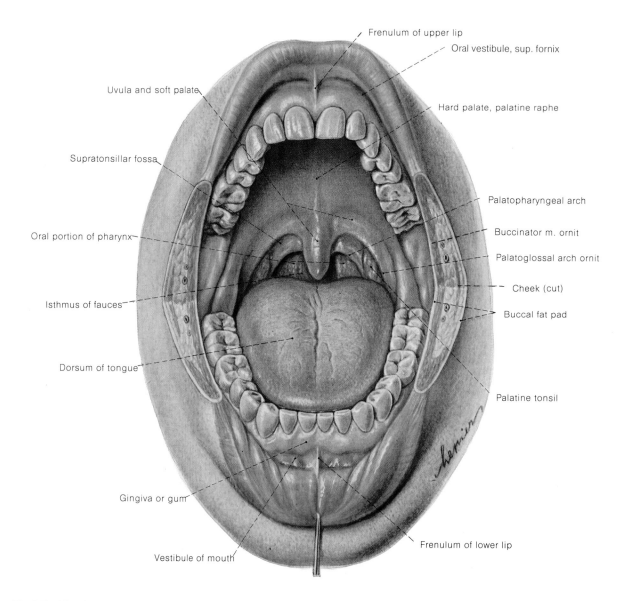

Frenulum of upper lip

Oral vestibule, sup. fornix

Uvula and soft palate

Hard palate, palatine raphe

Supratonsillar fossa

Palatopharyngeal arch

Oral portion of pharynx

Buccinator m. ornit

Palatoglossal arch ornit

Isthmus of fauces

Cheek (cut)

Buccal fat pad

Dorsum of tongue

Palatine tonsil

Gingiva or gum

Frenulum of lower lip

Vestibule of mouth

**Fig. 250.** View into oral cavity with wide open jaws. The cheeks have been cut, upper and lower lip reflected so as to expose the vestibule of the oral cavity. The isthmus faucium is bordered by the root of the tongue and the palatine arches; through the isthmus faucium one sees the posterior wall of the oropharynx. Between the two palatine arches are the palatine tonsils.

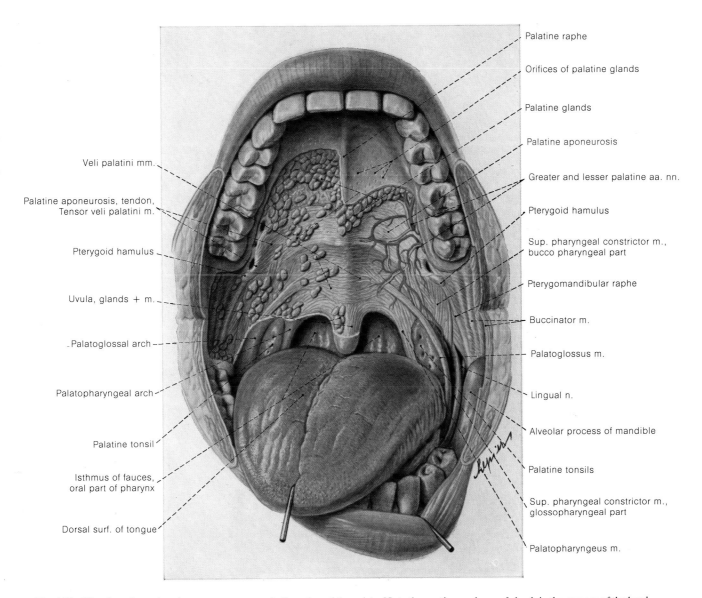

Palatine raphe

Orifices of palatine glands

Palatine glands

Palatine aponeurosis

Greater and lesser palatine aa. nn.

Pterygoid hamulus

Sup. pharyngeal constrictor m., bucco pharyngeal part

Pterygomandibular raphe

Buccinator m.

Palatoglossus m.

Lingual n.

Alveolar process of mandible

Palatine tonsils

Sup. pharyngeal constrictor m., glossopharyngeal part

Palatopharyngeus m.

Veli palatini mm.

Palatine aponeurosis, tendon, Tensor veli palatini m.

Pterygoid hamulus

Uvula, glands + m.

Palatoglossal arch

Palatopharyngeal arch

Palatine tonsil

Isthmus of fauces, oral part of pharynx

Dorsal surf. of tongue

**Fig. 251.** View into the oral cavity, tongue protracted, dissection of the palate. Note the continuous layer of glands in the mucosa of the hard palate and the muscles of the soft palate connected to the palatine aponeurosis. Blood vessels and nerves reach the palate through the palatine foramina; they run in bony sulci in the depth of the mucosa.

# Oral Cavity, Teeth, Masticatory System

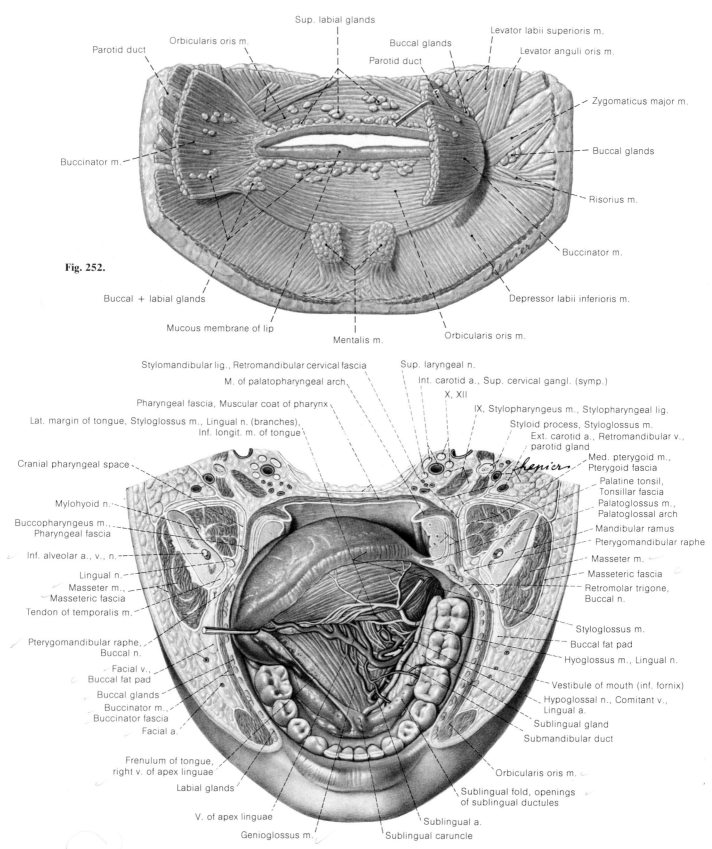

**Fig. 252.**

Labels for Fig. 252:
- Parotid duct
- Orbicularis oris m.
- Sup. labial glands
- Buccal glands
- Parotid duct
- Levator labii superioris m.
- Levator anguli oris m.
- Zygomaticus major m.
- Buccal glands
- Risorius m.
- Buccinator m.
- Buccinator m.
- Depressor labii inferioris m.
- Buccal + labial glands
- Mucous membrane of lip
- Mentalis m.
- Orbicularis oris m.

Labels for Fig. 253:
- Stylomandibular lig., Retromandibular cervical fascia
- M. of palatopharyngeal arch
- Pharyngeal fascia, Muscular coat of pharynx
- Lat. margin of tongue, Styloglossus m., Lingual n. (branches), Inf. longit. m. of tongue
- Cranial pharyngeal space
- Mylohyoid n.
- Buccopharyngeus m., Pharyngeal fascia
- Inf. alveolar a., v., n.
- Lingual n.
- Masseter m., Masseteric fascia
- Tendon of temporalis m.
- Pterygomandibular raphe, Buccal n.
- Facial v., Buccal fat pad
- Buccal glands
- Buccinator m., Buccinator fascia
- Facial a.
- Frenulum of tongue, right v. of apex linguae
- Labial glands
- V. of apex linguae
- Genioglossus m.
- Sublingual caruncle
- Sublingual a.
- Sublingual fold, openings of sublingual ductules
- Orbicularis oris m.
- Submandibular duct
- Sublingual gland
- Hypoglossal n., Comitant v., Lingual a.
- Vestibule of mouth (inf. fornix)
- Hyoglossus m., Lingual n.
- Buccal fat pad
- Styloglossus m.
- Retromolar trigone, Buccal n.
- Masseteric fascia
- Masseter m.
- Pterygomandibular raphe
- Mandibular ramus
- Palatoglossus m., Palatoglossal arch
- Palatine tonsil, Tonsillar fascia
- Med. pterygoid m., Pterygoid fascia
- Ext. carotid a., Retromandibular v., parotid gland
- Styloid process, Styloglossus m.
- IX, Stylopharyngeus m., Stylopharyngeal lig.
- Int. carotid a., Sup. cervical gangl. (symp.)
- X, XII
- Sup. laryngeal n.

**Fig. 253.** Blood vessels on the left side of the floor of the mouth and the tongue. Cross section through the walls of the mouth and pharynx. (From PERNKOPF: Atlas der topographischen und angewandten Anatomie des Menschen, Vol. 1, 2nd ed. [Ed. H. FERNER]. Urban & Schwarzenberg, Munich–Vienna–Baltimore 1980.)

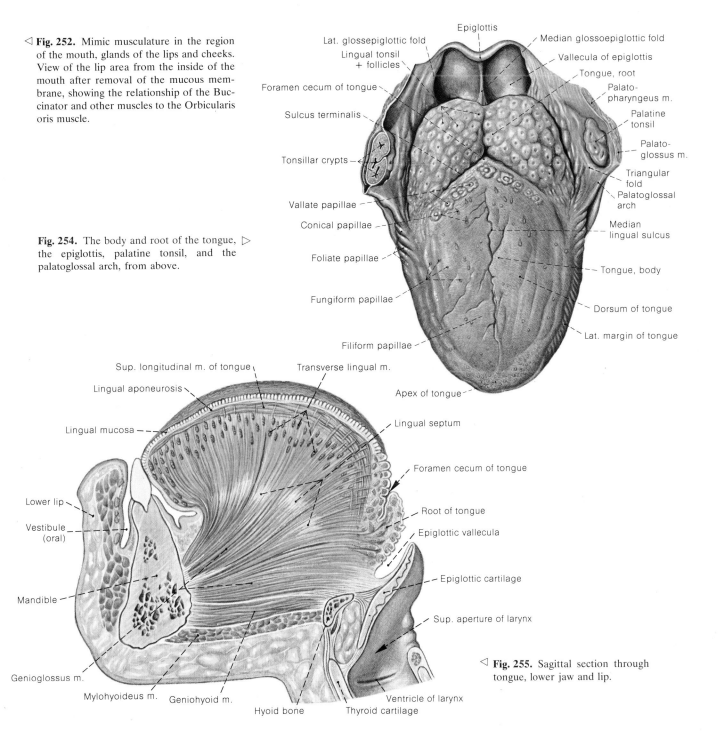

**Fig. 252.** Mimic musculature in the region of the mouth, glands of the lips and cheeks. View of the lip area from the inside of the mouth after removal of the mucous membrane, showing the relationship of the Buccinator and other muscles to the Orbicularis oris muscle.

**Fig. 254.** The body and root of the tongue, ▷ the epiglottis, palatine tonsil, and the palatoglossal arch, from above.

Epiglottis
Lat. glossepiglottic fold
Lingual tonsil + follicles
Foramen cecum of tongue
Sulcus terminalis
Tonsillar crypts
Vallate papillae
Conical papillae
Foliate papillae
Fungiform papillae
Filiform papillae

Median glossoepiglottic fold
Vallecula of epiglottis
Tongue, root
Palato-pharyngeus m.
Palatine tonsil
Palato-glossus m.
Triangular fold
Palatoglossal arch
Median lingual sulcus
Tongue, body
Dorsum of tongue
Lat. margin of tongue
Apex of tongue

Sup. longitudinal m. of tongue
Lingual aponeurosis
Lingual mucosa
Lower lip
Vestibule (oral)
Mandible
Genioglossus m.
Mylohyoideus m.
Geniohyoid m.
Hyoid bone

Transverse lingual m.
Lingual septum
Foramen cecum of tongue
Root of tongue
Epiglottic vallecula
Epiglottic cartilage
Sup. aperture of larynx
Ventricle of larynx
Thyroid cartilage

◁ **Fig. 255.** Sagittal section through tongue, lower jaw and lip.

### The intrinsic muscles of the tongue

1.  **Inferior longitudinal m.,** paired, flat-cylindrical muscle on the inferior surface of the tongue between genioglossus m. and hyoglossus m., reaching from the base to the tip of the tongue.

2.  **Superior longitudinal m.,** unpaired fiber strands in sagittal direction close under the upper surface of the surface of the tongue, not a well defined muscle of its own but extension of fibers stemming from the hypoglossus m. and styloglossus m.

3.  **Transverse muscle of the tongue,** transverse fiber strands from the lingual septum to the lateral margins of the tongue; unpaired in front of the anterior end of the septum; posteriorly they merge with the palatoglossus m. and the glossopharyngeal portion of the superior constrictor pharyngits m.

4.  **Vertical lingual m.,** collective name for the fibers running vertically from the upper to the lower surface of the tongue.

The function of these muscle strands corresponds to their course, they change form and position of the tongue.

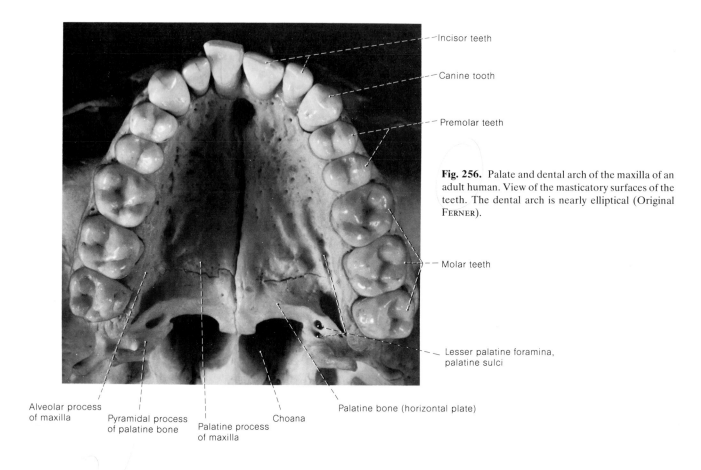

Incisor teeth

Canine tooth

Premolar teeth

Molar teeth

Lesser palatine foramina, palatine sulci

Palatine bone (horizontal plate)

Alveolar process of maxilla

Pyramidal process of palatine bone

Palatine process of maxilla

Choana

**Fig. 256.** Palate and dental arch of the maxilla of an adult human. View of the masticatory surfaces of the teeth. The dental arch is nearly elliptical (Original FERNER).

**Fig. 257.** Right half of a human lower jaw with the ▷ eight permanent teeth and horizontal section through the alveolar and root region. Explanation of form, number and position of the dental roots (Original FERNER).

NOTE: The row of teeth in the lower law is arranged in such a way that the more frontal teeth are closer to the vestibular side while the molars are standing more on the lingual side of the mandible. This is especially well seen in the section through the root region. The dental arch of the mandible resembles a parabola. The circumference of the occlusal surfaces of the lower molars is more rectangular (the upper ones are more rhomboid). The cusps are arranged vestibular and lingual. The lower molars have two roots, one mesial and one distal. The roots are surrounded by a thin shell of alveolar bone and are embedded between the strong cortical shells of the mandibular body (Original FERNER).

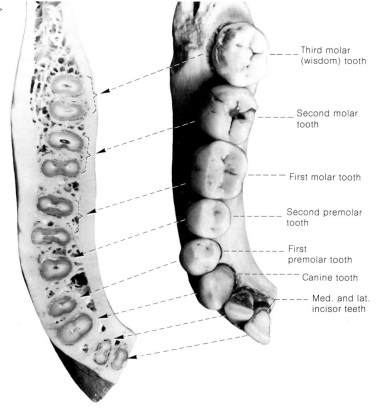

Third molar (wisdom) tooth

Second molar tooth

First molar tooth

Second premolar tooth

First premolar tooth

Canine tooth

Med. and lat. incisor teeth

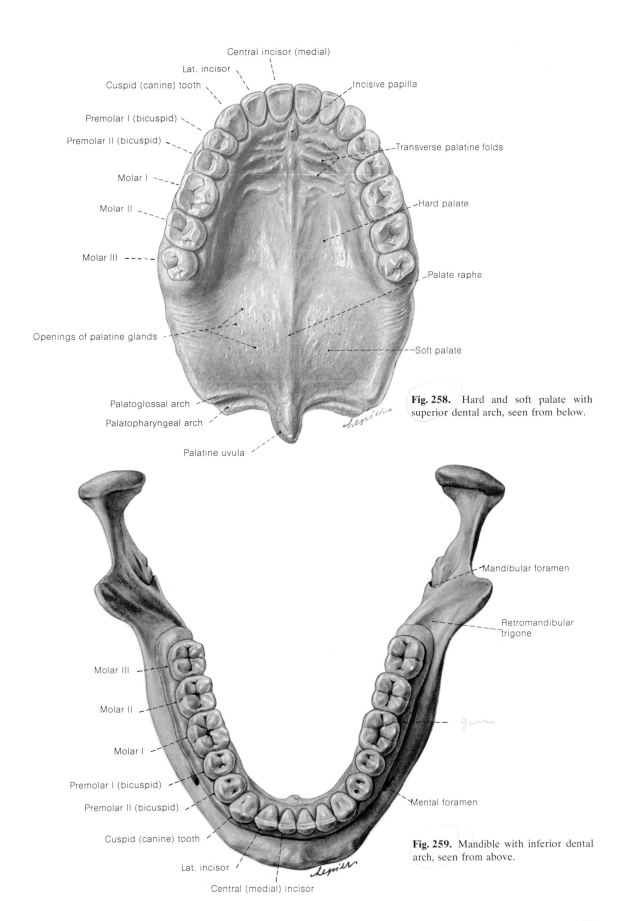

Central incisor (medial)

Lat. incisor

Cuspid (canine) tooth

Premolar I (bicuspid)

Premolar II (bicuspid)

Molar I

Molar II

Molar III

Openings of palatine glands

Palatoglossal arch

Palatopharyngeal arch

Palatine uvula

Incisive papilla

Transverse palatine folds

Hard palate

Palate raphe

Soft palate

**Fig. 258.** Hard and soft palate with superior dental arch, seen from below.

Mandibular foramen

Retromandibular trigone

Molar III

Molar II

Molar I

Premolar I (bicuspid)

Premolar II (bicuspid)

Cuspid (canine) tooth

Lat. incisor

Central (medial) incisor

Mental foramen

**Fig. 259.** Mandible with inferior dental arch, seen from above.

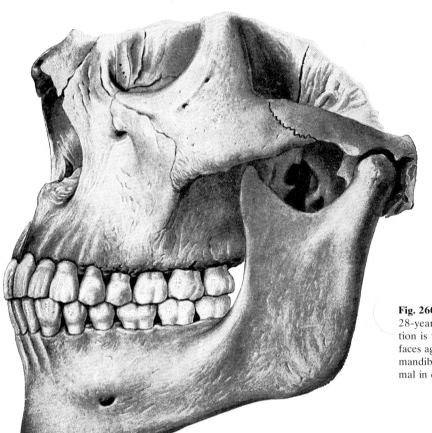

**Fig. 260.** Upper and lower dental arches of a 28-year old man in centric occlusion. Articulation is the sliding motion of the occluding surfaces against each other in conjunction with the mandibulotemporal joint during chewing. Optimal in eugnathic dentition. Dynamic process.

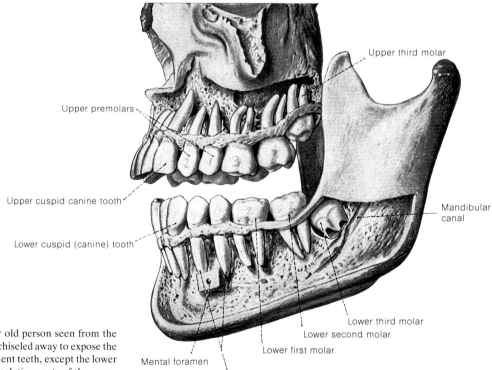

Upper third molar

Upper premolars

Upper cuspid canine tooth

Lower cuspid (canine) tooth

Mandibular canal

Lower third molar

Lower second molar

Lower first molar

Mental foramen

Lower premolars

**Fig. 261.** Dentition of a 20-year old person seen from the left side. The alveolar walls were chiseled away to expose the roots of the teeth. All the permanent teeth, except the lower third molars, have erupted. The palatine roots of the upper molars are not visible.

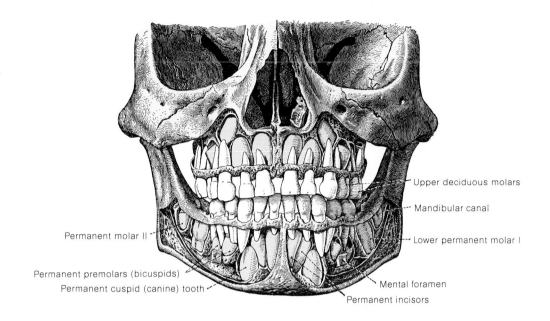

Upper deciduous molars

Mandibular canal

Lower permanent molar I

Permanent molar II

Permanent premolars (bicuspids)

Permanent cuspid (canine) tooth

Mental foramen

Permanent incisors

**Fig. 262 a.** Facial skeleton of a 5-year old child with 20 deciduous (milk) teeth. The rudiments of the permanent teeth (colored blue) have been exposed by chiseling off the alveolar processes.

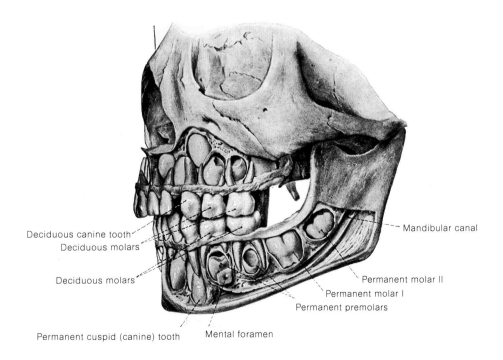

Deciduous canine tooth

Deciduous molars

Deciduous molars

Mandibular canal

Permanent molar II

Permanent molar I

Permanent premolars

Permanent cuspid (canine) tooth

Mental foramen

**Fig. 262 b.** Same preparation as in Fig. 262 a, seen from the left. Permanent teeth shown in blue.

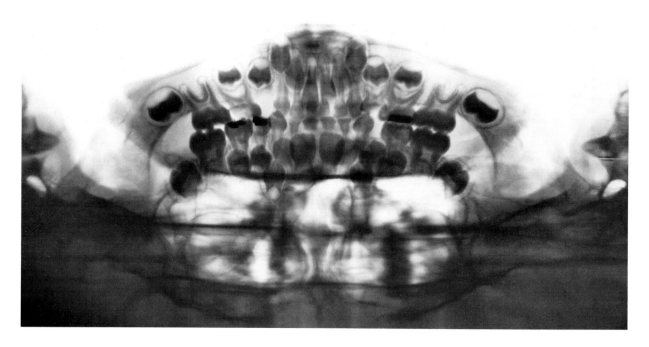

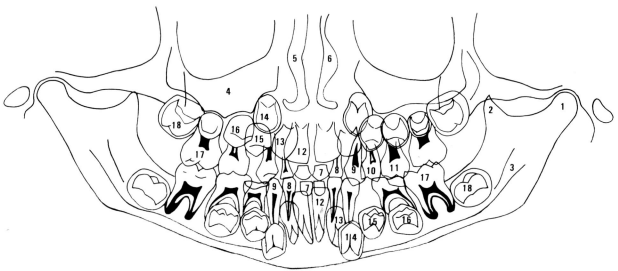

**Fig. 263.** X-ray film of the jaws in panoramic view. Changing dentition of a 7-year old child. Carious defects and fillings in deciduous molars.
(Photo: Priv.-Doz. Dr. Dr. J. DÜKER, Zentrum Zahn-, Mund- und Kieferheilkunde, University of Freiburg i. Brsg.)

| | | | |
|---|---|---|---|
| 1 Condylar process | 6 Nasal septum | 11 Second deciduous molar | 16 Second permanent premolar |
| 2 Coronoid process | 7 First deciduous incisor | 12 First permanent incisor | 17 First permanent molar |
| 3 Mandibular canal | 8 Second deciduous incisor | 13 Second permanent incisor | 18 Second permanent molar |
| 4 Maxillary sinus | 9 Deciduous canine | 14 Permanent canine | |
| 5 Nasal cavity | 10 First deciduous molar | 15 First permanent premolar | |

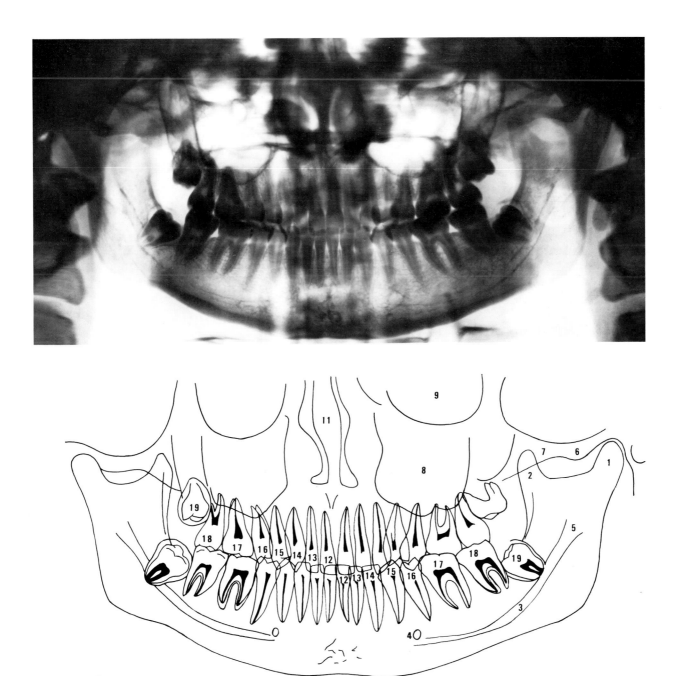

**Fig. 264.** X-ray film and explanatory diagram of the jaws in panoramic view. Complete dentition of an 18-year old woman with wisdom teeth, molars with fillings.
(Photo: Priv.-Doz. Dr. Dr. J. DÜKER, Zentrum Zahn-, Mund- und Kieferheilkunde, University of Freiburg i. Brsg.)

| | | | |
|---|---|---|---|
| 1 Condylar process | 6 Articular tubercle | 11 Nasal septum | 16 Permanent premolar II |
| 2 Coronoid process | 7 Zygomatic arch | 12 Permanent incisor I | 17 Permanent molar I |
| 3 Mandibular canal | 8 Maxillary sinus | 13 Permanent incisor II | 18 Permanent molar II |
| 4 Mental foramen | 9 Orbit | 14 Permanent canine | 19 Permanent molar III |
| 5 Mandibular foramen | 10 Nasal cavity | 15 Permanent premolar I | |

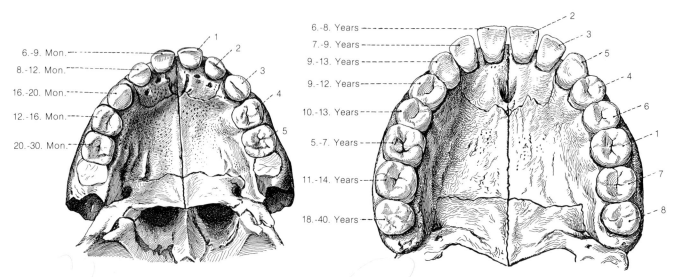

**Fig. 265.** Diagram showing the eruption schedule of deciduous teeth in the maxilla. On the left side of the illustration, the eruption times are given in months, on the right, the sequence in which the teeth appear is indicated by numbers.

**Fig. 266.** Diagram showing the eruption schedule of the permanent teeth in the maxilla. The left side of the illustration gives the time of eruption in years; the right, the order in which the teeth appear is indicated by numbers.

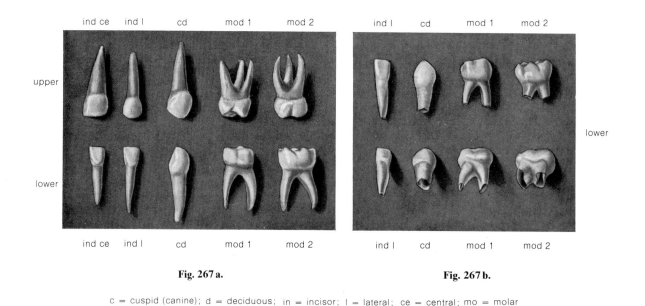

**Fig. 267 a.**                                    **Fig. 267 b.**

c = cuspid (canine); d = deciduous; in = incisor; l = lateral; ce = central; mo = molar

**Fig. 267 a.** Deciduous dentition of a 3-year old child, seen from the lingual (labial) or else facial (buccal) surface.

**Fig. 267 b.** Mandibular deciduous teeth of a 2-year old child. Lingual (labial) or else facial (buccal) side of the lateral incisor, cuspid (canine), and two molars in upper row. In the lower row, these teeth have been tilted to show that the roots are in different stages of calcification.

**Fig. 270.** Right lower permanent cuspid (canine) seen from the lingual side. The upper and lower cuspids have the longest roots. The roots ▷ of the lower cuspids (canine) are occasionally divided.

**Fig. 271.** Left lower permanent second molar tooth, seen from the (buccal) facial side. The chewing surface (masticatory surface) always has two facial and two lingual cusps. The two strong roots of this tooth develop slightly curved distally (typical root characteristic).

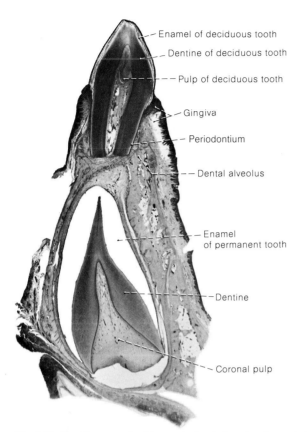

Enamel of deciduous tooth

Dentine of deciduous tooth

Pulp of deciduous tooth

Gingiva

Periodontium

Dental alveolus

Enamel of permanent tooth

Dentine

Coronal pulp

**Fig. 268.** Deciduous tooth with resorbed apical root region and absorbed deciduous alveolus of shallow depth. The resorption of the root of the deciduous tooth (dentine and cementum) will progress toward the neck so that only a hallow crown will remain. Below this is the permanent tooth of which only the crown but not the root has developed. The permanent tooth is located in a bony alveolus (Preparation FERNER).

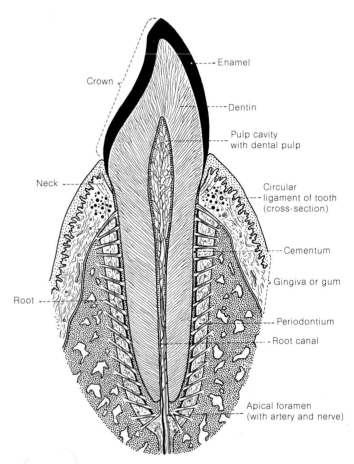

Crown

Neck

Root

Enamel

Dentin

Pulp cavity with dental pulp

Circular ligament of tooth (cross-section)

Cementum

Gingiva or gum

Periodontium

Root canal

Apical foramen (with artery and nerve)

**Fig. 269.** Diagram of a longitudinal section through a tooth in the alveolus.

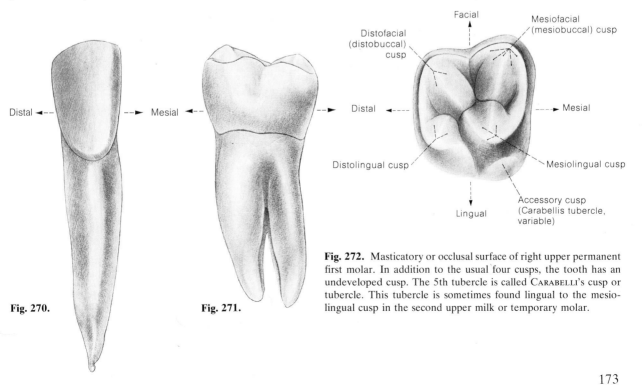

Distal — Mesial — Distal

Facial

Distofacial (distobuccal) cusp

Mesiofacial (mesiobuccal) cusp

Mesial

Distolingual cusp

Mesiolingual cusp

Accessory cusp (Carabellis tubercle, variable)

Lingual

**Fig. 270.**

**Fig. 271.**

**Fig. 272.** Masticatory or occlusal surface of right upper permanent first molar. In addition to the usual four cusps, the tooth has an undeveloped cusp. The 5th tubercle is called CARABELLI's cusp or tubercle. This tubercle is sometimes found lingual to the mesiolingual cusp in the second upper milk or temporary molar.

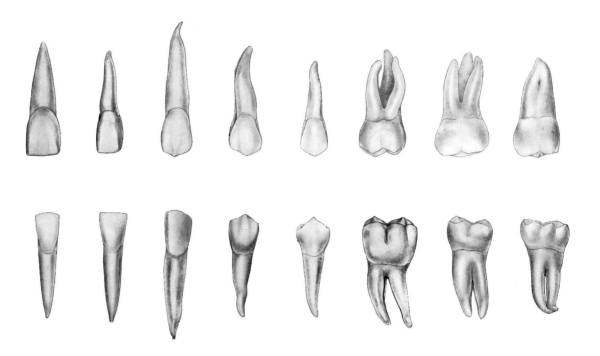

**Fig. 273.** Permanent teeth of the left maxilla, seen from the labial or buccal (facial) side. Teeth in order of succession from left: 2 incisors, 1 cuspid (canine), 2 (bicuspids) premolars, and 3 molars.

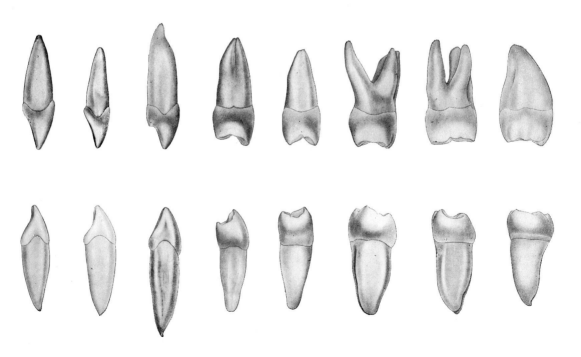

**Fig. 274.** Permanent teeth of the left maxilla and mandible, seen from medial side. Order of teeth the same as in Fig. 273.

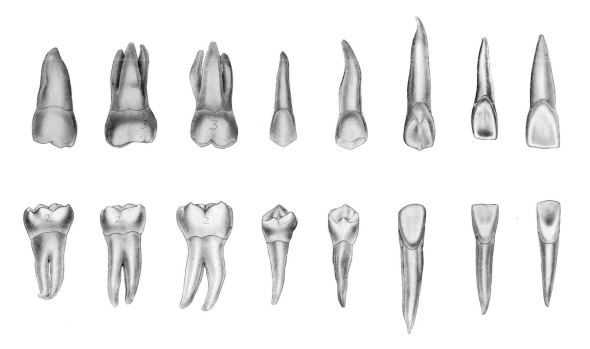

**Fig. 275.** Permanent teeth of the left maxilla and mandible, seen from oral side. Order of teeth in order of succession from right; 2 incisors, 1 cuspid (canine), 2 (bicuspids) premolars, 3 molars.

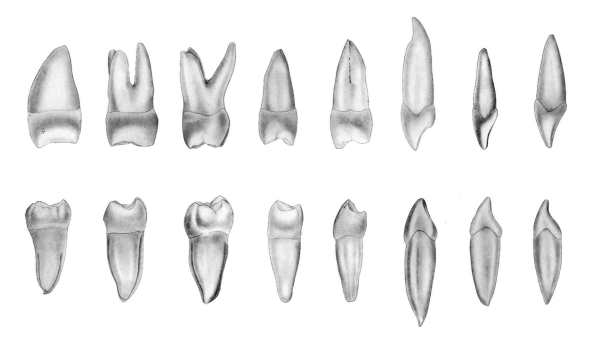

**Fig. 276.** Permanent teeth of the left maxilla and mandible, seen from distal. Same order as in Fig. 275.

175

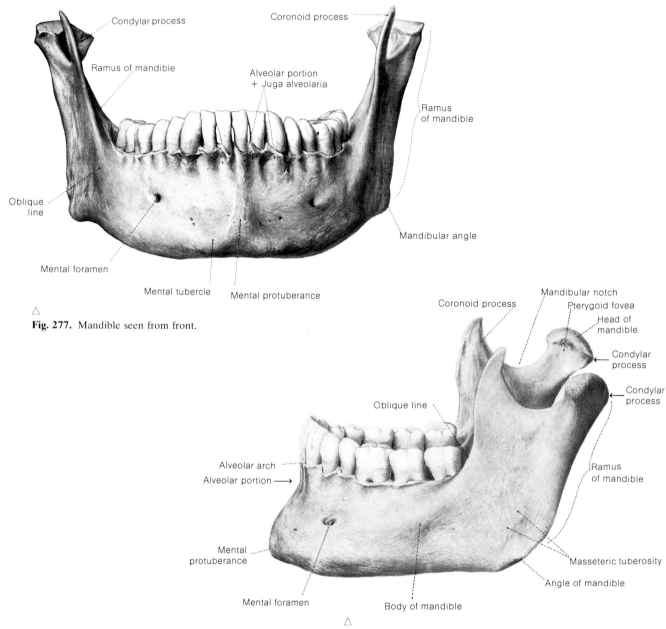

Condylar process

Coronoid process

Ramus of mandible

Alveolar portion + Juga alveolaria

Ramus of mandible

Oblique line

Mandibular angle

Mental foramen

Mental tubercle  Mental protuberance

**Fig. 277.** Mandible seen from front.

Coronoid process

Mandibular notch
Pterygoid fovea
Head of mandible
Condylar process
Condylar process

Oblique line

Alveolar arch
Alveolar portion →

Ramus of mandible

Mental protuberance

Masseteric tuberosity

Mental foramen  Body of mandible

Angle of mandible

**Fig. 278.** Mandible, seen from left lateral side.

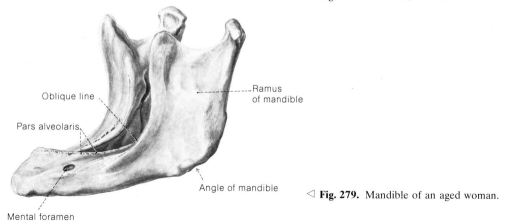

Oblique line

Ramus of mandible

Pars alveolaris

Angle of mandible

**Fig. 279.** Mandible of an aged woman.

Mental foramen

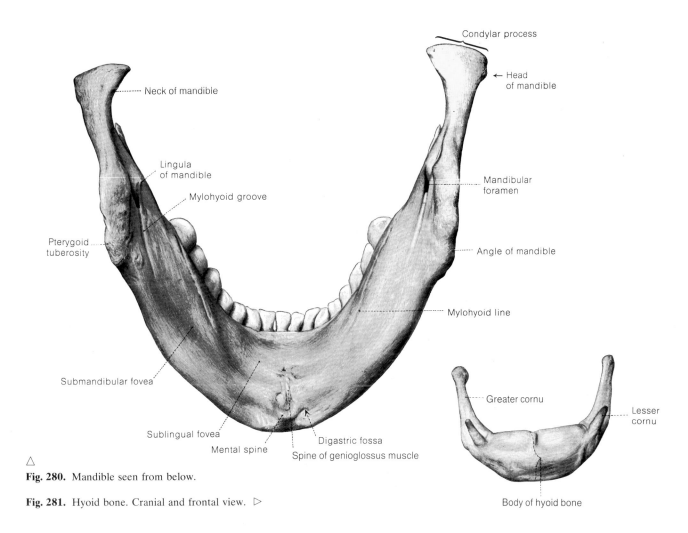

Fig. 280. Mandible seen from below.

Fig. 281. Hyoid bone. Cranial and frontal view.  ▷

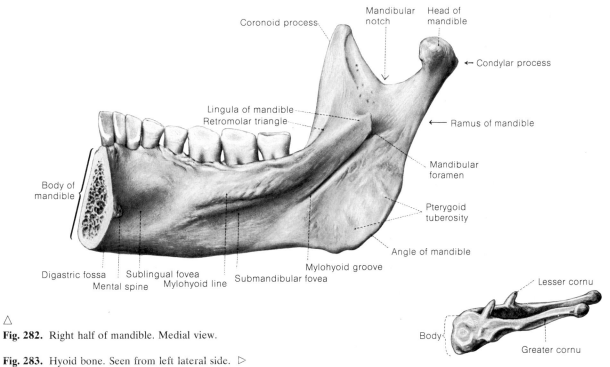

Fig. 282. Right half of mandible. Medial view.

Fig. 283. Hyoid bone. Seen from left lateral side.  ▷

177

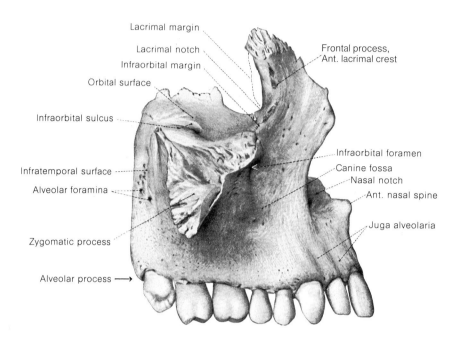

Lacrimal margin

Lacrimal notch

Infraorbital margin

Orbital surface

Infraorbital sulcus

Infratemporal surface

Alveolar foramina

Zygomatic process

Alveolar process ⟶

Frontal process,
Ant. lacrimal crest

Infraorbital foramen

Canine fossa

Nasal notch

Ant. nasal spine

Juga alveolaria

**Fig. 284.** Right maxilla. Lateral view.

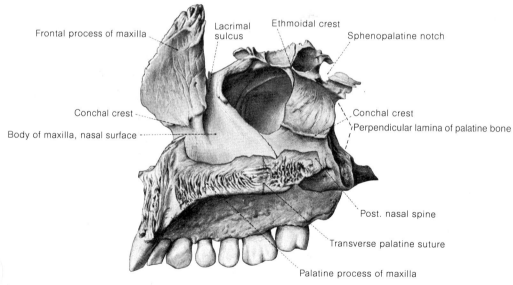

Frontal process of maxilla

Lacrimal sulcus

Ethmoidal crest

Sphenopalatine notch

Conchal crest

Body of maxilla, nasal surface

Conchal crest

Perpendicular lamina of palatine bone

Post. nasal spine

Transverse palatine suture

Palatine process of maxilla

**Fig. 285.** Right maxilla and palatine bones. Palatine, blue.

◁ **Fig. 288.** Innervation of the teeth by the second and third branch of the trigeminal nerve.

**Fig. 289.** Maxillary nerve, pterygopalatine ganglion, intracranial portion of facial nerve and tympanic nerve. The orbit has been opened laterally and its contents have been removed. The pterygoid canal, tympanic cavity and facial canal have been opened, the temporal bone has been sectioned obliquely and the trigeminal ganglion has been pulled upward. The labyrinthine wall of the tympanic cavity is exposed.

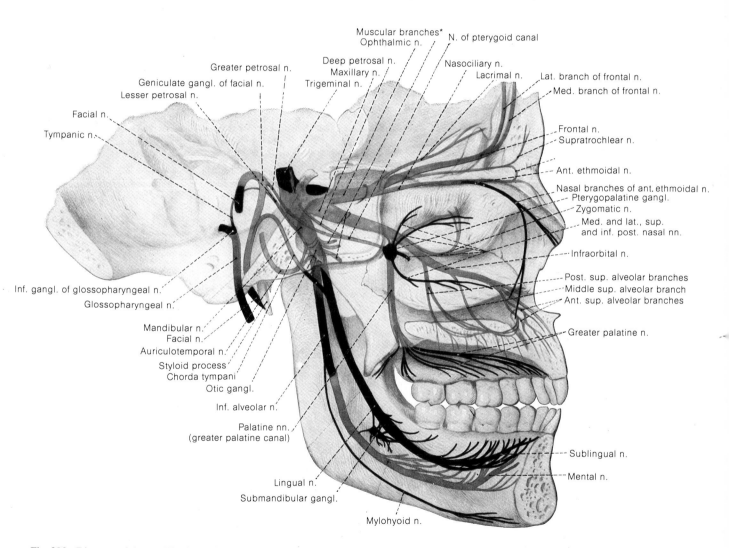

**Fig. 290.** Diagram of the ramifications of the trigeminal nerve and its connections with the facial and glossopharyngeal nerves (projected onto a median section of the skull). Black: exposed portions of nerves, gray: portions covered by bone. * = previously called masticatory nerve.

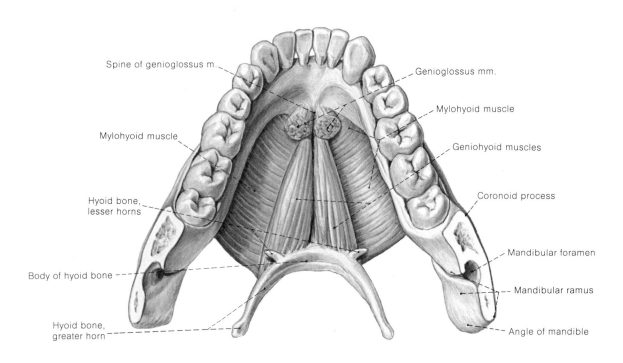

Spine of genioglossus m.

Genioglossus mm.

Mylohyoid muscle

Mylohyoid muscle

Geniohyoid muscles

Hyoid bone, lesser horns

Coronoid process

Mandibular foramen

Body of hyoid bone

Mandibular ramus

Hyoid bone, greater horn

Angle of mandible

**Fig. 291.** Teeth of the lower jaw, view of the occlusal surfaces, diaphragm of the oral cavity. Hyoid bone with greater and lesser bones, (cornua), mylohyoid and geniohyoid muscles seen from the oral side. Genioglossus muscle stumps of origin were preserved.

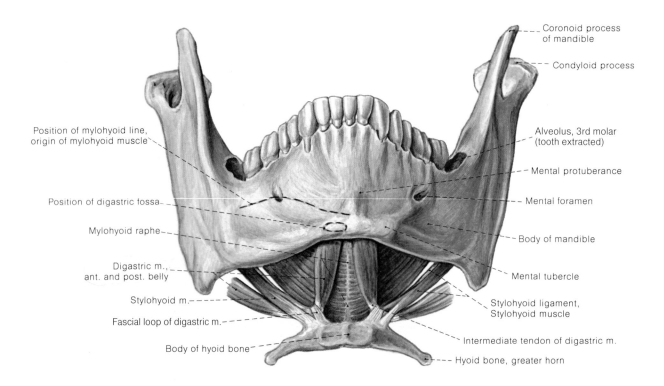

Coronoid process of mandible

Condyloid process

Position of mylohyoid line, origin of mylohyoid muscle

Alveolus, 3rd molar (tooth extracted)

Mental protuberance

Position of digastric fossa

Mental foramen

Mylohyoid raphe

Body of mandible

Digastric m., ant. and post. belly

Mental tubercle

Stylohyoid m.

Stylohyoid ligament, Stylohyoid muscle

Fascial loop of digastric m.

Intermediate tendon of digastric m.

Body of hyoid bone

Hyoid bone, greater horn

**Fig. 292.** Mandible, hyoid bone, muscles of the hyoid bone, seen from in front and below. The origin of the Mylohyoid muscle and the diagastric fossa on the inner surface of the mandible are indicated by interrupted lines.

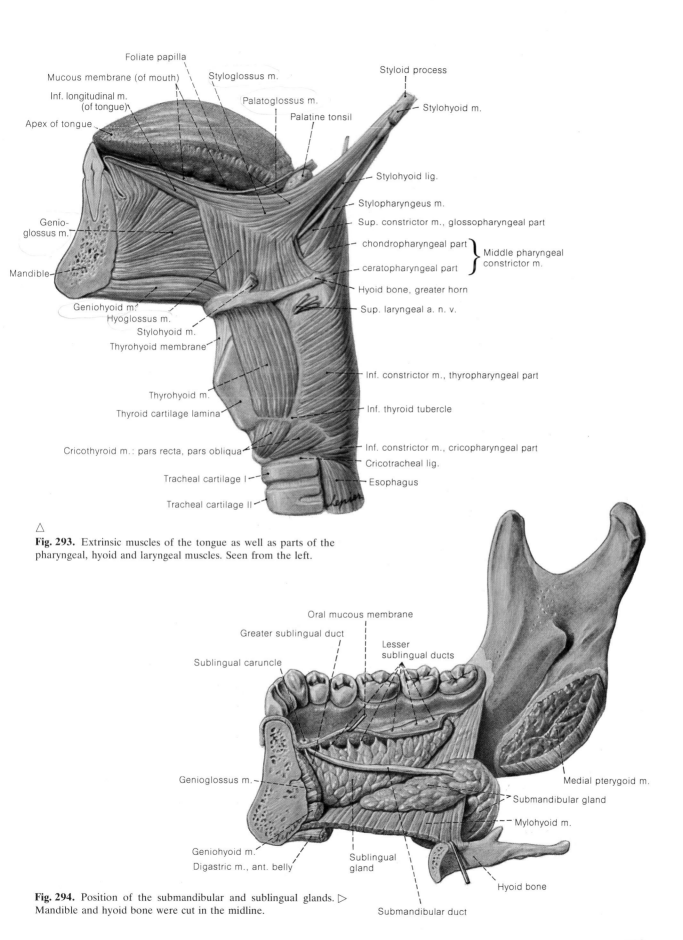

Foliate papilla
Mucous membrane (of mouth)
Inf. longitudinal m. (of tongue)
Apex of tongue
Styloglossus m.
Palatoglossus m.
Palatine tonsil
Styloid process
Stylohyoid m.
Stylohyoid lig.
Stylopharyngeus m.
Sup. constrictor m., glossopharyngeal part
chondropharyngeal part
ceratopharyngeal part
} Middle pharyngeal constrictor m.
Genio-glossus m.
Mandible
Geniohyoid m.
Hyoglossus m.
Stylohyoid m.
Thyrohyoid membrane
Thyrohyoid m.
Thyroid cartilage lamina
Cricothyroid m.: pars recta, pars obliqua
Tracheal cartilage I
Tracheal cartilage II
Hyoid bone, greater horn
Sup. laryngeal a. n. v.
Inf. constrictor m., thyropharyngeal part
Inf. thyroid tubercle
Inf. constrictor m., cricopharyngeal part
Cricotracheal lig.
Esophagus

**Fig. 293.** Extrinsic muscles of the tongue as well as parts of the pharyngeal, hyoid and laryngeal muscles. Seen from the left.

Oral mucous membrane
Greater sublingual duct
Sublingual caruncle
Lesser sublingual ducts
Genioglossus m.
Geniohyoid m.
Digastric m., ant. belly
Sublingual gland
Medial pterygoid m.
Submandibular gland
Mylohyoid m.
Hyoid bone
Submandibular duct

**Fig. 294.** Position of the submandibular and sublingual glands. ▷ Mandible and hyoid bone were cut in the midline.

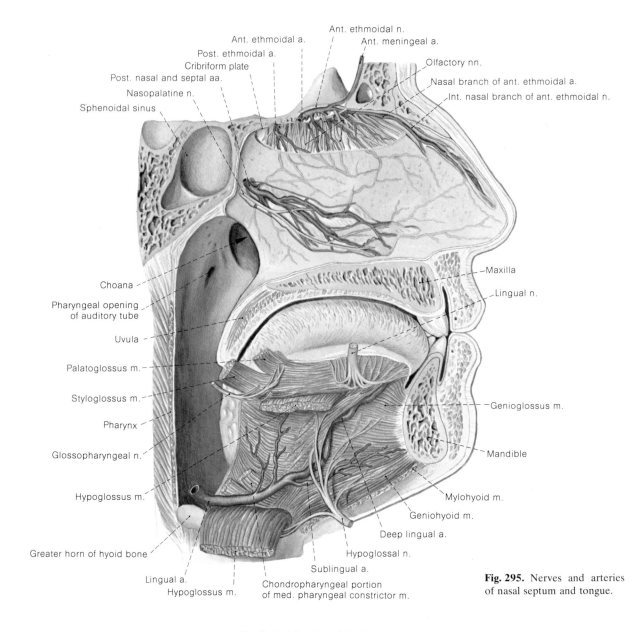

Ant. ethmoidal n.
Ant. ethmoidal a.
Ant. meningeal a.
Post. ethmoidal a.
Cribriform plate
Olfactory nn.
Post. nasal and septal aa.
Nasopalatine n.
Nasal branch of ant. ethmoidal a.
Int. nasal branch of ant. ethmoidal n.
Sphenoidal sinus
Maxilla
Lingual n.
Choana
Pharyngeal opening of auditory tube
Uvula
Palatoglossus m.
Genioglossus m.
Styloglossus m.
Pharynx
Mandible
Glossopharyngeal n.
Hypoglossus m.
Mylohyoid m.
Geniohyoid m.
Deep lingual a.
Greater horn of hyoid bone
Hypoglossal n.
Sublingual a.
Lingual a.
Hypoglossus m.
Chondropharyngeal portion of med. pharyngeal constrictor m.

**Fig. 295.** Nerves and arteries of nasal septum and tongue.

## Extrinsic Muscles of the Tongue

| Name | Origin | Insertion | Action |
|------|--------|-----------|--------|
| **1. Genioglossus m.** | Mental spine of mandible | Projections to body of tongue and lingual aponeurosis | Protrudes and depresses the tongue |
| **2. Hyoglossus m.** | Body of hyoid bone and and greater cornu | Lateral portions of tongue, lingual aponeurosis | Depresses and retracts tongue |
| **3. Chondroglossus m.** | Lesser cornu of hyoid bone | | |
| **4. Styloglossus m.** | Styloid process of temporal bone | Enters lateral portions of tongue from above and behind | Retracts and elevates the tongue (in sucking and swallowing |
| **5. Palatoglossus m.** | Palatal aponeurosis | Upper, posterior portion of tongue | Narrows isthmus of the fauces |

*Nerve:*  Hypoglossal nerve for all tongue muscles

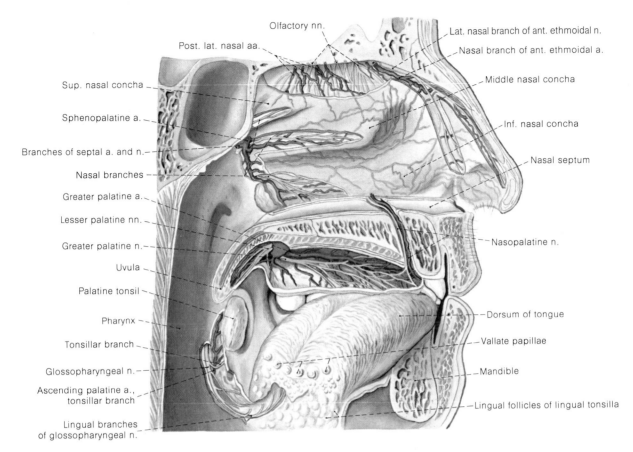

Olfactory nn.

Post. lat. nasal aa.

Lat. nasal branch of ant. ethmoidal n.

Nasal branch of ant. ethmoidal a.

Sup. nasal concha

Middle nasal concha

Sphenopalatine a.

Inf. nasal concha

Branches of septal a. and n.

Nasal septum

Nasal branches

Greater palatine a.

Lesser palatine nn.

Nasopalatine n.

Greater palatine n.

Uvula

Palatine tonsil

Dorsum of tongue

Pharynx

Vallate papillae

Tonsillar branch

Glossopharyngeal n.

Mandible

Ascending palatine a., tonsillar branch

Lingual follicles of lingual tonsilla

Lingual branches of glossopharyngeal n.

**Fig. 296.** Nerves and arteries of the lateral nasal wall and palate, superficial layer. The root of the tongue is pulled forward; the nasal septum has been removed with the exception of its lower portion; the mucous membrane of the isthmus of the fauces has been split along the glossopharyngeal nerve and the ascending palatine artery.

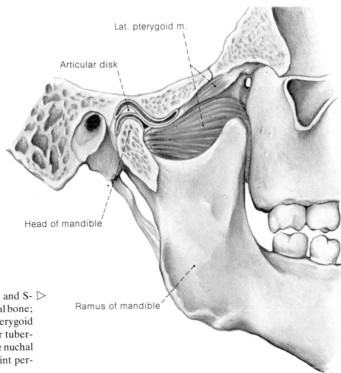

Lat. pterygoid m.

Articular disk

Head of mandible

Ramus of mandible

**Fig. 297.** Die temporomandibular joint with articular disk and S- ▷ shaped gliding surface of the mandibular fossa of the temporal bone; sagittal section. During opening of the jaws, the lateral pterygoid muscle pulls the condylar process forward onto the articular tubercle. With further opening, the head is moved backward by the nuchal muscles (e.g. during snapping). The temporomandibular joint permits rotation and gliding.

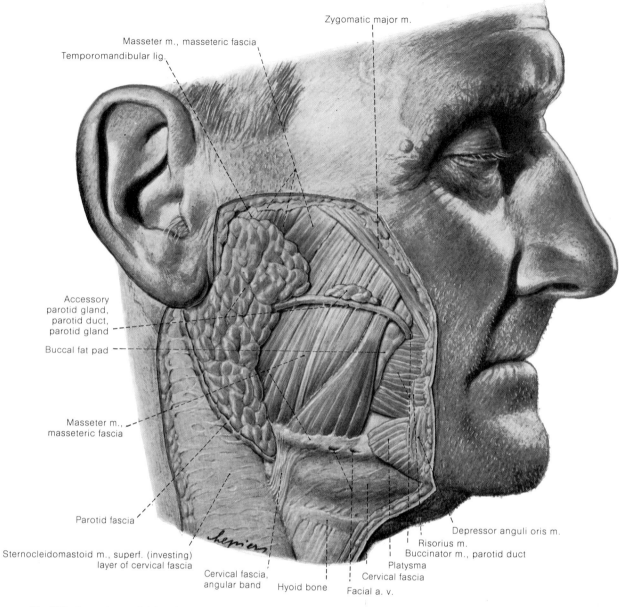

Zygomatic major m.

Masseter m., masseteric fascia

Temporomandibular lig.

Accessory
parotid gland,
parotid duct,
parotid gland

Buccal fat pad

Masseter m.,
masseteric fascia

Parotid fascia

Sternocleidomastoid m., superf. (investing)
layer of cervical fascia

Cervical fascia,
angular band

Hyoid bone

Facial a. v.

Cervical fascia

Platysma

Buccinator m., parotid duct

Risorius m.

Depressor anguli oris m.

**Fig. 298.** Lateral superficial region. Parotideomasseteric region after removal of its fascia. The parotid duct runs one fingers width below the zygomatic and across the masseter muscle, turns inward at its anterior margin and over the buccal fat pad, penetrates the buccinator muscle and opens into the oral vestibule opposite the second upper molar. The buccinator muscle is the core structure of the cheek (innervated by the facial nerve).

### Muscles of Mastication

The muscles of mastication are invested by fasciae. They are the only cranial muscles resembling the true skeletal muscles with distinct separate muscles with well defined fascia. These 4 muscles (Masseter, Temporal and both Pterygoid muscles) move the mandible in the temporomandibular articulation.

| Name | Origin | Insertion |
|---|---|---|
| **1. Masseter muscle** <br> Superficial portion | Zygomatic process of maxilla; lower margin of zygomatic arch | Angle and ramus of mandible; base of coronoid process |
| Deep portion | From posterior part of lower margin and medial surface of zygomatic arch | |

| | |
|---|---|
| *Nerve:* | Masseteric nerve from mandibular division of trigeminal nerve |
| *Function:* | Closes jaws, elevates mandible |

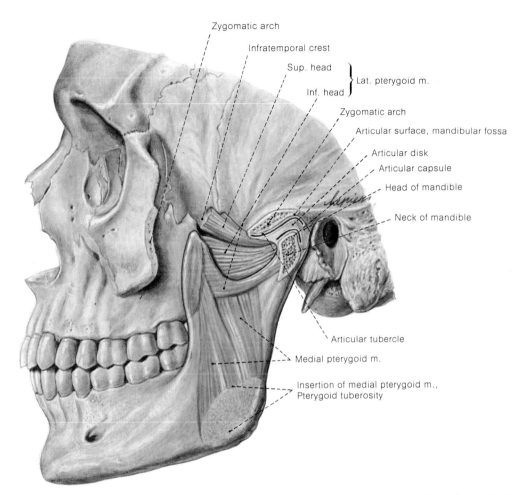

**Fig. 299.** Mandibular articulation. The temporomandibular joint was opened. The cut was made near the articular tubercle in a sagittal direction so that the neck of the mandible and the capsular ligament may be seen with the articular disk. The ramus of the mandible is displayed as being transparent in order to show the origin and course of the Lateral and Medial pterygoid muscles.

### Muscles of Mastication *(continued)*

| Name | Origin | Insertion |
|---|---|---|
| **2. Temporal muscle** | Temporal fossa and temporal fascia | Anterior border and medial surface of coronoid process of mandible |
| *Nerve:* Deep temporal nerves from mandibular division of trigeminal | | |
| *Function:* Elevates mandible (closes jaws); posterior fibers retract mandible | | |
| **3. Lateral pterygoid muscle** | *Main lower head:* Lateral surface of pterygoid lamina<br>*Accessory upper head:* Infratemporal surface of great wing of sphenoid | Pterygoid fova of condyloid process of mandible; articular disk of temporomandibular joint |
| **4. Medial pterygoid muscle** | Pterygoid fossa; pyramidal process of palatine bone; lateral lamina of pterygoid bone | Medial surface and angle of mandible; opposite the masseter muscle (on pterygoid tuberosity) |
| *Nerve:* Lateral and medial pterygoid nerves, respectively, from mandibular division of trigeminal | | |
| *Function:* Opens jaws, protrudes mandible, moves mandible from side to side, grinding motion (lateral); closes jaws (medial) | | |

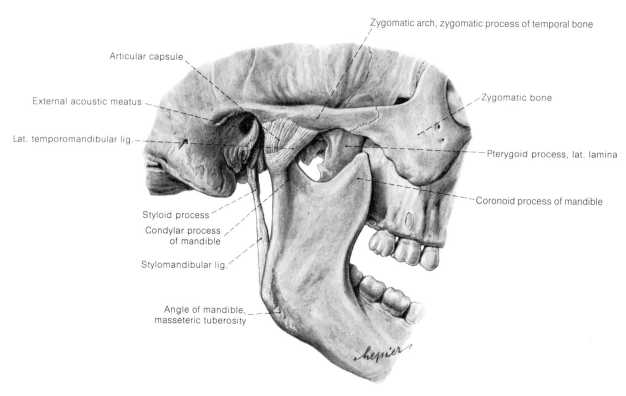

**Fig. 300.** The right temporomandibular joint with ligaments. Lateral view.

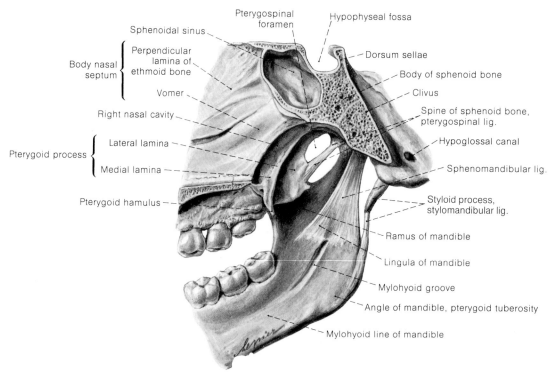

**Fig. 301.** The right temporomandibular joint with ligaments. Medial view.

**Fig. 302.** Median section through the face, head, and neck. The arrows I–V give operative accessibility to the pharynx, larynx, and trachea: ▷ I Subhyoid pharyngotomy; II Laryngotomy; III Coniotomy (intrathyroid laryngotomy) between the thyroid and cricoid cartilage, through the cricothyroid ligament; IV Superior tracheotomy below the cricocartilage arch and above the isthmus of the thyroid gland; V Inferior tracheotomy below the isthmus of the thyroid gland.

# Pharynx

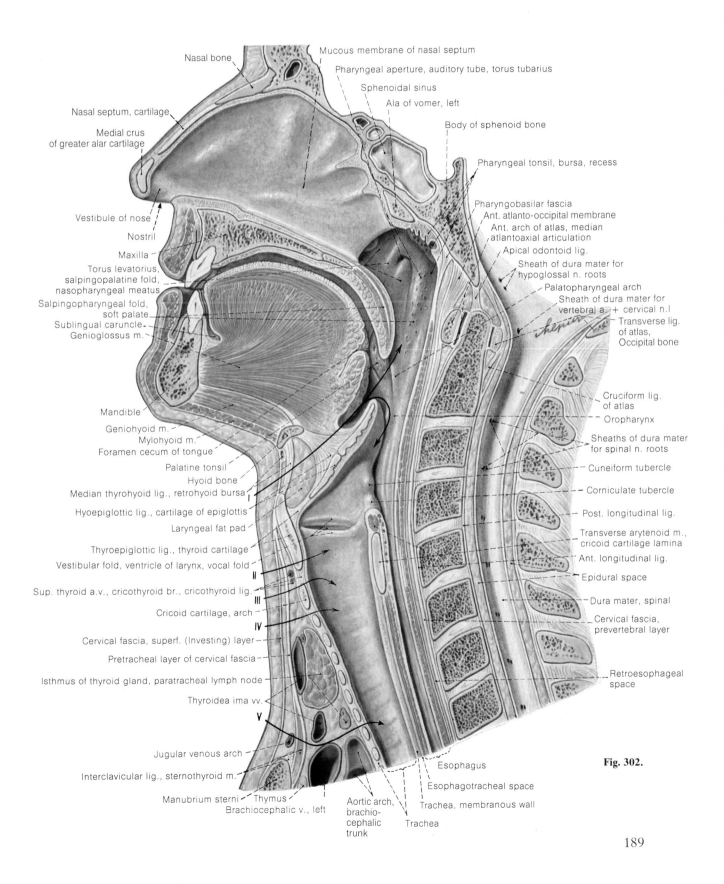

Nasal bone

Mucous membrane of nasal septum

Pharyngeal aperture, auditory tube, torus tubarius

Sphenoidal sinus

Ala of vomer, left

Body of sphenoid bone

Nasal septum, cartilage

Medial crus
of greater alar cartilage

Pharyngeal tonsil, bursa, recess

Pharyngobasilar fascia
Ant. atlanto-occipital membrane
Ant. arch of atlas, median
atlantoaxial articulation
Apical odontoid lig.
Sheath of dura mater for
hypoglossal n. roots

Vestibule of nose

Nostril

Maxilla

Torus levatorius,
salpingopalatine fold,
nasopharyngeal meatus
Salpingopharyngeal fold,
soft palate
Sublingual caruncle
Genioglossus m.

Palatopharyngeal arch
Sheath of dura mater for
vertebral a. + cervical n.I
Transverse lig.
of atlas,
Occipital bone

Mandible

Geniohyoid m.
Mylohyoid m.
Foramen cecum of tongue

Cruciform lig.
of atlas

Oropharynx

Sheaths of dura mater
for spinal n. roots

Cuneiform tubercle

Corniculate tubercle

Palatine tonsil
Hyoid bone
Median thyrohyoid lig., retrohyoid bursa
Hyoepiglottic lig., cartilage of epiglottis
Laryngeal fat pad

Post. longitudinal lig.

Transverse arytenoid m.,
cricoid cartilage lamina

Thyroepiglottic lig., thyroid cartilage
Vestibular fold, ventricle of larynx, vocal fold

Ant. longitudinal lig.

Epidural space

Sup. thyroid a.v., cricothyroid br., cricothyroid lig.

Cricoid cartilage, arch

Dura mater, spinal

Cervical fascia,
prevertebral layer

Cervical fascia, superf. (Investing) layer

Pretracheal layer of cervical fascia

Isthmus of thyroid gland, paratracheal lymph node

Thyroidea ima vv.

Retroesophageal
space

Jugular venous arch

Interclavicular lig., sternothyroid m.

Manubrium sterni  Thymus
Brachiocephalic v., left

Esophagus

Esophagotracheal space

Aortic arch,
brachio-
cephalic
trunk

Trachea, membranous wall

Trachea

**Fig. 302.**

189

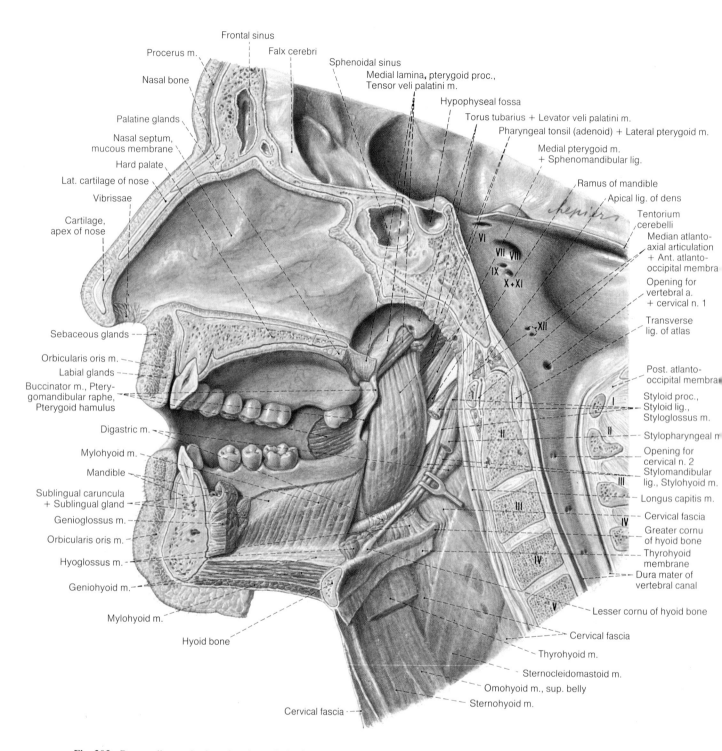

Frontal sinus
Procerus m.
Falx cerebri
Nasal bone
Sphenoidal sinus
Medial lamina, pterygoid proc.,
Tensor veli palatini m.
Hypophyseal fossa
Palatine glands
Torus tubarius + Levator veli palatini m.
Nasal septum,
mucous membrane
Pharyngeal tonsil (adenoid) + Lateral pterygoid m.
Hard palate
Medial pterygoid m.
+ Sphenomandibular lig.
Lat. cartilage of nose
Ramus of mandible
Vibrissae
Apical lig. of dens
Cartilage,
apex of nose
Tentorium
cerebelli
Median atlanto-
axial articulation
+ Ant. atlanto-
occipital membra
Opening for
vertebral a.
+ cervical n. 1
Sebaceous glands
Transverse
lig. of atlas
Orbicularis oris m.
Labial glands
Buccinator m., Ptery-
gomandibular raphe,
Pterygoid hamulus
Post. atlanto-
occipital membra
Digastric m.
Styloid proc.,
Styloid lig.,
Styloglossus m.
Mylohyoid m.
Stylopharyngeal m
Mandible
Opening for
cervical n. 2
Stylomandibular
lig., Stylohyoid m.
Sublingual caruncula
+ Sublingual gland
Longus capitis m.
Genioglossus m.
Cervical fascia
Orbicularis oris m.
Greater cornu
of hyoid bone
Hyoglossus m.
Thyrohyoid
membrane
Geniohyoid m.
Dura mater of
vertebral canal
Mylohyoid m.
Lesser cornu of hyoid bone
Hyoid bone
Cervical fascia
Thyrohyoid m.
Sternocleidomastoid m.
Omohyoid m., sup. belly
Cervical fascia
Sternohyoid m.

**Fig. 303.** Paramedian sagittal section through the face and neck. The nasal and oral cavities, as well as some muscles of the floor of the mouth and upper cervical region are displayed. Cervical vertebrae, I–V. The points of exits of the cranial nerves through the dura mater, VI–XII.

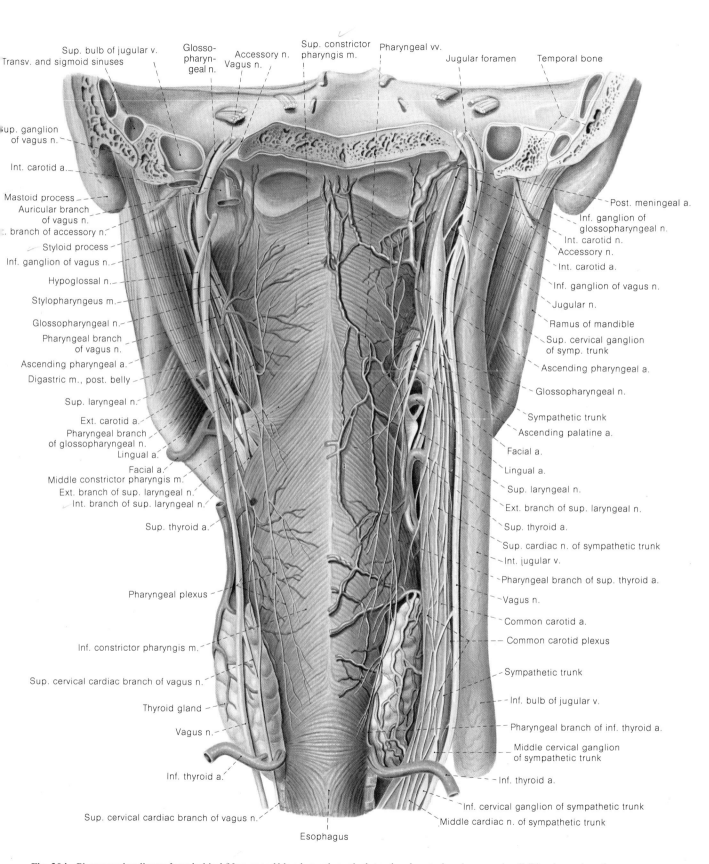

Sup. bulb of jugular v.
Transv. and sigmoid sinuses
Glosso-pharyn-geal n.
Accessory n.
Vagus n.
Sup. constrictor pharyngis m.
Pharyngeal vv.
Jugular foramen
Temporal bone

Sup. ganglion of vagus n.

Int. carotid a.

Mastoid process
Auricular branch of vagus n.
branch of accessory n.
Styloid process
Inf. ganglion of vagus n.
Hypoglossal n.
Stylopharyngeus m.
Glossopharyngeal n.
Pharyngeal branch of vagus n.
Ascending pharyngeal a.
Digastric m., post. belly
Sup. laryngeal n.
Ext. carotid a.
Pharyngeal branch of glossopharyngeal n.
Lingual a.
Facial a.
Middle constrictor pharyngis m.
Ext. branch of sup. laryngeal n.
Int. branch of sup. laryngeal n.
Sup. thyroid a.

Pharyngeal plexus

Inf. constrictor pharyngis m.

Sup. cervical cardiac branch of vagus n.

Thyroid gland

Vagus n.

Inf. thyroid a.

Sup. cervical cardiac branch of vagus n.

Esophagus

Post. meningeal a.
Inf. ganglion of glossopharyngeal n.
Int. carotid n.
Accessory n.
Int. carotid a.
Inf. ganglion of vagus n.
Jugular n.
Ramus of mandible
Sup. cervical ganglion of symp. trunk
Ascending pharyngeal a.
Glossopharyngeal n.
Sympathetic trunk
Ascending palatine a.
Facial a.
Lingual a.
Sup. laryngeal n.
Ext. branch of sup. laryngeal n.
Sup. thyroid a.
Sup. cardiac n. of sympathetic trunk
Int. jugular v.
Pharyngeal branch of sup. thyroid a.
Vagus n.
Common carotid a.
Common carotid plexus
Sympathetic trunk
Inf. bulb of jugular v.
Pharyngeal branch of inf. thyroid a.
Middle cervical ganglion of sympathetic trunk
Inf. thyroid a.
Inf. cervical ganglion of sympathetic trunk
Middle cardiac n. of sympathetic trunk

**Fig. 304.** Pharyngeal wall seen from behind. Nerves and blood vessels on the lateral and posterior pharyngeal wall. Blood vessels and nerves in the parapharyngeal space.

**The Constrictor Muscles of the Pharynx**

| Name | Origin | Insertion |
|------|--------|-----------|
| **1. Superior constrictor muscle of the pharynx** | | |
| *Pterygopharyngeal portion* | Pterygoid hamulus of sphenoid bone | |
| *Buccopharyngeal portion* | Pterygomandibular raphe | |
| *Mylopharyngeal portion* | Mylohyoid line of mandible | |
| *Glossopharyngeal portion* | Transversus muscle of the tongue | |
| **2. Middle constrictor muscle of the pharynx** | | Unites and interdigitates in the pharyngeal raphe |
| *Chondropharyngeal portion* | Lesser cornu of hyoid bone | |
| *Ceratopharyngeal portion* | Greater cornu of hyoid bone | |
| **3. Inferior constrictor muscle of the pharynx** | | |
| *Thyropharyngeal portion* | Oblique line of thyroid cartilage | |
| *Cricopharyngeal portion* | Lateral margin of cricoid cartilage | |
| **4. Stylopharyngeus muscle** | Styloid process of temporal bone | Between the Superior and Middle constrictor muscles of the pharynx |
| **5. Salpingopharyngeus muscle** | Cartilage of auditory tube | Lateral pharyngeal wall |

*Nerve:*   1, 2, 3, and 5 from pharyngeal plexus of the glossopharyngeal (IX), vagus (X), and accessory (XI) nerves.
4 from only the glossopharyngeal nerve (IX)

*Function:*   1–3 constricts the pharynx; on contraction, 1 conveys the food downward into the esophagus (by closing the nasopharynx by the soft palate); 4 elevates the pharynx

**Muscles of the Soft Palate: The Veli palatini muscles**

| Name | Origin | Insertion |
|------|--------|-----------|
| **1. Uvular muscle** | Palatine aponeurosis, posterior nasal spine of the palatine bone | Stroma of the palatine uvula |
| **2. Levator veli palatini muscle** (formed beneath the mucosa of the levator ridge) | Inferior surface of the petrous part of the temporal bone, and the cartilaginous auditory tube | The muscles on both sides interdigitate in the soft palate without a tendon |
| **3. Tensor veli palatini muscle** lies directly upon the fascia of the medial pterygoid muscle) | Scaphoid spine and fossa of sphenoid and cartilaginous auditory tube | It runs as a flattened tendon through the sulcus of the pterygoid hamulus forming, with the tendon of the opposite side, the palatine aponeurosis (in the oral aspect of the soft palate) |

*Nerve:*   1 and 2 from the glossopharyngeal IX and vagus X nerves (pharyngeal plexus).
3 from the third branch of the trigeminal nerve V.

*Function:*   1 raises the uvula; 2 elevates the soft palate against the dorsal pharyngeal wall; 3 tenses the soft palate, dilates the auditory tube (very important for swallowing)

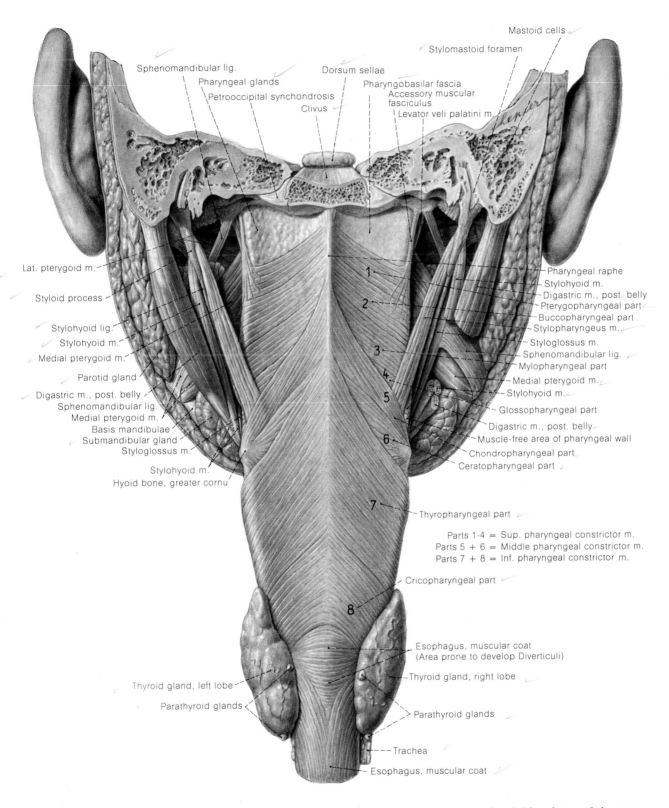

Mastoid cells
Stylomastoid foramen
Sphenomandibular lig.
Pharyngeal glands
Dorsum sellae
Pharyngobasilar fascia
Petrooccipital synchondrosis
Accessory muscular fasciculus
Clivus
Levator veli palatini m.

Lat. pterygoid m.
1 — Pharyngeal raphe
Styloid process
Stylohyoid m.
2 — Digastric m., post. belly
Stylohyoid lig.
Pterygopharyngeal part
Stylohyoid m.
Buccopharyngeal part
Medial pterygoid m.
Stylopharyngeus m.
3 — Styloglossus m.
Sphenomandibular lig.
Parotid gland
4 — Mylopharyngeal part
Digastric m., post. belly
Medial pterygoid m.
Sphenomandibular lig.
5 — Stylohyoid m.
Medial pterygoid m.
Glossopharyngeal part
Basis mandibulae
Digastric m., post. belly
Submandibular gland
6 — Muscle-free area of pharyngeal wall
Styloglossus m.
Chondropharyngeal part
Ceratopharyngeal part
Stylohyoid m.
Hyoid bone, greater cornu

7 — Thyropharyngeal part

Parts 1-4 = Sup. pharyngeal constrictor m.
Parts 5 + 6 = Middle pharyngeal constrictor m.
Parts 7 + 8 = Inf. pharyngeal constrictor m.

Cricopharyngeal part

8

Esophagus, muscular coat
(Area prone to develop Diverticuli)
Thyroid gland, left lobe
Thyroid gland, right lobe
Parathyroid glands
Parathyroid glands
Trachea
Esophagus, muscular coat

**Fig. 305.** The muscular wall of the pharynx after removal of the pharyngeal fascia, seen from dorsal. Musculature of the upper parapharyngeal space. The numerals are explained by indicator lines. Note the weak triangle at the beginning of the esophagus (LAIMER's triangle) (Pulsation diverticulum).

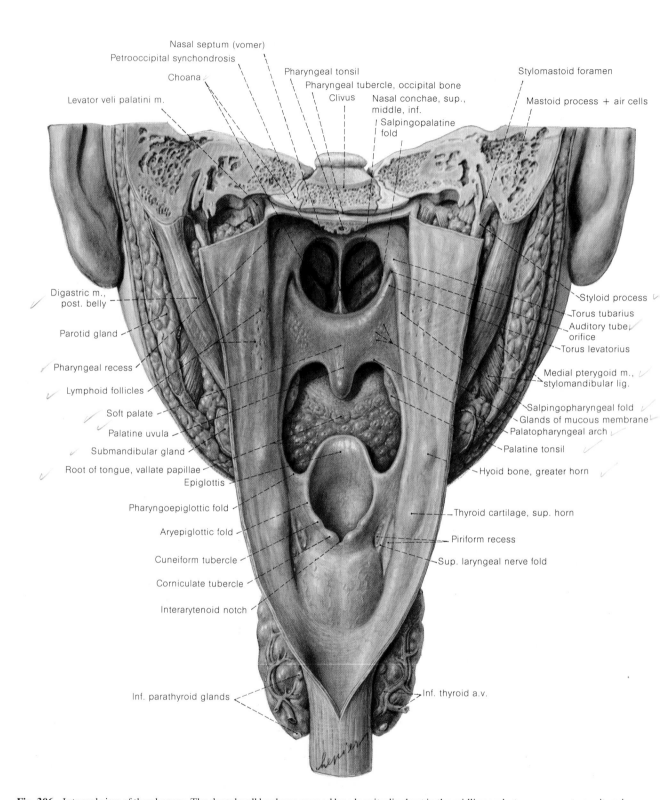

Nasal septum (vomer)
Petrooccipital synchondrosis
Choana
Levator veli palatini m.

Pharyngeal tonsil
Pharyngeal tubercle, occipital bone
Clivus
Nasal conchae, sup.,
middle, inf.
Salpingopalatine
fold

Stylomastoid foramen
Mastoid process + air cells

Digastric m.,
post. belly
Parotid gland
Pharyngeal recess
Lymphoid follicles
Soft palate
Palatine uvula
Submandibular gland
Root of tongue, vallate papillae
Epiglottis
Pharyngoepiglottic fold
Aryepiglottic fold
Cuneiform tubercle
Corniculate tubercle
Interarytenoid notch

Styloid process
Torus tubarius
Auditory tube,
orifice
Torus levatorius
Medial pterygoid m.,
stylomandibular lig.
Salpingopharyngeal fold
Glands of mucous membrane
Palatopharyngeal arch
Palatine tonsil
Hyoid bone, greater horn
Thyroid cartilage, sup. horn
Piriform recess
Sup. laryngeal nerve fold

Inf. parathyroid glands

Inf. thyroid a.v.

**Fig. 306.** Internal view of the pharynx. The dorsal wall has been opened by a longitudinal cut in the midline and a transverse cut near its origin on the base of the skull. The skull has been cut in the plane of the mastoid process and the clivus, and the occipital portion was removed.

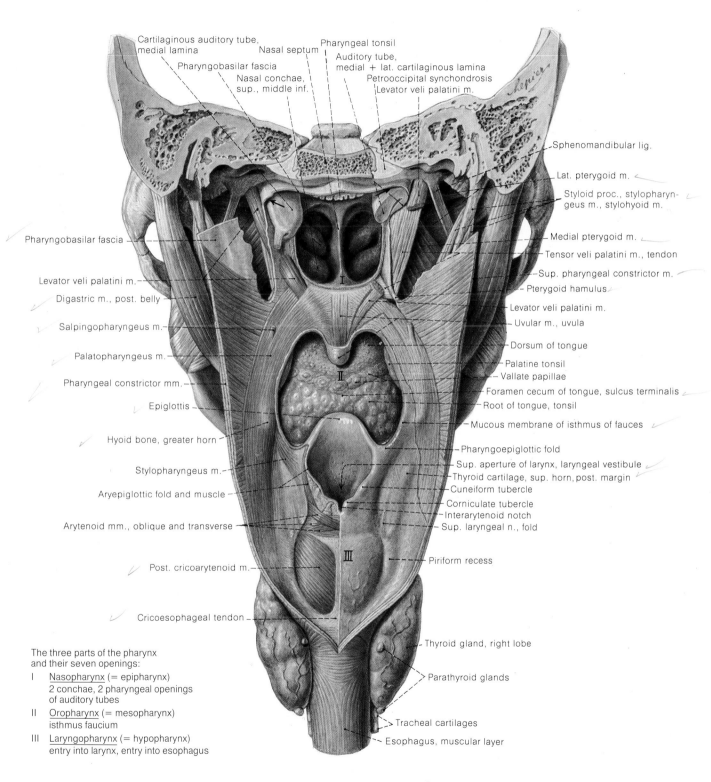

Cartilaginous auditory tube, medial lamina
Nasal septum
Pharyngeal tonsil
Pharyngobasilar fascia
Auditory tube, medial + lat. cartilaginous lamina
Nasal conchae, sup., middle inf.
Petrooccipital synchondrosis
Levator veli palatini m.

Sphenomandibular lig.

Pharyngobasilar fascia
Lat. pterygoid m.
Styloid proc., stylopharyngeus m., stylohyoid m.

Levator veli palatini m.
Medial pterygoid m.
Digastric m., post. belly
Tensor veli palatini m., tendon
Salpingopharyngeus m.
Sup. pharyngeal constrictor m.
Pterygoid hamulus
Palatopharyngeus m.
Levator veli palatini m.
Pharyngeal constrictor mm.
Uvular m., uvula
Epiglottis
Dorsum of tongue
Hyoid bone, greater horn
Palatine tonsil
Stylopharyngeus m.
Vallate papillae
Foramen cecum of tongue, sulcus terminalis
Aryepiglottic fold and muscle
Root of tongue, tonsil
Arytenoid mm., oblique and transverse
Mucous membrane of isthmus of fauces
Pharyngoepiglottic fold
Sup. aperture of larynx, laryngeal vestibule
Thyroid cartilage, sup. horn, post. margin
Cuneiform tubercle
Corniculate tubercle
Interarytenoid notch
Sup. laryngeal n., fold
Post. cricoarytenoid m.
Piriform recess

Cricoesophageal tendon

Thyroid gland, right lobe

The three parts of the pharynx and their seven openings:
I   Nasopharynx (= epipharynx)
    2 conchae, 2 pharyngeal openings of auditory tubes
II  Oropharynx (= mesopharynx)
    isthmus faucium
III Laryngopharynx (= hypopharynx)
    entry into larynx, entry into esophagus

Parathyroid glands

Tracheal cartilages
Esophagus, muscular layer

**Fig. 307.** The same preparation as in Fig. 306, after extensive removal of the pharyngeal mucous membrane. Through the opening of the dorsal wall of the pharynx, the three stages are visible with their boundaries and openings. The muscles of the soft palate, the pharynx, and the dorsal side of the larynx are displayed. The auditory tube is cut on the right side, so that the lateral and medial lamina of the tubal cartilage, as well as the slit-like opening of the auditory tube may be seen. The right and left arrows on the roof of the pharynx show the paired pharyngeal recesses (ROSENMÜLLER).

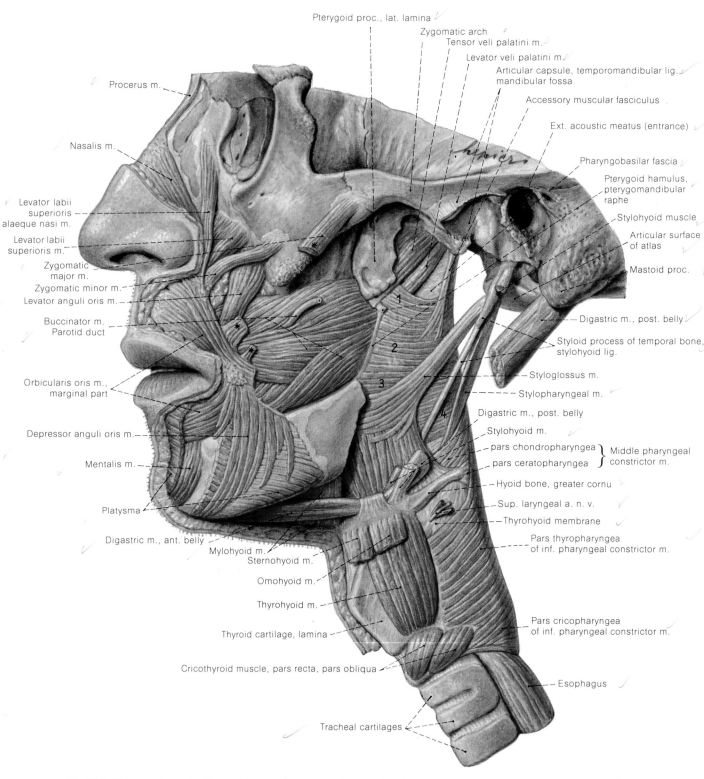

Pterygoid proc., lat. lamina

Zygomatic arch

Tensor veli palatini m.

Levator veli palatini m.

Articular capsule, temporomandibular lig., mandibular fossa

Accessory muscular fasciculus

Ext. acoustic meatus (entrance)

Pharyngobasilar fascia

Pterygoid hamulus, pterygomandibular raphe

Stylohyoid muscle

Articular surface of atlas

Mastoid proc.

Digastric m., post. belly

Styloid process of temporal bone, stylohyoid lig.

Styloglossus m.

Stylopharyngeal m.

Digastric m., post. belly

Stylohyoid m.

pars chondropharyngea ⎫ Middle pharyngeal
pars ceratopharyngea ⎬ constrictor m.

Hyoid bone, greater cornu

Sup. laryngeal a. n. v.

Thyrohyoid membrane

Pars thyropharyngea of inf. pharyngeal constrictor m.

Pars cricopharyngea of inf. pharyngeal constrictor m.

Esophagus

Procerus m.

Nasalis m.

Levator labii superioris alaeque nasi m.

Levator labii superioris m.

Zygomatic major m.

Zygomatic minor m.

Levator anguli oris m.

Buccinator m.
Parotid duct

Orbicularis oris m., marginal part

Depressor anguli oris m.

Mentalis m.

Platysma

Digastric m., ant. belly

Mylohyoid m.

Sternohyoid m.

Omohyoid m.

Thyrohyoid m.

Thyroid cartilage, lamina

Cricothyroid muscle, pars recta, pars obliqua

Tracheal cartilages

**Fig. 308.** Pharyngeal muscles, External laryngeal muscles, and a part of the facial musculature of the left side. 1, 2, 3, 4 are numbered parts of the Superior pharyngeal constrictor muscles: Pterygopharyngeal, Buccopharyngeal, Mylopharyngeal, and Glossopharyngeal muscles, * Greater and lesser zygomatic muscles.

# Larynx

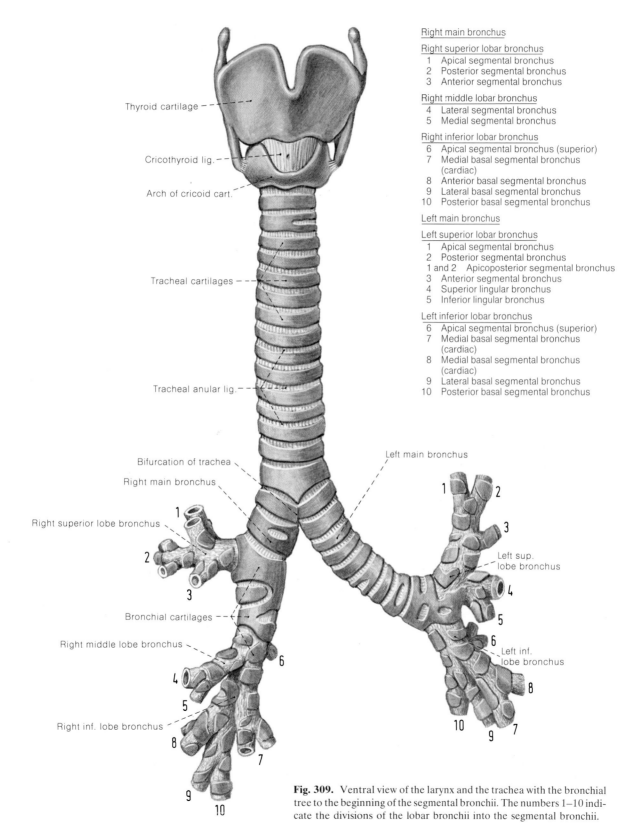

Right main bronchus

Right superior lobar bronchus
1 Apical segmental bronchus
2 Posterior segmental bronchus
3 Anterior segmental bronchus

Right middle lobar bronchus
4 Lateral segmental bronchus
5 Medial segmental bronchus

Right inferior lobar bronchus
6 Apical segmental bronchus (superior)
7 Medial basal segmental bronchus (cardiac)
8 Anterior basal segmental bronchus
9 Lateral basal segmental bronchus
10 Posterior basal segmental bronchus

Left main bronchus

Left superior lobar bronchus
1 Apical segmental bronchus
2 Posterior segmental bronchus
1 and 2 Apicoposterior segmental bronchus
3 Anterior segmental bronchus
4 Superior lingular bronchus
5 Inferior lingular bronchus

Left inferior lobar bronchus
6 Apical segmental bronchus (superior)
7 Medial basal segmental bronchus (cardiac)
8 Medial basal segmental bronchus (cardiac)
9 Lateral basal segmental bronchus
10 Posterior basal segmental bronchus

Thyroid cartilage

Cricothyroid lig.

Arch of cricoid cart.

Tracheal cartilages

Tracheal anular lig.

Bifurcation of trachea

Right main bronchus

Right superior lobe bronchus

Bronchial cartilages

Right middle lobe bronchus

Right inf. lobe bronchus

Left main bronchus

Left sup. lobe bronchus

Left inf. lobe bronchus

**Fig. 309.** Ventral view of the larynx and the trachea with the bronchial tree to the beginning of the segmental bronchii. The numbers 1–10 indicate the divisions of the lobar bronchii into the segmental bronchii.

197

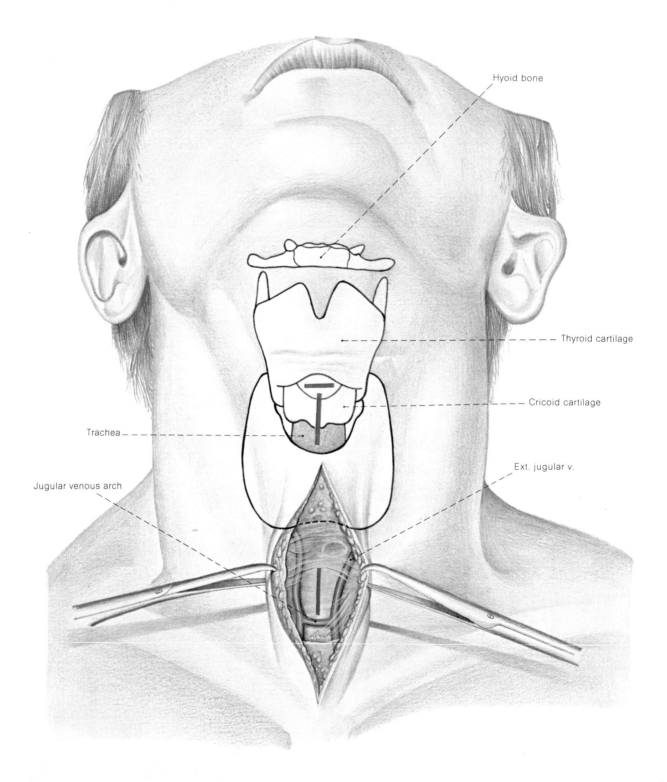

Hyoid bone

Thyroid cartilage

Cricoid cartilage

Trachea

Ext. jugular v.

Jugular venous arch

**Fig. 310.** Projection of the larynx, hyoid bone and thyroid gland onto the anterior surface of the neck. The skin over the jugular notch has been opened by a longitudinal cut to gain access to the suprasternal space with the jugular venous arch and the external jugular vein on each side (first layer for the inferior tracheotomy). The trachea lies, in the area of the jugular notch, in a depth of about 4–5 cm. Shown also is the transverse cut for the laryngotomy in the area of the cricothyroid ligament (conus elasticus, thus also coniotomy). Longitudinal cut through the area of the cricoid cartilage. Cricotomy. In coniotomy the trachea is entered about 1 cm below the vocal cords. All three accesses to the trachea are marked in red.

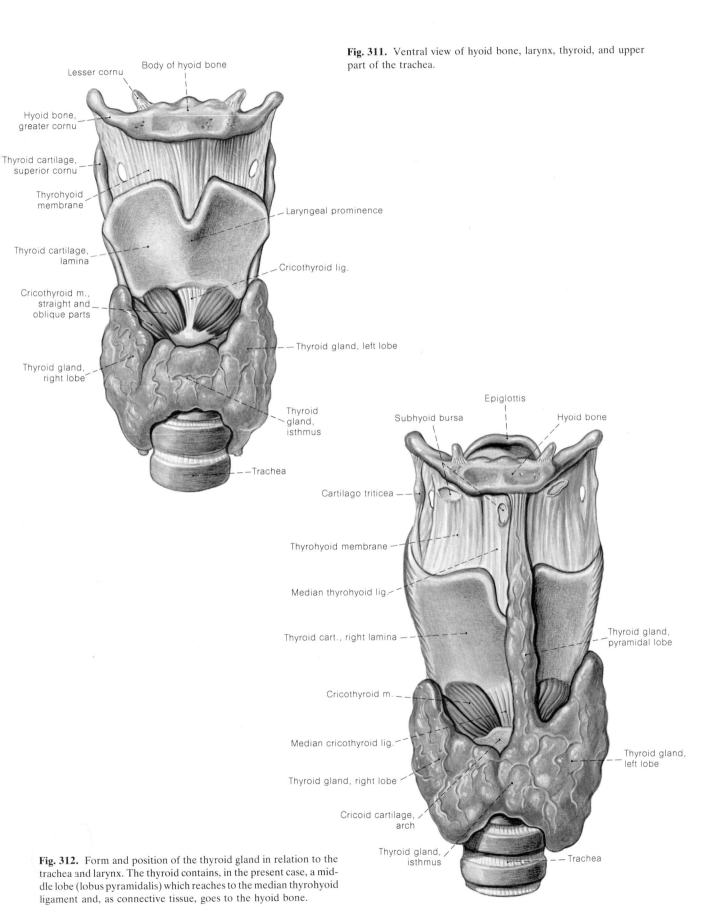

Lesser cornu

Body of hyoid bone

Hyoid bone, greater cornu

Thyroid cartilage, superior cornu

Thyrohyoid membrane

Thyroid cartilage, lamina

Cricothyroid m., straight and oblique parts

Thyroid gland, right lobe

Laryngeal prominence

Cricothyroid lig.

Thyroid gland, left lobe

Thyroid gland, isthmus

Trachea

**Fig. 311.** Ventral view of hyoid bone, larynx, thyroid, and upper part of the trachea.

Epiglottis

Subhyoid bursa

Hyoid bone

Cartilago triticea

Thyrohyoid membrane

Median thyrohyoid lig.

Thyroid cart., right lamina

Cricothyroid m.

Median cricothyroid lig.

Thyroid gland, right lobe

Cricoid cartilage, arch

Thyroid gland, isthmus

Thyroid gland, pyramidal lobe

Thyroid gland, left lobe

Trachea

**Fig. 312.** Form and position of the thyroid gland in relation to the trachea and larynx. The thyroid contains, in the present case, a middle lobe (lobus pyramidalis) which reaches to the median thyrohyoid ligament and, as connective tissue, goes to the hyoid bone.

199

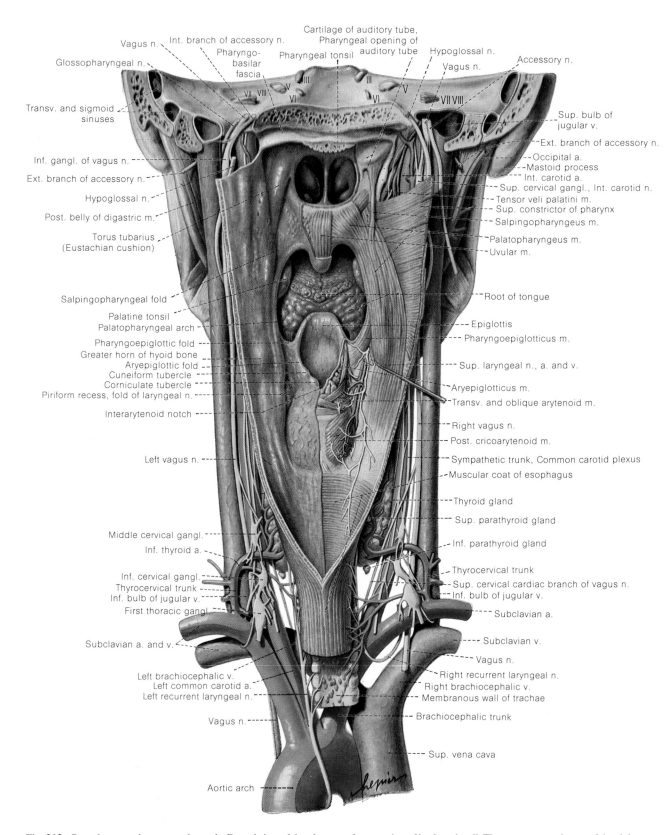

**Fig. 313.** Parapharyngeal nerves and vessels. Dorsal view of the pharynx after opening of its dorsal wall. The mucous membrane of the right side of the pharynx has been removed. The posterior portion of the cranium has been removed at the plane of the jugular foramina.

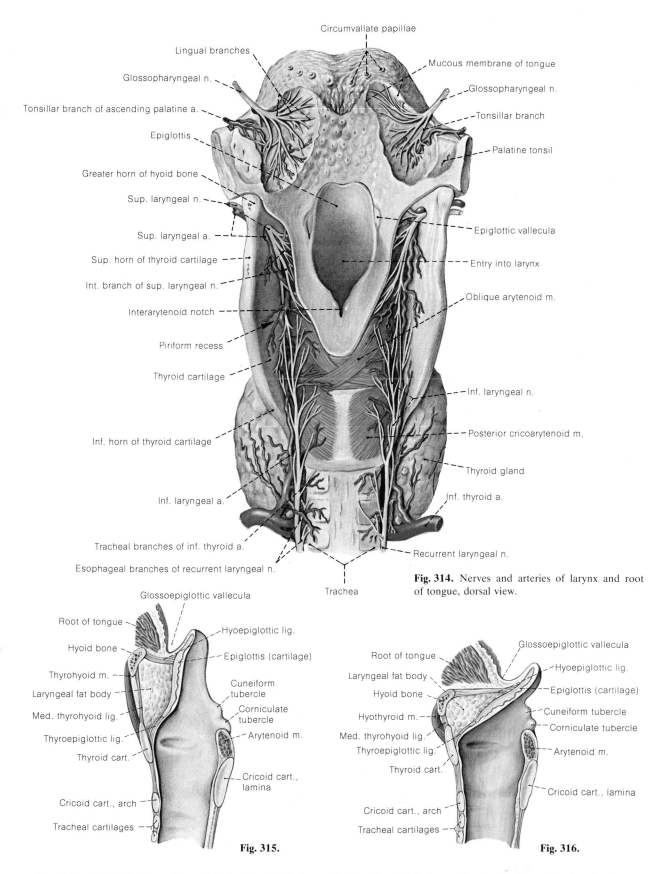

Circumvallate papillae

Lingual branches

Glossopharyngeal n.

Tonsillar branch of ascending palatine a.

Epiglottis

Greater horn of hyoid bone

Sup. laryngeal n.

Sup. laryngeal a.

Sup. horn of thyroid cartilage

Int. branch of sup. laryngeal n.

Interarytenoid notch

Piriform recess

Thyroid cartilage

Inf. horn of thyroid cartilage

Inf. laryngeal a.

Tracheal branches of inf. thyroid a.

Esophageal branches of recurrent laryngeal n.

Mucous membrane of tongue

Glossopharyngeal n.

Tonsillar branch

Palatine tonsil

Epiglottic vallecula

Entry into larynx

Oblique arytenoid m.

Inf. laryngeal n.

Posterior cricoarytenoid m.

Thyroid gland

Inf. thyroid a.

Recurrent laryngeal n.

Trachea

**Fig. 314.** Nerves and arteries of larynx and root of tongue, dorsal view.

Glossoepiglottic vallecula

Root of tongue

Hyoid bone

Thyrohyoid m.

Laryngeal fat body

Med. thyrohyoid lig.

Thyroepiglottic lig.

Thyroid cart.

Cricoid cart., arch

Tracheal cartilages

Hyoepiglottic lig.

Epiglottis (cartilage)

Cuneiform tubercle

Corniculate tubercle

Arytenoid m.

Cricoid cart., lamina

**Fig. 315.**

Root of tongue

Laryngeal fat body

Hyoid bone

Hyothyroid m.

Med. thyrohyoid lig.

Thyroepiglottic lig.

Thyroid cart.

Cricoid cart., arch

Tracheal cartilages

Glossoepiglottic vallecula

Hyoepiglottic lig.

Epiglottis (cartilage)

Cuneiform tubercle

Corniculate tubercle

Arytenoid m.

Cricoid cart., lamina

**Fig. 316.**

**Figs. 315 and 316.** Position of the epiglottis: Fig. 315 during respiration, Fig. 316 during swallowing. During swallowing, the distance between the hyoid bone and the thyroid cartilage is decreased and the adipose tissue pushes the epiglottis downward.

201

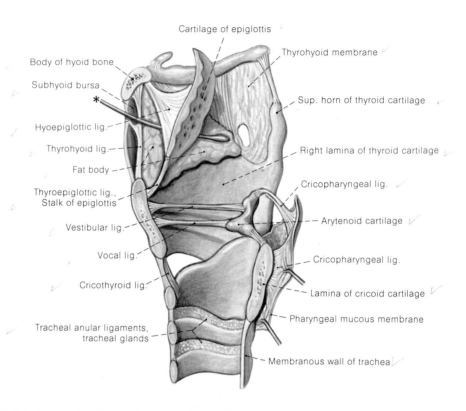

**Fig. 317.** Right half of the laryngeal cartilage and ligaments in a midsagittal section. * Probe between epiglottis and the fat body.

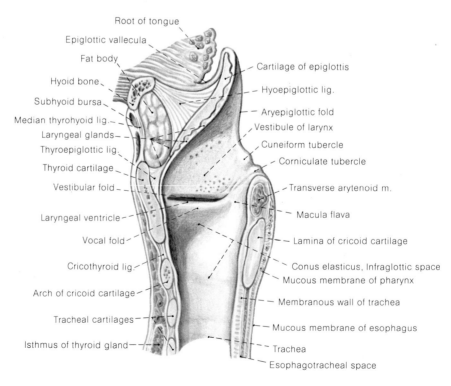

**Fig. 318.** Midsagittal section of larynx. View of inside and cut surface of right half.

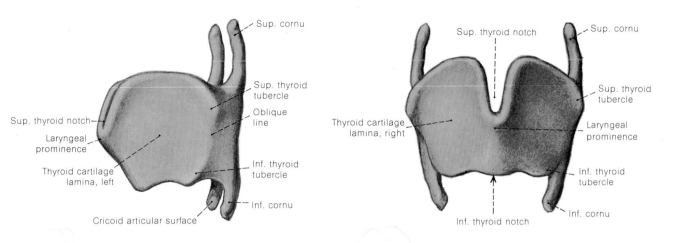

**Fig. 319.** Thyroid cartilage, seen from left side.

**Fig. 320.** Thyroid cartilage, seen from ventral.

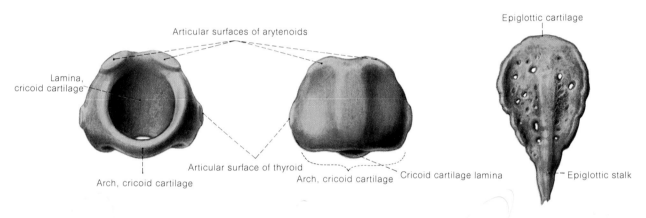

**Fig. 321.** Cricoid cartilage, seen from cranial and ventral.

**Fig. 322.** Cricoid cartilage, seen from dorsal.

**Fig. 323.** Epiglottic cartilage, seen from dorsal.

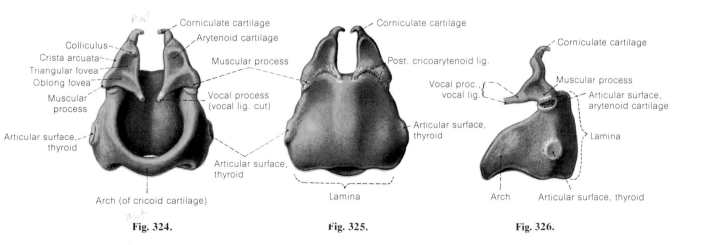

**Fig. 324.**

**Fig. 325.**

**Fig. 326.**

**Figs. 324–326.** Articulated cricoid, arytenoid and corniculate cartilages. Fig. 324 from above, Fig. 325 from dorsal, Fig. 326 from left side.

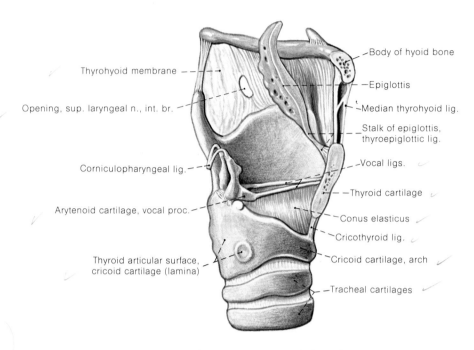

Body of hyoid bone

Thyrohyoid membrane

Epiglottis

Opening, sup. laryngeal n., int. br.

Median thyrohyoid lig.

Stalk of epiglottis, thyroepiglottic lig.

Corniculopharyngeal lig.

Vocal ligs.

Thyroid cartilage

Arytenoid cartilage, vocal proc.

Conus elasticus

Cricothyroid lig.

Thyroid articular surface, cricoid cartilage (lamina)

Cricoid cartilage, arch

Tracheal cartilages

**Fig. 327.** Median section through the upper part of the larynx. Right half of hyoid bone, the epiglottis, and the thyroid cartilage were removed. Both arytenoid cartilages, the cricoid cartilage and the two upper tracheal cartilages remain. The conus elasticus spreads itself between the vocal ligament, the vocal process of the arytenoid (on one side) and the angle of the thyroid cartilage and the cricothyroid ligament (on the other).

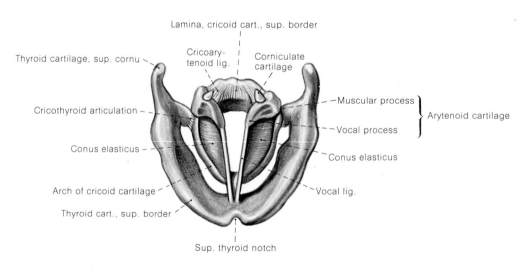

Lamina, cricoid cart., sup. border

Thyroid cartilage, sup. cornu

Cricoary-tenoid lig.

Corniculate cartilage

Cricothyroid articulation

Muscular process

Arytenoid cartilage

Vocal process

Conus elasticus

Conus elasticus

Arch of cricoid cartilage

Vocal lig.

Thyroid cart., sup. border

Sup. thyroid notch

**Fig. 328.** The laryngeal cartilages from above, with the vocal ligament and conus elasticus.

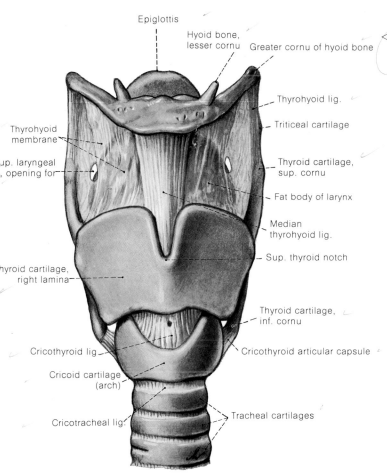

Epiglottis

Hyoid bone, lesser cornu

Greater cornu of hyoid bone

Thyrohyoid lig.

Triticeal cartilage

Thyroid cartilage, sup. cornu

Fat body of larynx

Median thyrohyoid lig.

Sup. thyroid notch

Thyrohyoid membrane

up. laryngeal, opening for

hyroid cartilage, right lamina

Thyroid cartilage, inf. cornu

Cricothyroid lig

Cricoid cartilage (arch)

Cricothyroid articular capsule

Cricotracheal lig.

Tracheal cartilages

**Fig. 329.** Laryngeal cartilages, ligaments, and articulations, including the hyoid bone and the upper part of the trachea. Ventral view. Hyaline cartilage, blue; bony part of the hyoid bone, yellow. Note the fat body (corpus adiposum laryngis) between the layers of the thyrohyoid membrane.

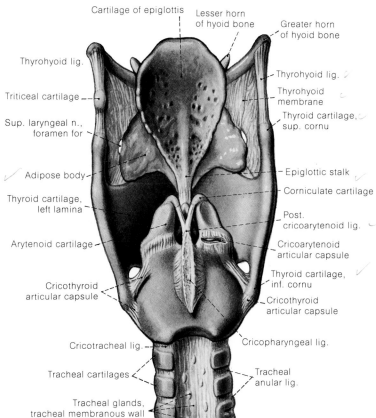

Cartilage of epiglottis

Lesser horn of hyoid bone

Greater horn of hyoid bone

Thyrohyoid lig.

Thyrohyoid lig.

Triticeal cartilage

Thyrohyoid membrane

Sup. laryngeal n., foramen for

Thyroid cartilage, sup. cornu

Adipose body

Epiglottic stalk

Corniculate cartilage

Thyroid cartilage, left lamina

Post. cricoarytenoid lig.

Arytenoid cartilage

Cricoarytenoid articular capsule

Thyroid cartilage, inf. cornu

Cricothyroid articular capsule

Cricothyroid articular capsule

Cricotracheal lig.

Cricopharyngeal lig.

Tracheal cartilages

Tracheal anular lig.

Tracheal glands, tracheal membranous wall

**Fig. 330.** Laryngeal cartilages, ligaments, and articulations, including the hyoid bone and the upper part of the trachea. Dorsal view. Ossified part of the hyoid bone and the fat body between the thyrohyoid membrane and epiglottis is yellow. The larynx shown in Figs. 329 and 330 is of a juvenile individual. After puberty there is an increasing calcification and ossification of the laryngeal cartilages.

# Larynx

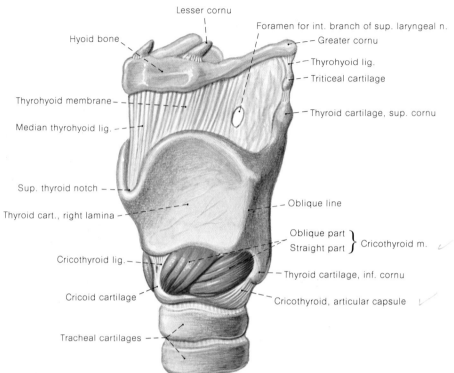

Lesser cornu

Hyoid bone

Foramen for int. branch of sup. laryngeal n.

Greater cornu

Thyrohyoid lig.

Triticeal cartilage

Thyrohyoid membrane

Median thyrohyoid lig.

Thyroid cartilage, sup. cornu

Sup. thyroid notch

Oblique line

Thyroid cart., right lamina

Oblique part ⎫
Straight part ⎭ Cricothyroid m.

Cricothyroid lig.

Thyroid cartilage, inf. cornu

Cricoid cartilage

Cricothyroid, articular capsule

Tracheal cartilages

**Fig. 331.** Larynx. Left ventrolateral view.

## Muscles of the Larynx

| Name | Origin | Insertion |
|---|---|---|
| **Cricothyroid muscle** superficial: *pars recta* deep: *pars obliqua* | Outer surface of the cricoid cartilage | Caudal margin and inferior cornu of thyroid cartilage |
| **Posterior cricoarytenoid muscle** | Dorsal surface of cricoid cartilage | Muscular process of arytenoid cartilage |
| **Lateral cricoarytenoid muscle** | Cranial margin of lateral part of cricoid cartilage | |
| **Transverse arytenoid muscle** | Lateral edge and dorsal surface of arytenoid cartilage | To the same part on the opposite side (crosses transversely between the 2 cartilages) |
| **Oblique arytenoid muscle** | Muscular process in one arytenoid cartilage | Apex of opposite arytenoid cartilage |
| **Aryepiglottic muscle** | Variable fibers of the Oblique arytenoid muscle in the aryepiglottic folds | |
| **Thyroarytenoid muscle** | Inner surface of angle of thyroid cartilage | Muscular process and lateral surface of arytenoid cartilage |
| **Vocalis muscle** | From medial fibers of thyroarytenoid m. adherent to the vocal lig. | Along vocal lig. extending to the vocal process of arytenoid cartilage |
| **Thyroepiglottic muscle** | Continuation of thyroarytenoid muscle in the aryepiglottic fold | |

*Nerve:* Cricothyroid muscle: external branch of the superior laryngeal; the remaining laryngeal muscles: from the recurrent laryngeal nerve.

*Function:* Cricothyroid muscle tenses the vocal cords. Posterior cricoarytenoid muscle dilates, and the Lateral cricoarytenoid muscle narrows the glottis. The remaining are essentially sphincter muscles for the entrance of the larynx and the rima glottidis or the the regulation of the tension in the Vocalis muscle.

**Fig. 332.** Muscles of the dorsal laryngeal surface. ▷

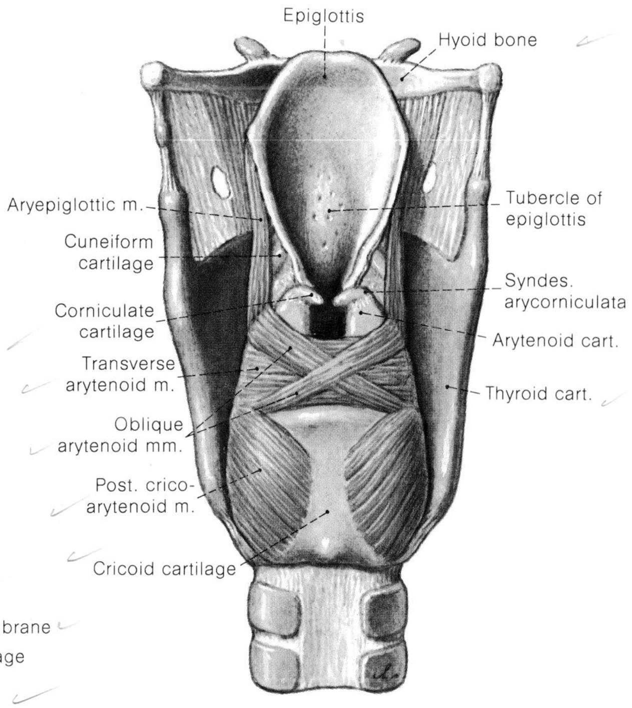

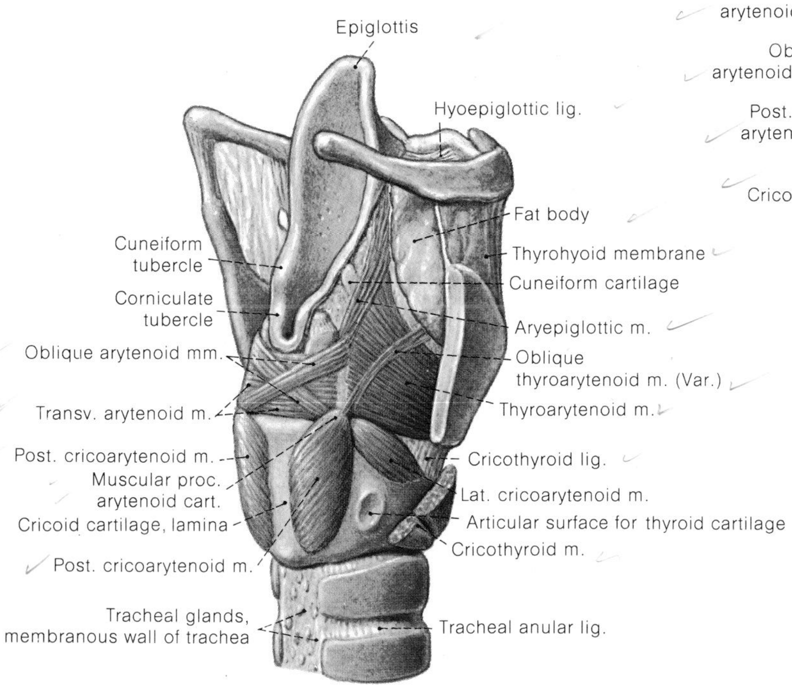

Epiglottis

Hyoid bone

Aryepiglottic m.

Tubercle of epiglottis

Cuneiform cartilage

Syndes. arycorniculata

Corniculate cartilage

Arytenoid cart.

Transverse arytenoid m.

Thyroid cart.

Oblique arytenoid mm.

Post. crico-arytenoid m.

Cricoid cartilage

Epiglottis

Hyoepiglottic lig.

Fat body

Cuneiform tubercle

Thyrohyoid membrane

Corniculate tubercle

Cuneiform cartilage

Oblique arytenoid mm.

Aryepiglottic m.

Oblique thyroarytenoid m. (Var.)

Transv. arytenoid m.

Thyroarytenoid m.

Post. cricoarytenoid m.

Muscular proc. arytenoid cart.

Cricothyroid lig.

Lat. cricoarytenoid m.

Cricoid cartilage, lamina

Articular surface for thyroid cartilage

Post. cricoarytenoid m.

Cricothyroid m.

Tracheal glands, membranous wall of trachea

Tracheal anular lig.

**Fig. 333.** Laryngeal musculature. Oblique, dorso-lateral view.

Epiglottis

Hyoid bone, greater cornu

Thyrohyoid lig.

Aryepiglottic fold

Triticeal cartilage

Epiglottic tubercle

Cuneiform tubercle

Thyroid cartilage, sup. cornu

Corniculate tubercle

Laryngeal glands to moisten vocal folds

Vestibular fold

Transverse arytenoid m.

Oblique arytenoid m.

Ventricle of larynx

Conus elasticus

Vocal fold

Vocalis m.

Post. cricoarytenoid m.

Cricothyroid m., straight part

Inferior cornu, thyroid cart.

Lat. crico-arytenoid m.

Crico-thyroid lig.

**Fig. 334.** Larynx held open with hooks. Cut in dorsal midline. Below the vocal fold, the mucous membrane and conus elasticus were removed to display the laryngeal muscles on the left from inside the larynx. ▷

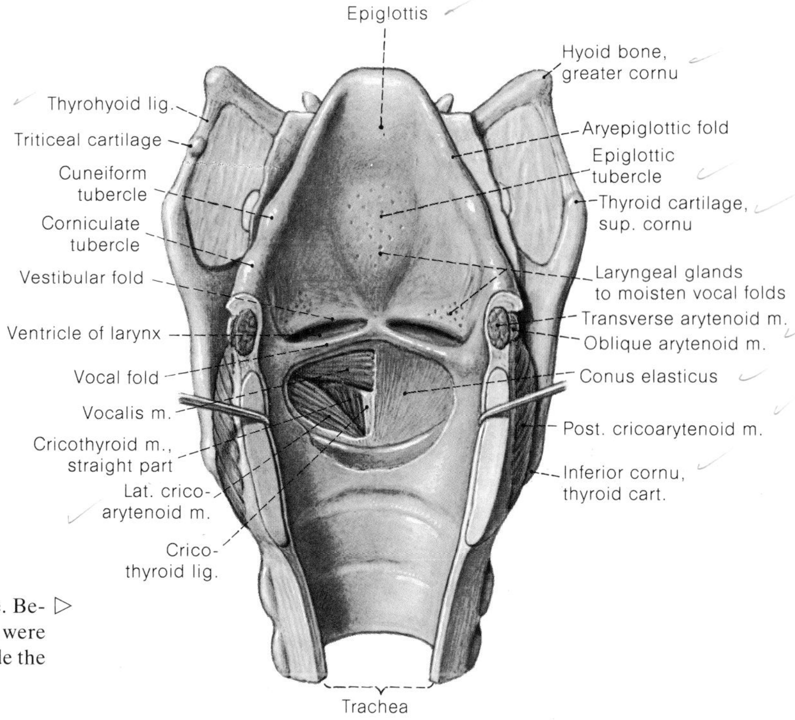

Trachea

207

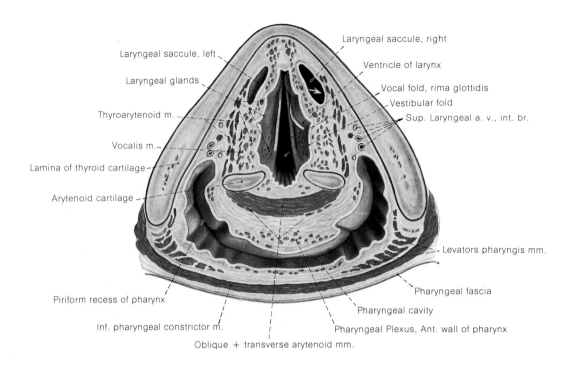

Laryngeal saccule, left
Laryngeal glands
Thyroarytenoid m.
Vocalis m.
Lamina of thyroid cartilage
Arytenoid cartilage

Laryngeal saccule, right
Ventricle of larynx
Vocal fold, rima glottidis
Vestibular fold
Sup. Laryngeal a. v., int. br.

Levators pharyngis mm.
Pharyngeal fascia
Piriform recess of pharynx
Pharyngeal cavity
Inf. pharyngeal constrictor m.
Pharyngeal Plexus, Ant. wall of pharynx
Oblique + transverse arytenoid mm.

**Fig. 335.** Horizontal section of the larynx at the level of the vestibular fold. A white arrow indicates the connection between the laryngeal ventricle and the saccule.

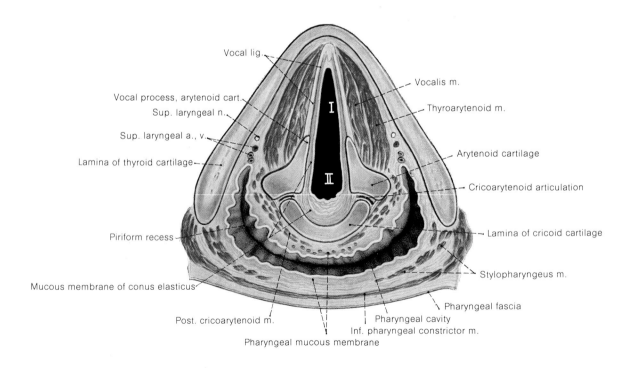

Vocal lig.
Vocal process, arytenoid cart.
Sup. laryngeal n.
Sup. laryngeal a., v.
Lamina of thyroid cartilage

Vocalis m.
Thyroarytenoid m.
Arytenoid cartilage
Cricoarytenoid articulation
Lamina of cricoid cartilage

Piriform recess
Stylopharyngeus m.
Mucous membrane of conus elasticus
Pharyngeal fascia
Post. cricoarytenoid m.
Pharyngeal cavity
Inf. pharyngeal constrictor m.
Pharyngeal mucous membrane

**Fig. 336.** Horizontal section of larynx at the level of the rima glottidis and through the laryngopharynx.

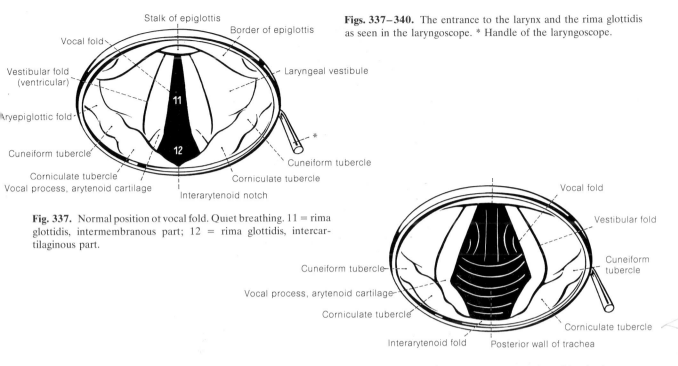

**Figs. 337–340.** The entrance to the larynx and the rima glottidis as seen in the laryngoscope. * Handle of the laryngoscope.

**Fig. 337.** Normal position of vocal fold. Quiet breathing. 11 = rima glottidis, intermembranous part; 12 = rima glottidis, intercartilaginous part.

**Fig. 338.** Rima glottidis in deep or forced inspiration.

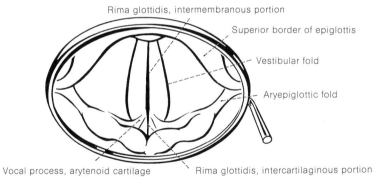

**Fig. 339.** During phonation, emitting shrill tones (narrow rima, tense vocal cords).

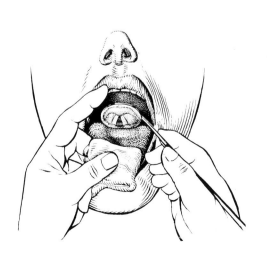

**Fig. 340.** Position during phonation by whispering.

◁ **Fig. 341.** Laryngoscopy with tongue pulled forward. View of the vocal folds.

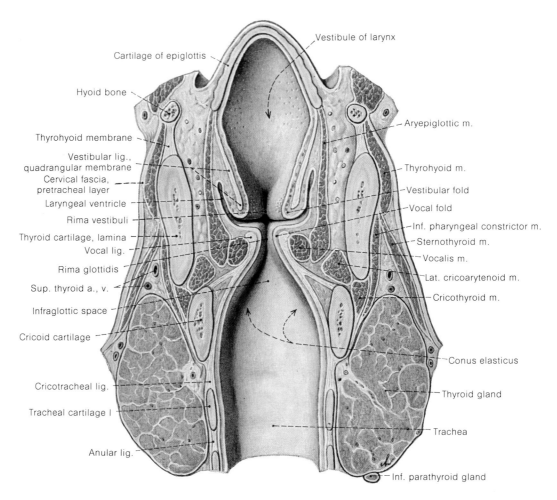

Cartilage of epiglottis

Hyoid bone

Thyrohyoid membrane

Vestibular lig., quadrangular membrane

Cervical fascia, pretracheal layer

Laryngeal ventricle

Rima vestibuli

Thyroid cartilage, lamina

Vocal lig.

Rima glottidis

Sup. thyroid a., v.

Infraglottic space

Cricoid cartilage

Cricotracheal lig.

Tracheal cartilage I

Anular lig.

Vestibule of larynx

Aryepiglottic m.

Thyrohyoid m.

Vestibular fold

Vocal fold

Inf. pharyngeal constrictor m.

Sternothyroid m.

Vocalis m.

Lat. cricoarytenoid m.

Cricothyroid m.

Conus elasticus

Thyroid gland

Trachea

Inf. parathyroid gland

**Fig. 342.** Frontal section through the larynx, thyroid gland and related cervical structures. Seen from dorsal aspect.

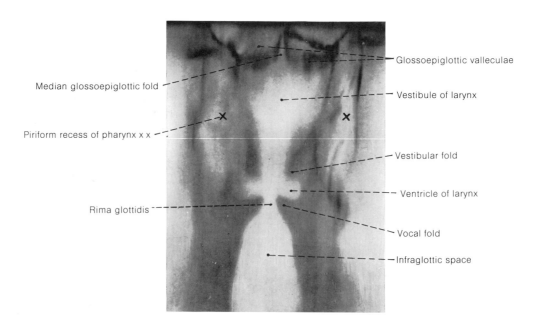

Median glossoepiglottic fold

Piriform recess of pharynx x x

Rima glottidis

Glossoepiglottic valleculae

Vestibule of larynx

Vestibular fold

Ventricle of larynx

Vocal fold

Infraglottic space

**Fig. 343.** X-ray film of larynx; sagittal projection.

# Eye and Orbit

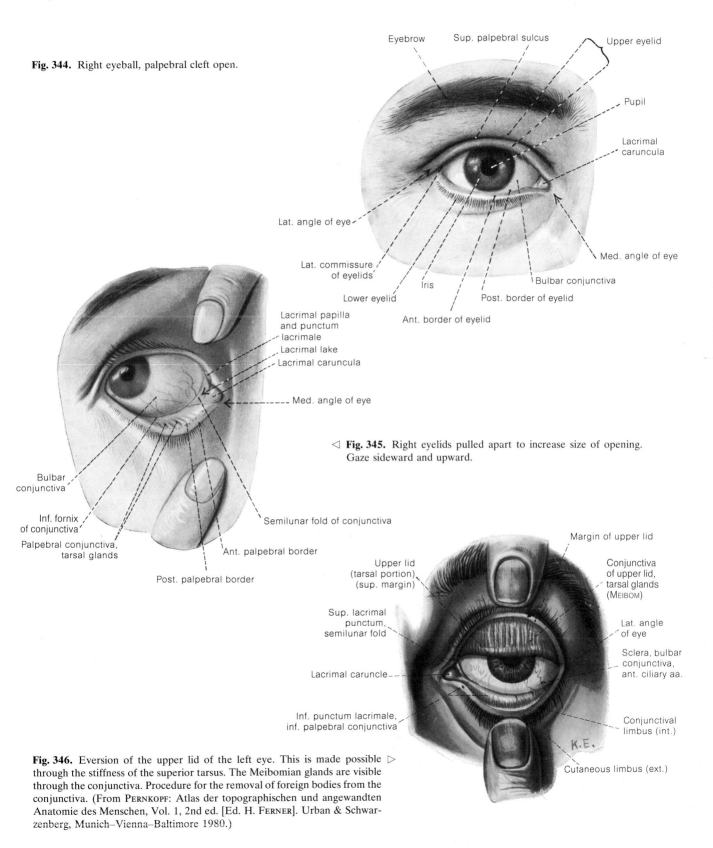

**Fig. 344.** Right eyeball, palpebral cleft open.

Eyebrow

Sup. palpebral sulcus

Upper eyelid

Pupil

Lacrimal caruncula

Lat. angle of eye

Lat. commissure of eyelids

Lower eyelid

Iris

Ant. border of eyelid

Post. border of eyelid

Bulbar conjunctiva

Med. angle of eye

Lacrimal papilla and punctum lacrimale

Lacrimal lake

Lacrimal caruncula

Med. angle of eye

Bulbar conjunctiva

Inf. fornix of conjunctiva

Palpebral conjunctiva, tarsal glands

Ant. palpebral border

Post. palpebral border

Semilunar fold of conjunctiva

◁ **Fig. 345.** Right eyelids pulled apart to increase size of opening. Gaze sideward and upward.

Margin of upper lid

Conjunctiva of upper lid, tarsal glands (MEIBOM)

Upper lid (tarsal portion) (sup. margin)

Lat. angle of eye

Sup. lacrimal punctum, semilunar fold

Sclera, bulbar conjunctiva, ant. ciliary aa.

Lacrimal caruncle

Inf. punctum lacrimale, inf. palpebral conjunctiva

Conjunctival limbus (int.)

Cutaneous limbus (ext.)

K.E.

**Fig. 346.** Eversion of the upper lid of the left eye. This is made possible ▷ through the stiffness of the superior tarsus. The Meibomian glands are visible through the conjunctiva. Procedure for the removal of foreign bodies from the conjunctiva. (From PERNKOPF: Atlas der topographischen und angewandten Anatomie des Menschen, Vol. 1, 2nd ed. [Ed. H. FERNER]. Urban & Schwarzenberg, Munich–Vienna–Baltimore 1980.)

211

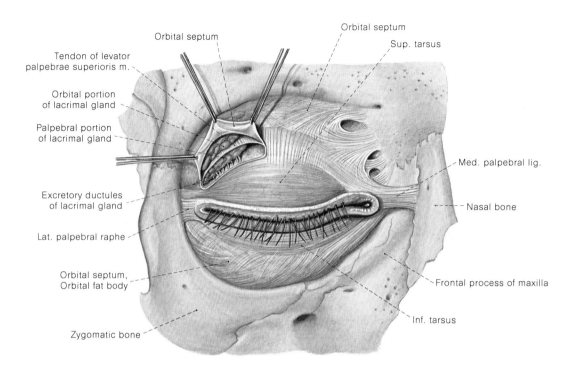

Orbital septum

Orbital septum

Sup. tarsus

Tendon of levator
palpebrae superioris m.

Orbital portion
of lacrimal gland

Palpebral portion
of lacrimal gland

Med. palpebral lig.

Excretory ductules
of lacrimal gland

Nasal bone

Lat. palpebral raphe

Orbital septum,
Orbital fat body

Frontal process of maxilla

Zygomatic bone

Inf. tarsus

**Fig. 347.** The orbital septum of the right eye in anterior view. In the lateral part of the upper lid the orbital septum is sectioned and reflected to expose the orbital and palpebral portions of the lacrimal gland. Between these two portions one sees the tendon of the levator palpebrae superioris muscle.

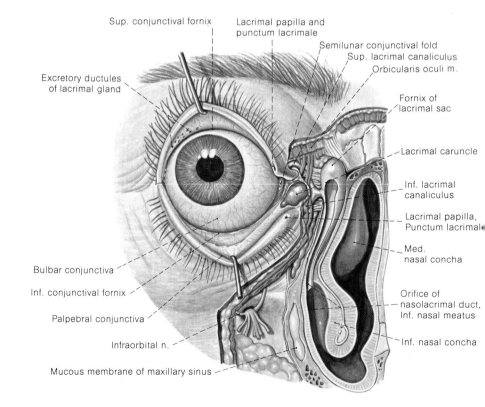

Sup. conjunctival fornix

Lacrimal papilla and
punctum lacrimale

Semilunar conjunctival fold
Sup. lacrimal canaliculus
Orbicularis oculi m.

Excretory ductules
of lacrimal gland

Fornix of
lacrimal sac

Lacrimal caruncle

Inf. lacrimal
canaliculus

Lacrimal papilla,
Punctum lacrimale

Med.
nasal concha

Bulbar conjunctiva

Inf. conjunctival fornix

Palpebral conjunctiva

Orifice of
nasolacrimal duct,
Inf. nasal meatus

Inf. nasal concha

Infraorbital n.

Mucous membrane of maxillary sinus

**Fig. 348.** The lacrimal apparatus. The eyelids have been pulled away from the eyeball to expose the conjunctival sac. At the medial palpebral angle the lacrimal canaliculi and their entry into the lacrimal sac can be seen. Note the small muscle bundles from the orbicularis oculi muscle that surround the lacrimal canaliculi; their contraction causes tear fluid to enter the canaliculi. The lacrimal sac and the nasolacrimal duct have been opened and its orifice under the inferior nasal concha is shown. Part of the outer nose and of the inferior concha have been removed.

212

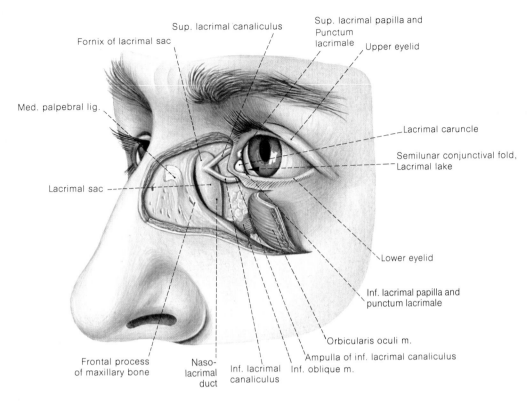

**Fig. 349.** Lacrimal sac and canaliculi seen from ventral and lateral. Skin and musculature are partially removed and the medial palpebral ligament has been transected.

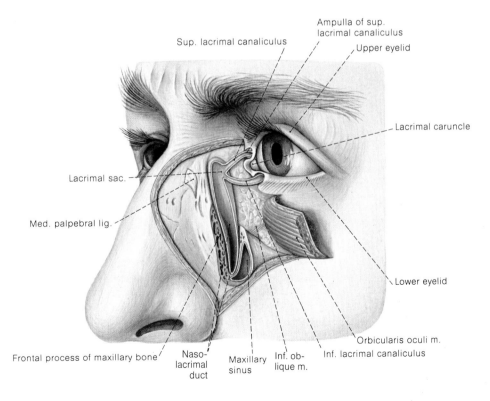

**Fig. 350.** Lacrimal canaliculi, lacrimal sac and nasolacrimal duct opened and viewed from ventral and lateral. Nasolacrimal duct within the nasolacrimal canal, entering the inferior nasal meatus.

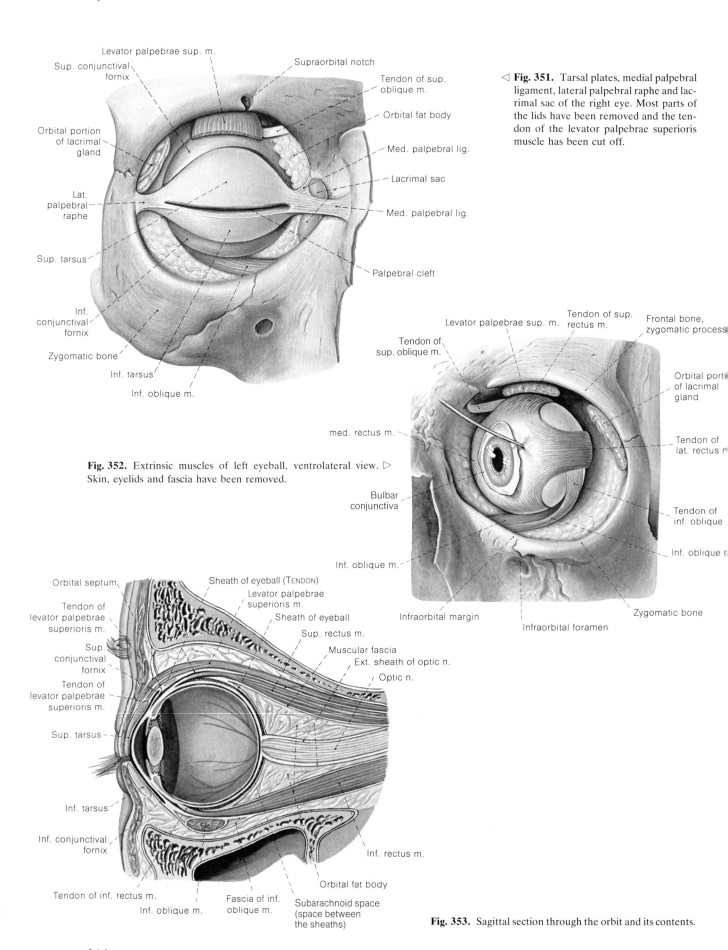

Levator palpebrae sup. m.

Sup. conjunctival fornix

Supraorbital notch

Tendon of sup. oblique m.

Orbital fat body

Orbital portion of lacrimal gland

Med. palpebral lig.

Lacrimal sac

Lat. palpebral raphe

Med. palpebral lig.

Sup. tarsus

Palpebral cleft

Inf. conjunctival fornix

Zygomatic bone

Inf. tarsus

Inf. oblique m.

◁ **Fig. 351.** Tarsal plates, medial palpebral ligament, lateral palpebral raphe and lacrimal sac of the right eye. Most parts of the lids have been removed and the tendon of the levator palpebrae superioris muscle has been cut off.

**Fig. 352.** Extrinsic muscles of left eyeball, ventrolateral view. ▷ Skin, eyelids and fascia have been removed.

Levator palpebrae sup. m.

Tendon of sup. rectus m.

Frontal bone, zygomatic process

Tendon of sup. oblique m.

med. rectus m.

Orbital port of lacrimal gland

Tendon of lat. rectus m

Bulbar conjunctiva

Tendon of inf. oblique

Inf. oblique m.

Inf. oblique r

Infraorbital margin

Zygomatic bone

Infraorbital foramen

Orbital septum

Sheath of eyeball (Tendon)

Tendon of levator palpebrae superioris m.

Levator palpebrae superioris m.

Sheath of eyeball

Sup. rectus m.

Sup. conjunctival fornix

Muscular fascia

Ext. sheath of optic n.

Tendon of levator palpebrae superioris m.

Optic n.

Sup. tarsus

Inf. tarsus

Inf. conjunctival fornix

Inf. rectus m.

Tendon of inf. rectus m.

Inf. oblique m.

Fascia of inf. oblique m.

Subarachnoid space (space between the sheaths)

Orbital fat body

**Fig. 353.** Sagittal section through the orbit and its contents.

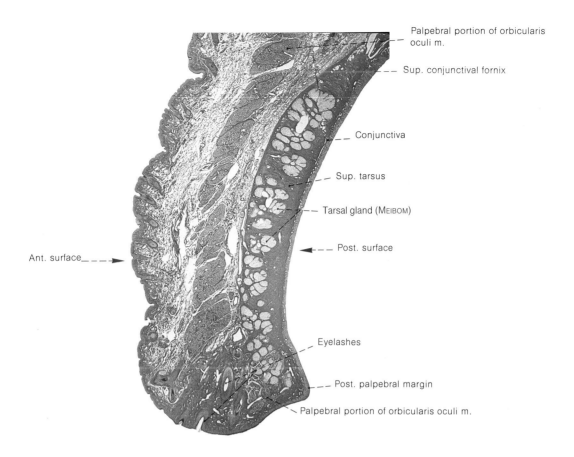

Palpebral portion of orbicularis oculi m.

Sup. conjunctival fornix

Conjunctiva

Sup. tarsus

Tarsal gland (MEIBOM)

Post. surface

Ant. surface

Eyelashes

Post. palpebral margin

Palpebral portion of orbicularis oculi m.

**Fig. 354.** Sagittal section through the upper eyelid; low magnification.

**Fig. 355.** Dorsal view of the eyelids made transparent by treatment with sodium hydroxide-glycerin to demonstrate the tarsal glands (MEIBOM). ▽

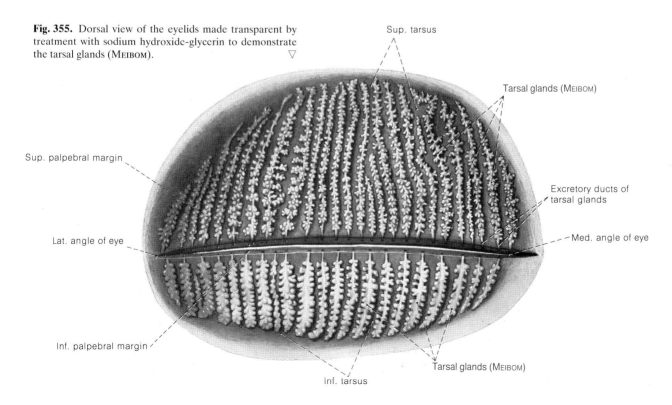

Sup. tarsus

Tarsal glands (MEIBOM)

Sup. palpebral margin

Excretory ducts of tarsal glands

Med. angle of eye

Lat. angle of eye

Inf. palpebral margin

Tarsal glands (MEIBOM)

Inf. tarsus

215

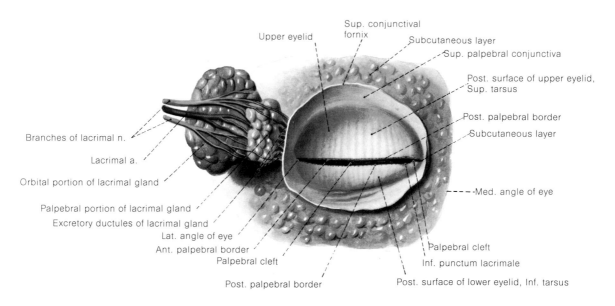

**Fig. 356.** Eyelids and lacrimal gland; dorsal aspect, left side.

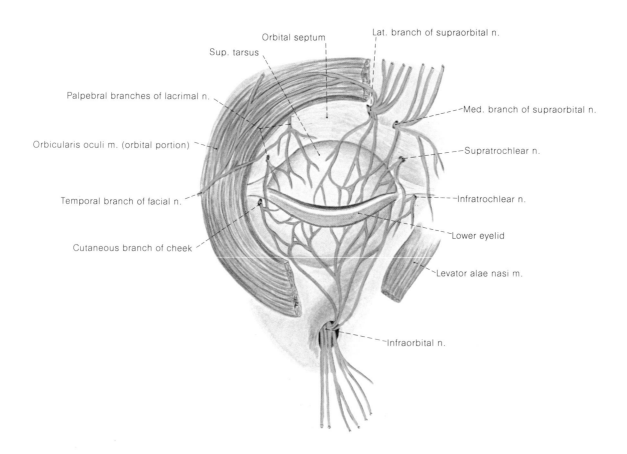

**Fig. 357.** The extensive and multiple innervation of the eyelids (right eye).

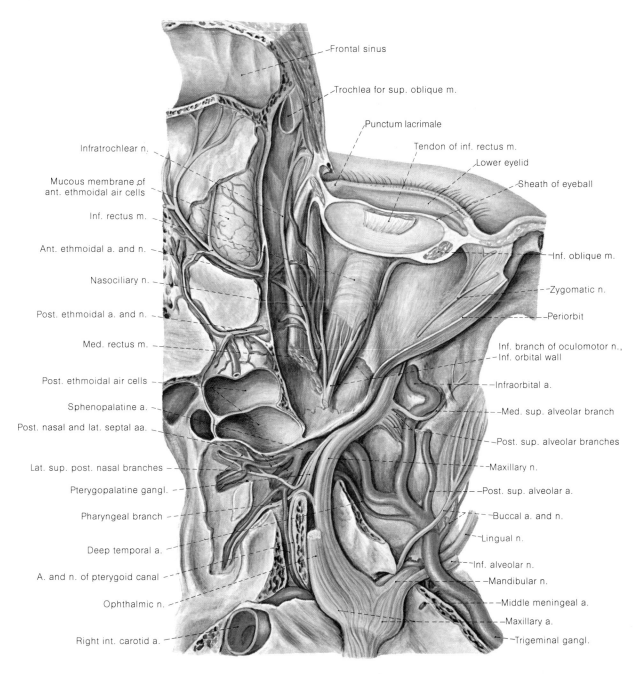

Frontal sinus

Trochlea for sup. oblique m.

Punctum lacrimale

Tendon of inf. rectus m.

Lower eyelid

Sheath of eyeball

Infratrochlear n.

Mucous membrane of ant. ethmoidal air cells

Inf. rectus m.

Ant. ethmoidal a. and n.

Nasociliary n.

Post. ethmoidal a. and n.

Med. rectus m.

Post. ethmoidal air cells

Sphenopalatine a.

Post. nasal and lat. septal aa.

Lat. sup. post. nasal branches

Pterygopalatine gangl.

Pharyngeal branch

Deep temporal a.

A. and n. of pterygoid canal

Ophthalmic n.

Right int. carotid a.

Inf. oblique m.

Zygomatic n.

Periorbit

Inf. branch of oculomotor n., Inf. orbital wall

Infraorbital a.

Med. sup. alveolar branch

Post. sup. alveolar branches

Maxillary n.

Post. sup. alveolar a.

Buccal a. and n.

Lingual n.

Inf. alveolar n.

Mandibular n.

Middle meningeal a.

Maxillary a.

Trigeminal gangl.

**Fig. 358.** Dissection of the orbit, of the trigeminal ganglion with its three main branches and of the end branches of the maxillary artery. Note the arterial and nervous supply of the paranasal sinuses through the branches of the ophthalmic artery and the nasociliary nerve (anterior and posterior ethmoidal artery and nerve), as well as branches from the area of the pterygopalatine ganglion (posterior nasal nerves). The terminations of the maxillary artery: toward the left the sphenopalatine artery into the nose and toward rostral the infraorbital artery and the superior posterior alveolar artery. Note the origin of the middle meningeal artery.

217

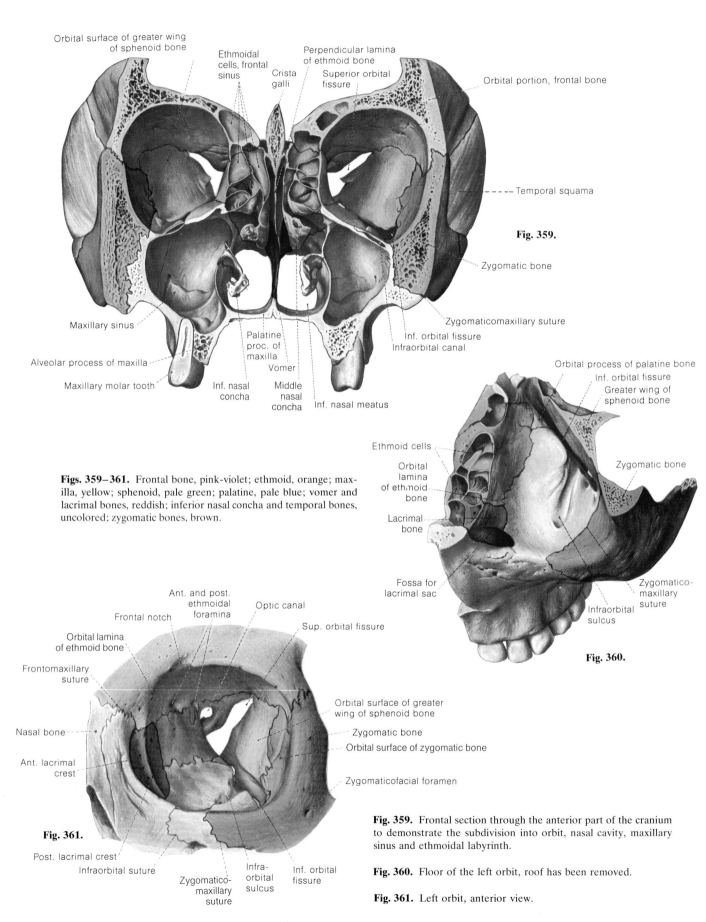

Orbital surface of greater wing of sphenoid bone

Ethmoidal cells, frontal sinus

Crista galli

Perpendicular lamina of ethmoid bone

Superior orbital fissure

Orbital portion, frontal bone

Temporal squama

Fig. 359.

Zygomatic bone

Zygomaticomaxillary suture

Inf. orbital fissure
Infraorbital canal

Maxillary sinus

Alveolar process of maxilla

Maxillary molar tooth

Palatine proc. of maxilla

Vomer

Inf. nasal concha

Middle nasal concha

Inf. nasal meatus

**Figs. 359–361.** Frontal bone, pink-violet; ethmoid, orange; maxilla, yellow; sphenoid, pale green; palatine, pale blue; vomer and lacrimal bones, reddish; inferior nasal concha and temporal bones, uncolored; zygomatic bones, brown.

Orbital process of palatine bone
Inf. orbital fissure
Greater wing of sphenoid bone

Ethmoid cells

Orbital lamina of ethmoid bone

Lacrimal bone

Zygomatic bone

Fossa for lacrimal sac

Zygomatico-maxillary suture

Infraorbital sulcus

Fig. 360.

Ant. and post. ethmoidal foramina

Frontal notch

Optic canal

Sup. orbital fissure

Orbital lamina of ethmoid bone

Frontomaxillary suture

Nasal bone

Ant. lacrimal crest

Orbital surface of greater wing of sphenoid bone

Zygomatic bone

Orbital surface of zygomatic bone

Zygomaticofacial foramen

Fig. 361.

Post. lacrimal crest

Infraorbital suture

Zygomatico-maxillary suture

Infra-orbital sulcus

Inf. orbital fissure

**Fig. 359.** Frontal section through the anterior part of the cranium to demonstrate the subdivision into orbit, nasal cavity, maxillary sinus and ethmoidal labyrinth.

**Fig. 360.** Floor of the left orbit, roof has been removed.

**Fig. 361.** Left orbit, anterior view.

**Fig. 362.** Medial wall of left orbit and pterygopalatine fossa. ▷

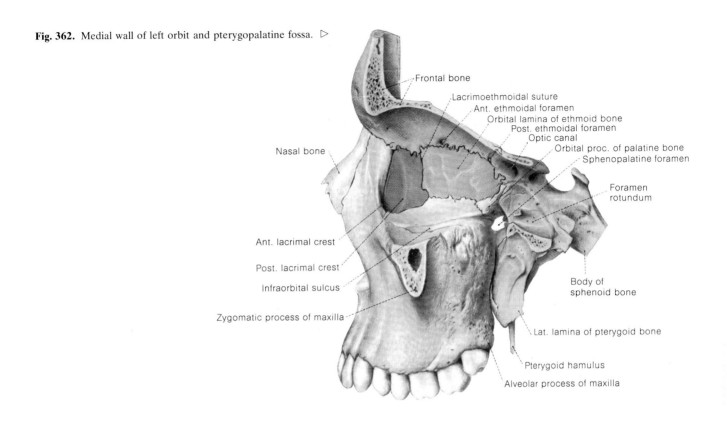

Frontal bone
Lacrimoethmoidal suture
Ant. ethmoidal foramen
Orbital lamina of ethmoid bone
Post. ethmoidal foramen
Optic canal
Orbital proc. of palatine bone
Sphenopalatine foramen
Nasal bone
Foramen rotundum
Ant. lacrimal crest
Post. lacrimal crest
Infraorbital sulcus
Body of sphenoid bone
Zygomatic process of maxilla
Lat. lamina of pterygoid bone
Pterygoid hamulus
Alveolar process of maxilla

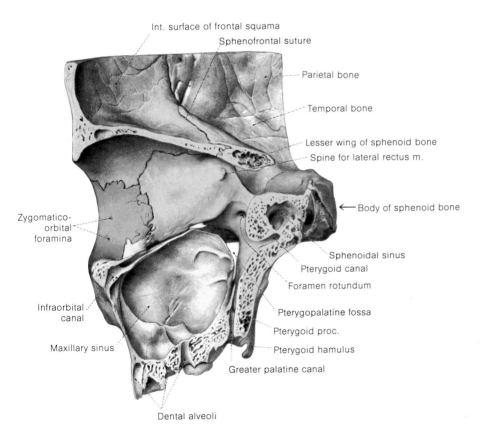

Int. surface of frontal squama
Sphenofrontal suture
Parietal bone
Temporal bone
Lesser wing of sphenoid bone
Spine for lateral rectus m.
Zygomatico-orbital foramina
Body of sphenoid bone
Sphenoidal sinus
Pterygoid canal
Foramen rotundum
Infraorbital canal
Pterygopalatine fossa
Pterygoid proc.
Maxillary sinus
Pterygoid hamulus
Greater palatine canal
Dental alveoli

**Fig. 363.** Lateral wall of right orbit, maxillary sinus, and the pterygopalatine fossa.

219

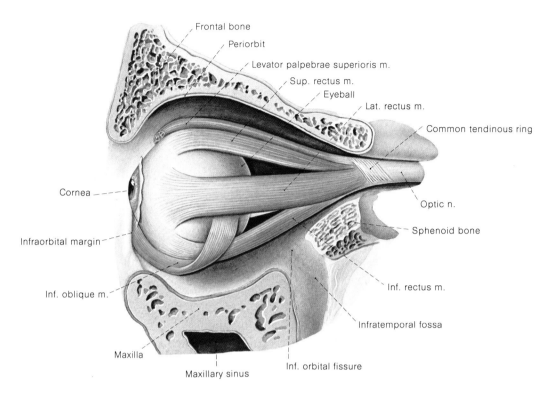

**Fig. 364.** The extrinsic muscles of the left eye in lateral view. The lateral wall of the left orbit and most of the contents of the orbit including the fascia, the eyelids and the anterior end of the levator palpebrae superioris muscle have been removed.

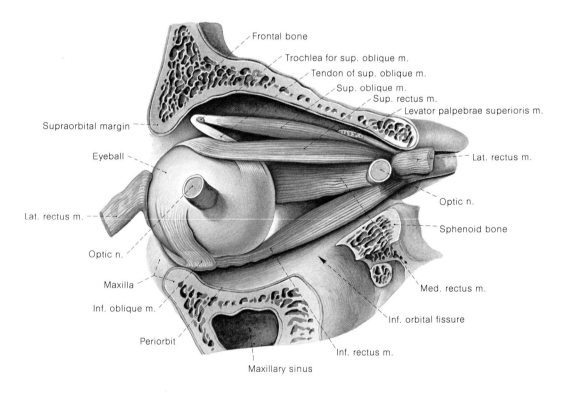

**Fig. 365.** The extrinsic muscles of the left eyeball in lateral view. The lateral rectus muscle and the optic nerve have been divided. The eyeball has been rotated to expose the dorsal pole with the stump of the optic nerve. Most of the levator palpebrae superioris muscle has been removed.

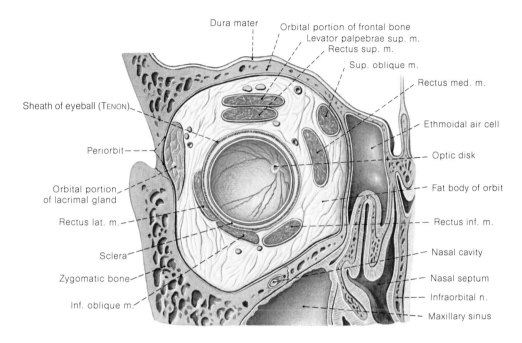

**Fig. 366.** Frontal section of the right orbit through the dorsal third of the eyeball. Anterior view.

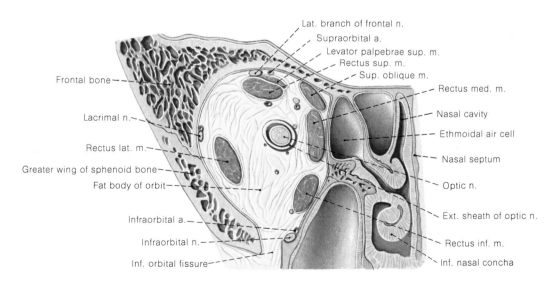

**Fig. 367.** Frontal section through the right orbit behind the eyeball. Ventral view.

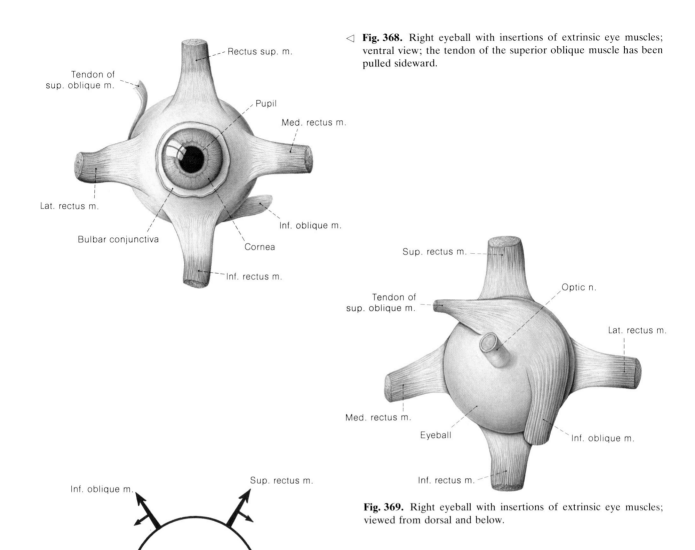

◁ **Fig. 368.** Right eyeball with insertions of extrinsic eye muscles; ventral view; the tendon of the superior oblique muscle has been pulled sideward.

Rectus sup. m.

Tendon of sup. oblique m.

Pupil

Med. rectus m.

Lat. rectus m.

Bulbar conjunctiva

Cornea

Inf. oblique m.

Inf. rectus m.

Sup. rectus m.

Tendon of sup. oblique m.

Optic n.

Lat. rectus m.

Med. rectus m.

Eyeball

Inf. oblique m.

Inf. rectus m.

**Fig. 369.** Right eyeball with insertions of extrinsic eye muscles; viewed from dorsal and below.

Inf. oblique m.

Sup. rectus m.

Lat. rectus m.

Med. rectus m.

Sup. oblique m.

Inf. rectus m.

**Fig. 370.** Diagram to illustrate the direction of traction of the extrinsic eye muscles; right eye.

Sup. rectus m.

Tendon of sup. oblique m.

Lat. rectus m.

Med. rectus m.

Inf. oblique m.

Inf. rectus m.

Optic n.

**Fig. 371.** Right eyeball with insertions of extrinsic eye muscles; viewed from behind and above. The inferior oblique muscle has been deflected from the eyeball.

222

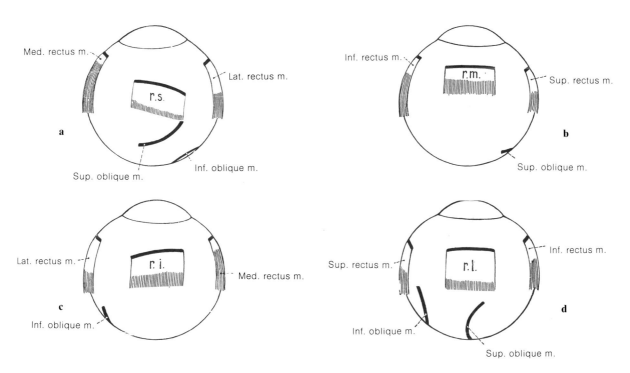

**Fig. 372.** Diagram to illustrate the insertions of the six extrinsic eye muscles on the right eye. a = seen from above, b = from medial, c = from below, d = from lateral. r.c. = inferior rectus muscle, r.l. = lateral rectus muscle, r.m. = medial rectus muscle, r.s. = superior rectus muscle.

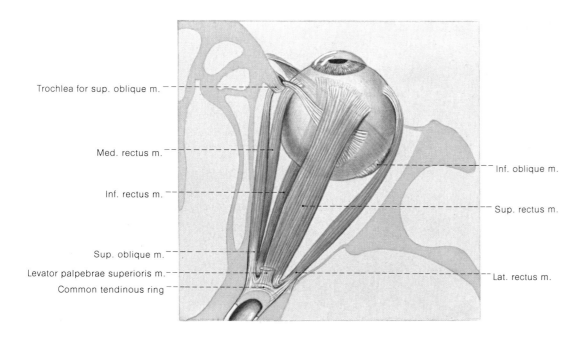

**Fig. 373.** Diagram of the extrinsic muscles of the right eyeball seen from above; muscles partially transparent. (From PERNKOPF: Atlas der topographischen und angewandten Anatomie des Menschen, Vol. 1, 2nd ed. [Ed. H. FERNER]. Urban & Schwarzenberg, Munich–Vienna–Baltimore 1980.)

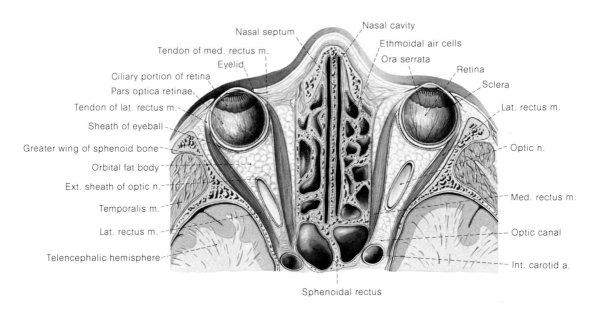

Fig. 374. Horizontal section through both orbits and the nasal cavity. Note the angle between the axis of the eyeball and the extrinsic muscles.

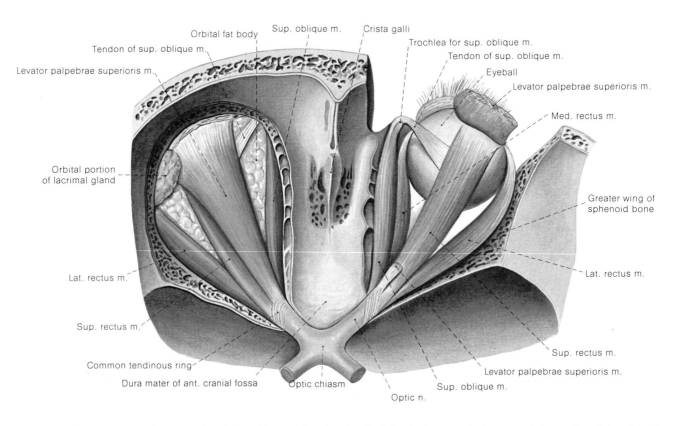

Fig. 375. The extrinsic eye muscles, their position and direction. On the right, the levator palpebrae superioris muscle and the orbital fat body have been removed. The fat body forms the bearing for the movements of the eyeball with the help of the capsule of Tenon, bulbar sheath.

224

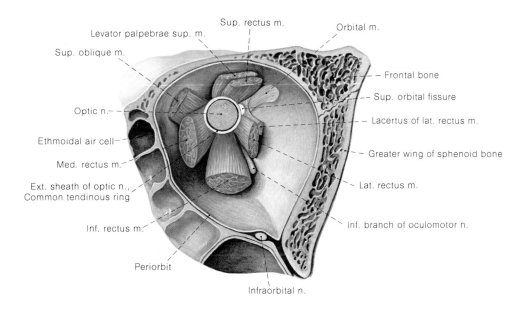

**Fig. 376.** The origins of the extrinsic ocular muscles from the common tendinous ring; frontal section through the orbit viewed from ventral. The optic nerve has been cut off close to the optic canal. The stumps of the muscles as well as the lower branch of the oculomotor nerve have been retained.

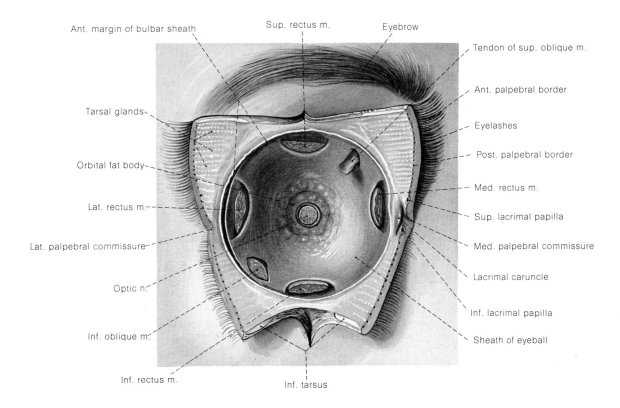

**Fig. 377.** The bulbar sheath (TENON's capsule) of the right eye with its openings for the extrinsic eye muscles that then insert on the sclera. The bulbar sheath acts like a joint capsule for movements of the eyeball.

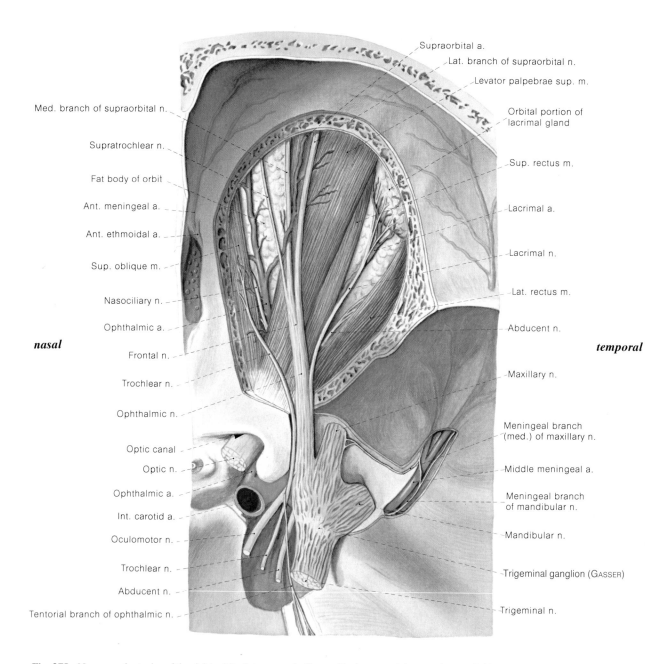

Supraorbital a.

Lat. branch of supraorbital n.

Levator palpebrae sup. m.

Med. branch of supraorbital n.

Orbital portion of
lacrimal gland

Supratrochlear n.

Sup. rectus m.

Fat body of orbit

Ant. meningeal a.

Lacrimal a.

Ant. ethmoidal a.

Lacrimal n.

Sup. oblique m.

Nasociliary n.

Lat. rectus m.

Ophthalmic a.

Abducent n.

*nasal*

*temporal*

Frontal n.

Maxillary n.

Trochlear n.

Ophthalmic n.

Meningeal branch
(med.) of maxillary n.

Optic canal

Optic n.

Middle meningeal a.

Ophthalmic a.

Meningeal branch
of mandibular n.

Int. carotid a.

Oculomotor n.

Mandibular n.

Trochlear n.

Trigeminal ganglion (GASSER)

Abducent n.

Tentorial branch of ophthalmic n.

Trigeminal n.

**Fig. 378.** Nerves and arteries of the right orbit after removal of its roof in the area of the anterior cranial fossa. The dura mater has been split along the middle meningeal artery and has been removed over the trigeminal ganglion and the nerves to the extrinsic eye muscles.

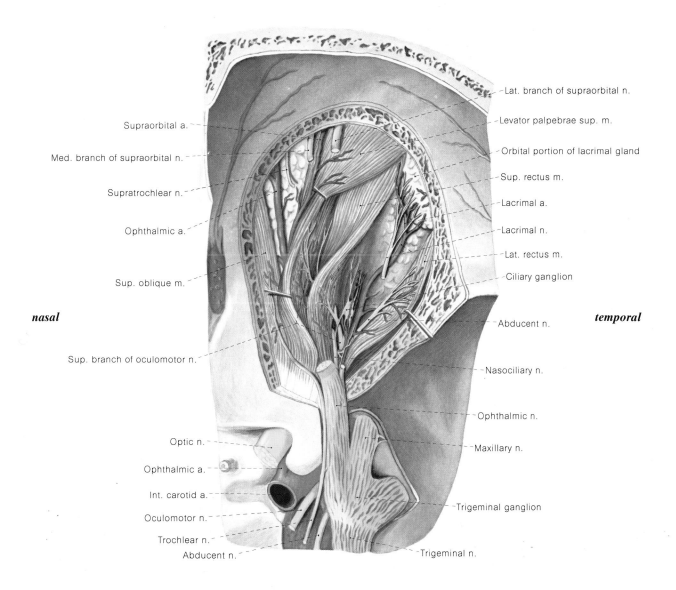

Lat. branch of supraorbital n.

Levator palpebrae sup. m.

Orbital portion of lacrimal gland

Sup. rectus m.

Lacrimal a.

Lacrimal n.

Lat. rectus m.

Ciliary ganglion

Abducent n.

Nasociliary n.

Ophthalmic n.

Maxillary n.

Trigeminal ganglion

Trigeminal n.

Supraorbital a.

Med. branch of supraorbital n.

Supratrochlear n.

Ophthalmic a.

Sup. oblique m.

*nasal*

Sup. branch of oculomotor n.

Optic n.

Ophthalmic a.

Int. carotid a.

Oculomotor n.

Trochlear n.

Abducent n.

*temporal*

**Fig. 379.** Nerves and arteries of the right orbit, second layer. Preparation similar to the one in Fig. 378. Major part of frontal nerve and a part of the temporal portion of the orbital fat body have been removed, the superior rectus muscle and the levator palpebrae superioris muscle have been pulled medially, the lateral rectus muscle laterally.

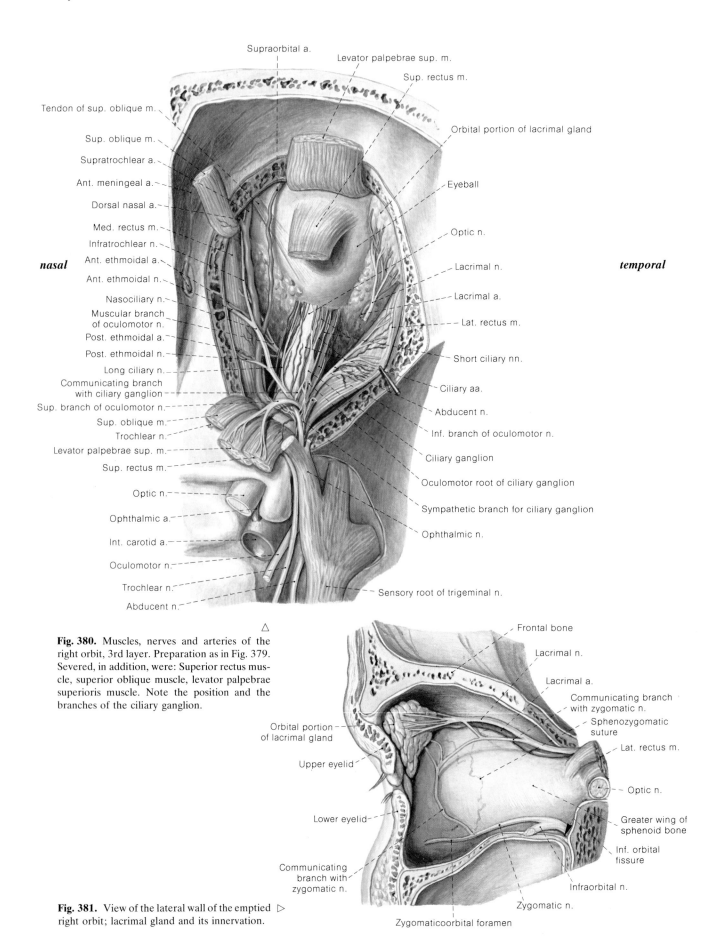

Supraorbital a.

Levator palpebrae sup. m.

Sup. rectus m.

Tendon of sup. oblique m.

Sup. oblique m.

Supratrochlear a.

Ant. meningeal a.

Dorsal nasal a.

Med. rectus m.

Infratrochlear n.

**nasal** Ant. ethmoidal a.

Ant. ethmoidal n.

Nasociliary n.

Muscular branch of oculomotor n.

Post. ethmoidal a.

Post. ethmoidal n.

Long ciliary n.

Communicating branch with ciliary ganglion

Sup. branch of oculomotor n.

Sup. oblique m.

Trochlear n.

Levator palpebrae sup. m.

Sup. rectus m.

Optic n.

Ophthalmic a.

Int. carotid a.

Oculomotor n.

Trochlear n.

Abducent n.

Orbital portion of lacrimal gland

Eyeball

Optic n.

Lacrimal n.

Lacrimal a.

Lat. rectus m.

Short ciliary nn.

Ciliary aa.

Abducent n.

Inf. branch of oculomotor n.

Ciliary ganglion

Oculomotor root of ciliary ganglion

Sympathetic branch for ciliary ganglion

Ophthalmic n.

Sensory root of trigeminal n.

**temporal**

**Fig. 380.** Muscles, nerves and arteries of the right orbit, 3rd layer. Preparation as in Fig. 379. Severed, in addition, were: Superior rectus muscle, superior oblique muscle, levator palpebrae superioris muscle. Note the position and the branches of the ciliary ganglion.

Frontal bone

Lacrimal n.

Lacrimal a.

Communicating branch with zygomatic n.

Sphenozygomatic suture

Lat. rectus m.

Optic n.

Greater wing of sphenoid bone

Inf. orbital fissure

Infraorbital n.

Orbital portion of lacrimal gland

Upper eyelid

Lower eyelid

Communicating branch with zygomatic n.

Zygomatic n.

Zygomaticoorbital foramen

**Fig. 381.** View of the lateral wall of the emptied ▷ right orbit; lacrimal gland and its innervation.

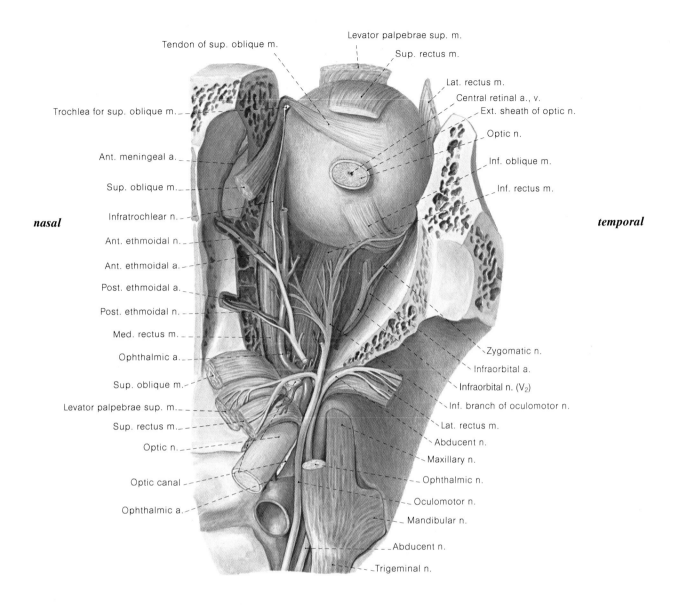

Tendon of sup. oblique m.

Levator palpebrae sup. m.

Sup. rectus m.

Lat. rectus m.

Central retinal a., v.

Ext. sheath of optic n.

Trochlea for sup. oblique m.

Optic n.

Ant. meningeal a.

Inf. oblique m.

Sup. oblique m.

Inf. rectus m.

**nasal**

**temporal**

Infratrochlear n.

Ant. ethmoidal n.

Ant. ethmoidal a.

Post. ethmoidal a.

Post. ethmoidal n.

Med. rectus m.

Ophthalmic a.

Zygomatic n.

Infraorbital a.

Infraorbital n. (V₂)

Sup. oblique m.

Inf. branch of oculomotor n.

Levator palpebrae sup. m.

Sup. rectus m.

Lat. rectus m.

Optic n.

Abducent n.

Maxillary n.

Optic canal

Ophthalmic n.

Oculomotor n.

Ophthalmic a.

Mandibular n.

Abducent n.

Trigeminal n.

**Fig. 382.** Nerves, arteries and muscles of the right orbit. The optic nerve and parts of the extrinsic muscles have been removed. Demonstrated is especially the course and the ramifications of the oculomotor n.

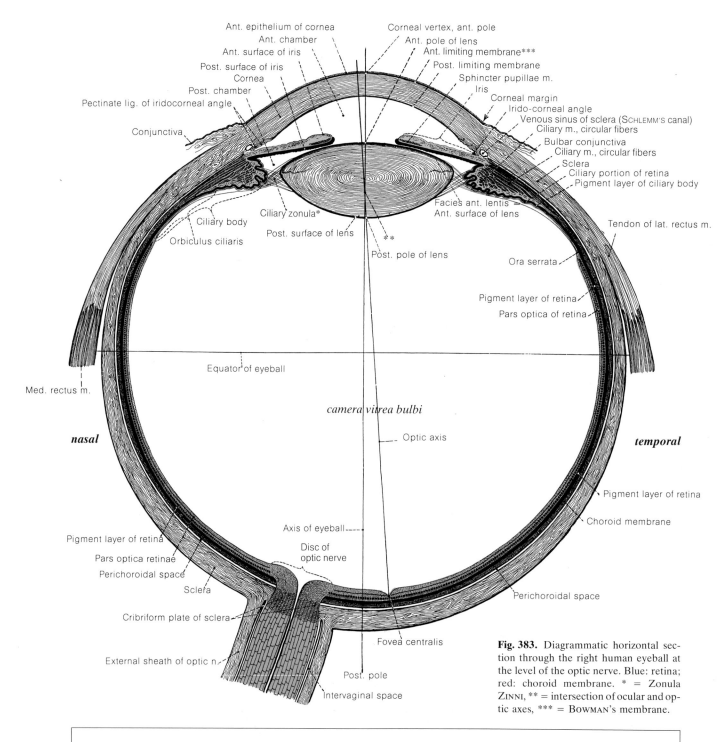

Ant. epithelium of cornea
Ant. chamber
Ant. surface of iris
Post. surface of iris
Cornea
Post. chamber
Pectinate lig. of iridocorneal angle
Conjunctiva

Corneal vertex, ant. pole
Ant. pole of lens
Ant. limiting membrane***
Post. limiting membrane
Sphincter pupillae m.
Iris
Corneal margin
Irido-corneal angle
Venous sinus of sclera (Schlemm's canal)
Ciliary m., circular fibers
Bulbar conjunctiva
Ciliary m., circular fibers
Sclera
Ciliary portion of retina
Pigment layer of ciliary body

Ciliary body
Orbiculus ciliaris
Ciliary zonula*
Post. surface of lens

Facies ant. lentis
Ant. surface of lens
**
Post. pole of lens

Tendon of lat. rectus m.

Ora serrata

Pigment layer of retina
Pars optica of retina

Equator of eyeball

Med. rectus m.

*nasal*

*camera vitrea bulbi*

Optic axis

*temporal*

Pigment layer of retina

Choroid membrane

Axis of eyeball
Disc of optic nerve

Pigment layer of retina
Pars optica retinae
Perichoroidal space
Sclera
Cribriform plate of sclera
External sheath of optic n.

Perichoroidal space

Fovea centralis

Post. pole

Intervaginal space

**Fig. 383.** Diagrammatic horizontal section through the right human eyeball at the level of the optic nerve. Blue: retina; red: choroid membrane. * = Zonula Zinni, ** = intersection of ocular and optic axes, *** = Bowman's membrane.

**Measurements of the human eyeball** (average values from the anatomical and ophthalmological literature):

⇕ outer diameter (axis) 24.27 mm,
✗ inner diameter (axis) 21.74 mm,
diameter at equator 24.32 mm,
vertical diameter 23.60 mm,
radius of scleral curvature 12.70 mm,
radius of corneal curvature 7.75 mm,
depth of anterior chamber 3 mm,

sagittal axis of lens 3 mm,
diameter of lens at equator 9–10 mm,
distance from lens to retina 14.5 mm,
interpupillary distance right ⟵⟶ left
   56–61 mm,
horizontal diameter of cornea 11.9 mm,
vertical diamenter of cornea 11.0 mm.

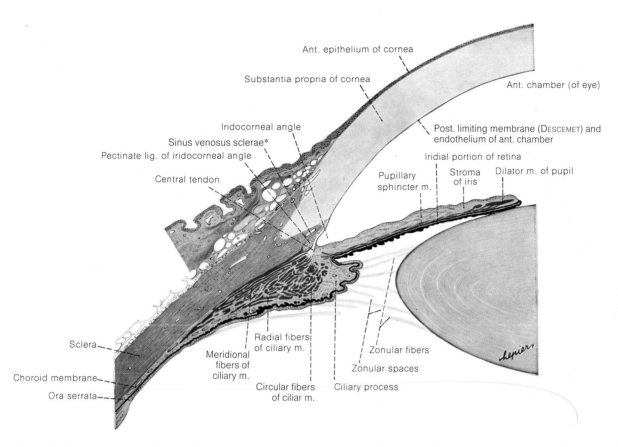

Ant. epithelium of cornea

Substantia propria of cornea

Ant. chamber (of eye)

Iridocorneal angle

Sinus venosus sclerae*

Pectinate lig. of iridocorneal angle

Central tendon

Post. limiting membrane (DESCEMET) and endothelium of ant. chamber

Iridial portion of retina

Pupillary sphincter m.

Stroma of iris

Dilator m. of pupil

Sclera

Meridional fibers of ciliary m.

Radial fibers of ciliary m.

Zonular fibers

Zonular spaces

Choroid membrane

Circular fibers of ciliar m.

Ciliary process

Ora serrata

**Fig. 384.** Horizontal section through the anterior part of the eyeball. (From PERNKOPF: Atlas der topographischen und angewandten Anatomie des Menschen, Vol. 1, 2nd ed. [Ed. H. FERNER]. Urban & Schwarzenberg, Munich–Vienna–Baltimore 1980.) * canal of SCHLEMM.

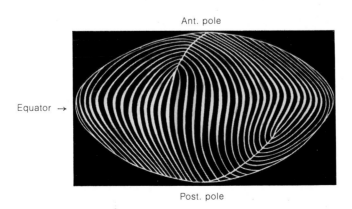

Ant. pole

Equator →

Post. pole

**Fig. 385.** Diagramm of the lens of a newborn; equatorial view. Course of the lens fibers. Note their beginning and ending at the anterior and posterior lens star, respectively. Compare Fig. 402. The anterior and posterior lens stars are shifted against each other for 120°. The lens of the adult has stars with multiple rays (comp. Fig. 399).

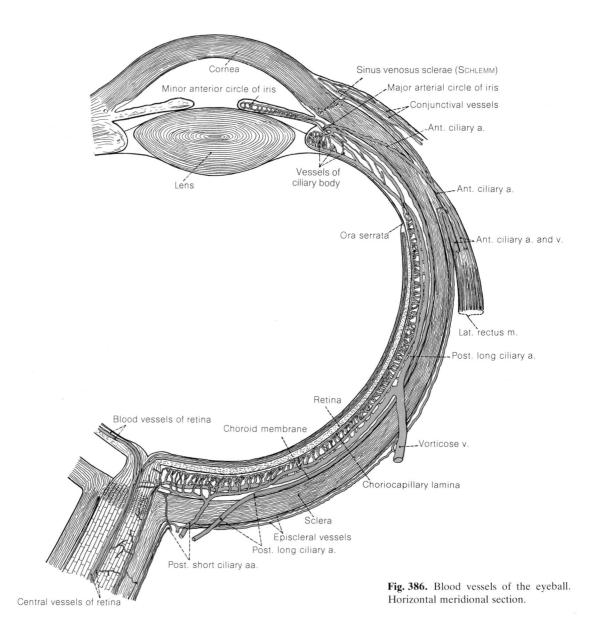

Fig. 386. Blood vessels of the eyeball. Horizontal meridional section.

**The Tunics of the Eyeball**

**I. Fibrous tunic** *(corneo-scleral coat)*

a) Cornea, anterior smaller portion (¹/₅), pronounced curvature, transparent.

b) Sclera, white appearance, larger portion (⁴/₅), less pronounced curvature, opaque, in infancy bluish-white, in senescence yellowish-white (in icteric conditions yellow).

**II. Middle, vascular tunic** *(uvea)*

a) iris with central, round opening = pupil

b) ciliary body with ciliary muscles, ciliary process, ciliary zonule (ZINN's)

c) choroid membrane

**III. Innermost tunic,** *retina proper* (inner layer of optic cup)

a) pars caeca, from pupillary margin of iris to ora serrata
   1. iridial portion of retina; simple, low, pigmented epithelium
   2. ciliary portion of retina; simple, non-pigmented epithelium

b) pars optica, stratified. Three-neuron-system. 1st neuron, outward location, bordering on pigment layer, neuro-epithelium, rod cells, cone cells, avascular. 2nd and 3rd neuron, inward location, vascularized. Specialized areas in the posterior segment of eyeball: macula lutea with central fovea (area of most acute vision), papilla of optic nerve (blind spot, exit of optic nerve containing central vessels).

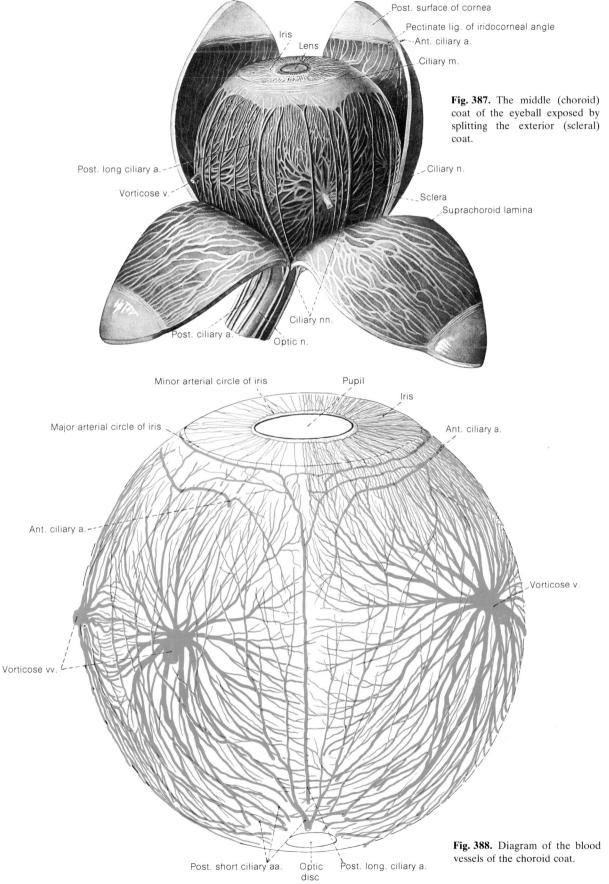

Iris
Lens
Post. surface of cornea
Pectinate lig. of iridocorneal angle
Ant. ciliary a.
Ciliary m.

**Fig. 387.** The middle (choroid) coat of the eyeball exposed by splitting the exterior (scleral) coat.

Post. long ciliary a.
Vorticose v.
Ciliary n.
Sclera
Suprachoroid lamina

Ciliary nn.
Post. ciliary a.
Optic n.

Minor arterial circle of iris
Pupil
Iris
Major arterial circle of iris
Ant. ciliary a.

Ant. ciliary a.
Vorticose v.

Vorticose vv.

Post. short ciliary aa.
Optic disc
Post. long. ciliary a.

**Fig. 388.** Diagram of the blood vessels of the choroid coat.

233

Fovea centralis    Sup. temporal v.    Sup. temporal a.

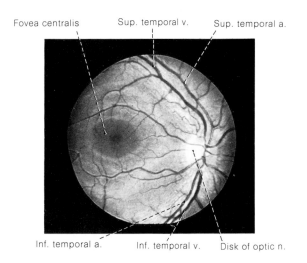

Inf. temporal a.    Inf. temporal v.    Disk of optic n.

**Fig. 389.** Normal central fundus of the right eye. Ophthalmoscopic picture. Originals of the Figs. 389–392 by Priv.-Doz. Dr. med. R. Unsöld, Univ.-Augenklinik Freiburg i. Brsg.

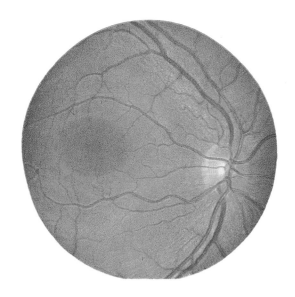

**Fig. 390.** Same as 389.

Disk of optic n.    Sup. temporal a.    Sup. temporal v.

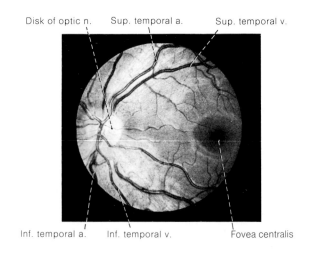

Inf. temporal a.    Inf. temporal v.    Fovea centralis

**Fig. 391.** Normal central fundus of the left eye. Ophthalmoscopic picture.

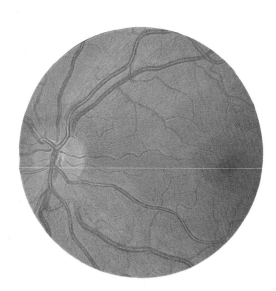

**Fig. 392.** Same as 391.

234

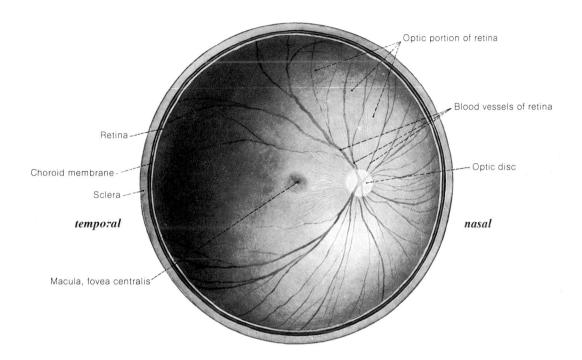

Optic portion of retina

Blood vessels of retina

Retina

Optic disc

Choroid membrane

Sclera

*temporal*

*nasal*

Macula, fovea centralis

**Fig. 393.** Posterior half of an equatorially sectioned right human eyeball. Anterior view of the optic disk (white "blind spot") and the fovea centralis (gray). Vitreous body has been removed.

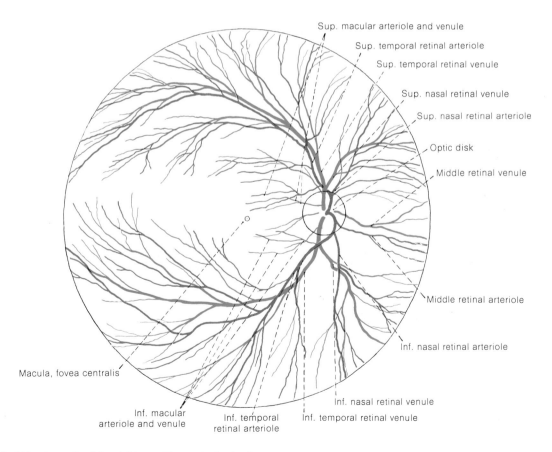

Sup. macular arteriole and venule

Sup. temporal retinal arteriole

Sup. temporal retinal venule

Sup. nasal retinal venule

Sup. nasal retinal arteriole

Optic disk

Middle retinal venule

Middle retinal arteriole

Inf. nasal retinal arteriole

Macula, fovea centralis

Inf. nasal retinal venule

Inf. macular arteriole and venule

Inf. temporal retinal arteriole

Inf. temporal retinal venule

**Fig. 394.** Retinal blood vessels of the right eye. View onto the fundus.

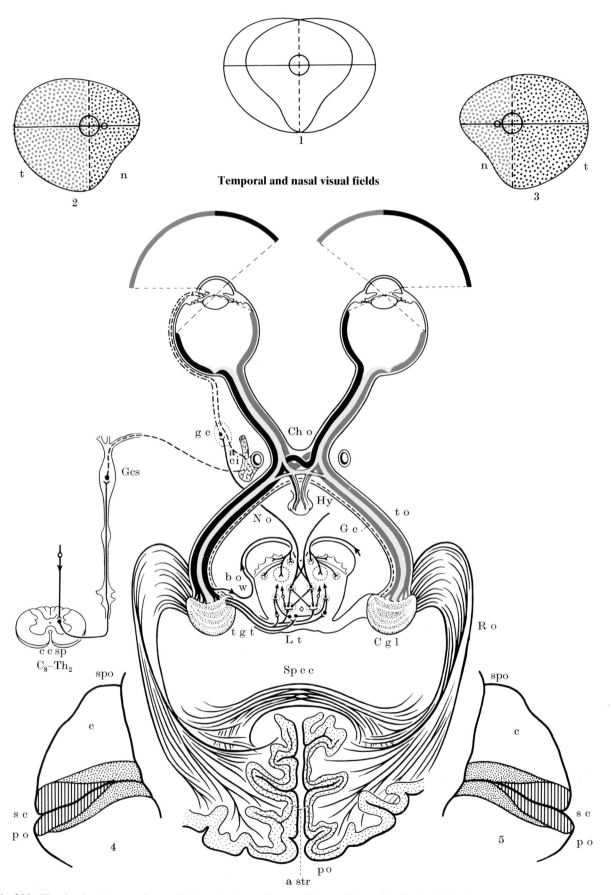

**Temporal and nasal visual fields**

**Fig. 395.** The visual pathway, retino-geniculo-cortical tract. Course of the pupillary reflex via the midbrain, oculomotor nerve and ciliary ganglion.

**The visual pathway**

light

↓

*pars optica of retina*

1. Light sensitive cells (rod cells and cone cells) = photo-receptor cells.

2. *Retinal ganglion;* relay and integration system of predominantly bipolar neurons.

3. *Ganglion of optic nerve;* multipolar neurons whose axons pass through the optic disc into the optic nerve. The disc corresponds to the blind spot. The area of the most acute vision is the central fovea with its immediate vicinity, the macula lutea. Light rays from an object in the visual axis reach the fovea centralis which contains only cone cells.

↓

*optic nerves*

↓

*optic chiasm*

Partial decussation of fibers. About 60% do cross, 40% remain uncrossed. Nasal fibers decussate, temporal fibers remain uncrossed; fibers from the central fovea are crossed or uncrossed.

↓

*optic tract*

↓

↓

secondary visual centers

1. *Lateral geniculate body.* Connection of both lateral geniculate bodies via GUDDEN's commissure.
2. *Pulvinar of thalamus*
3. *Nucleus of superior colliculus*

↓

Connections to extrinsic ocular muscle nuclei, muscle of accommodation, sphincter pupillae muscle and cilio-spinal center (pupillary reflex).

*Optic radiation.* This large fiber system, fan-shaped and spiraled, courses through the posterior limb of the internal capsule, above the amygdala, lateral to the posterior horn of the lateral ventricle to the *visual cortex* in the occipital lobe, the *striate cortex* around the *calcarine sulcus.* The retina is represented in the striate area of the cortex with exact point-to-point projection (17 and 18 after BRODMAN). The representation of the central fovea occupies the largest part of the striate area. Furthermore, the optic region expands into the area of the cuneus and the medial occipitotemporal gyrus as well as the lateral surface of the occipital lobe. The optic radiations and the striate areas of both hemispheres may be interconnected through the splenium of the corpus callosum.

---

◁ **Fig. 395.** Diagram of the visual pathway and its stations.

| | |
|---|---|
| 1 | binocular visual field |
| 2 | visual field of the left eye |
| 3 | visual field of the right eye |
| n | nasal |
| t | temporal |
| 4, 5 | medial aspect of the occipital lobe of the telencephalon |
| Ch o | optic chiasm |
| a c i | internal carotid artery with sympathetic carotid plexus |
| g c | ciliary ganglion |
| Hy | hypophysis |
| t o | optic tract |
| G c | GUDDEN's commissure = connection of the lateral geniculate bodies |
| b o w | basal optic root = reflex pathway to the nuclear areas of the midbrain |

| | |
|---|---|
| L t | lamina tecti (quadrigemina) |
| t g t | geniculo-tectal tract |
| N o | oculomotor nerve |
| C g l | lateral geniculate body |
| R o | optic radiation (GRATIOLET) |
| Sp c c | splenium of corpus callosum with possible connections of the optic radiations of both hemispheres |
| a str | striate cortex |
| p o | occipital pole |
| s c | calcarine sulcus; vertical hatching: projection area of the central fovea, the papillomacular bundle of the upper and lower half of the contralateral optic radiation; stippled area: projection area of the retinal periphery of the upper and lower quadrant |
| c | cuneus |
| spo | parieto-occipital sulcus |
| Gcs | superior cervical ganglion |
| c c sp | ciliospinal center C 8 – Th 2 (dilatation of pupil) |

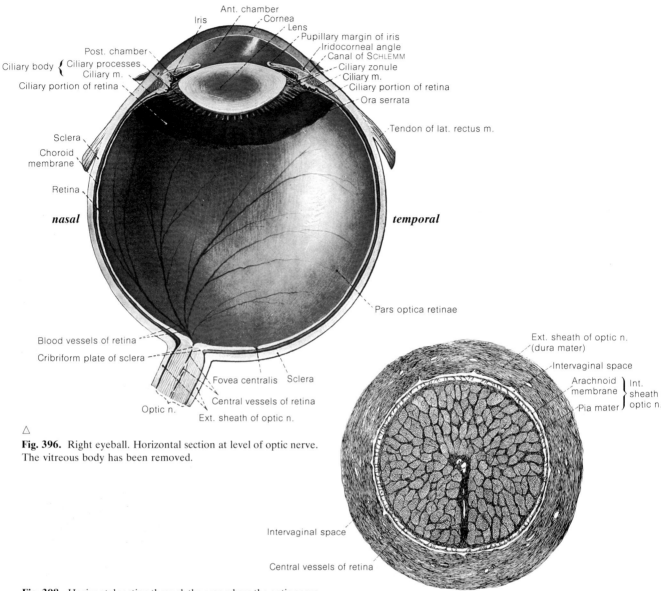

Iris
Ant. chamber
Cornea
Lens
Pupillary margin of iris
Iridocorneal angle
Canal of SCHLEMM
Ciliary zonule
Ciliary m.
Ciliary portion of retina
Ora serrata

Post. chamber
Ciliary body { Ciliary processes
Ciliary m.
Ciliary portion of retina

Tendon of lat. rectus m.

Sclera
Choroid
membrane

Retina

**nasal**

**temporal**

Pars optica retinae

Blood vessels of retina
Cribriform plate of sclera

Fovea centralis    Sclera
Central vessels of retina
Optic n.
Ext. sheath of optic n.

△

**Fig. 396.** Right eyeball. Horizontal section at level of optic nerve. The vitreous body has been removed.

Ext. sheath of optic n. (dura mater)
Intervaginal space
Arachnoid membrane } Int.
Pia mater } sheath optic n.

Intervaginal space

Central vessels of retina

**Fig. 398.** Horizontal section through the area where the optic nerve exits from the eyeball. The three coats of the eyeball are rendered in different colors. (From PERNKOPF: Atlas der topographischen und angewandten Anatomie des Menschen, Vol. 1, 2nd ed. [Ed. H. FERNER]. Urban & Schwarzenberg, Munich–Vienna–Baltimore 1980.)

△

**Fig. 397.** Cross section through the optic nerve near the eyeball.

▽

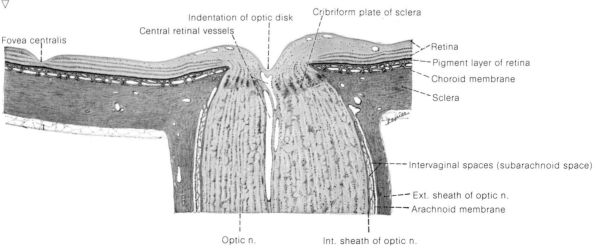

Indentation of optic disk
Central retinal vessels
Cribriform plate of sclera

Fovea centralis

Retina
Pigment layer of retina
Choroid membrane
Sclera

Intervaginal spaces (subarachnoid space)

Ext. sheath of optic n.
Arachnoid membrane

Optic n.    Int. sheath of optic n.

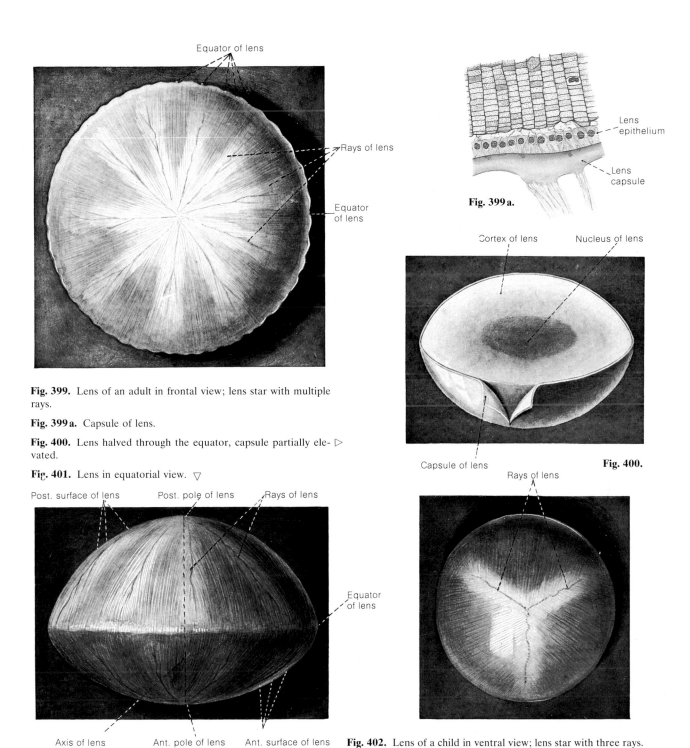

Equator of lens

Rays of lens

Equator of lens

Lens epithelium

Lens capsule

**Fig. 399 a.**

Cortex of lens    Nucleus of lens

Capsule of lens

Rays of lens

**Fig. 400.**

Post. surface of lens    Post. pole of lens    Rays of lens

Equator of lens

Axis of lens    Ant. pole of lens    Ant. surface of lens

**Fig. 399.** Lens of an adult in frontal view; lens star with multiple rays.

**Fig. 399 a.** Capsule of lens.

**Fig. 400.** Lens halved through the equator, capsule partially ele- ▷ vated.

**Fig. 401.** Lens in equatorial view. ▽

**Fig. 402.** Lens of a child in ventral view; lens star with three rays.

NOTE: The ring-shaped suspensory apparatus of the lens, the zonula, consists of meridionally arranged very fine, yet rigid fibrils, the zonular fibers. They originate from the ciliary orbiculus and the valleys between the ciliary processes. These fine fibers are grouped into dense bundles. They course in the valleys between the ciliary processes toward the lens where, in the area of the equator, they insert in the lens capsule thereby causing small, yet distinct notches on the equatorial surface. Fine interstices, spatia zonularia, exist between the main fiber bundles.

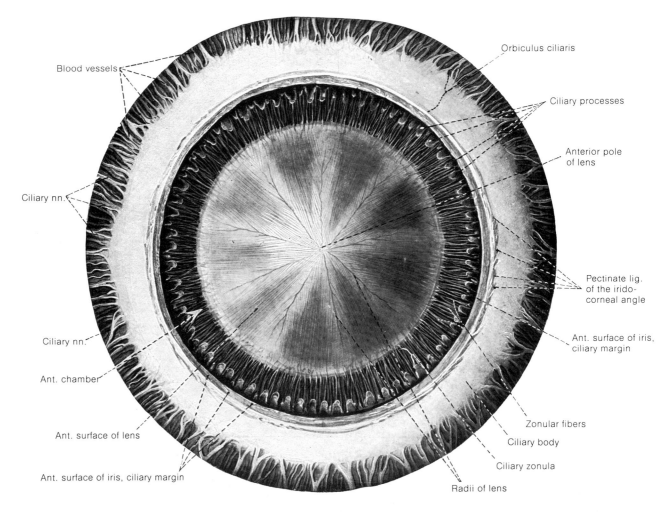

Blood vessels

Ciliary nn.

Ciliary nn.

Ant. chamber

Ant. surface of lens

Ant. surface of iris, ciliary margin

Orbiculus ciliaris

Ciliary processes

Anterior pole of lens

Pectinate lig. of the irido-corneal angle

Ant. surface of iris, ciliary margin

Zonular fibers

Ciliary body

Ciliary zonula

Radii of lens

**Fig. 403.** Suspensory apparatus of the lens, anterior view. Cornea and iris have been removed. The anterior ends of the ciliary processes can be seen. Between them are the zonular fibers of the suspensory apparatus of the lens. They insert at the equator of the lens as well as at the anterior and posterior surface of the lens capsule. The lens star and lens fibers are also illustrated.

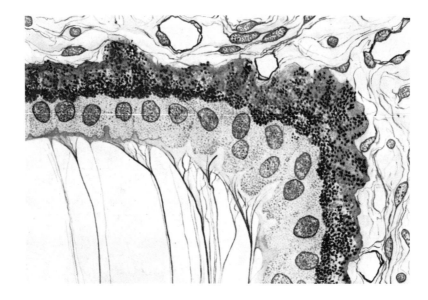

**Fig. 404.** Origin of the zonular fibers from the epithelium of the ciliary body. Beginning on the cuticle of the inner epithelium (after FERNER: Zschr. Zellforschg. 45, 1957).

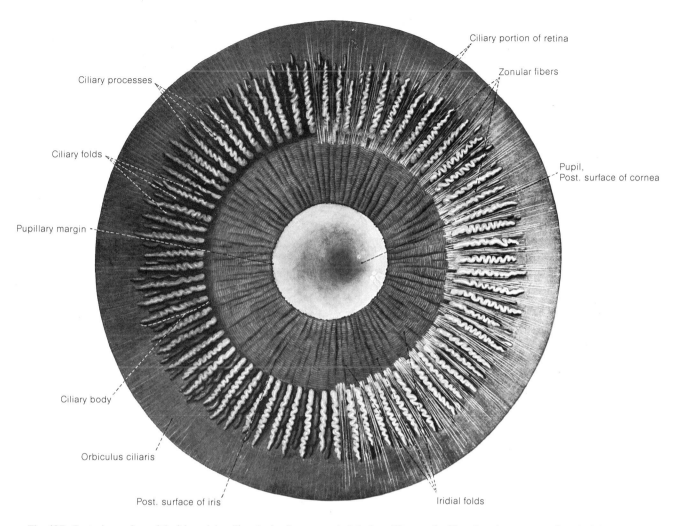

Ciliary portion of retina

Zonular fibers

Ciliary processes

Pupil,
Post. surface of cornea

Ciliary folds

Pupillary margin

Ciliary body

Orbiculus ciliaris

Post. surface of iris

Iridial folds

**Fig. 405.** Posterior surface of the iris and the ciliary body after removal of the lens. The zonular fibers have been removed on the left side, on the right they are sectioned close to the ciliary body; through the pupil one looks onto the posterior surface of the cornea.

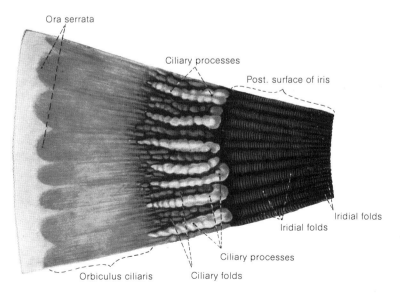

Ora serrata

Ciliary processes

Post. surface of iris

Iridial folds

Iridial folds

Orbiculus ciliaris

Ciliary processes

Ciliary folds

**Fig. 406.** Enlarged portion of Fig. 405. From left to right: ora serrata, orbiculus ciliaris, ciliary corona with ciliary processes and folds, dark posterior surface of iris with its relief.

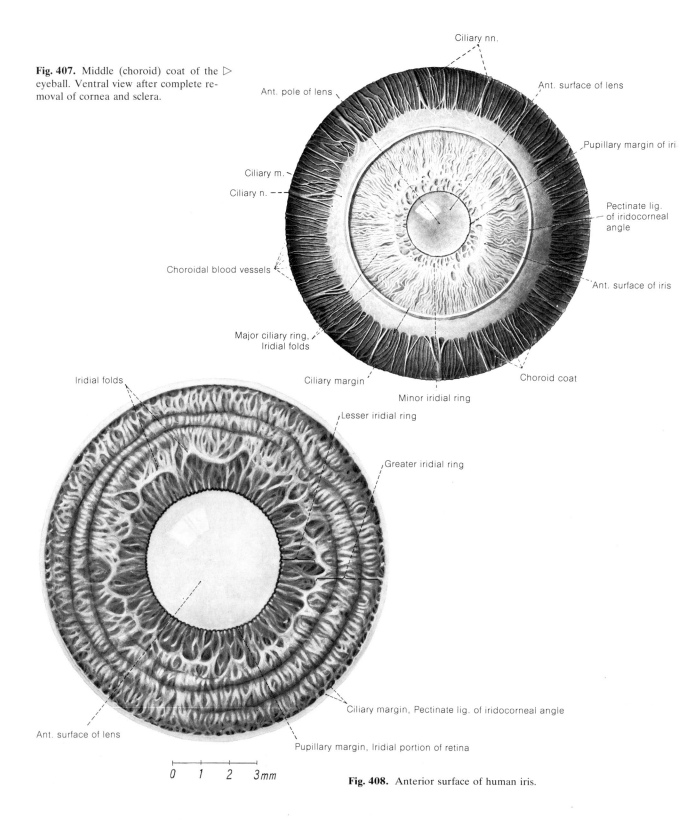

**Fig. 407.** Middle (choroid) coat of the ▷ eyeball. Ventral view after complete removal of cornea and sclera.

Ciliary nn.

Ant. pole of lens

Ant. surface of lens

Pupillary margin of iri

Ciliary m.

Ciliary n.

Pectinate lig. of iridocorneal angle

Choroidal blood vessels

Ant. surface of iris

Major ciliary ring, Iridial folds

Ciliary margin

Choroid coat

Minor iridial ring

Lesser iridial ring

Iridial folds

Greater iridial ring

Ciliary margin, Pectinate lig. of iridocorneal angle

Ant. surface of lens

Pupillary margin, Iridial portion of retina

0   1   2   3mm

**Fig. 408.** Anterior surface of human iris.

**Fig. 410.** The compartments of the middle ear. 1. Tympanic cavity, 2. Auditory tube, 3. Mastoid air cells. (From PERNKOPF: Atlas der topo- ▷ graphischen und angewandten Anatomie des Menschen, Vol. 1, 2nd ed. [Ed. H. FERNER]. Urban & Schwarzenberg, Munich–Vienna–Baltimore 1980.)

**Fig. 411.** Topographical survey of the portions of the vestibulocochlear organ located within the temporal bone of the right side. Red: external acoustic meatus; green: tympanic cavity, canalis musculotubarius, mastoid antrum, mastoid air cells, auditory ossicles; blue: internal ear = membranous labyrinth, cochlear duct. (From PERNKOPF: Atlas der topographischen und angewandten Anatomie des Menschen, Vol. 1, 2nd ed. [Ed. H. FERNER]. Urban & Schwarzenberg, Munich–Vienna–Baltimore 1980.)

242

# Organ of Hearing and Equilibrium

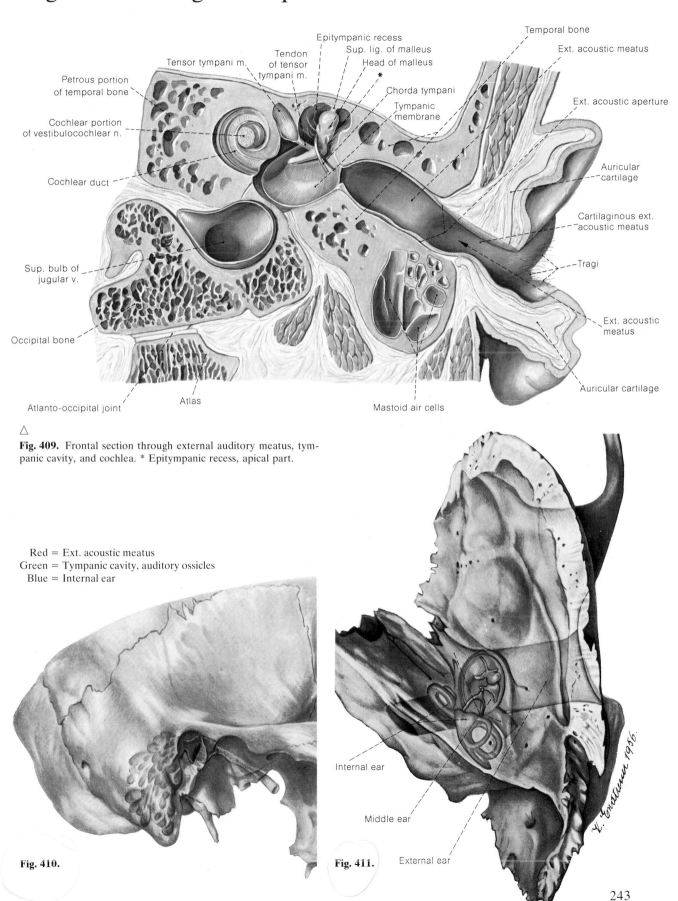

Tensor tympani m.
Tendon of tensor tympani m.
Epitympanic recess
Sup. lig. of malleus
Head of malleus
*
Temporal bone
Ext. acoustic meatus

Petrous portion of temporal bone
Chorda tympani
Tympanic membrane
Ext. acoustic aperture

Cochlear portion of vestibulocochlear n.
Auricular cartilage

Cochlear duct
Cartilaginous ext. acoustic meatus

Tragi

Sup. bulb of jugular v.
Ext. acoustic meatus

Occipital bone
Auricular cartilage

Atlanto-occipital joint
Atlas
Mastoid air cells

**Fig. 409.** Frontal section through external auditory meatus, tympanic cavity, and cochlea. * Epitympanic recess, apical part.

Red = Ext. acoustic meatus
Green = Tympanic cavity, auditory ossicles
Blue = Internal ear

Internal ear

Middle ear

**Fig. 410.**

**Fig. 411.**
External ear

# Organ of Hearing and Equilibrium

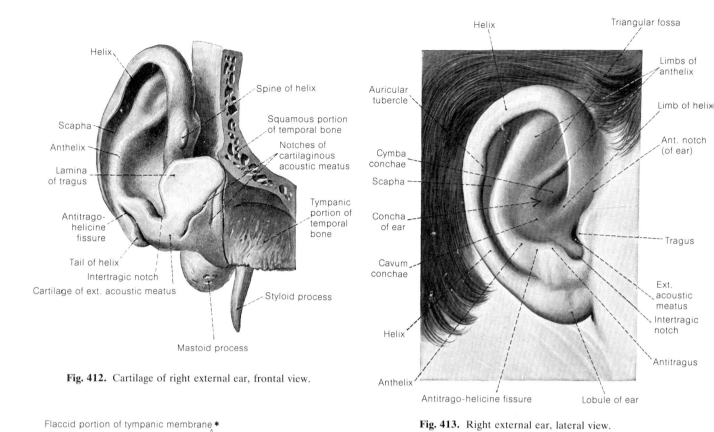

Helix

Scapha

Anthelix

Lamina of tragus

Antitrago-helicine fissure

Tail of helix

Intertragic notch

Cartilage of ext. acoustic meatus

Spine of helix

Squamous portion of temporal bone

Notches of cartilaginous acoustic meatus

Tympanic portion of temporal bone

Styloid process

Mastoid process

**Fig. 412.** Cartilage of right external ear, frontal view.

Helix

Triangular fossa

Limbs of anthelix

Limb of helix

Auricular tubercle

Cymba conchae

Scapha

Concha of ear

Cavum conchae

Helix

Anthelix

Ant. notch (of ear)

Tragus

Ext. acoustic meatus

Intertragic notch

Antitragus

Antitrago-helicine fissure

Lobule of ear

**Fig. 413.** Right external ear, lateral view.

Flaccid portion of tympanic membrane *

Post. mallear fold

Long. limb of incus

Post. limb of stapes

Promotory

Fossula of cochlear (round) window

Ant. mallear fold

Mallear prominence (lat. process of malleus)

Mallear stria (handle of malleus)

Ant. wall of ext. acoustic meatus

Umbo of tympanic membrane

Tense portion of tympanic membrane

Tympanic ring

Fibrocartilaginous ring

**Fig. 414.** Labeled line diagram for Fig. 415. For practical reasons the surface of the tympanic membrane is subdivided into four quadrants (I–IV). In the otoscopic picture of the normal tympanic membrane a glistening light reflection extends from the umbo toward the second quadrant (**). * = SHRAPNELL's membrane = flaccid portion of tympanic membrane.

10–11 mm

9 mm

cm     1     2

Natural size and orientation of right tympanic membrane.

**Fig. 415.** Right tympanic membrane as seen through an otoscope in a living person. Magnification about 6 ×.

244

**Fig. 416.** Right external ear, removed from head, medial view. ▷

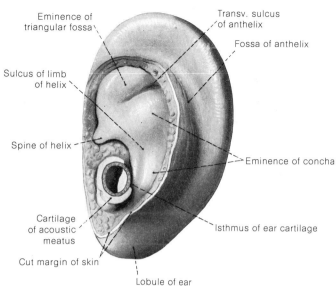

Eminence of triangular fossa

Sulcus of limb of helix

Spine of helix

Transv. sulcus of anthelix

Fossa of anthelix

Eminence of concha

Isthmus of ear cartilage

Cartilage of acoustic meatus

Cut margin of skin

Lobule of ear

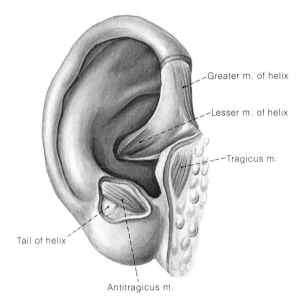

Greater m. of helix

Lesser m. of helix

Tragicus m.

Tail of helix

Antitragicus m.

**Fig. 417.** Muscles of the lateral surface of the right external ear.

Sup. auricular m.

Oblique auricular m.

Transv. auricular m.

Ext. acoustic meatus

Post. auricular m.

**Fig. 418.** Muscles of the medial surface of the right external ear. Ligaments may be present instead of superior and posterior auricular muscles.

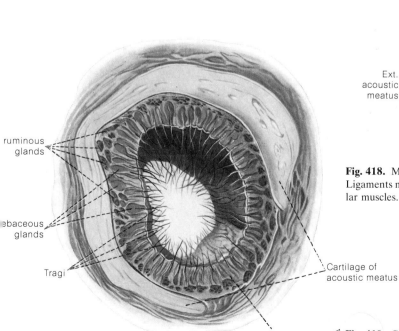

ruminous glands

ebaceous glands

Tragi

Cartilage of acoustic meatus

Skin of ext. acoustic meatus

◁ **Fig. 419.** Cross section through cartilaginous portion of external acoustic meatus. Enlarged about 8×.

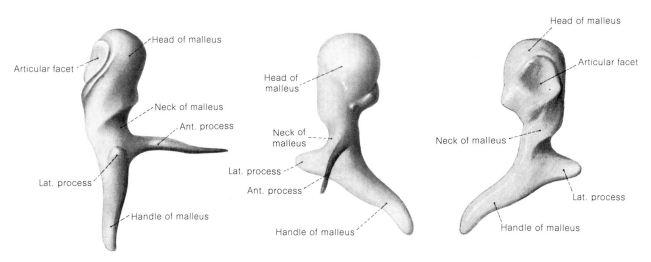

**Fig. 420.** Right malleus, lateral view.

**Fig. 421.** Right malleus, anterior view.

**Fig. 422.** Right malleus, dorsal view.

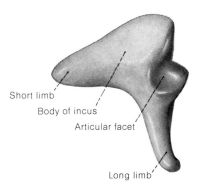

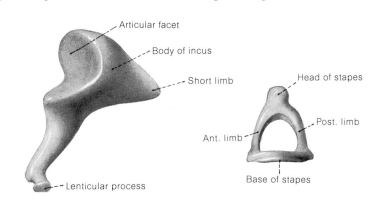

**Fig. 423.** Right incus, lateral view.

**Fig. 424.** Right incus, medial view.

**Fig. 425.** Right stapes, seen from above.

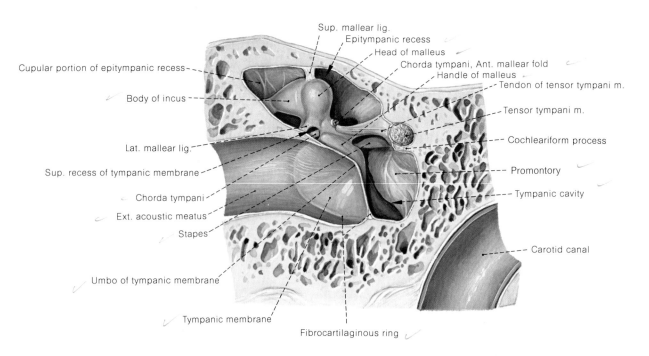

**Fig. 426.** Frontal section through right external auditory meatus, tympanic membrane and tympanic cavity. Note the narrowest area of the tympanic membrane. The epitympanic cupular recess is the highest point of the tympanic cavity. The surgical access to the upper tympanic cavity is through that portion of the temporal squama that reaches as "mur de la loguette" to the flaccid portion of the tympanic membrane.

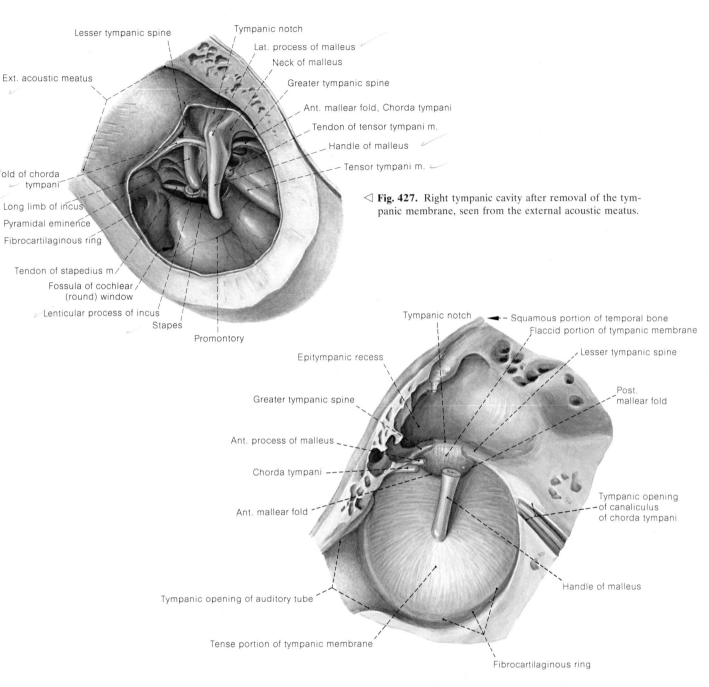

Lesser tympanic spine
Tympanic notch
Lat. process of malleus
Neck of malleus
Ext. acoustic meatus
Greater tympanic spine
Ant. mallear fold, Chorda tympani
Tendon of tensor tympani m.
Handle of malleus
Tensor tympani m.
old of chorda tympani
Long limb of incus
Pyramidal eminence
Fibrocartilaginous ring
Tendon of stapedius m.
Fossula of cochlear (round) window
Lenticular process of incus
Stapes
Promontory

◁ **Fig. 427.** Right tympanic cavity after removal of the tympanic membrane, seen from the external acoustic meatus.

Tympanic notch
Squamous portion of temporal bone
Flaccid portion of tympanic membrane
Lesser tympanic spine
Epitympanic recess
Post. mallear fold
Greater tympanic spine
Ant. process of malleus
Chorda tympani
Tympanic opening of canaliculus of chorda tympani
Ant. mallear fold
Handle of malleus
Tympanic opening of auditory tube
Tense portion of tympanic membrane
Fibrocartilaginous ring

**Fig. 428.** Lateral (membranous) wall of the tympanic cavity and the tympanic surface of the tympanic membrane, medial view (from the tympanic cavity). The bone has been sectioned parallel to the tympanic membrane. The contents of the tympanic cavity including the mucous membrane have been removed. Only the handle of the malleus has been left in place on the tympanic membrane.

NOTE: There are three stories in the tympanic cavity (Figs. 426, 431).

Upper story: epitympanic recess with mastoid antrum extending to the neck of the malleus and the anterior and posterior mallear folds.

Middle story: area of the tympanic membrane and the tympanic opening of the auditory tube.

Lower story: hypotympanic recess extending to the jugular wall (floor) of the tympanic cavity.

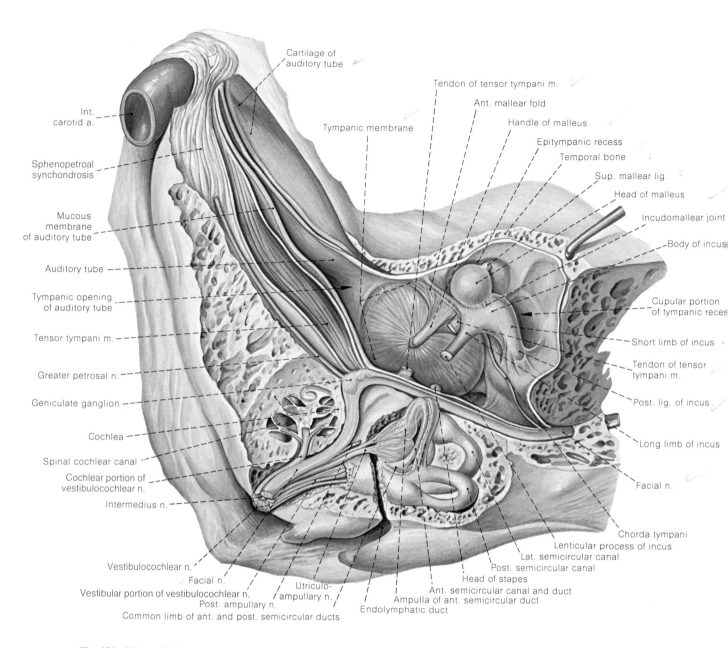

Int. carotid a.

Sphenopetroal synchondrosis

Mucous membrane of auditory tube

Auditory tube

Tympanic opening of auditory tube

Tensor tympani m.

Greater petrosal n.

Geniculate ganglion

Cochlea

Spinal cochlear canal

Cochlear portion of vestibulocochlear n.

Intermedius n.

Vestibulocochlear n.

Facial n.

Vestibular portion of vestibulocochlear n.

Post. ampullary n.

Common limb of ant. and post. semicircular ducts

Cartilage of auditory tube

Tympanic membrane

Tendon of tensor tympani m.

Ant. mallear fold

Handle of malleus

Epitympanic recess

Temporal bone

Sup. mallear lig.

Head of malleus

Incudomallear joint

Body of incus

Cupular portion of tympanic reces

Short limb of incus

Tendon of tensor tympani m.

Post. lig. of incus

Long limb of incus

Facial n.

Chorda tympani

Lenticular process of incus

Lat. semicircular canal

Post. semicircular canal

Head of stapes

Ant. semicircular canal and duct

Ampulla of ant. semicircular duct

Endolymphatic duct

Utriculo-ampullary n.

**Fig. 429.** Right middle and inner ear, survey preparation of a decalcified temporal bone. The tendon of the tensor tympani muscle has been cut and the joint between stapes and incus has been divided. Both halves of the preparation have been bent and pulled up and down in the arc of the section through the tympanic cavity. Note the course of the facial and vestibulocochlear nerves as well as the relationship of the labyrinth to the tympanic cavity and its walls.

NOTE: Curtailment of the motility of the middle ear ossicles leads to hearing impairment (hypacusis). In the condition, stapes ankylosis, the motility of the stapedial footplate within the oval window is impaired or completely blocked by newly formed bone (otosclerosis).

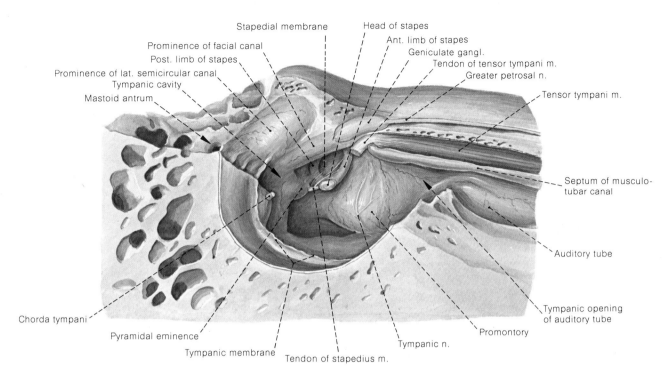

Stapedial membrane
Prominence of facial canal
Post. limb of stapes
Prominence of lat. semicircular canal
Tympanic cavity
Mastoid antrum
Head of stapes
Ant. limb of stapes
Geniculate gangl.
Tendon of tensor tympani m.
Greater petrosal n.
Tensor tympani m.
Septum of musculo-tubar canal
Auditory tube
Chorda tympani
Pyramidal eminence
Tympanic membrane
Tendon of stapedius m.
Tympanic n.
Promontory
Tympanic opening of auditory tube

**Fig. 430.** Medial (labyrinthine) wall of right tympanic cavity, lateral view. The lateral and superior wall of the tympanic cavity, malleus and incus as well as the major portion of the external auditory meatus have been removed. A small rim of tympanic membrane has been retained. The chorda tympani has been severed where it enters the tympanic cavity through the tympanic orifice of its canaliculus. The septum of the musculotubar canal has been partially cut off in order to expose the tensor tympani muscle, the tendon of which is sectioned close to the cochleariform process. The facial nerve has been exposed for a short distance near the geniculate ganglion, and the greater petrosal nerve was dissected where it emerges from the hiatus of the facial canal and enters the middle cranial fossa.

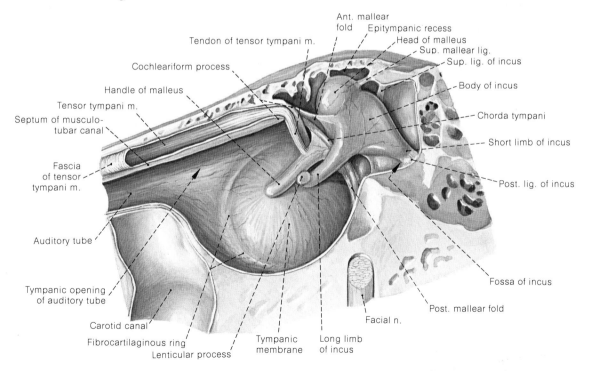

Tendon of tensor tympani m.
Cochleariform process
Handle of malleus
Tensor tympani m.
Septum of musculo-tubar canal
Fascia of tensor tympani m.
Auditory tube
Tympanic opening of auditory tube
Carotid canal
Fibrocartilaginous ring
Lenticular process
Ant. mallear fold
Epitympanic recess
Head of malleus
Sup. mallear lig.
Sup. lig. of incus
Body of incus
Chorda tympani
Short limb of incus
Post. lig. of incus
Fossa of incus
Post. mallear fold
Facial n.
Tympanic membrane
Long limb of incus

**Fig. 431.** Lateral (membranous) wall of the right tympanic cavity, medial view. The tensor tympani muscle is made visible by removal of the major portion of the septum of the musculotubar canal up to the cochleariform process. Note the insertion of the tendon of the muscle on the handle of the malleus and its course within a mucosal fold. The dense fascia surrounding the muscle has been partially retained.

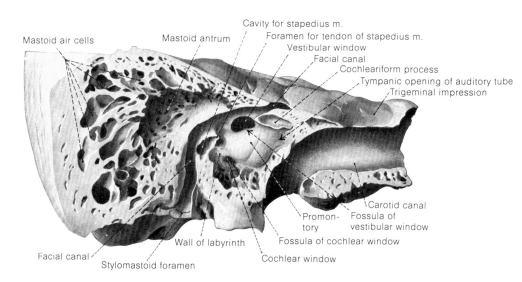

Mastoid air cells

Mastoid antrum

Cavity for stapedius m.

Foramen for tendon of stapedius m.

Vestibular window

Facial canal

Cochleariform process

Tympanic opening of auditory tube

Trigeminal impression

Carotid canal

Promontory

Fossula of vestibular window

Wall of labyrinth

Facial canal

Stylomastoid foramen

Fossula of cochlear window

Cochlear window

**Fig. 432.** Longitudinal section through the right petrous bone to demonstrate the labyrinthine wall of the tympanic cavity with the oval window. The facial and carotid canals are opened lengthwise. On the left are the mastoid air cells and their entry from the mastoid antrum.

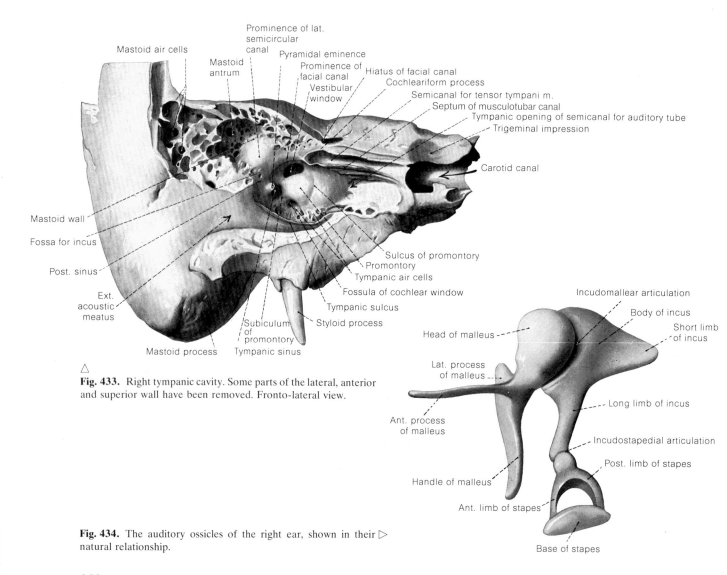

Mastoid air cells

Mastoid antrum

Prominence of lat. semicircular canal

Pyramidal eminence

Prominence of facial canal

Hiatus of facial canal

Cochleariform process

Vestibular window

Semicanal for tensor tympani m.

Septum of musculotubar canal

Tympanic opening of semicanal for auditory tube

Trigeminal impression

Carotid canal

Mastoid wall

Fossa for incus

Post. sinus

Ext. acoustic meatus

Mastoid process

Subiculum of promontory

Tympanic sinus

Styloid process

Tympanic sulcus

Fossula of cochlear window

Tympanic air cells

Promontory

Sulcus of promontory

**Fig. 433.** Right tympanic cavity. Some parts of the lateral, anterior and superior wall have been removed. Fronto-lateral view.

Incudomallear articulation

Body of incus

Short limb of incus

Head of malleus

Lat. process of malleus

Long limb of incus

Ant. process of malleus

Incudostapedial articulation

Post. limb of stapes

Handle of malleus

Ant. limb of stapes

Base of stapes

**Fig. 434.** The auditory ossicles of the right ear, shown in their ▷ natural relationship.

250

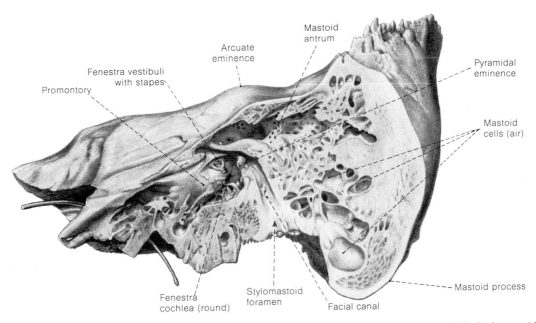

**Fig. 435.** Longitudinal section through the petrous bone. View of the labyrinthine wall with the promontory. Probe in the carotid canal. Note the extensive pneumatization of the mastoid process and the nearby bone.

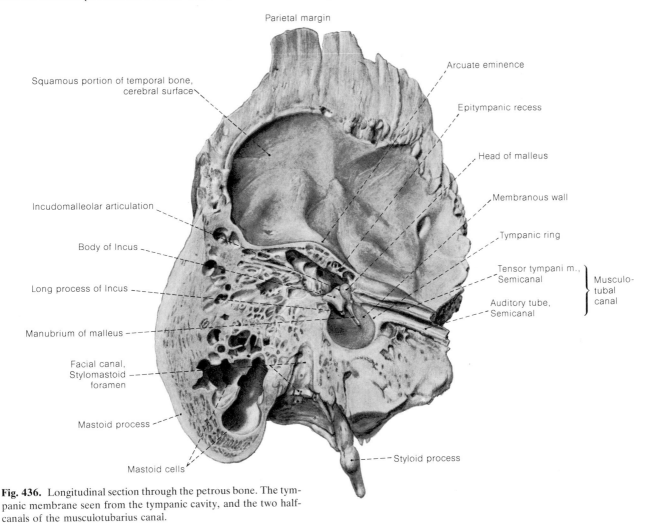

**Fig. 436.** Longitudinal section through the petrous bone. The tympanic membrane seen from the tympanic cavity, and the two half-canals of the musculotubarius canal.

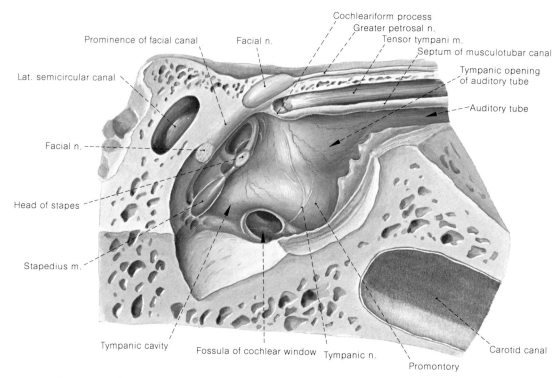

Cochleariform process
Greater petrosal n.
Tensor tympani m.
Septum of musculotubar canal

Prominence of facial canal

Facial n.

Tympanic opening
of auditory tube

Lat. semicircular canal

Auditory tube

Facial n.

Head of stapes

Stapedius m.

Tympanic cavity

Fossula of cochlear window

Tympanic n.

Promontory

Carotid canal

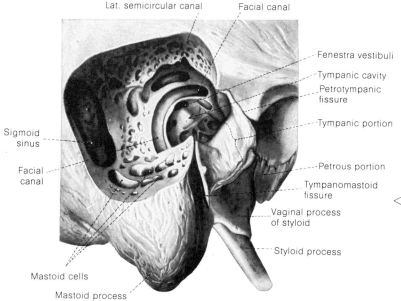

Lat. semicircular canal

Facial canal

Fenestra vestibuli

Tympanic cavity

Petrotympanic
fissure

Tympanic portion

Petrous portion

Tympanomastoid
fissure

Vaginal process
of styloid

Styloid process

Sigmoid
sinus

Facial
canal

Mastoid cells

Mastoid process

**Fig. 437.** Medial (labyrinthine) wall of the right tympanic cavity, lateral view. The posterior wall of the tympanic cavity has been partially removed, the stapedius muscle has been partially exposed by removal of the bony wall of the pyramidal eminence. The lower portion of the facial canal has been removed; the lateral semicircular canal and the carotid canal have been opened.

◁ **Fig. 438.** Right temporal bone. Opened and dissected from lateral side, revealing the inner space with the relative positions between the sigmoid sinus, facial canal, and bony configuration of the organs of equilibrium and hearing.

## The boundaries of the tympanic cavity with reference to their clinical significance (after O. GROSSER)

| Name | Constituents | Neighboring organs | Peculiarities | Clinical complications |
|------|-------------|-------------------|---------------|----------------------|
| roof | epitympanic recess, tegmen tympani of temporal bone, petrosquamous suture | middle cranial fossa, meninges, temporal lobe of telencephalon | vascular channels in the roof and suture: route for infections | meningitis, abscess of temporal lobe |
| floor | floor of tympanic cavity, jugular air cells, styloid prominence | jugular fossa, superior bulb of jugular vein | variable form and size of air cells, bony lamina may be partially absent | septic thrombosis of internal jugular vein → pyemia |

**Fig. 439.** Intracranial extent of facial nerve. Facial canal ▷ and tympanic cavity have been opened form behind.

**Fig. 440.** Intracranial course of the facial nerve and its connections, projected onto the temporal bone. ▽

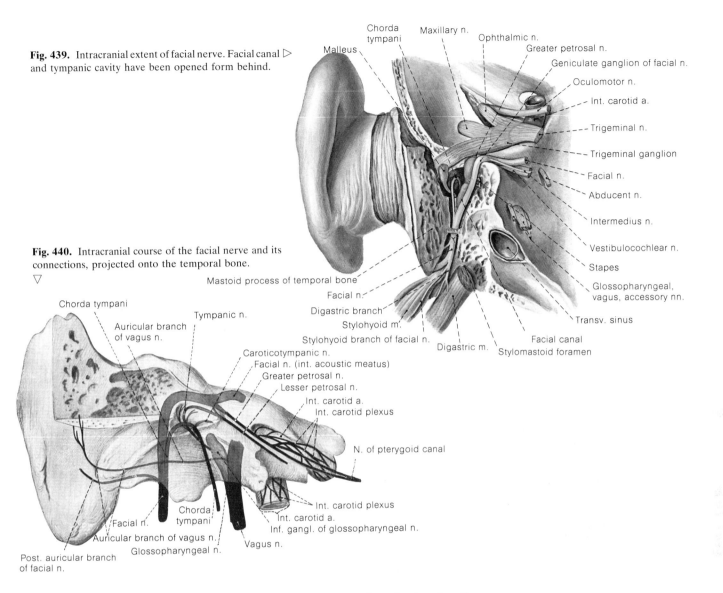

Chorda tympani
Maxillary n.
Ophthalmic n.
Greater petrosal n.
Geniculate ganglion of facial n.
Oculomotor n.
Int. carotid a.
Trigeminal n.
Trigeminal ganglion
Facial n.
Abducent n.
Intermedius n.
Vestibulocochlear n.
Stapes
Glossopharyngeal, vagus, accessory nn.
Transv. sinus
Facial canal
Stylomastoid foramen
Malleus

Mastoid process of temporal bone
Facial n.
Digastric branch
Stylohyoid m.
Stylohyoid branch of facial n.
Caroticotympanic n.
Facial n. (int. acoustic meatus)
Greater petrosal n.
Lesser petrosal n.
Int. carotid a.
Int. carotid plexus
N. of pterygoid canal
Digastric m.

Chorda tympani
Auricular branch of vagus n.
Tympanic n.
Int. carotid plexus
Int. carotid a.
Inf. gangl. of glossopharyngeal n.
Facial n.
Chorda tympani
Auricular branch of vagus n.
Glossopharyngeal n.
Vagus n.
Post. auricular branch of facial n.

**The boundaries of the tympanic cavity** *(continued)*

| Name | Constituents | Neighboring organs | Pecularities | Clinical complications |
|---|---|---|---|---|
| medial (labyrinthine) wall | promontory, oval and round window, prominence of facial canal, tympanic nervous plexus | membranous labyrinth, facial nerve | — | infections of the labyrinth (deafness), facial paresis |
| lateral (membranous) wall | tympanic membrane, manubrium of malleus, (chorda tympani) | external acoustic meatus | — | perforation of tympanic membrane |
| posterior (mastoid) wall | mastoid antrum, mastoid air cells, prominence of lat. semicircular canal, facial canal | facial nerve, sigmoid sinus, posterior cranial fossa, cerebellum | variable pneumatization of the mastoid process | sinus thrombosis, meningitis, cerebellar abscess, facial paresis |
| anterior (carotid) wall | tympanic opening of auditory tube, musculo-tubular canal | carotid canal, cavernous sinus, abducent nerve, trigeminal ganglion | apical pneumatization of the pyramid | auditory tube as route for infections, infection of apical air cells, abducent paresis |

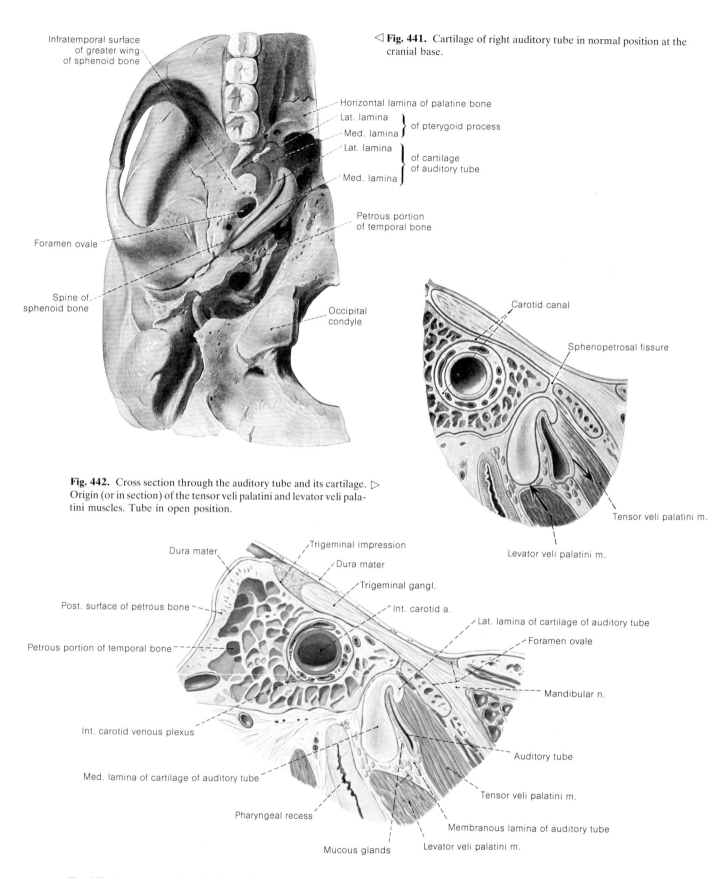

Infratemporal surface of greater wing of sphenoid bone

Horizontal lamina of palatine bone

Lat. lamina
Med. lamina } of pterygoid process

Lat. lamina
Med. lamina } of cartilage of auditory tube

Petrous portion of temporal bone

Foramen ovale

Spine of sphenoid bone

Occipital condyle

◁ **Fig. 441.** Cartilage of right auditory tube in normal position at the cranial base.

Carotid canal

Sphenopetrosal fissure

Tensor veli palatini m.

Levator veli palatini m.

**Fig. 442.** Cross section through the auditory tube and its cartilage. ▷ Origin (or in section) of the tensor veli palatini and levator veli palatini muscles. Tube in open position.

Dura mater

Trigeminal impression

Dura mater

Post. surface of petrous bone

Trigeminal gangl.

Int. carotid a.

Petrous portion of temporal bone

Lat. lamina of cartilage of auditory tube

Foramen ovale

Mandibular n.

Int. carotid venous plexus

Auditory tube

Med. lamina of cartilage of auditory tube

Tensor veli palatini m.

Pharyngeal recess

Membranous lamina of auditory tube

Mucous glands

Levator veli palatini m.

**Fig. 443.** Cross section through the cartilaginous portion of the left auditory tube near the pharyngeal opening. Tube in closed position.

254

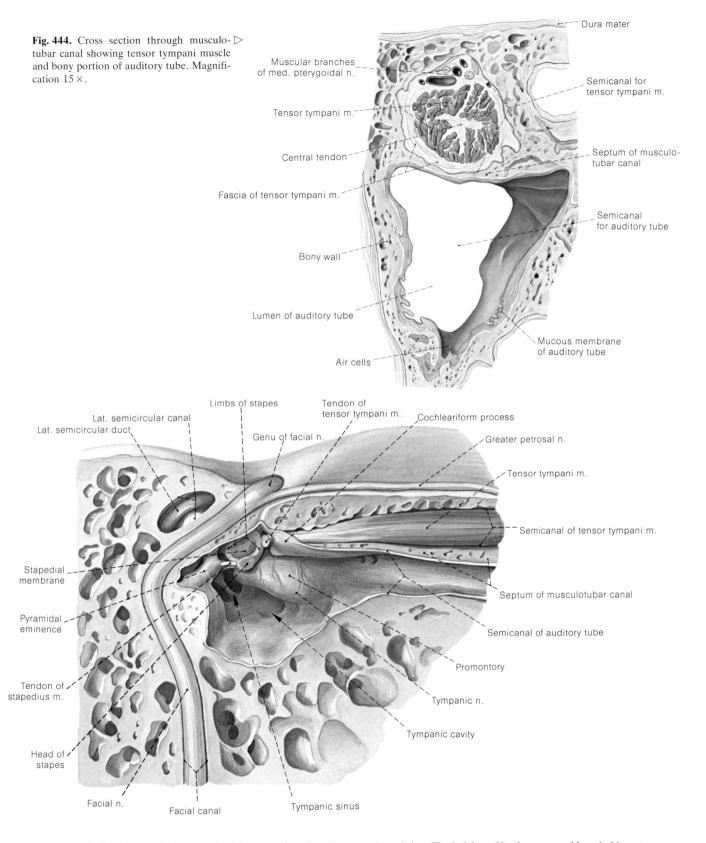

**Fig. 444.** Cross section through musculo-▷ tubar canal showing tensor tympani muscle and bony portion of auditory tube. Magnification 15 ×.

Dura mater

Muscular branches of med. pterygoidal n.

Semicanal for tensor tympani m.

Tensor tympani m.

Central tendon

Septum of musculotubar canal

Fascia of tensor tympani m.

Semicanal for auditory tube

Bony wall

Lumen of auditory tube

Mucous membrane of auditory tube

Air cells

Limbs of stapes

Tendon of tensor tympani m.

Cochleariform process

Lat. semicircular canal

Lat. semicircular duct

Genu of facial n.

Greater petrosal n.

Tensor tympani m.

Semicanal of tensor tympani m.

Stapedial membrane

Septum of musculotubar canal

Pyramidal eminence

Semicanal of auditory tube

Promontory

Tendon of stapedius m.

Tympanic n.

Tympanic cavity

Head of stapes

Facial n.

Facial canal

Tympanic sinus

**Fig. 445.** Medial (labyrinthine) wall of the right tympanic cavity with stapes, lateral view. The facial canal has been opened from its hiatus to near the stylomastoid foramen in order to expose the facial nerve. The tympanic cavity has been divided by a section approximately parallel to the long axis of the petrous bone; the lateral wall including tympanic membrane, malleus and incus have been removed. The tendon of the tensor tympani muscle has been cut off near the cochleariform process; the musculotubar canal has been opened.

255

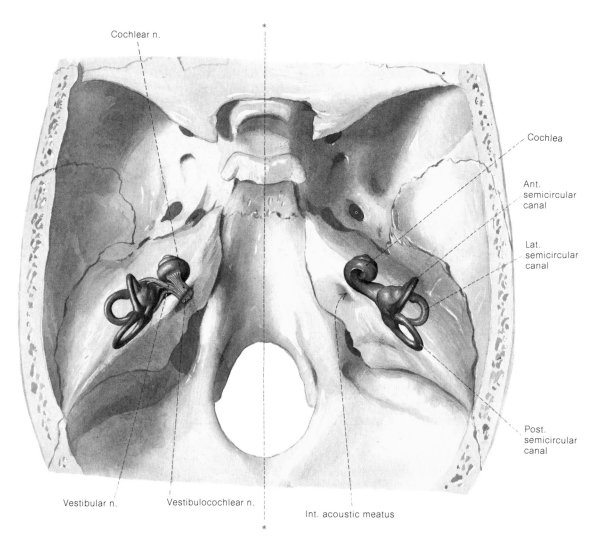

Cochlear n.

Cochlea

Ant. semicircular canal

Lat. semicircular canal

Post. semicircular canal

Vestibular n.

Vestibulocochlear n.

Int. acoustic meatus

**Fig. 446.** Phantom view of osseous labyrinths in natural position projected onto the inside of the cranial base with nerve supply on the left. Note the oblique orientation of the cochlear axis. The cochlea points in the lateral anterior caudal direction. * = median line.

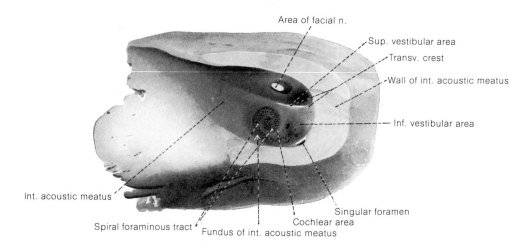

Area of facial n.

Sup. vestibular area

Transv. crest

Wall of int. acoustic meatus

Inf. vestibular area

Int. acoustic meatus

Singular foramen

Spiral foraminous tract

Cochlear area

Fundus of int. acoustic meatus

**Fig. 447.** The right internal acoustic meatus after partial removal of its posterior wall. Note the beginning of the facial canal at a right angle from the axis of the pyramid (area of facial nerve).

256

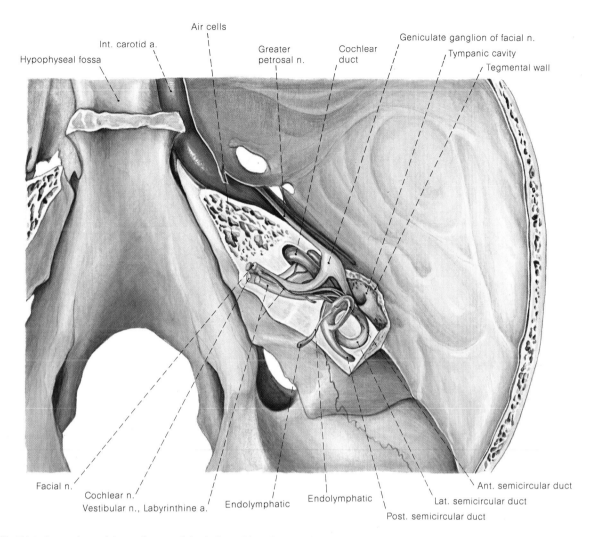

Hypophyseal fossa

Int. carotid a.

Air cells

Greater
petrosal n.

Cochlear
duct

Geniculate ganglion of facial n.

Tympanic cavity

Tegmental wall

Facial n.

Cochlear n.

Vestibular n., Labyrinthine a.

Endolymphatic

Endolymphatic

Post. semicircular duct

Lat. semicircular duct

Ant. semicircular duct

**Fig. 448.** Right internal ear with membranous labyrinth, cochlear duct, vestibulocochlear nerve and facial nerve within the petrous part of temporal bone. The upper portion of the petrous bone has been removed. (From PERNKOPF: Atlas der topographischen und angewandten Anatomie des Menschen, Vol. 1, 2nd ed. [Ed. H. FERNER]. Urban & Schwarzenberg, Munich–Vienna–Baltimore 1980.)

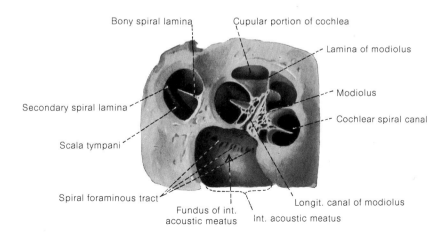

Bony spiral lamina

Cupular portion of cochlea

Lamina of modiolus

Secondary spiral lamina

Modiolus

Cochlear spiral canal

Scala tympani

Spiral foraminous tract

Fundus of int.
acoustic meatus

Int. acoustic meatus

Longit. canal of modiolus

**Fig. 449.** Left bony cochlea sectioned along the axis of the modiolus.

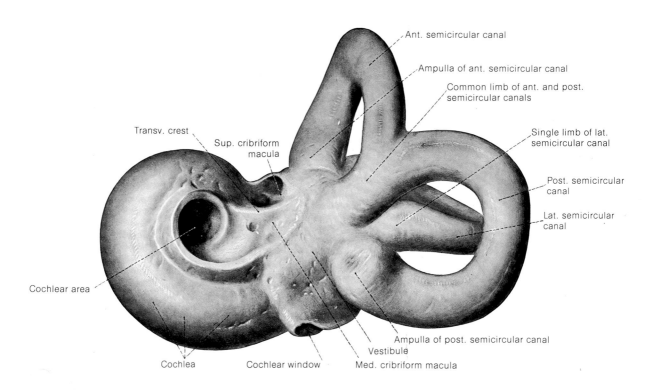

Ant. semicircular canal

Ampulla of ant. semicircular canal

Common limb of ant. and post. semicircular canals

Single limb of lat. semicircular canal

Post. semicircular canal

Lat. semicircular canal

Transv. crest

Sup. cribriform macula

Cochlear area

Cochlea

Cochlear window

Ampulla of post. semicircular canal

Vestibule

Med. cribriform macula

**Fig. 450.** Right bony labyrinth, seen from medial and behind. Carved out of the petrous bone. The cavities are surrounded by cortical bone.

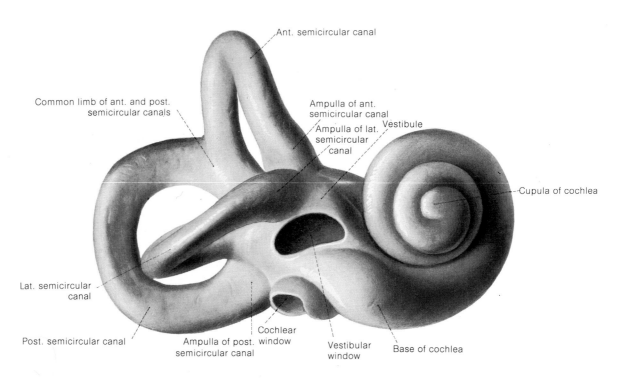

Ant. semicircular canal

Common limb of ant. and post. semicircular canals

Ampulla of ant. semicircular canal

Ampulla of lat. semicircular canal

Vestibule

Cupula of cochlea

Lat. semicircular canal

Post. semicircular canal

Ampulla of post. semicircular canal

Cochlear window

Vestibular window

Base of cochlea

**Fig. 451.** Right bony labyrinth, carved out of the petrous bone; antero-lateral view.

258

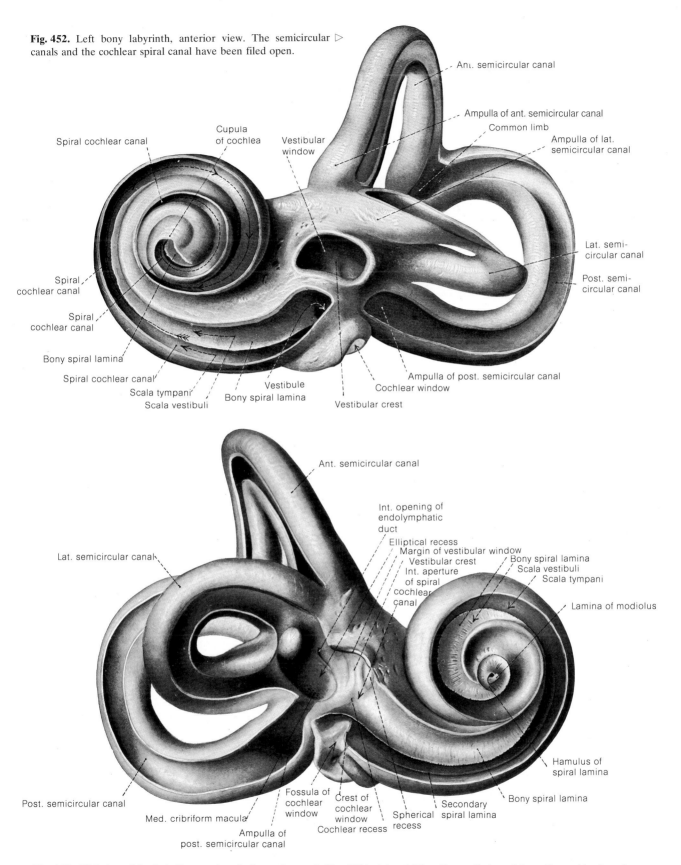

**Fig. 452.** Left bony labyrinth, anterior view. The semicircular ▷ canals and the cochlear spiral canal have been filed open.

Ant. semicircular canal

Ampulla of ant. semicircular canal

Common limb

Ampulla of lat. semicircular canal

Cupula of cochlea

Spiral cochlear canal

Vestibular window

Lat. semicircular canal

Post. semicircular canal

Spiral cochlear canal

Spiral cochlear canal

Bony spiral lamina

Spiral cochlear canal

Scala tympani

Scala vestibuli

Vestibule

Bony spiral lamina

Vestibular crest

Cochlear window

Ampulla of post. semicircular canal

Ant. semicircular canal

Int. opening of endolymphatic duct

Elliptical recess

Margin of vestibular window

Vestibular crest

Int. aperture of spiral cochlear canal

Bony spiral lamina

Scala vestibuli

Scala tympani

Lamina of modiolus

Lat. semicircular canal

Hamulus of spiral lamina

Bony spiral lamina

Secondary spiral lamina

Post. semicircular canal

Med. cribriform macula

Fossula of cochlear window

Crest of cochlear window

Spherical recess

Ampulla of post. semicircular canal

Cochlear recess

**Fig. 453.** Right bony labyrinth. Preparation similar to the one in Fig. 452 but, in addition, the vestibule and the entire cochlea have been filed open.

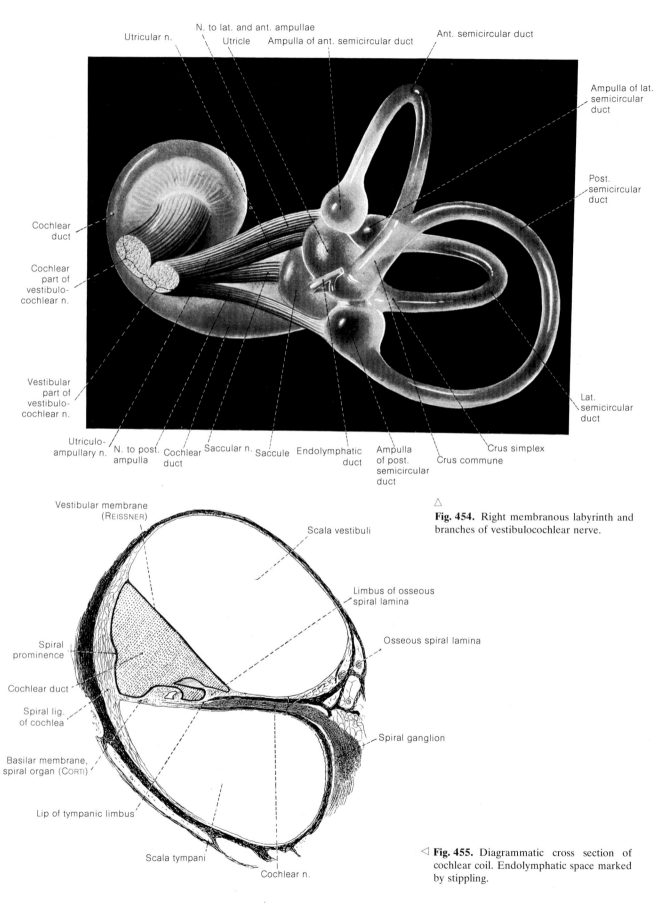

Utricular n.

N. to lat. and ant. ampullae

Utricle    Ampulla of ant. semicircular duct

Ant. semicircular duct

Ampulla of lat. semicircular duct

Post. semicircular duct

Cochlear duct

Cochlear part of vestibulocochlear n.

Vestibular part of vestibulocochlear n.

Lat. semicircular duct

Utriculoampullary n.    N. to post. ampulla    Cochlear duct    Saccular n.    Saccule    Endolymphatic duct    Ampulla of post. semicircular duct    Crus commune    Crus simplex

**Fig. 454.** Right membranous labyrinth and branches of vestibulocochlear nerve.

Vestibular membrane (REISSNER)

Scala vestibuli

Limbus of osseous spiral lamina

Osseous spiral lamina

Spiral prominence

Cochlear duct

Spiral lig. of cochlea

Spiral ganglion

Basilar membrane, spiral organ (CORTI)

Lip of tympanic limbus

Scala tympani

Cochlear n.

◁ **Fig. 455.** Diagrammatic cross section of cochlear coil. Endolymphatic space marked by stippling.

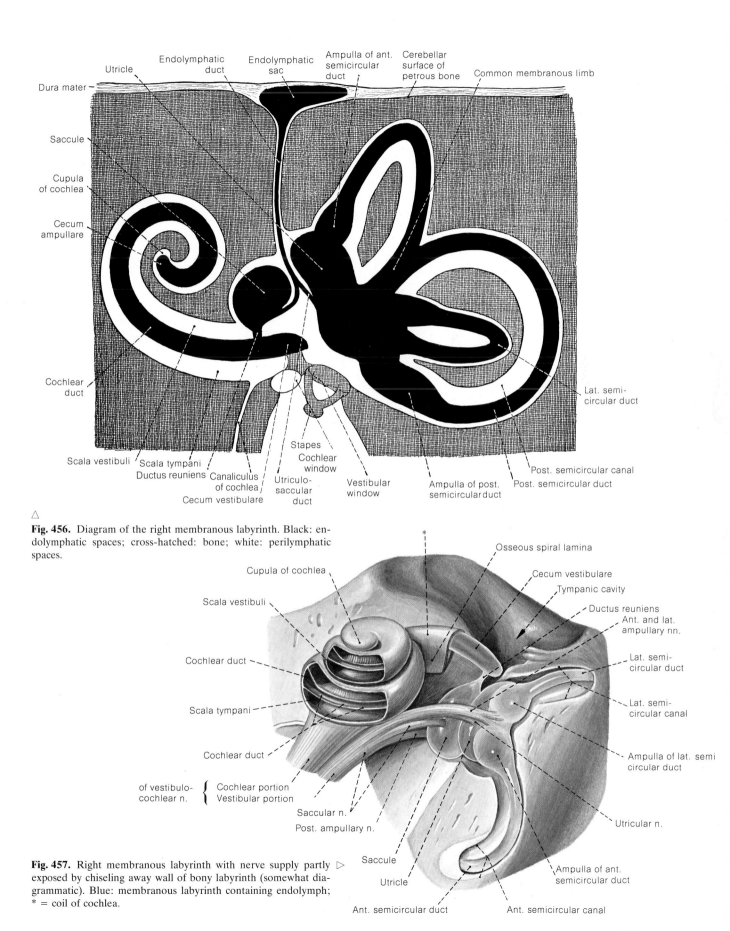

**Fig. 456.** Diagram of the right membranous labyrinth. Black: endolymphatic spaces; cross-hatched: bone; white: perilymphatic spaces.

Labels for Fig. 456:
Dura mater
Utricle
Endolymphatic duct
Endolymphatic sac
Ampulla of ant. semicircular duct
Cerebellar surface of petrous bone
Common membranous limb
Saccule
Cupula of cochlea
Cecum ampullare
Cochlear duct
Lat. semicircular duct
Scala vestibuli
Scala tympani
Ductus reuniens
Canaliculus of cochlea
Cecum vestibulare
Utriculo-saccular duct
Stapes
Cochlear window
Vestibular window
Ampulla of post. semicircular duct
Post. semicircular canal
Post. semicircular duct

**Fig. 457.** Right membranous labyrinth with nerve supply partly ▷ exposed by chiseling away wall of bony labyrinth (somewhat diagrammatic). Blue: membranous labyrinth containing endolymph; * = coil of cochlea.

Labels for Fig. 457:
Osseous spiral lamina
Cecum vestibulare
Tympanic cavity
Ductus reuniens
Ant. and lat. ampullary nn.
Cupula of cochlea
Scala vestibuli
Cochlear duct
Lat. semicircular duct
Lat. semicircular canal
Scala tympani
Ampulla of lat. semi circular duct
Cochlear duct
of vestibulo-cochlear n. { Cochlear portion / Vestibular portion
Saccular n.
Post. ampullary n.
Utricular n.
Saccule
Utricle
Ampulla of ant. semicircular duct
Ant. semicircular duct
Ant. semicircular canal

261

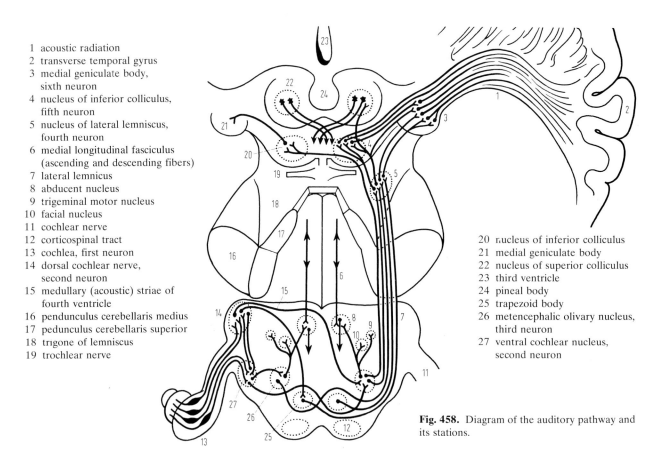

1  acoustic radiation
2  transverse temporal gyrus
3  medial geniculate body,
   sixth neuron
4  nucleus of inferior colliculus,
   fifth neuron
5  nucleus of lateral lemniscus,
   fourth neuron
6  medial longitudinal fasciculus
   (ascending and descending fibers)
7  lateral lemnicus
8  abducent nucleus
9  trigeminal motor nucleus
10 facial nucleus
11 cochlear nerve
12 corticospinal tract
13 cochlea, first neuron
14 dorsal cochlear nerve,
   second neuron
15 medullary (acoustic) striae of
   fourth ventricle
16 pedunculus cerebellaris medius
17 pedunculus cerebellaris superior
18 trigone of lemniscus
19 trochlear nerve

20 nucleus of inferior colliculus
21 medial geniculate body
22 nucleus of superior colliculus
23 third ventricle
24 pineal body
25 trapezoid body
26 metencephalic olivary nucleus,
   third neuron
27 ventral cochlear nucleus,
   second neuron

**Fig. 458.** Diagram of the auditory pathway and its stations.

## Auditory Pathway

The basilar lamina of the organ of CORTI bears the auditory receptor cells. They are surrounded by supporting cells. The receptor cells are capable of responding to frequencies from about 16 Hz to 21 000 Hz. They are arranged in three to four rows of outer hair cells and one row of inner hair cells on both sides of the inner tunnel space.

Neurons

1.  The hair cells are contacted by the peripheral extensions of neurons of the *spinal ganglion* of the *cochlea*. Their central extensions form the *cochlear portion* of the *vestibulocochlear nerve* which runs to the
    ↓

2.  *dorsal cochlear nucleus* ⟵⟶ *ventral cochlear nucleus* (lateral region of the rhombic fossa)
    ↓

3.  { *superior olivary nucleus* ⟶ *med. longit. fasciculus* and *motor nuclei of trigeminal, abducent and facial nerves*
    ↓
    { *nucleus of trapezoid body*
    ↓
    *lateral leminiscus* with
    ↓

4.  *nucleus of lateral lemniscus* ⟶ *superior colliculus*
    ↓

5.  *nucleus of inferior colliculus*
    ↓

6.  *medial geniculate body*
    ↓

*acoustic radiation.* Through sublenticular portion of the posterior limb of the internal capsule

cortical auditory center, *transverse temporal gyri* and parts of the *superior temporal gyrus.*

**Fig. 459.** Head, neck, and upper thorax, showing triangles of the neck. The facial muscles for expression and part of the muscles of mastica- ▷ tion, cervical muscles, the Deltoid, Pectoralis major, carotid triangle, and brachial plexus. The lower part of the parotid gland is pulled forward with a hook.

# Neck and Nucha

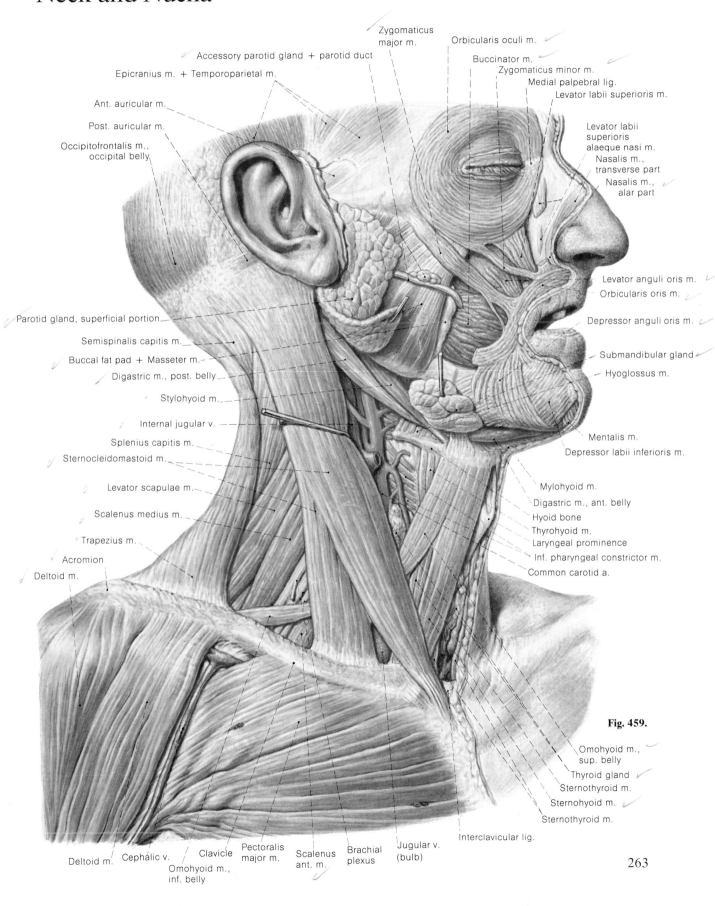

Zygomaticus major m.

Orbicularis oculi m.

Accessory parotid gland + parotid duct

Buccinator m.

Zygomaticus minor m.

Epicranius m. + Temporoparietal m.

Medial palpebral lig.

Levator labii superioris m.

Ant. auricular m.

Levator labii superioris alaeque nasi m.

Post. auricular m.

Nasalis m., transverse part

Occipitofrontalis m., occipital belly

Nasalis m., alar part

Levator anguli oris m.

Orbicularis oris m.

Parotid gland, superficial portion

Depressor anguli oris m.

Semispinalis capitis m.

Submandibular gland

Buccal fat pad + Masseter m.

Hyoglossus m.

Digastric m., post. belly

Stylohyoid m.

Internal jugular v.

Mentalis m.

Splenius capitis m.

Depressor labii inferioris m.

Sternocleidomastoid m.

Mylohyoid m.

Levator scapulae m.

Digastric m., ant. belly

Hyoid bone

Scalenus medius m.

Thyrohyoid m.

Laryngeal prominence

Trapezius m.

Inf. pharyngeal constrictor m.

Acromion

Common carotid a.

Deltoid m.

**Fig. 459.**

Omohyoid m., sup. belly

Thyroid gland

Sternothyroid m.

Sternohyoid m.

Sternothyroid m.

Interclavicular lig.

Deltoid m.    Cephalic v.    Clavicle    Pectoralis major m.    Scalenus ant. m.    Brachial plexus    Jugular v. (bulb)

Omohyoid m., inf. belly

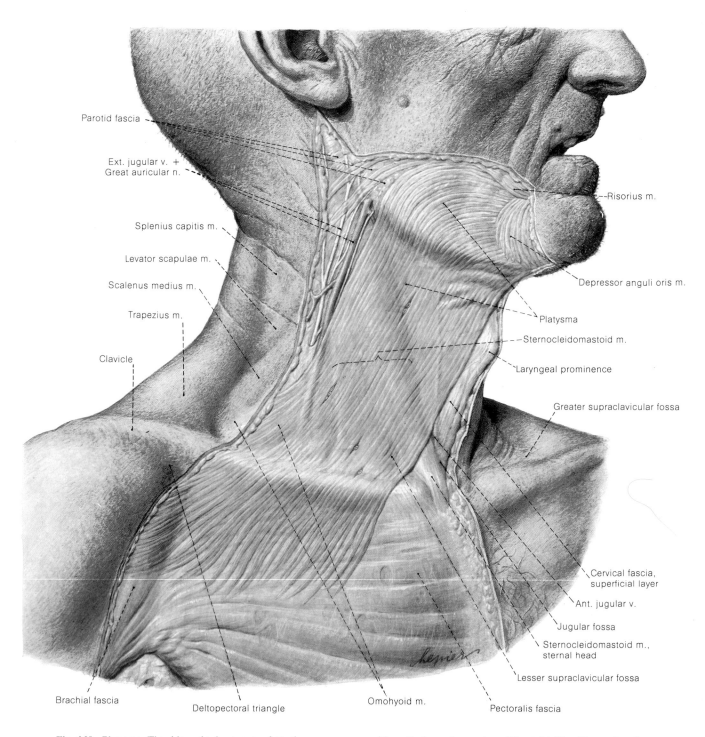

Parotid fascia

Ext. jugular v. +
Great auricular n.

Splenius capitis m.

Levator scapulae m.

Scalenus medius m.

Trapezius m.

Clavicle

Risorius m.

Depressor anguli oris m.

Platysma

Sternocleidomastoid m.

Laryngeal prominence

Greater supraclavicular fossa

Cervical fascia,
superficial layer

Ant. jugular v.

Jugular fossa

Sternocleidomastoid m.,
sternal head

Lesser supraclavicular fossa

Brachial fascia

Deltopectoral triangle

Omohyoid m.

Pectoralis fascia

**Fig. 460.** Platysma. The skin and subcutaneous fatty tissue were removed from the lower jaw region of the right side of the neck and upper thorax.

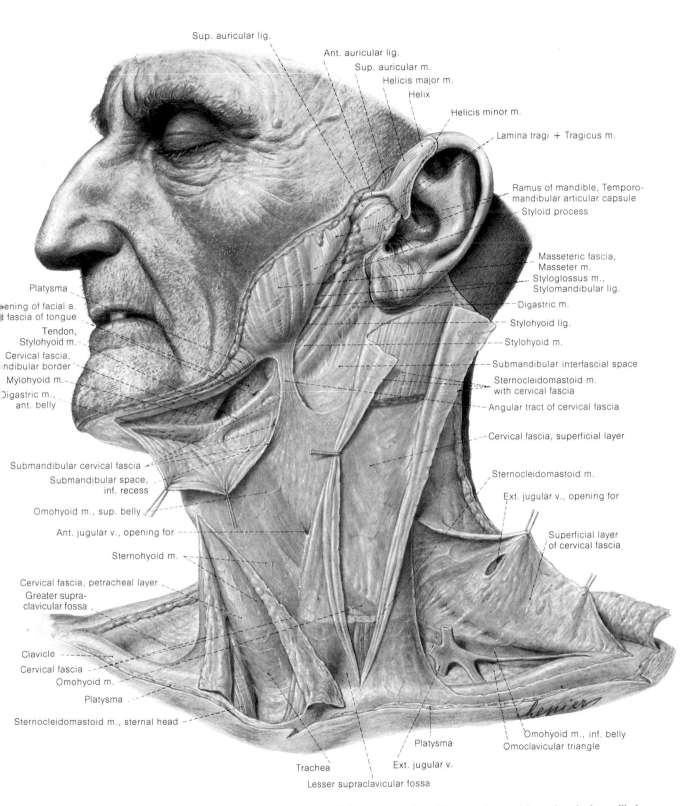

Sup. auricular lig.

Ant. auricular lig.

Sup. auricular m.

Helicis major m.

Helix

Helicis minor m.

Lamina tragi + Tragicus m.

Ramus of mandible, Temporomandibular articular capsule

Styloid process

Masseteric fascia,
Masseter m.

Styloglossus m.,
Stylomandibular lig.

Digastric m.

Stylohyoid lig.

Stylohyoid m.

Submandibular interfascial space

Sternocleidomastoid m.
with cervical fascia

Angular tract of cervical fascia

Cervical fascia, superficial layer

Sternocleidomastoid m.

Ext. jugular v., opening for

Superficial layer
of cervical fascia

Platysma

ening of facial a.
l fascia of tongue

Tendon,
Stylohyoid m.

Cervical fascia,
ndibular border

Mylohyoid m.

Digastric m.,
ant. belly

Submandibular cervical fascia

Submandibular space,
inf. recess

Omohyoid m., sup. belly

Ant. jugular v., opening for

Sternohyoid m.

Cervical fascia, petracheal layer

Greater supra-
clavicular fossa

Clavicle

Cervical fascia

Omohyoid m.

Platysma

Sternocleidomastoid m., sternal head

Omohyoid m., inf. belly
Omoclavicular triangle

Platysma

Trachea

Ext. jugular v.

Lesser supraclavicular fossa

**Fig. 461.** The cervical fascia and the exposed areas after the removal of a greater portion of the musculature of the neck and submandibular region, including the vessels and nerves. Ventrolateral view.

265

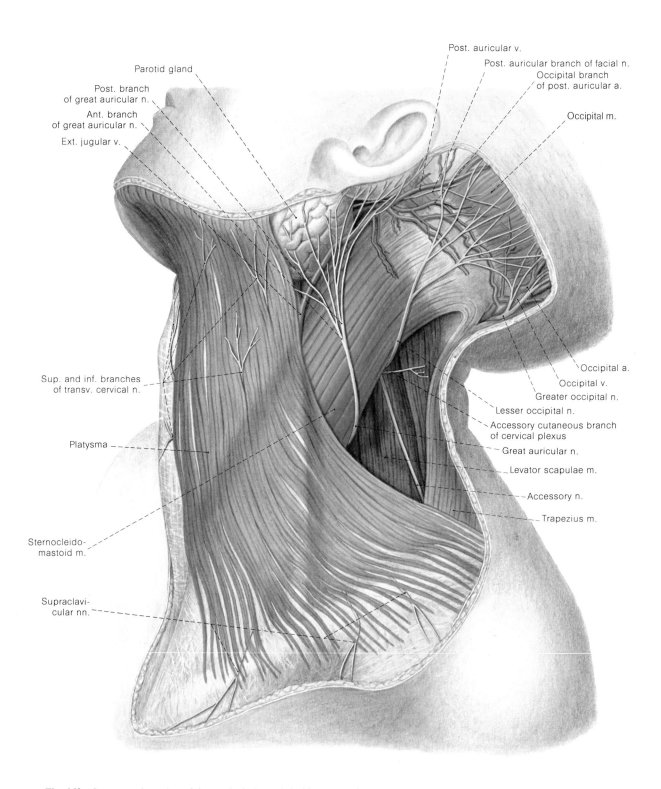

Parotid gland

Post. auricular v.

Post. auricular branch of facial n.

Occipital branch
of post. auricular a.

Post. branch
of great auricular n.

Ant. branch
of great auricular n.

Occipital m.

Ext. jugular v.

Sup. and inf. branches
of transv. cervical n.

Occipital a.

Occipital v.

Greater occipital n.

Lesser occipital n.

Accessory cutaneous branch
of cervical plexus

Platysma

Great auricular n.

Levator scapulae m.

Accessory n.

Trapezius m.

Sternocleido-
mastoid m.

Supraclavi-
cular nn.

**Fig. 462.** Cutaneous branches of the cervical plexus, left side. That point at the posterior margin of the sternocleidomastoid muscle at the level of the third cervical vertebra where the cutaneous nerves of the cervical plexus exit is designated as punctum nervosum.

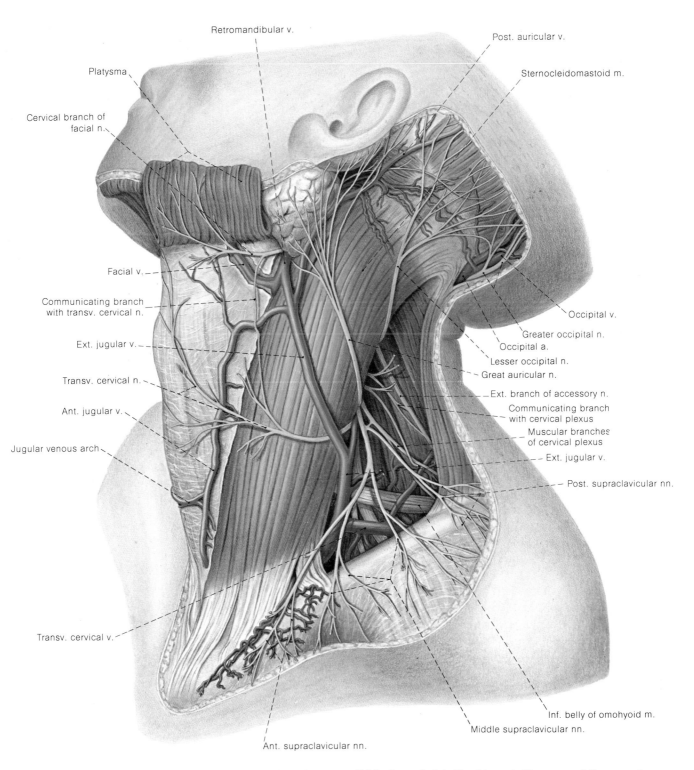

Retromandibular v.

Post. auricular v.

Platysma

Sternocleidomastoid m.

Cervical branch of
facial n.

Facial v.

Communicating branch
with transv. cervical n.

Occipital v.

Ext. jugular v.

Greater occipital n.
Occipital a.

Transv. cervical n.

Lesser occipital n.
Great auricular n.

Ant. jugular v.

Ext. branch of accessory n.
Communicating branch
with cervical plexus
Muscular branches
of cervical plexus

Jugular venous arch

Ext. jugular v.

Post. supraclavicular nn.

Transv. cervical v.

Inf. belly of omohyoid m.
Middle supraclavicular nn.

Ant. supraclavicular nn.

**Fig. 463.** Cutaneous and muscular branches of the cervical plexus, superficial veins on the left side of the neck. Platysma partially removed, its upper portion reflected upward. Superficial lamina of cervical fascia anterior to the sternocleidomastoid muscle has been retained and split along the facial vein.

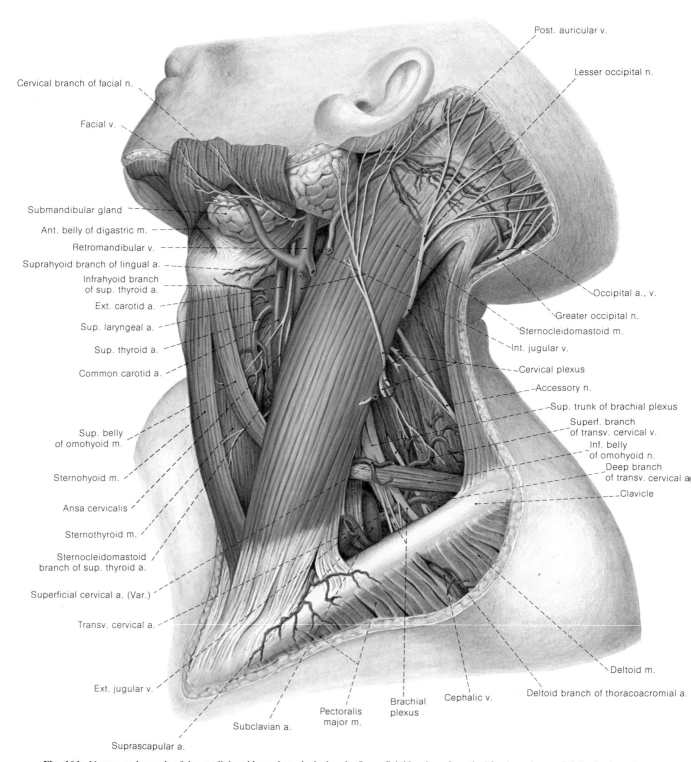

**Fig. 464.** Nerves and vessels of the medial and lateral cervical triangle. Superficial lamina of cervical fascia and superficial veins have been removed.

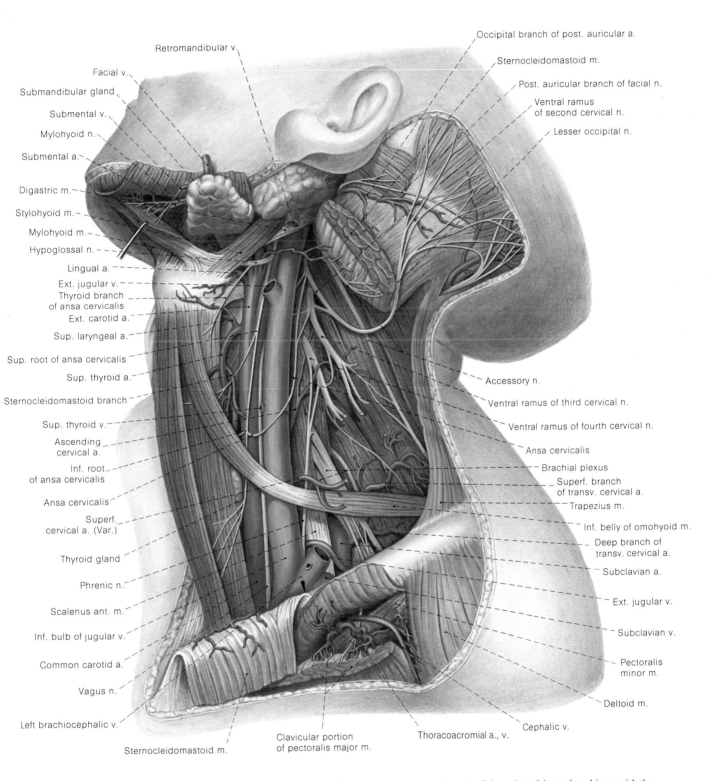

Retromandibular v.
Occipital branch of post. auricular a.
Sternocleidomastoid m.
Facial v.
Post. auricular branch of facial n.
Submandibular gland
Ventral ramus of second cervical n.
Submental v.
Mylohyoid n.
Lesser occipital n.
Submental a.
Digastric m.
Stylohyoid m.
Mylohyoid m.
Hypoglossal n.
Lingual a.
Ext. jugular v.
Thyroid branch of ansa cervicalis
Ext. carotid a.
Sup. laryngeal a.
Sup. root of ansa cervicalis
Accessory n.
Sup. thyroid a.
Ventral ramus of third cervical n.
Sternocleidomastoid branch
Ventral ramus of fourth cervical n.
Sup. thyroid v.
Ansa cervicalis
Ascending cervical a.
Inf. root of ansa cervicalis
Brachial plexus
Ansa cervicalis
Superf. branch of transv. cervical a.
Superf. cervical a. (Var.)
Trapezius m.
Thyroid gland
Inf. belly of omohyoid m.
Deep branch of transv. cervical a.
Phrenic n.
Subclavian a.
Scalenus ant. m.
Ext. jugular v.
Inf. bulb of jugular v.
Subclavian v.
Common carotid a.
Pectoralis minor m.
Vagus n.
Deltoid m.
Left brachiocephalic v.
Cephalic v.
Sternocleidomastoid m.
Clavicular portion of pectoralis major m.
Thoracoacromial a., v.

**Fig. 465.** The deep layer of the left cervical region after removal of the sternocleidomastoid muscle. Dissection of the scalene hiatus with the subclavian vessels und the cervical plexus.

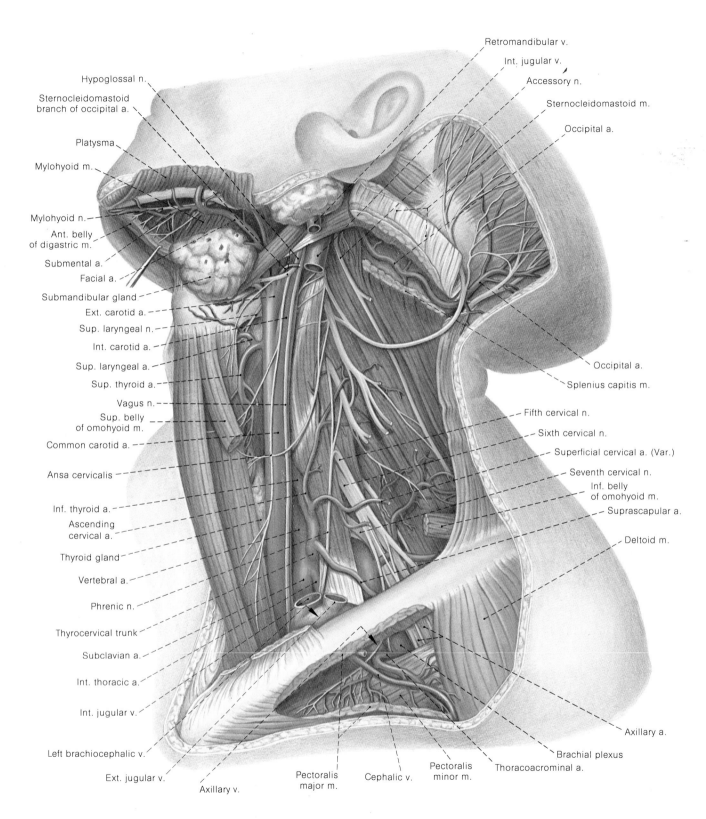

**Fig. 466.** Intermediate layer of nerves and arteries of the left side of the neck in the area of the deltoideopectoral triangle.

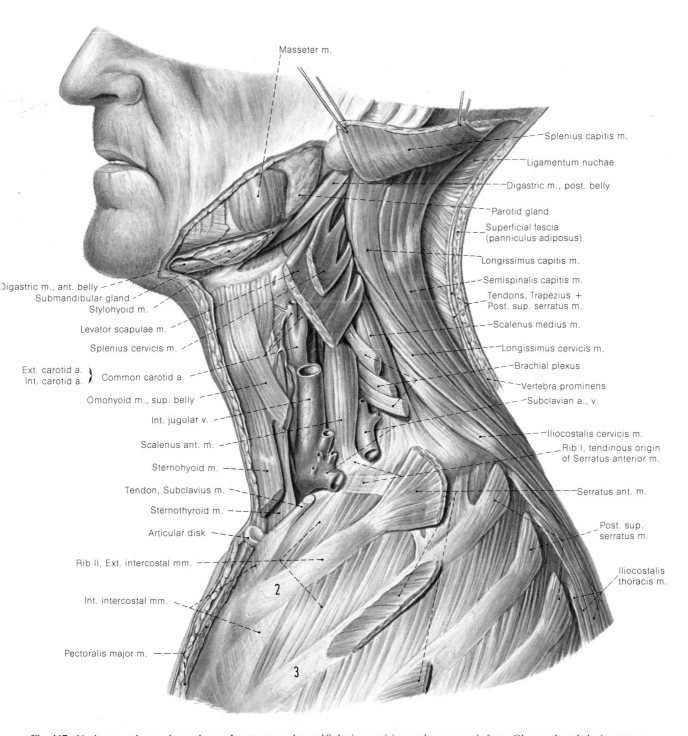

Masseter m.

Splenius capitis m.

Ligamentum nuchae

Digastric m., post. belly

Parotid gland

Superficial fascia
(panniculus adiposus)

Longissimus capitis m.

Semispinalis capitis m.

Tendons, Trapezius +
Post. sup. serratus m.

Scalenus medius m.

Longissimus cervicis m.

Brachial plexus

Vertebra prominens

Subclavian a., v.

Iliocostalis cervicis m.

Rib I, tendinous origin
of Serratus anterior m.

Serratus ant. m.

Post. sup.
serratus m.

Iliocostalis
thoracis m.

Digastric m., ant. belly
Submandibular gland
Stylohyoid m.

Levator scapulae m.

Splenius cervicis m.

Ext. carotid a.
Int. carotid a. } Common carotid a.

Omohyoid m., sup. belly

Int. jugular v.

Scalenus ant. m.

Sternohyoid m.

Tendon, Subclavius m.

Sternothyroid m.

Articular disk

Rib II, Ext. intercostal mm.

Int. intercostal mm.

Pectoralis major m.

2

3

**Fig. 467.** Neck, upper thorax, deeper layers. Levator scapulae and Splenius cervicis muscles were cut in front. Observe the subclavian artery and brachial plexus in the scalene hiatus.

**The Suprahyoid Muscles***

| Name | Origin | Insertion |
|---|---|---|
| **1. Digastric muscle**<br>Divided into 2 bellies by a tendon. These are fastened through a short tendon to the margin of the hyoid bone | Mastoid notch of temporal bone (posterior belly) | Digastric fossa of mandible (anterior belly) |
| *Nerve:*   Anterior belly: mylohyoid nerve. Posterior belly: facial nerve | | |
| *Function:*   Opens jaws (depresses lower jaw); elevates (fixes) the hyoid bone | | |
| **2. Stylohyoid muscle**<br>Passes on either side of tendon of the Digastric muscle | Styloid process of temporal bone | Lateral margin of the body of the hyoid bone near the greater cornu |
| *Nerve:*   Facial nerve | | |
| *Function:*   Fixes hyoid bone; it pulls the hyoid bone backward and upward during deglutition | | |
| **3. Mylohyoid muscle**<br>The muscles of both sides in midline are united by a raphe | Mylohyoid line of the mandible. The muscles form a fleshy plate across the mandibular arch | Mylohyoid raphe and cranial margin of body of hyoid bone |
| *Nerve:*   Mylohyoid nerve from mandibular division of trigeminal nerve | | |
| *Function:*   Elevates oral floor and tongue during deglutition; depresses mandible, or elevates hyoid bone | | |
| **4. Geniohyoid muscle**<br>It borders directly on the tongue muscles, especially the Genioglossus | Inferior mental spine of the mandible, short tendon | Ventral margin of body of hyoid bone |
| | Muscles on both sides lie close together, a thin connective tissue-like septum separates them in the midline | |
| *Nerve:*   Hypoglossal nerve | | |
| *Function:*   Supports the action of Mylohyoid muscle (elevates the tongue); elevates and fixes hyoid bone, depresses mandible | | |

* In contrast to the Infrahyoid muscles, the Suprahyoid muscles belong to the muscles of the head, since they connect only bones of the head. The Digastric muscle is not a true Hyoid muscle, since it is only indirectly connected with the hyoid bone.

**Fig. 468.** The submandibular trigone and its contents.
Boundaries: Body of mandible, digastric muscle with intermediate tendon. Submandibular gland on the mylohoid muscle. Facial vein superficially, Facial artery ascending from deep toward the mandibular margin. Skin and superficial cervical fascia, wich forms a capsule for the gland, have been removed.  ▷

**Fig. 469.** Submandibular and sublingual regions.
Reflexion of the mylohyoid muscle toward the left permits view of the sublingual region from below. One sees the sublingual gland, the submandibular duct, the lingual nerve with the autonomic submandibular ganglion which sends off the secretory fibers for the salivary glands mentioned. Below it lies the hypoglossal nerve with the lingual vein. Note the lingual trigone bounded by the intermediate tendon of the digastric muscle below and the hypoglossal nerve above. Here, the lingual artery lies below the hypoglossus muscle (point for ligature!).

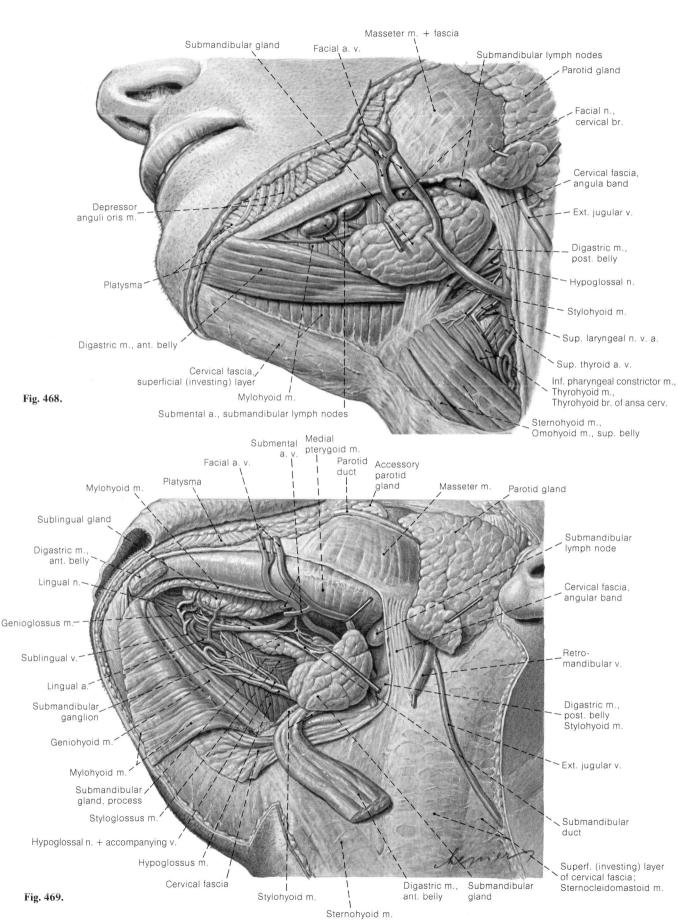

Fig. 468.

Submandibular gland — Facial a. v. — Masseter m. + fascia — Submandibular lymph nodes — Parotid gland

Facial n., cervical br.

Cervical fascia, angula band

Depressor anguli oris m.

Ext. jugular v.

Digastric m., post. belly

Platysma

Hypoglossal n.

Stylohyoid m.

Sup. laryngeal n. v. a.

Digastric m., ant. belly

Sup. thyroid a. v.

Cervical fascia, superficial (investing) layer

Inf. pharyngeal constrictor m., Thyrohyoid m., Thyrohyoid br. of ansa cerv.

Mylohyoid m.

Submental a., submandibular lymph nodes

Sternohyoid m., Omohyoid m., sup. belly

Fig. 469.

Submental a. v. — Medial pterygoid m. — Parotid duct — Accessory parotid gland

Mylohyoid m. — Platysma — Facial a. v. — Masseter m. — Parotid gland

Sublingual gland

Submandibular lymph node

Digastric m., ant. belly

Cervical fascia, angular band

Lingual n.

Genioglossus m.

Retro-mandibular v.

Sublingual v.

Lingual a.

Digastric m., post. belly Stylohyoid m.

Submandibular ganglion

Geniohyoid m.

Ext. jugular v.

Mylohyoid m.

Submandibular gland, process

Styloglossus m.

Submandibular duct

Hypoglossal n. + accompanying v.

Hypoglossus m.

Superf. (investing) layer of cervical fascia; Sternocleidomastoid m.

Cervical fascia

Stylohyoid m.

Sternohyoid m.

Digastric m., ant. belly

Submandibular gland

273

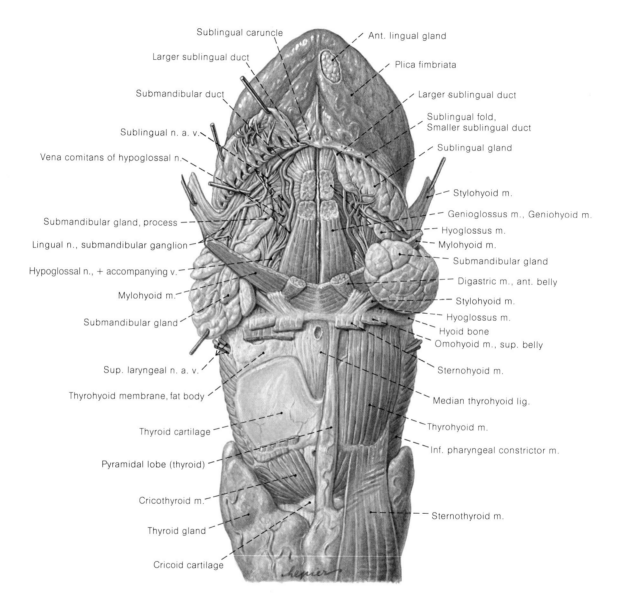

Sublingual caruncle

Larger sublingual duct

Submandibular duct

Sublingual n. a. v.

Vena comitans of hypoglossal n.

Submandibular gland, process

Lingual n., submandibular ganglion

Hypoglossal n., + accompanying v.

Mylohyoid m.

Submandibular gland

Sup. laryngeal n. a. v.

Thyrohyoid membrane, fat body

Thyroid cartilage

Pyramidal lobe (thyroid)

Cricothyroid m.

Thyroid gland

Cricoid cartilage

Ant. lingual gland

Plica fimbriata

Larger sublingual duct

Sublingual fold, Smaller sublingual duct

Sublingual gland

Stylohyoid m.

Genioglossus m., Geniohyoid m.

Hyoglossus m.

Mylohyoid m.

Submandibular gland

Digastric m., ant. belly

Stylohyoid m.

Hyoglossus m.

Hyoid bone

Omohyoid m., sup. belly

Sternohyoid m.

Median thyrohyoid lig.

Thyrohyoid m.

Inf. pharyngeal constrictor m.

Sternothyroid m.

**Fig. 470.** Oral and cervical viscera. Ventral part seen from below, after amputation of the tongue muscle from the mandible and the base of the skull. Demonstration of the salivary glands. On the left of the illustration, the sublingual gland is pulled upward, to display the submandibular duct. On the right, near the tip of the tongue, the lingual gland has been exposed.

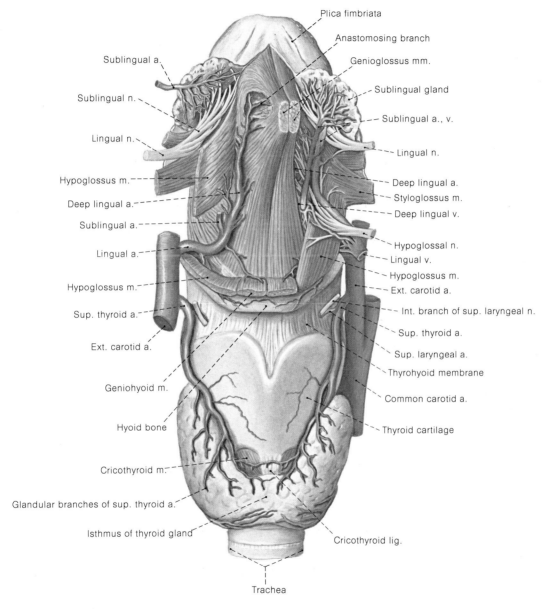

Plica fimbriata

Anastomosing branch

Sublingual a.

Genioglossus mm.

Sublingual n.

Sublingual gland

Lingual n.

Sublingual a., v.

Lingual n.

Hypoglossus m.

Deep lingual a.

Deep lingual a.

Styloglossus m.

Sublingual a.

Deep lingual v.

Lingual a.

Hypoglossal n.

Lingual v.

Hypoglossus m.

Hypoglossus m.

Ext. carotid a.

Sup. thyroid a.

Int. branch of sup. laryngeal n.

Ext. carotid a.

Sup. thyroid a.

Sup. laryngeal a.

Geniohyoid m.

Thyrohyoid membrane

Common carotid a.

Hyoid bone

Thyroid cartilage

Cricothyroid m.

Glandular branches of sup. thyroid a.

Isthmus of thyroid gland

Cricothyroid lig.

Trachea

**Fig. 471.** Nerves and arteries of tongue and larynx, ventral view. On the left side, also the veins of the tongue are shown, the hypoglossus muscle is transected on the right side.

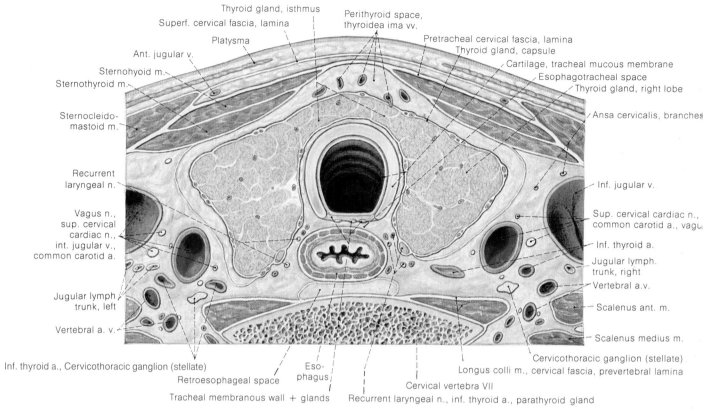

Thyroid gland, isthmus
Superf. cervical fascia, lamina
Platysma
Ant. jugular v.
Sternohyoid m.
Sternothyroid m.
Sternocleido-mastoid m.
Recurrent laryngeal n.
Vagus n., sup. cervical cardiac n., int. jugular v., common carotid a.
Jugular lymph trunk, left
Vertebral a. v.
Perithyroid space, thyroidea ima vv.
Pretracheal cervical fascia, lamina
Thyroid gland, capsule
Cartilage, tracheal mucous membrane
Esophagotracheal space
Thyroid gland, right lobe
Ansa cervicalis, branches
Inf. jugular v.
Sup. cervical cardiac n., common carotid a., vagu
Inf. thyroid a.
Jugular lymph. trunk, right
Vertebral a.v.
Scalenus ant. m.
Scalenus medius m.
Cervicothoracic ganglion (stellate)
Longus colli m., cervical fascia, prevertebral lamina
Inf. thyroid a., Cervicothoracic ganglion (stellate)
Retroesophageal space
Eso-phagus
Tracheal membranous wall + glands
Recurrent laryngeal n., inf. thyroid a., parathyroid gland
Cervical vertebra VII

**Fig. 472.** Horizontal section through the cervical viscera at the level of the second tracheal cartilage.

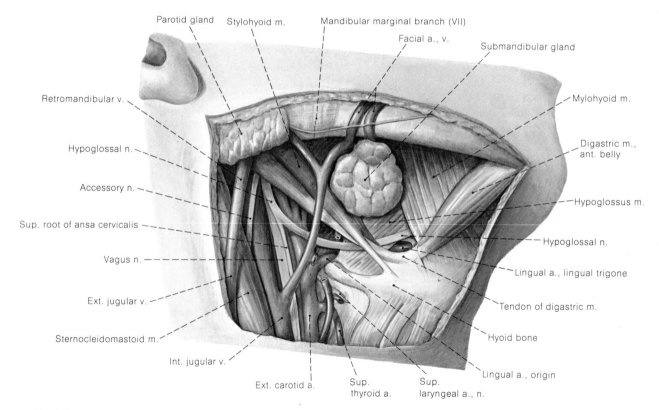

Parotid gland
Stylohyoid m.
Mandibular marginal branch (VII)
Facial a., v.
Submandibular gland
Retromandibular v.
Hypoglossal n.
Accessory n.
Sup. root of ansa cervicalis
Vagus n.
Ext. jugular v.
Sternocleidomastoid m.
Int. jugular v.
Ext. carotid a.
Sup. thyroid a.
Sup. laryngeal a., n.
Mylohyoid m.
Digastric m., ant. belly
Hypoglossus m.
Hypoglossal n.
Lingual a., lingual trigone
Tendon of digastric m.
Hyoid bone
Lingual a., origin

**Fig. 473.** The submandibular trigone. Topography. The "lingual trigone" is bounded by the hypoglossal nerve above, by the intermediate tendon of the digastric muscle below, and by the margin of the mylohyoid muscle on the medial side.

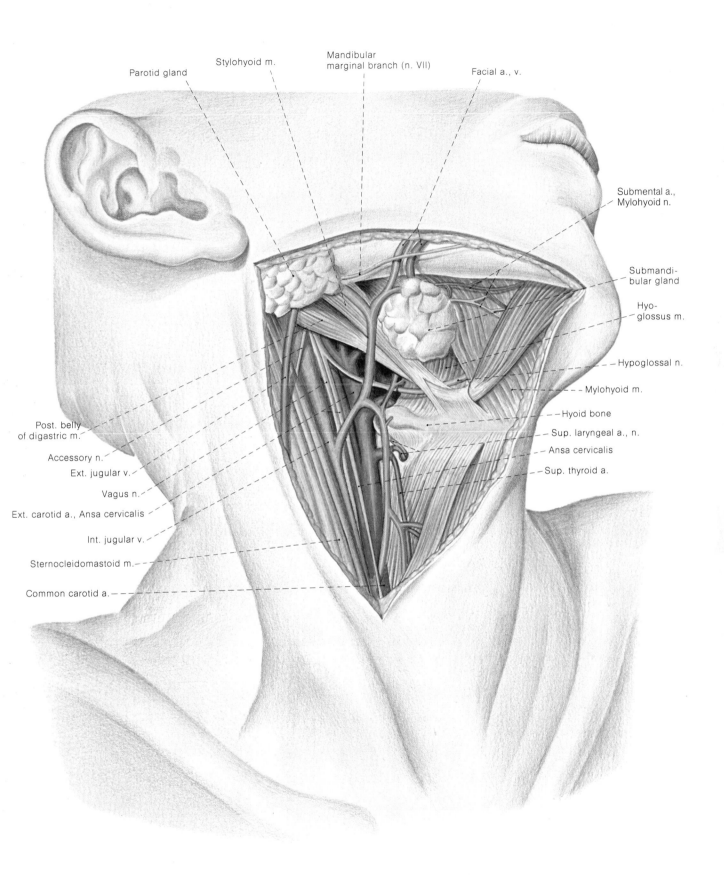

Parotid gland

Stylohyoid m.

Mandibular
marginal branch (n. VII)

Facial a., v.

Submental a.,
Mylohyoid n.

Submandi-
bular gland

Hyo-
glossus m.

Hypoglossal n.

Mylohyoid m.

Hyoid bone

Sup. laryngeal a., n.

Ansa cervicalis

Sup. thyroid a.

Post. belly
of digastric m.

Accessory n.

Ext. jugular v.

Vagus n.

Ext. carotid a., Ansa cervicalis

Int. jugular v.

Sternocleidomastoid m.

Common carotid a.

**Fig. 474.** Dissection of the anterior cervical triangle with submandibular trigone and carotid fossa (from J. TANDLER: Topographische Anatomie dringlicher Operationen. Springer-Verlag, Berlin 1923).

277

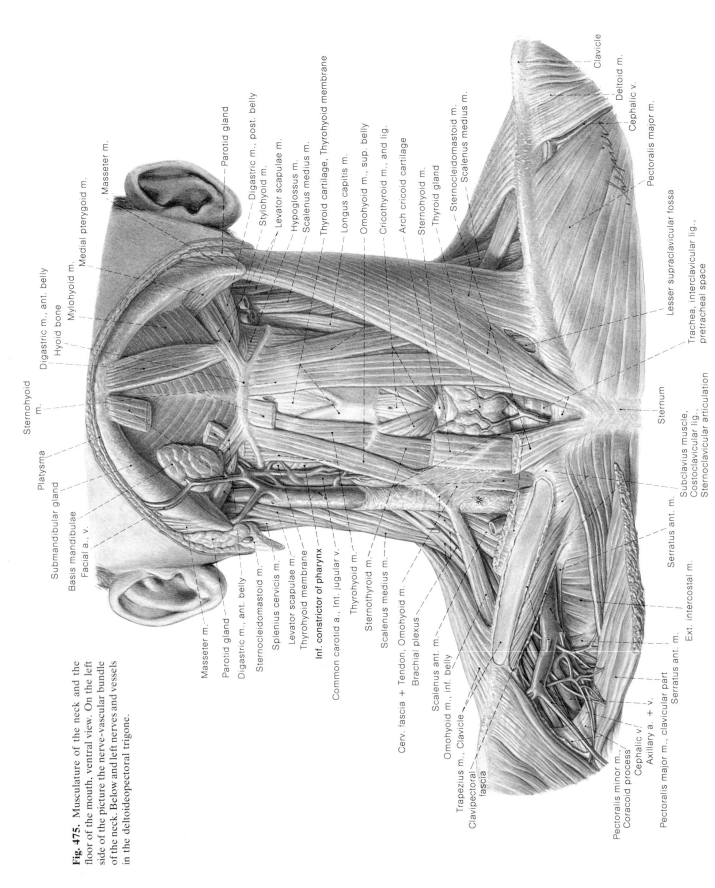

**Fig. 475.** Musculature of the neck and the floor of the mouth, ventral view. On the left side of the picture the nerve-vascular bundle of the neck. Below and left nerves and vessels in the deltoideopectoral trigone.

Sternohyoid m.

Platysma

Submandibular gland

Basis mandibulae

Facial a., v.

Masseter m.

Parotid gland

Digastric m., ant. belly

Sternocleidomastoid m.

Splenius cervicis m.

Levator scapulae m.

Thyrohyoid membrane

Common carotid a., Int. jugular v.

Thyrohyoid m.

Sternothyroid m.

Scalenus medius m.

Cerv. fascia + Tendon. Omohyoid m.

Brachial plexus

Scalenus ant. m.

Omohyoid m., inf. belly

Trapezius m., Clavicle

Clavipectoral fascia

Pectoralis minor m.,
Coracoid process

Cephalic v.

Axillary a. + v.

Pectoralis major m., clavicular part

Serratus ant. m.

**Inf. constrictor of pharynx**

Digastric m., ant. belly

Hyoid bone

Mylohyoid m.

Medial pterygoid m.

Masseter m.

Parotid gland

Digastric m., post. belly

Stylohyoid m.

Levator scapulae m.

Hypoglossus m.

Scalenus medius m.

Thyroid cartilage, Thyrohyoid membrane

Longus capitis m.

Omohyoid m., sup. belly

Cricothyroid m., and lig.

Arch cricoid cartilage

Sternohyoid m.

Thyroid gland

Sternocleidomastoid m.

Scalenus medius m.

Clavicle

Deltoid m.

Cephalic v.

Pectoralis major m.

Lesser supraclavicular fossa

Trachea, interclavicular lig.,
pretracheal space

Sternum

Subclavius muscle,
Costoclavicular lig.,
Sternoclavicular articulation

Serratus ant. m.

Ext. intercostal m.

278

| Name | | Origin | Insertion |
|---|---|---|---|
| **1. Sternocleidomastoid muscle** | | | |
| | Sternal head: | Ventral surface of the manubrium sterni | Lateral surface of mastoid process; superior nuchal line of occipital bone |
| | Clavicular head: | Cranial surface of medial third of clavicle | |

*Nerve:* Spinal accessory nerve; fibers from second cervical nerve

*Function:* Various: Both sides together, hold head, move chin upward and pull back of head down. One side alone, turns chin upward and to opposite side. The understanding of this muscle clarifies the anatomy of the neck

## Infrahyoid muscles

| Name | Origin | Insertion |
|---|---|---|
| **1. Sternohyoid muscle** (thin, narrow muscles) | Inner surface of manubrium sterni and sternoclavicular joint | Body of hyoid bone |
| **2. Sternothyroid muscle** (shorter, wider muscle) | 1st costal cartilage; dorsal surface of manubrium sterni, caudal to Sternohyoid muscle | Outer surface of thyroid cartilage (opposite the origin of Thyrohyoid muscle) |
| **3. Thyrohyoid muscle** (small quadrilateral muscle) | Outer surface of the thyroid cartilage | Inferior border of greater cornu of hyoid bone |
| **4. Omohyoid muscle** (two fleshy bellies united in middle by a single tendon | Superior margin of scapula between superior angle and scapular notch (inferior belly) | Caudal border of lateral section of body of hyoid bone (superior belly) |

*Nerve:* Ansa cervicalis

*Function:* Fixes hyoid bone firmly; with Suprahyoid muscles, assists in movements of tongue, hyoid bone, and larynx in swallowing and phonation. With the Tyhrohyoid muscle (and hyoid bone fixed) elevates larynx in act of swallowing and production of high notes. The Sternothyroid muscle does the opposite in drawing down the larynx to produce low notes. Muscles assist in respiration (pull sternum cranially in inspiration)

## Auricular muscles

| Name | Origin | Insertion |
|---|---|---|
| **Anterior auricular muscle** | Temporal fascia, superficial lamina | Base of cartilaginous external ear |
| **Posterior auricular muscle** | Tendon of insertion of Sternocleidomastoid muscle | |

*Nerve:* Facial nerve

*Function:* Moves the external ear (pinna)

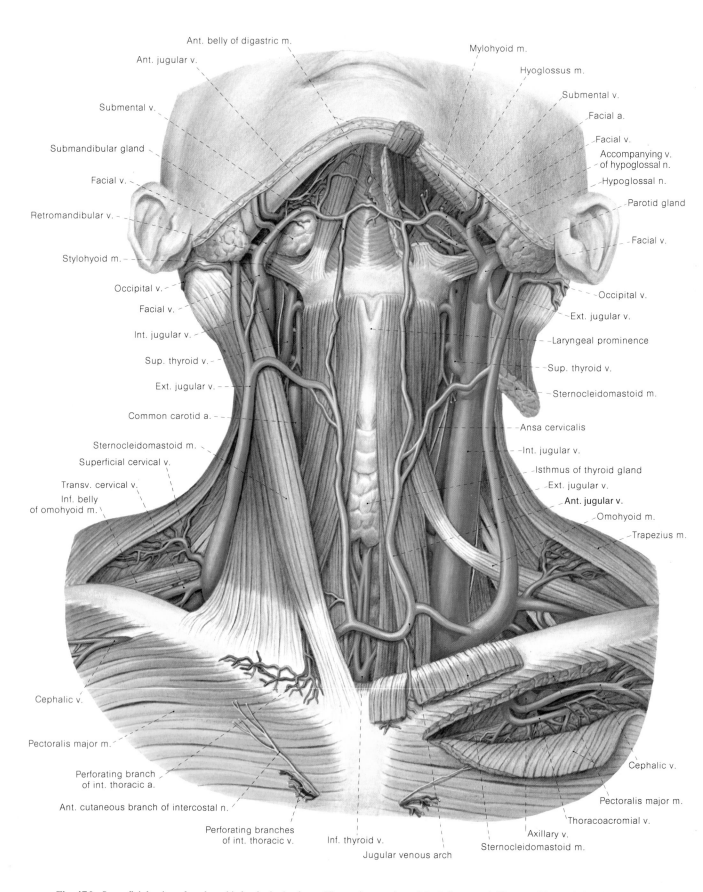

Ant. belly of digastric m.

Ant. jugular v.

Submental v.

Submandibular gland

Facial v.

Retromandibular v.

Stylohyoid m.

Occipital v.

Facial v.

Int. jugular v.

Sup. thyroid v.

Ext. jugular v.

Common carotid a.

Sternocleidomastoid m.

Superficial cervical v.

Transv. cervical v.

Inf. belly
of omohyoid m.

Cephalic v.

Pectoralis major m.

Perforating branch
of int. thoracic a.

Ant. cutaneous branch of intercostal n.

Perforating branches
of int. thoracic v.

Inf. thyroid v.

Jugular venous arch

Mylohyoid m.

Hyoglossus m.

Submental v.

Facial a.

Facial v.

Accompanying v.
of hypoglossal n.

Hypoglossal n.

Parotid gland

Facial v.

Occipital v.

Ext. jugular v.

Laryngeal prominence

Sup. thyroid v.

Sternocleidomastoid m.

Ansa cervicalis

Int. jugular v.

Isthmus of thyroid gland

Ext. jugular v.

Ant. jugular v.

Omohyoid m.

Trapezius m.

Cephalic v.

Pectoralis major m.

Thoracoacromial v.

Axillary v.

Sternocleidomastoid m.

**Fig. 476.** Superficial veins of neck and infraclavicular fossa. The major portion of the left sternocleidomastoid muscle has been removed.

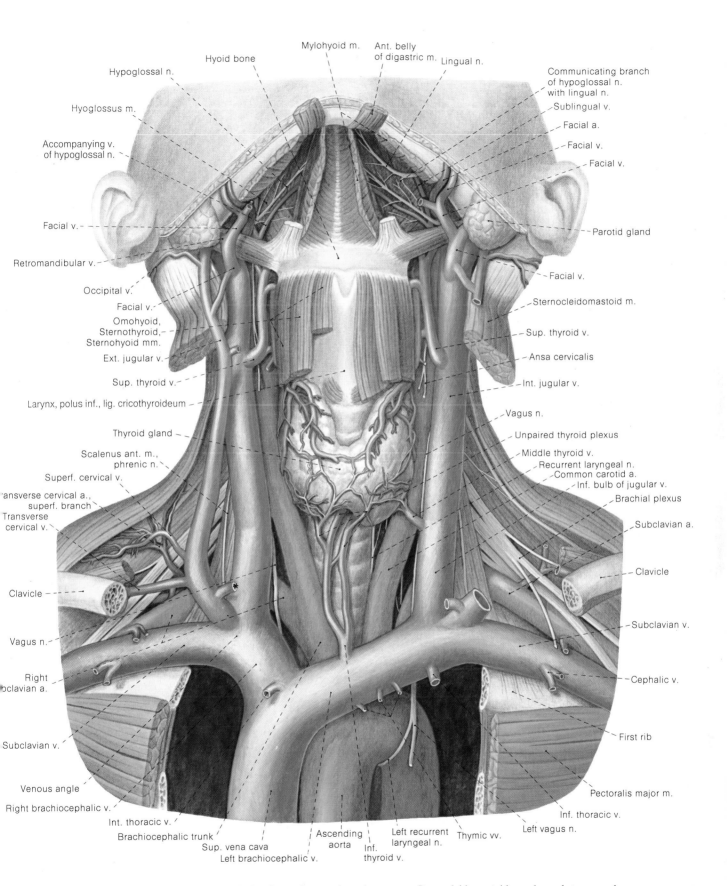

Hyoid bone
Mylohyoid m.
Ant. belly of digastric m.
Lingual n.
Hypoglossal n.
Communicating branch of hypoglossal n. with lingual n.
Hyoglossus m.
Sublingual v.
Facial a.
Facial v.
Accompanying v. of hypoglossal n.
Facial v.
Facial v.
Parotid gland
Retromandibular v.
Facial v.
Occipital v.
Sternocleidomastoid m.
Facial v.
Omohyoid, Sternothyroid, Sternohyoid mm.
Sup. thyroid v.
Ansa cervicalis
Ext. jugular v.
Int. jugular v.
Sup. thyroid v.
Larynx, polus inf., lig. cricothyroideum
Vagus n.
Thyroid gland
Unpaired thyroid plexus
Scalenus ant. m., phrenic n.
Middle thyroid v.
Recurrent laryngeal n.
Common carotid a.
Superf. cervical v.
Inf. bulb of jugular v.
Transverse cervical a., superf. branch
Brachial plexus
Transverse cervical v.
Subclavian a.
Clavicle
Clavicle
Subclavian v.
Vagus n.
Cephalic v.
Right subclavian a.
Subclavian v.
First rib
Venous angle
Pectoralis major m.
Right brachiocephalic v.
Inf. thoracic v.
Int. thoracic v.
Left vagus n.
Brachiocephalic trunk
Ascending aorta
Left recurrent laryngeal n.
Thymic vv.
Sup. vena cava
Inf. thyroid v.
Left brachiocephalic v.

**Fig. 477.** Nerves and vessels of the deep cervical region and upper thoracic aperture. Sternocleidomastoid muscles and strap muscles partially removed. Mylohyoid and digastric muscles sectioned. Sternum and anterior portions of first and second rib removed. Veins maximally filled. * = anterior jugular vein.

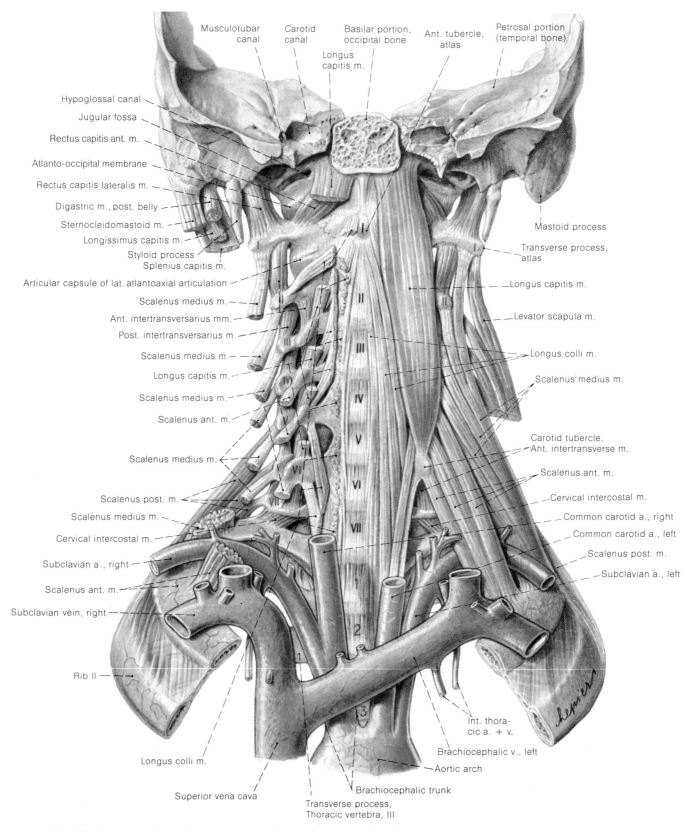

Musculotubar canal · Carotid canal · Basilar portion, occipital bone · Longus capitis m. · Ant. tubercle, atlas · Petrosal portion (temporal bone)

Hypoglossal canal
Jugular fossa
Rectus capitis ant. m.
Atlanto-occipital membrane
Rectus capitis lateralis m.
Digastric m., post. belly
Sternocleidomastoid m.
Longissimus capitis m.
Styloid process
Splenius capitis m.
Articular capsule of lat. atlantoaxial articulation
Scalenus medius m.
Ant. intertransversarius mm.
Post. intertransversarius m.
Scalenus medius m.
Longus capitis m.
Scalenus medius m.
Scalenus ant. m.
Scalenus medius m.
Scalenus post. m.
Scalenus medius m.
Cervical intercostal m.
Subclavian a., right
Scalenus ant. m.
Subclavian vein, right
Rib II
Longus colli m.
Superior vena cava

Mastoid process
Transverse process, atlas
Longus capitis m.
Levator scapula m.
Longus colli m.
Scalenus medius m.
Carotid tubercle, Ant. intertransverse m.
Scalenus ant. m.
Cervical intercostal m.
Common carotid a., right
Common carotid a., left
Scalenus post. m.
Subclavian a., left
Int. thoracic a. + v.
Brachiocephalic v., left
Aortic arch
Brachiocephalic trunk
Transverse process, Thoracic vertebra, III

**Fig. 478.** Deep cervical muscles after removal of the cervical viscera. Ventral view. Cervical vertebrae: I–VII; upper thoracic vertebrae: 1–3. The base of the skull cut off almost frontally near the level of the basilar portion. First and second ribs were cut near the bone-cartilage junction. The superior vena cava and arch of the aorta are shown with their large trunks: the brachiocephalic trunk, the common carotid artery, the left subclavian artery with its passage through the scalene hiatus.

### Lateral Vertebral Group of Deep Cervical Muscles

| Name | Origin | Insertion |
|---|---|---|
| 1. Scalenus anterior muscle | Anterior tubercles of transverse processes of 3rd to 6th cervical vertebrae | Scalene tubercle on 1st rib |
| 2. Scalenus medius muscle | Posterior tubercles of transverse processes of last six cervical vertebrae | Cranial surface of 1st rib, dorsal to subclavian groove |
| 3. Scalenus posterior muscle | Posterior tubercles of transverse processes of last three cervical vertebrae | Outer surface of 2nd rib |

*Nerve:* Cervical plexus (and brachial plexus)

*Function:* Scalene muscles, acting together, elevate 1st and 2nd ribs or flex the vertebral column (muscles of inspiration); acting one side at a time, they bend neck to side

### Anterior Vertebral Group of Deep Cervical Muscles

| Name | Origin | Insertion |
|---|---|---|
| 1. Longus colli muscle | | |
| Vertical portion | Body of first 3 thoracic and last 3 cervical vertebrae | Bodies of cervical vertebrae $C_2 - C_4$ |
| Superior oblique | Anterior tubercle of transverse process of cervical vertebrae $C_3 - C_5$ | Tubercle on anterior arch of the atlas and body of next cervical vertebra |
| Inferior oblique | Anterior surface of bodies of first 2 or 3 thoracic vertebrae | Anterior tubercles of the transverse processes of 5th and 6th cervical vertebrae |
| 2. Longus capitis muscle | Anterior tubercle of transverse processes of 3rd – 6th cervical vertebrae | Inferior border of basilar part of occipital bone |
| 3. Rectus capitis anterior muscle | Lateral mass of atlas and root of its transverse process | as above |

*Nerve:* Cervical plexus

*Function:* Bend the cervical vertebral column or the head forward, by unilateral innervation, incline and rotate the head toward the same side

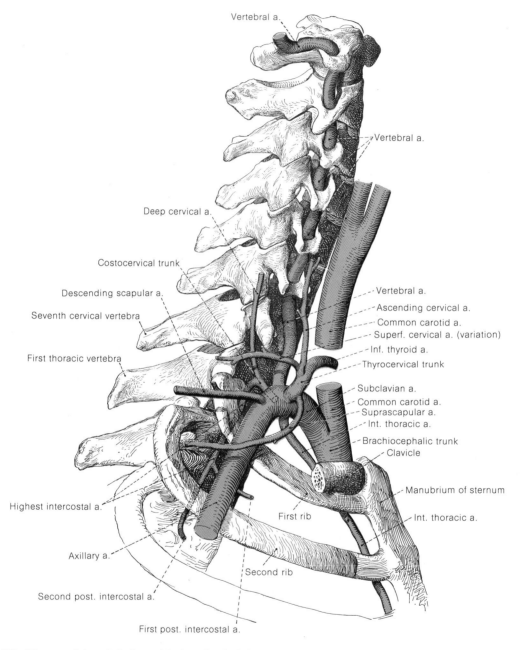

**Fig. 479.** Diagram of the subclavian and its branches and the course of the vertebral artery.

Vertebral a.

Vertebral a.

Deep cervical a.

Costocervical trunk

Descending scapular a.

Seventh cervical vertebra

First thoracic vertebra

Vertebral a.

Ascending cervical a.

Common carotid a.

Superf. cervical a. (variation)

Inf. thyroid a.

Thyrocervical trunk

Subclavian a.

Common carotid a.

Suprascapular a.

Int. thoracic a.

Brachiocephalic trunk

Clavicle

Manubrium of sternum

Highest intercostal a.

Int. thoracic a.

First rib

Axillary a.

Second rib

Second post. intercostal a.

First post. intercostal a.

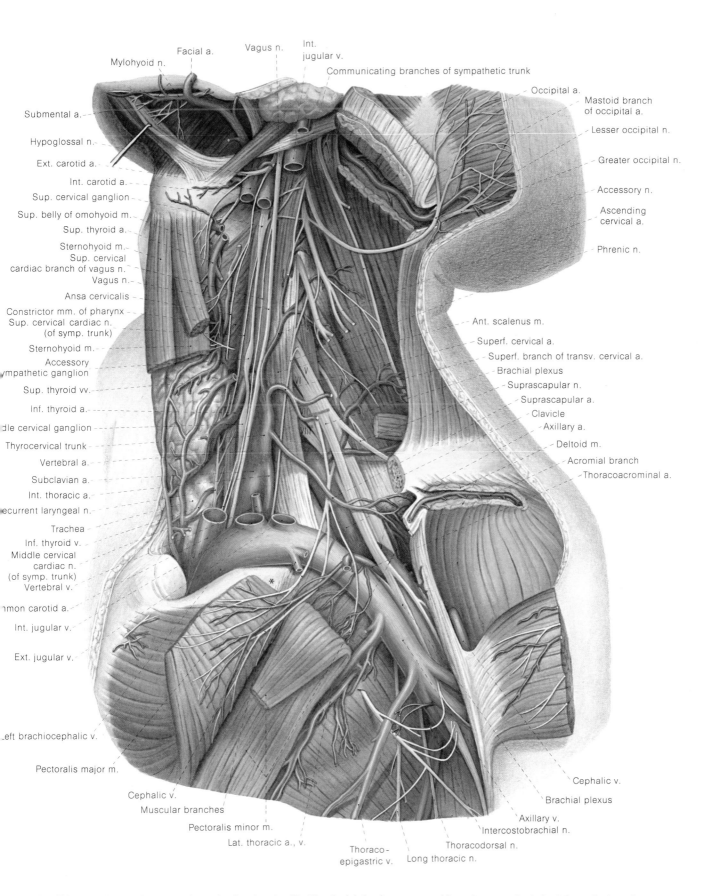

Facial a. · Vagus n. · Int. jugular v.
Mylohyoid n.
Communicating branches of sympathetic trunk
Submental a.
Occipital a.
Mastoid branch of occipital a.
Hypoglossal n.
Lesser occipital n.
Ext. carotid a.
Greater occipital n.
Int. carotid a.
Accessory n.
Sup. cervical ganglion
Ascending cervical a.
Sup. belly of omohyoid m.
Sup. thyroid a.
Phrenic n.
Sternohyoid m.
Sup. cervical cardiac branch of vagus n.
Vagus n.
Ansa cervicalis
Ant. scalenus m.
Constrictor mm. of pharynx
Sup. cervical cardiac n. (of symp. trunk)
Superf. cervical a.
Sternohyoid m.
Superf. branch of transv. cervical a.
Accessory sympathetic ganglion
Brachial plexus
Suprascapular n.
Sup. thyroid vv.
Suprascapular a.
Inf. thyroid a.
Clavicle
Middle cervical ganglion
Axillary a.
Thyrocervical trunk
Deltoid m.
Vertebral a.
Acromial branch
Subclavian a.
Thoracoacromial a.
Int. thoracic a.
Recurrent laryngeal n.
Trachea
Inf. thyroid v.
Middle cervical cardiac n. (of symp. trunk)
Vertebral v.
Common carotid a.
Int. jugular v.
Ext. jugular v.
Left brachiocephalic v.
Pectoralis major m.
Cephalic v.
Muscular branches
Pectoralis minor m.
Lat. thoracic a., v.
Cephalic v.
Brachial plexus
Axillary v.
Intercostobrachial n.
Thoracodorsal n.
Thoraco-epigastric v.
Long thoracic n.

**Fig. 480.** Deep layers of nerves and vessels of neck and axilla. The clavicle has been removed from the sternoclavicular joint to the insertion of the trapazius muscle. Strap muscles, sternocleidomastoid muscle and major cervical vessels have been mostly removed. * = first rib.

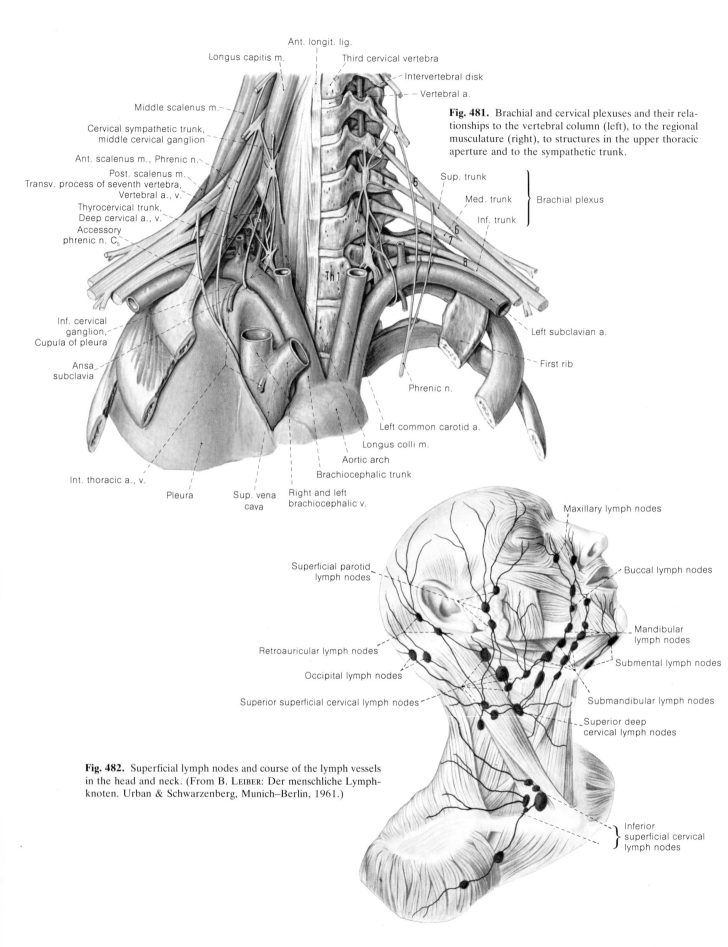

Ant. longit. lig.

Longus capitis m.

Third cervical vertebra

Intervertebral disk

Vertebral a.

Middle scalenus m.

Cervical sympathetic trunk, middle cervical ganglion

Ant. scalenus m., Phrenic n.

Post. scalenus m.

Transv. process of seventh vertebra, Vertebral a., v.

Thyrocervical trunk, Deep cervical a., v.

Accessory phrenic n. C₅

Inf. cervical ganglion, Cupula of pleura

Ansa subclavia

Int. thoracic a., v.

Pleura

Sup. vena cava

Right and left brachiocephalic v.

Brachiocephalic trunk

Aortic arch

Longus colli m.

Left common carotid a.

Phrenic n.

First rib

Left subclavian a.

Sup. trunk

Med. trunk

Inf. trunk

} Brachial plexus

**Fig. 481.** Brachial and cervical plexuses and their relationships to the vertebral column (left), to the regional musculature (right), to structures in the upper thoracic aperture and to the sympathetic trunk.

Maxillary lymph nodes

Buccal lymph nodes

Mandibular lymph nodes

Submental lymph nodes

Submandibular lymph nodes

Superior deep cervical lymph nodes

Inferior superficial cervical lymph nodes

Superficial parotid lymph nodes

Retroauricular lymph nodes

Occipital lymph nodes

Superior superficial cervical lymph nodes

**Fig. 482.** Superficial lymph nodes and course of the lymph vessels in the head and neck. (From B. LEIBER: Der menschliche Lymphknoten. Urban & Schwarzenberg, Munich–Berlin, 1961.)

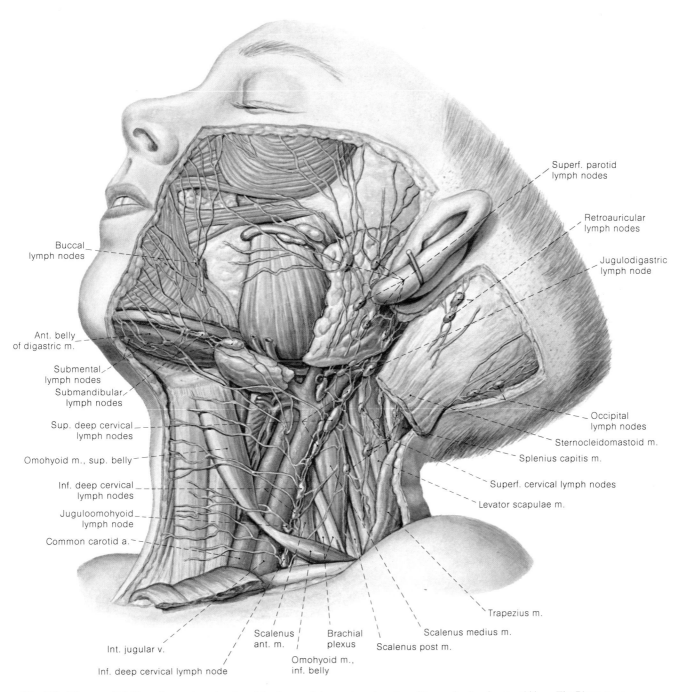

Superf. parotid
lymph nodes

Retroauricular
lymph nodes

Jugulodigastric
lymph node

Buccal
lymph nodes

Ant. belly
of digastric m.

Submental
lymph nodes

Submandibular
lymph nodes

Sup. deep cervical
lymph nodes

Omohyoid m., sup. belly

Inf. deep cervical
lymph nodes

Juguloomohyoid
lymph node

Common carotid a.

Occipital
lymph nodes

Sternocleidomastoid m.

Splenius capitis m.

Superf. cervical lymph nodes

Levator scapulae m.

Trapezius m.

Int. jugular v.

Inf. deep cervical lymph node

Scalenus
ant. m.

Brachial
plexus

Omohyoid m.,
inf. belly

Scalenus post. m.

Scalenus medius m.

**Fig. 483.** The superficial lymph vessels and nodes of the face and deeper lymph nodes of the neck of an 8-year old boy. The Platysma was resected and the Sternocleidomastoid muscle was cut. The lymph nodes along the large cervical vessels form the chains of the so-called cervical glands.

287

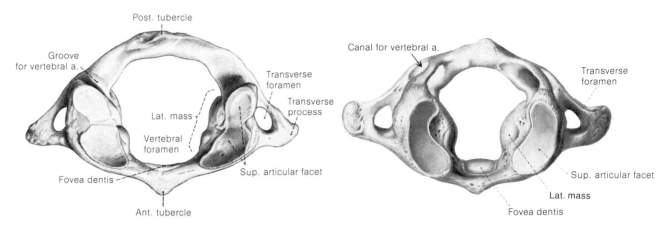

**Fig. 484.** Atlas. Cranial view.

**Fig. 485.** Atlas. Cranial view, with closed sulcus for vertebral artery (Variation).

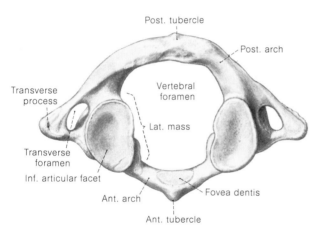

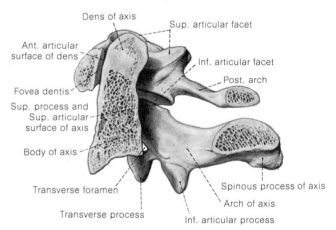

**Fig. 486.** Atlas. Caudal view.

**Fig. 487.** Atlas and axis. Median sagittal section.

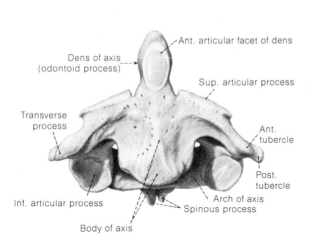

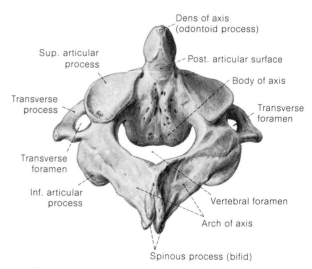

**Fig. 488.** Axis. Ventral view.

**Fig. 489.** Axis. Dorsal view.

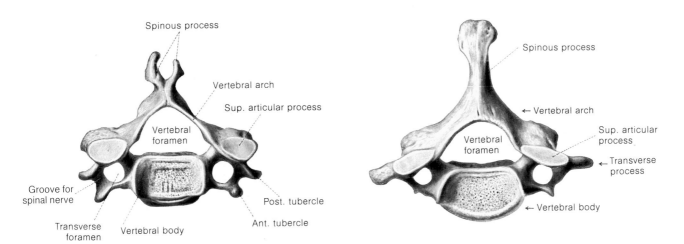

**Fig. 490.** Fifth cervical vertebra. Cranial view.

**Fig. 491.** Seventh cervical vertebra (vertebra prominens). Cranial view.

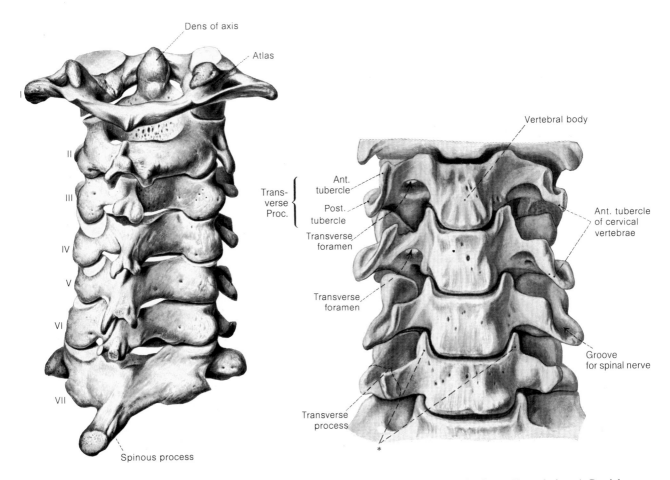

**Fig. 492.** Cervical spinal column. Dorsal view, somewhat from right side. Roman numerals indicate the number of the cervical vertebra.

**Fig. 493.** Lower cervical spinal column. Ventral view. * Cranial flanges of lateral borders of vertebral bodies.

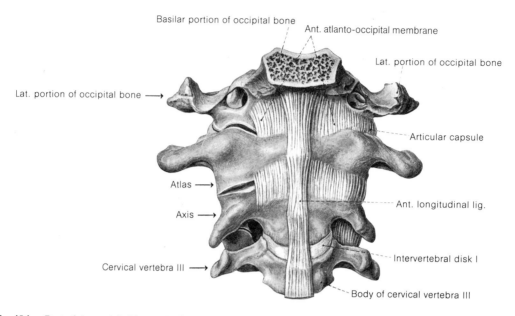

**Fig. 494.** Part of the occipital bone, the first three vertebrae, the anterior atlantooccipital membrane, and the cranial end of the anterior longitudinal ligament. Articular capsules are removed on the right. Ventral view.

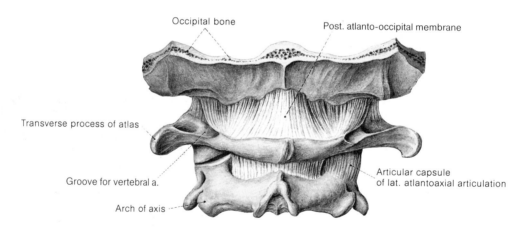

**Fig. 495.** Part of the occipital bone, atlas, and axis with their ligaments, and the posterior atlanto-occipital membrane. The articular capsule of the lateral atlantoaxial articulation removed on left. Dorsal view.

NOTE: The atlanto-occipital, lateral atlantoaxial, and median atlantoaxial articulations form a functional unit with the effect of a ball and socket joint. The subdivision of these articular portions forms a safeguard against dislocation.

**Fig. 496.** Tectorial membrane. Dorsal view. The dorsal section of ▷
the occipital bone and the arches of the three cranial cervical vertebrae are sawed off. The articular capsules of the intervertebral joints
are removed on the right.

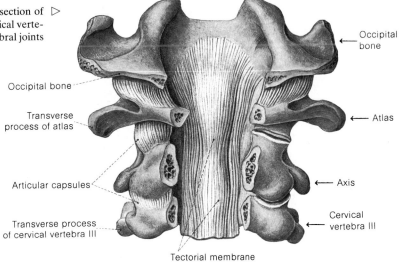

Occipital bone

Transverse
process of atlas

Occipital bone

Atlas

Articular capsules

Axis

Transverse process
of cervical vertebra III

Cervical
vertebra III

Tectorial membrane

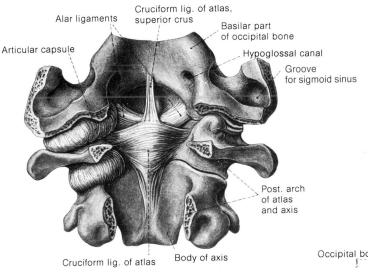

Alar ligaments

Cruciform lig. of atlas,
superior crus

Basilar part
of occipital bone

Articular capsule

Hypoglossal canal

Groove
for sigmoid sinus

Post. arch
of atlas
and axis

Cruciform lig. of atlas

Body of axis

△

**Fig. 497.** Cruciform ligament of the atlas after removal of the tectorial membrane. Seen from dorsal. Prepared as in Figure 496.

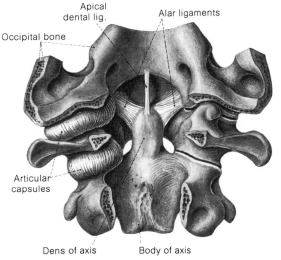

Apical
dental lig.

Alar ligaments

Occipital bone

Articular
capsules

Dens of axis

Body of axis

△

**Fig. 498.** Alar and apical ligaments after removal of the cruciform
ligament of the atlas. Seen from dorsal. Prepared as in Fig. 496.

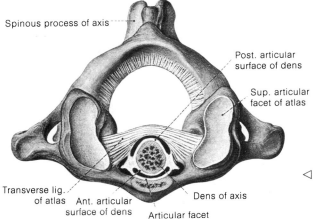

Spinous process of axis

Post. articular
surface of dens

Sup. articular
facet of atlas

Transverse lig.
of atlas

Ant. articular
surface of dens

Dens of axis

Articular facet

◁ **Fig. 499.** Median atlantoaxial articulation. The atlas is removed
from the atlantooccipital articulation. The dens of the axis and the
ventral arch of the atlas are sawed through horizontally. Cranial
view.

291

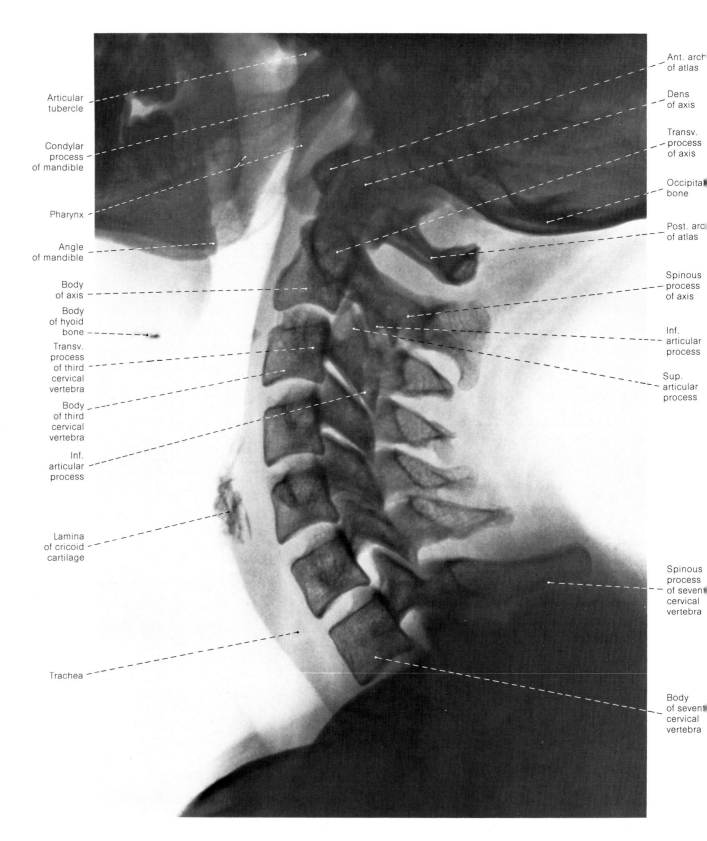

Articular tubercle

Condylar process of mandible

Pharynx

Angle of mandible

Body of axis

Body of hyoid bone

Transv. process of third cervical vertebra

Body of third cervical vertebra

Inf. articular process

Lamina of cricoid cartilage

Trachea

Ant. arch of atlas

Dens of axis

Transv. process of axis

Occipital bone

Post. arch of atlas

Spinous process of axis

Inf. articular process

Sup. articular process

Spinous process of seventh cervical vertebra

Body of seventh cervical vertebra

**Fig. 500.** X-ray film of the cervical vertebral column in lateral projection. (From L. Wicke: Atlas der Röntgenanatomie, 2nd ed. Urban & Schwarzenberg, Munich–Vienna–Baltimore 1980.)

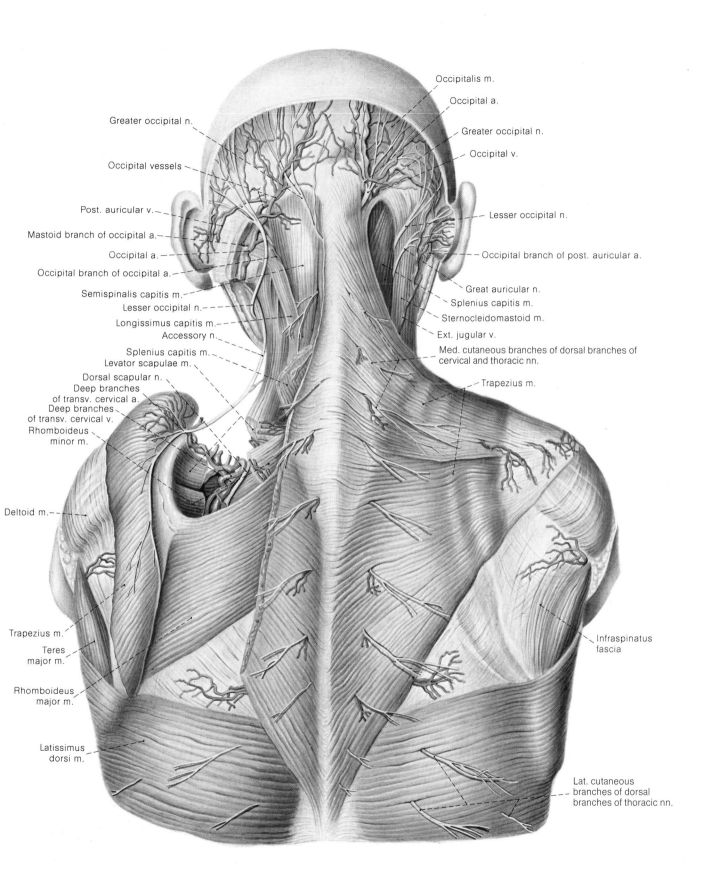

Occipitalis m.

Occipital a.

Greater occipital n.

Greater occipital n.

Occipital v.

Occipital vessels

Post. auricular v.

Lesser occipital n.

Mastoid branch of occipital a.

Occipital a.

Occipital branch of post. auricular a.

Occipital branch of occipital a.

Great auricular n.

Semispinalis capitis m.

Splenius capitis m.

Lesser occipital n.

Sternocleidomastoid m.

Longissimus capitis m.

Ext. jugular v.

Accessory n.

Med. cutaneous branches of dorsal branches of cervical and thoracic nn.

Splenius capitis m.

Levator scapulae m.

Trapezius m.

Dorsal scapular n.
Deep branches
of transv. cervical a.
Deep branches
of transv. cervical v.
Rhomboideus
minor m.

Deltoid m.

Infraspinatus
fascia

Trapezius m.

Teres
major m.

Rhomboideus
major m.

Latissimus
dorsi m.

Lat. cutaneous
branches of dorsal
branches of thoracic nn.

**Fig. 501.** Superficial and middle layer of nerves and vessels of the upper back and neck. On the left side, the trapezius, sternocleidomastoid, splenius capitis and levator scapulae muscles were divided.

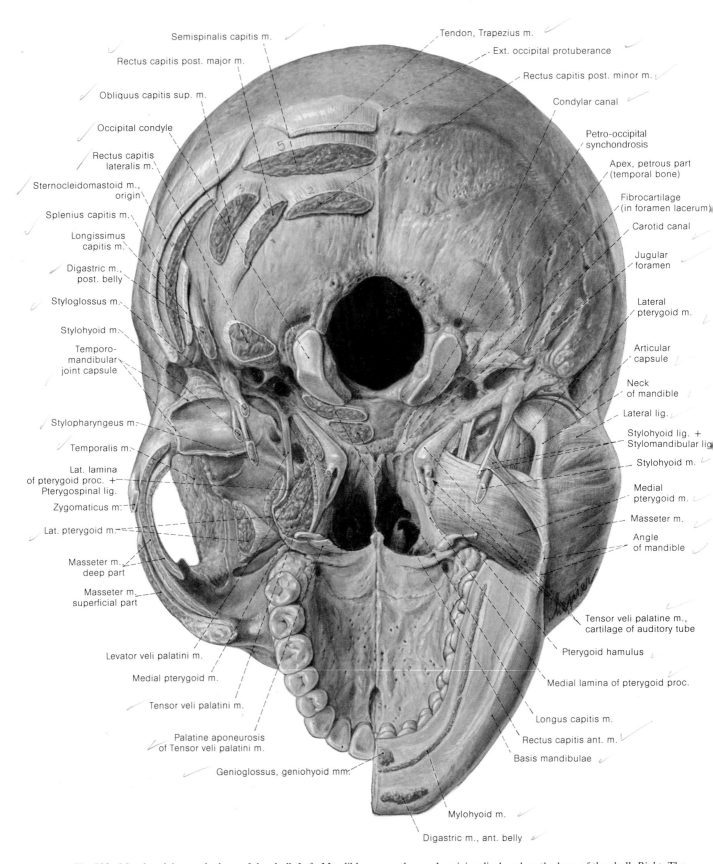

Semispinalis capitis m.

Rectus capitis post. major m.

Obliquus capitis sup. m.

Occipital condyle

Rectus capitis
lateralis m.

Sternocleidomastoid m.,
origin

Splenius capitis m.

Longissimus
capitis m.

Digastric m.,
post. belly

Styloglossus m.

Stylohyoid m.

Temporo-
mandibular
joint capsule

Stylopharyngeus m.

Temporalis m.

Lat. lamina
of pterygoid proc. +
Pterygospinal lig.

Zygomaticus m.

Lat. pterygoid m.

Masseter m.
deep part

Masseter m.
superficial part

Levator veli palatini m.

Medial pterygoid m.

Tensor veli palatini m.

Palatine aponeurosis
of Tensor veli palatini m.

Genioglossus, geniohyoid mm.

Tendon, Trapezius m.

Ext. occipital protuberance

Rectus capitis post. minor m.

Condylar canal

Petro-occipital
synchondrosis

Apex, petrous part
(temporal bone)

Fibrocartilage
(in foramen lacerum)

Carotid canal

Jugular
foramen

Lateral
pterygoid m.

Articular
capsule

Neck
of mandible

Lateral lig.

Stylohyoid lig. +
Stylomandibular lig.

Stylohyoid m.

Medial
pterygoid m.

Masseter m.

Angle
of mandible

Tensor veli palatine m.,
cartilage of auditory tube

Pterygoid hamulus

Medial lamina of pterygoid proc.

Longus capitis m.

Rectus capitis ant. m.

Basis mandibulae

Mylohyoid m.

Digastric m., ant. belly

**Fig. 502.** Muscle origins on the base of the skull. *Left:* Mandible removed; muscle origins displayed on the base of the skull. *Right:* The masticator muscles retained.

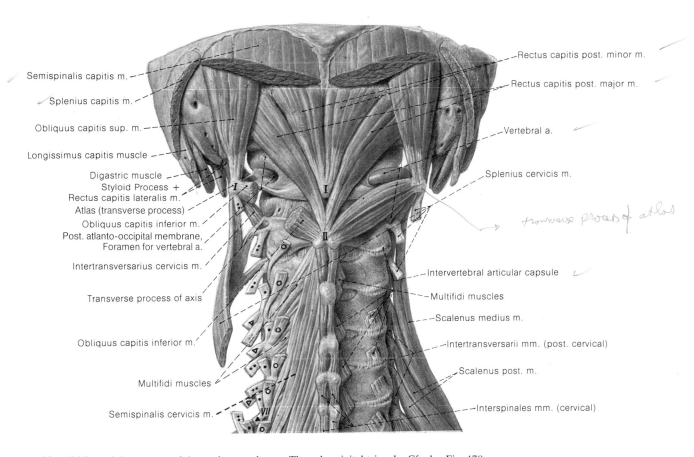

Semispinalis capitis m.
Splenius capitis m.
Obliquus capitis sup. m.
Longissimus capitis muscle
Digastric muscle
Styloid Process +
Rectus capitis lateralis m.
Atlas (transverse process)
Obliquus capitis inferior m.
Post. atlanto-occipital membrane,
Foramen for vertebral a.
Intertransversarius cervicis m.
Transverse process of axis
Obliquus capitis inferior m.
Multifidi muscles
Semispinalis cervicis m.

Rectus capitis post. minor m.
Rectus capitis post. major m.
Vertebral a.
Splenius cervicis m.
transverse process of atlas
Intervertebral articular capsule
Multifidi muscles
Scalenus medius m.
Intertransversarii mm. (post. cervical)
Scalenus post. m.
Interspinales mm. (cervical)

**Fig. 503.** Middle and deep layers of the neck musculature. The suboccipital triangle. Cf. also Fig. 479.

## Anterior Vertebral Group of Deep Cervical Muscles

| Name | Origin | Insertion |
|---|---|---|
| **1. Longus colli muscle** | | |
| Vertical portion | Body of first 3 thoracic and last 3 cervical vertebrae | Bodies of cervical vertebrae $C_2 - C_4$ |
| Superior oblique | Anterior tubercle of transverse process of cervical vertebrae $C_3 - C_5$ | Tubercle on anterior arch of the atlas and body of next cervical vertebra |
| Inferior oblique | Anterior surface of bodies of first 2 or 3 thoracic vertebrae | Anterior tubercles of the transverse processes of 5th and 6th cervical vertebrae |
| **2. Longus capitis muscle** | Anterior tubercle of transverse processes of 3rd – 6th cervical vertebrae | Inferior border of basilar part of occipital bone |
| **3. Rectus capitis anterior muscle** | Lateral mass of atlas and root of its transverse process | as above |

*Nerve:* Cervical plexus

*Function:* Bend the cervical vertebral column or the head forward, by unilateral innervation, incline and rotate the head toward the same side

### Splenius capitis and cervicis muscles

The two muscles are close together at their origin (from the spinous processes). Gradually as they approach their indivual insertions, they become separated into two specific muscles.

| Name | Origin | Insertion |
| --- | --- | --- |
| **1. Splenius capitis muscle**<br>The splenius muscles get their innervations from the true back muscles | Nuchal ligament, spinous processes of 3rd (4th) to 7th cervical and first 3 thoracic vertebrae | Lateral third of the superior nuchal line (and the mastoid process of the temporal bone) |

*Nerve:* Dorsal rami of nerves C 2–5, lateral branches

*Function:* Muscles of both sides, acting together, extend the head and neck; one side acting alone, rotates the head to the same side

| | | |
| --- | --- | --- |
| **2. Splenius cervicis muscle** | Spines of 3rd (or 4th) to 6th thoracic vertebrae | Posterior tubercles of the transverse processes of the first 3 cervical vertebrae |

*Nerve:* Dorsal rami of nerves C 2–5, lateral branches (same as Splenius capitis muscle)

*Function:* Muscles of both sides acting together extend the neck and head. Muscles of one side rotates the upper cervical vertebrae and, by its action on the atlas, rotates the head to the same side

### Short suboccipital muscles

| Name | Origin | Insertion |
| --- | --- | --- |
| **1. Rectus capitis posterior major muscle** | Spinous process of the axis (II) | Inferior nuchal line (of occipital bone) |
| **2. Rectus capitis posterior minor muscle** | Posterior tubercle of atlas (I) | Medial part of the inferior nuchal line of the occipital bone |
| **3. Rectus capitis lateralis muscle** | Transverse process of the atlas | Jugular process of the occipital bone |
| **4. Obliquus capitis superior muscle** | Transverse process of the atlas | Occipital bone, above the inferior nuchal line |
| **5. Obliquus capitis inferior muscle** | Spinous process of the axis (II) | Transverse process of the atlas |

*Nerve:* Suboccipital nerve (dorsal ramus of the first cervical nerve)

*Function:* Extend and rotate head. The Rectus capitis posterior major and Obliquus capitis inferior muscles turn the head to the same side; the Rectus capitis lateralis muscle bends the head laterally (unilateral innervation)

---

NOTE: The vertebral artery (Fig. 503) is deep in the suboccipital triangle, bounded by the Obliquus capitis superior and inferior muscles and the Rectus capitis posterior major muscle. After passing through the transverse foramen of the atlas, the vertebral artery runs directly medial in its groove in the atlas, and passes through the posterior atlanto-occipital membrane and the dura, through the large occipital foramen to supply part of the brain.

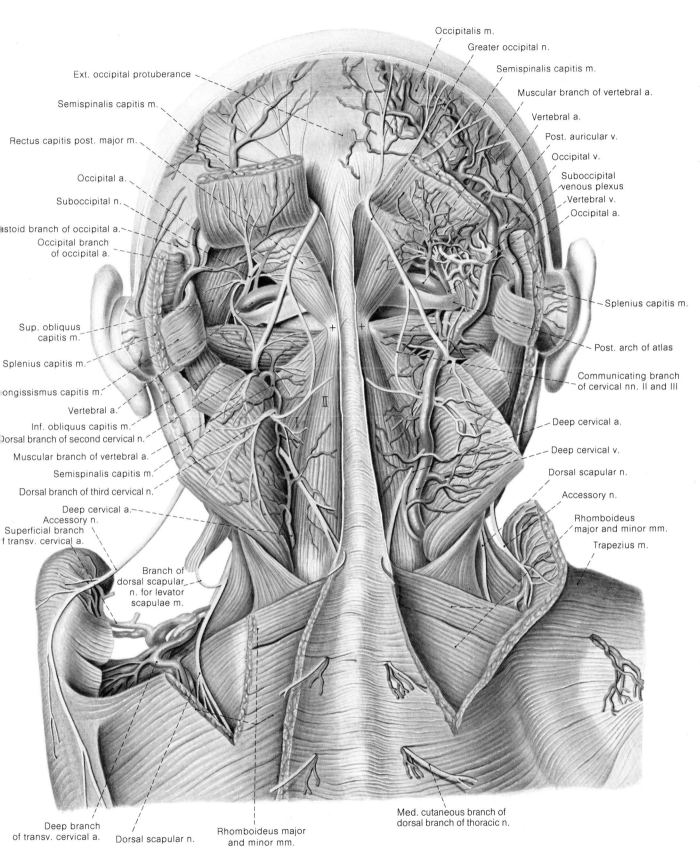

Occipitalis m.

Greater occipital n.

Semispinalis capitis m.

Muscular branch of vertebral a.

Vertebral a.

Post. auricular v.

Occipital v.

Suboccipital venous plexus

Vertebral v.

Occipital a.

Ext. occipital protuberance

Semispinalis capitis m.

Rectus capitis post. major m.

Occipital a.

Suboccipital n.

astoid branch of occipital a.

Occipital branch of occipital a.

Sup. obliquus capitis m.

Splenius capitis m.

ongissimus capitis m.

Vertebral a.

Inf. obliquus capitis m.

Dorsal branch of second cervical n.

Muscular branch of vertebral a.

Semispinalis capitis m.

Dorsal branch of third cervical n.

Deep cervical a.

Accessory n.

Superficial branch f transv. cervical a.

Branch of dorsal scapular n. for levator scapulae m.

Splenius capitis m.

Post. arch of atlas

Communicating branch of cervical nn. II and III

Deep cervical a.

Deep cervical v.

Dorsal scapular n.

Accessory n.

Rhomboideus major and minor mm.

Trapezius m.

Deep branch of transv. cervical a.

Dorsal scapular n.

Rhomboideus major and minor mm.

Med. cutaneous branch of dorsal branch of thoracic n.

**Fig. 504.** Nerves and vessels of the occipital and nuchal regions. Deep layer, I = Multifidus m., II = Semispinalis cervicis m., + + = Spinous process of axis.

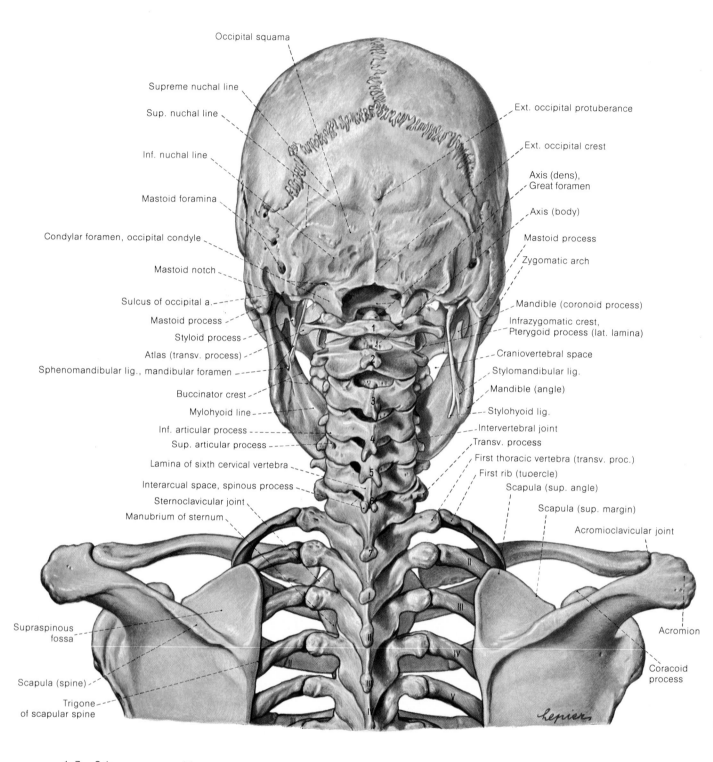

Occipital squama

Supreme nuchal line

Sup. nuchal line

Inf. nuchal line

Mastoid foramina

Condylar foramen, occipital condyle

Mastoid notch

Sulcus of occipital a.

Mastoid process

Styloid process

Atlas (transv. process)

Sphenomandibular lig., mandibular foramen

Buccinator crest

Mylohyoid line

Inf. articular process

Sup. articular process

Lamina of sixth cervical vertebra

Interarcual space, spinous process

Sternoclavicular joint

Manubrium of sternum

Supraspinous fossa

Scapula (spine)

Trigone of scapular spine

Ext. occipital protuberance

Ext. occipital crest

Axis (dens), Great foramen

Axis (body)

Mastoid process

Zygomatic arch

Mandible (coronoid process)

Infrazygomatic crest, Pterygoid process (lat. lamina)

Craniovertebral space

Stylomandibular lig.

Mandible (angle)

Stylohyoid lig.

Intervertebral joint

Transv. process

First thoracic vertebra (transv. proc.)

First rib (tubercle)

Scapula (sup. angle)

Scapula (sup. margin)

Acromioclavicular joint

Acromion

Coracoid process

1−7 = Spinous processes of the seven cervical vertebrae
I−V = Spinous processes of the upper four thoracic vertebrae and the five upper ribs, respectively

**Fig. 505.** The skeleton of the occiput and the neck. Dorsal view. (From PERNKOPF: Atlas der topographischen und angewandten Anatomie des Menschen, Vol. 1, 2nd ed. [Ed. H. FERNER]. Urban & Schwarzenberg, Munich–Vienna–Baltimore 1980.)

# Upper Extremity

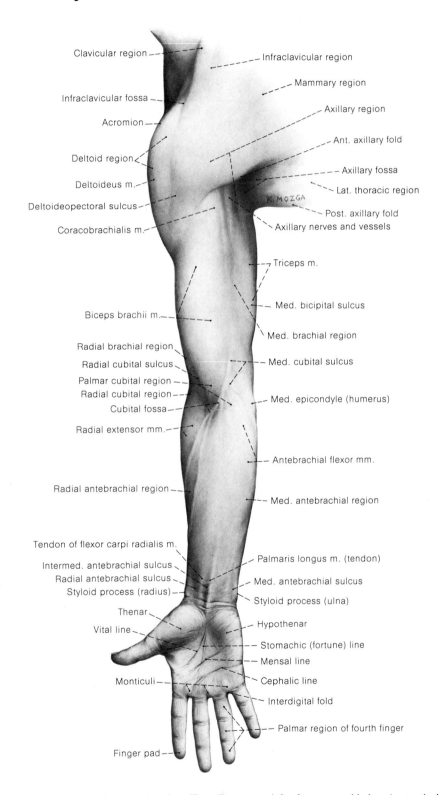

Clavicular region — Infraclavicular region

Mammary region

Infraclavicular fossa — Axillary region

Acromion — Ant. axillary fold

Deltoid region — Axillary fossa

Deltoideus m. — Lat. thoracic region

Deltoideopectoral sulcus — K. MOZGA

Post. axillary fold

Coracobrachialis m. — Axillary nerves and vessels

Triceps m.

Med. bicipital sulcus

Biceps brachii m. — Med. brachial region

Radial brachial region — Med. cubital sulcus

Radial cubital sulcus

Palmar cubital region — Med. epicondyle (humerus)

Radial cubital region

Cubital fossa

Radial extensor mm. — Antebrachial flexor mm.

Radial antebrachial region — Med. antebrachial region

Tendon of flexor carpi radialis m. — Palmaris longus m. (tendon)

Intermed. antebrachial sulcus — Med. antebrachial sulcus

Radial antebrachial sulcus — Styloid process (ulna)

Styloid process (radius)

Thenar — Hypothenar

Vital line — Stomachic (fortune) line

Mensal line

Cephalic line

Monticuli — Interdigital fold

Palmar region of fourth finger

Finger pad

**Fig. 506.** Surface relief of the upper extremity. Anterior view. (From PERNKOPF: Atlas der topographischen Anatomie des Menschen, Vol. 4, 2nd Half. Urban & Schwarzenberg, Vienna 1937–1941.)
The subdivisions of the regions and their names are not contained in the Nomina anatomica of 1977.

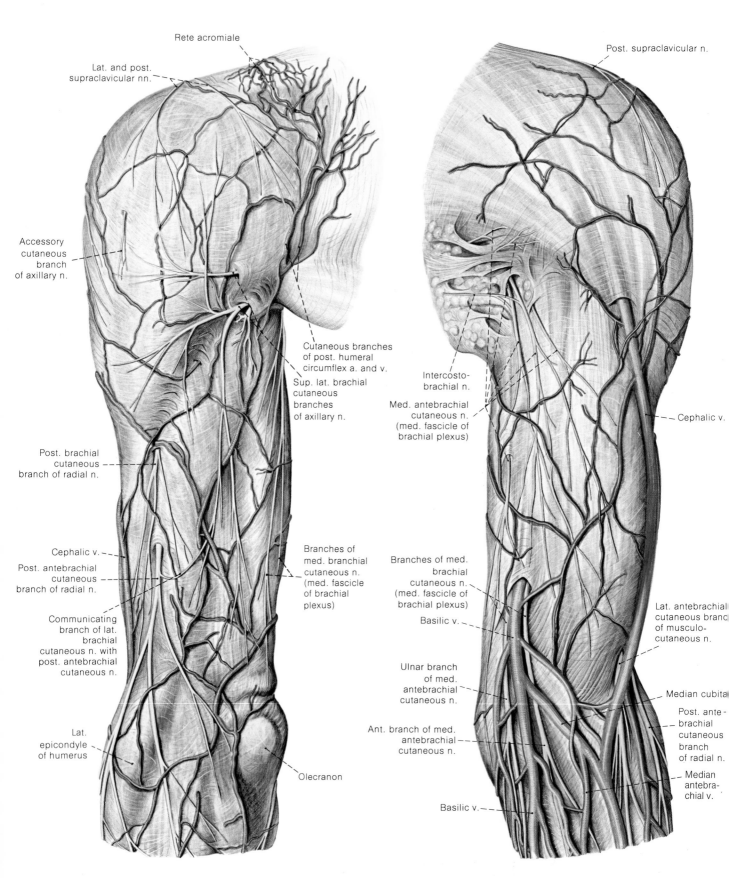

Rete acromiale

Lat. and post.
supraclavicular nn.

Accessory
cutaneous
branch
of axillary n.

Post. brachial
cutaneous
branch of radial n.

Cephalic v.

Post. antebrachial
cutaneous
branch of radial n.

Communicating
branch of lat.
brachial
cutaneous n. with
post. antebrachial
cutaneous n.

Lat.
epicondyle
of humerus

Cutaneous branches
of post. humeral
circumflex a. and v.

Sup. lat. brachial
cutaneous
branches
of axillary n.

Branches of
med. branchial
cutaneous n.
(med. fascicle
of brachial
plexus)

Olecranon

Post. supraclavicular n.

Intercosto-
brachial n.

Med. antebrachial
cutaneous n.
(med. fascicle of
brachial plexus)

Cephalic v.

Branches of med.
brachial
cutaneous n.
(med. fascicle
of brachial plexus)

Basilic v.

Ulnar branch
of med.
antebrachial
cutaneous n.

Ant. branch of med.
antebrachial
cutaneous n.

Basilic v.

Lat. antebrachial
cutaneous branch
of musculo-
cutaneous n.

Median cubital

Post. ante-
brachial
cutaneous
branch
of radial n.

Median
antebra-
chial v.

**Fig. 507.** Cutaneous nerves and veins of the posterior brachial surface.

**Fig. 508.** Cutaneous nerves and veins of the flexor surface of the left brachium. Skin and subcutaneous fat have been removed, the fascia has been retained.

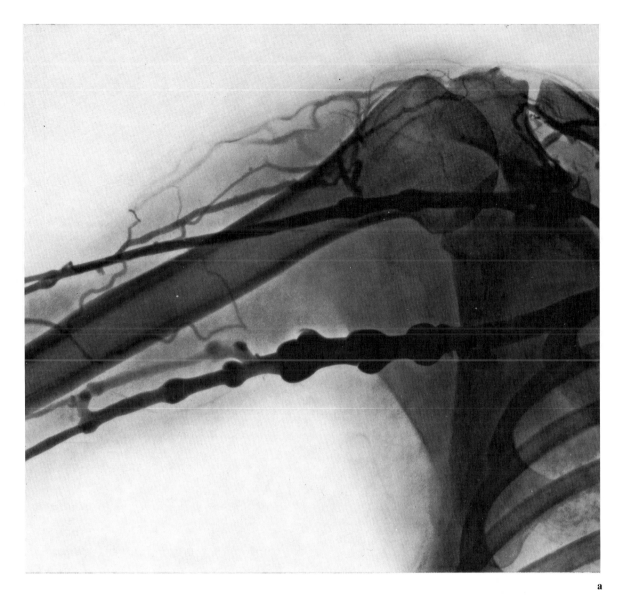

a

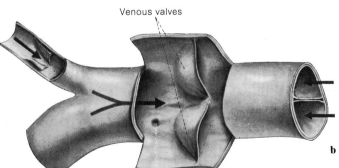

Venous valves

b

**Figs. 509 a and b.** (a) X-ray (veno- or phlebogram) of the brachial vein → axillary vein, as well as the cephalic vein, and some of their tributaries. Note the valvular segments of the axillary vein, clearly seen one after another in succession. (b) Schematic venous valve. The arrows on left indicate the normal blood flow which keeps the venous valves open. The opposing arrows on the right indicate the back pressure to close the valves to prevent the blood from flowing backwards.

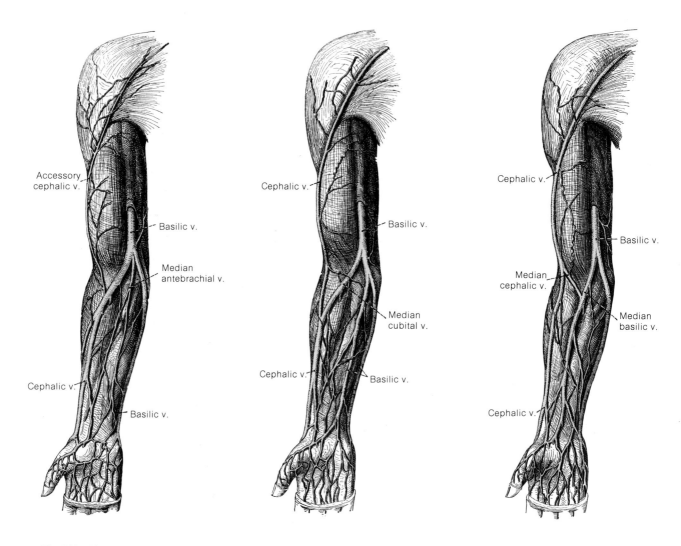

**Fig. 510.** The most common variations in the venous pattern of the upper extremity.

**Cutaneous veins of the upper extremity**

1. *Cephalic vein;* it begins at the radial half of the back of the hand from tributaries of the venous network; it receives blood from the palm of the hand via the intercapital veins; it courses proximally on the radial side of the antebrachium toward the cubital fossa where it anastomoses with the basilic vein. It continues through the lateral bicipital sulcus toward the deltoideopectoral triangle where it penetrates the fascia and empties into the axillary vein.

2. *Basilic vein;* it originates from the ulnar side of the back of the hand and courses over the ulnar flexor side of the antebrachium toward the cubital fossa where it connects to the cephalic vein via the median cubital vein. In the brachial area it is, in most cases, larger than the cephalic vein. It runs in the medial bicipital sulcus to approximately the middle of the brachium where it penetrates the fascia and continues proximally as medial brachial vein.

3. *Median cubital vein;* it is an oblique, highly variable, anastomosis between the basilic and cephalic veins and receives, in most instances, the median antebrachial vein which originates from veins of the palmar surface of hand and antebrachium.

4. *Median basilic vein* and 5. *Median cephalic vein;* these are very variable and, if present, form connections between cephalic, basilic and median cubital veins.

Clinical significance of the cutaneous veins in the cubital fossa; to draw blood or make intravenous injections.

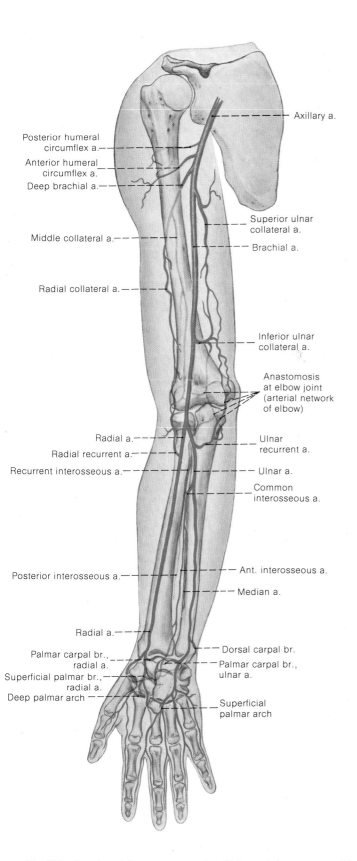

Axillary a.

Posterior humeral circumflex a.

Anterior humeral circumflex a.

Deep brachial a.

Superior ulnar collateral a.

Middle collateral a.

Brachial a.

Radial collateral a.

Inferior ulnar collateral a.

Anastomosis at elbow joint (arterial network of elbow)

Radial a.

Ulnar recurrent a.

Radial recurrent a.

Recurrent interosseous a.

Ulnar a.

Common interosseous a.

Posterior interosseous a.

Ant. interosseous a.

Median a.

Radial a.

Palmar carpal br., radial a.

Dorsal carpal br.

Palmar carpal br., ulnar a.

Superficial palmar br., radial a.

Deep palmar arch

Superficial palmar arch

**Fig. 511.** Arteries of the upper extremity. (Schematic.)

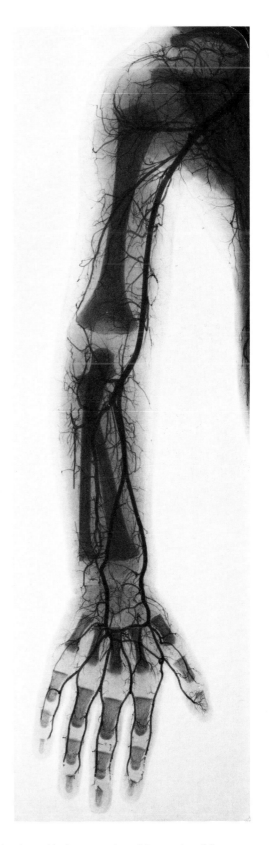

**Fig. 512.** Angiographic demonstration of the arteries of the upper extremity of an infant (stillborn). Original: Prof. Dr. G. W. KAUFF-MANN, Zentrum Radiologie des Klinikums Freiburg i. Brsg.

303

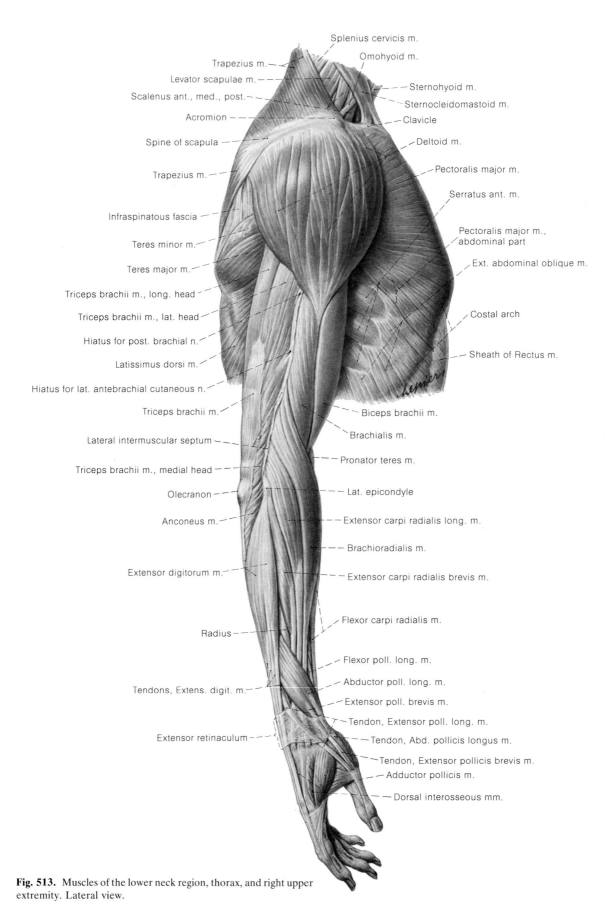

Splenius cervicis m.

Omohyoid m.

Trapezius m.

Levator scapulae m.

Scalenus ant., med., post.

Sternohyoid m.

Sternocleidomastoid m.

Acromion

Clavicle

Spine of scapula

Deltoid m.

Trapezius m.

Pectoralis major m.

Serratus ant. m.

Infraspinatous fascia

Pectoralis major m., abdominal part

Teres minor m.

Ext. abdominal oblique m.

Teres major m.

Triceps brachii m., long. head

Costal arch

Triceps brachii m., lat. head

Hiatus for post. brachial n.

Sheath of Rectus m.

Latissimus dorsi m.

Hiatus for lat. antebrachial cutaneous n.

Triceps brachii m.

Biceps brachii m.

Brachialis m.

Lateral intermuscular septum

Pronator teres m.

Triceps brachii m., medial head

Olecranon

Lat. epicondyle

Anconeus m.

Extensor carpi radialis long. m.

Brachioradialis m.

Extensor digitorum m.

Extensor carpi radialis brevis m.

Flexor carpi radialis m.

Radius

Flexor poll. long. m.

Abductor poll. long. m.

Tendons, Extens. digit. m.

Extensor poll. brevis m.

Tendon, Extensor poll. long. m.

Extensor retinaculum

Tendon, Abd. pollicis longus m.

Tendon, Extensor pollicis brevis m.

Adductor pollicis m.

Dorsal interosseous mm.

**Fig. 513.** Muscles of the lower neck region, thorax, and right upper extremity. Lateral view.

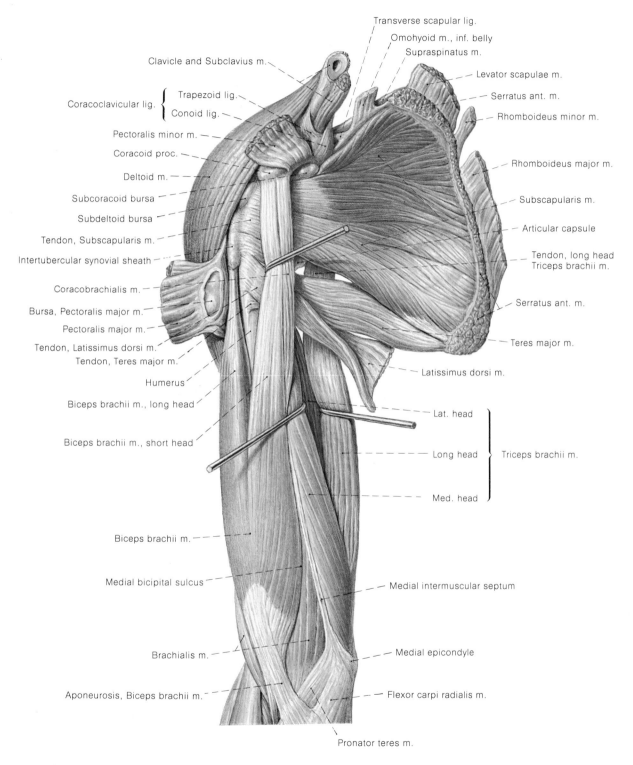

Transverse scapular lig.

Omohyoid m., inf. belly

Supraspinatus m.

Clavicle and Subclavius m.

Levator scapulae m.

Serratus ant. m.

Coracoclavicular lig. { Trapezoid lig.

Conoid lig.

Rhomboideus minor m.

Pectoralis minor m.

Coracoid proc.

Rhomboideus major m.

Deltoid m.

Subcoracoid bursa

Subscapularis m.

Subdeltoid bursa

Articular capsule

Tendon, Subscapularis m.

Tendon, long head
Triceps brachii m.

Intertubercular synovial sheath

Coracobrachialis m.

Serratus ant. m.

Bursa, Pectoralis major m.

Pectoralis major m.

Teres major m.

Tendon, Latissimus dorsi m.

Tendon, Teres major m.

Latissimus dorsi m.

Humerus

Biceps brachii m., long head

Lat. head

Biceps brachii m., short head

Long head        Triceps brachii m.

Med. head

Biceps brachii m.

Medial bicipital sulcus

Medial intermuscular septum

Brachialis m.

Medial epicondyle

Aponeurosis, Biceps brachii m.

Flexor carpi radialis m.

Pronator teres m.

**Fig. 514.** The muscles of the costal surface of the scapula and muscles of the flexor side of the upper arm. Superficial layer.

**Joints of the Upper Extremity**

| Joint | Type of Joint | Possibility of Movement |
|-------|---------------|-------------------------|
| *Shoulder joint* | Ball and socket joint | Flexion        Abduction<br>Extension     Adduction<br>Inward rotation<br>Outward rotation |
| *Elbow joint*<br>a) Humeroulnar<br>    articulation<br>b) Humeroradial<br>    articulation<br><br>c) Proximal radioulnar<br>    articulation<br><br>Distal radioulnar<br>articulation | Hinge joint<br><br>Ball and socket joint<br>(functionally restricted)<br><br>Pivot joint | Flexion<br>Extension<br>Flexion<br>Extension<br>Rotation<br><br>Pronation<br>Supination |
| *Carpal joints*<br>a) Radio-carpal<br>    articulation<br>b) Mediocarpal<br>    articulation | Ellipsoidal joints | Ulnarduction<br>Radialduction<br>(palmar-) Flexion<br>(dorsal-) Extension |
| *Carpometacarpal*<br>articulation of thumb | Saddle joint | Flexion, Extension<br>Abduction, Adduction<br>Opposition |
| *Metacarpophalangeal*<br>articulations | Ball and socket joints<br>(functionally restricted) | Flexion, Extension<br>Abduction, Adduction |
| *Finger joints*<br>(interphalangeal articulations) | Hinge joints | Flexion, Extension |

**Shoulder Muscles**

| Name | Origin | Insertion |
|---|---|---|
| **1. Supraspinatus muscle** | Supraspinatous fossa of the scapula | Highest facet of greater tubercle of humerus (tendinous) |
| **2. Infraspinatus muscle** | Caudal margin of the spine of the scapula, infraspinatous fossa and fascia | Middle facet of greater tubercle of humerus (tendinous) |

*Nerve:*   Suprascapular nerve from brachial plexus (C 4, 5, 6)

*Function:*   Supraspinatus muscle abducts humerus; starts abduction and assists the deltoid muscle.
Infraspinatus muscle rotates humerus laterally; assists in holding head of humerus in glenoid cavity

| | | |
|---|---|---|
| **3. Teres minor muscle** | Caudal section of infraspinatous fossa and lateral margin (²/₃) of scapula, infraspinatous fascia | Lower facet of greater tubercle of humerus (tendinous) |

*Nerve:*   Axillary nerve from brachial plexus (C 4, 5)

*Function:*   Lateral rotator and adductor of humerus

| | | |
|---|---|---|
| **4. Teres major muscle** | Lateral border of scapula near inferior angle (medial third) | Tendon on crest of lesser tubercle of humerus, dorsal to that of the Latissimus dorsi muscle (the 2 tendons separated by bursa) |

*Nerve:*   Subscapular nerves (C 5, 6, 7) of the brachial plexus

*Function:*   Adductor, medial rotator and extensor of arm

| | | |
|---|---|---|
| **5. Subscapularis muscle** (under the insertion: the subscapular bursa) | Costal surface of scapula; subscapular fossa | Short, broad tendon into the lesser tubercle and its adjacent crest; blends with capsule of shoulder joint |

*Nerve:*   Subscapular nerves (C 5, 6, 7) from brachial plexus

*Function:*   Adductor and medial rotator of arm; assists in flexion and extension

| | | |
|---|---|---|
| **6. Deltoid muscle** | Acromial third of clavicle, the acromion, and spine of scapula | Deltoid tuberosity of humerus (subdeltoid bursa between muscle and greater tubercle) |

*Nerve:*   Axillary nerve (C 5, 6)

*Function:*   Ventral (clavicular) fibers assist in flexion and medial rotation of humerus. Dorsal (scapular) fibers assist in extension and lateral rotation of humerus. Middle or central part is a powerful abductor of humerus, lifting it to the horizontal

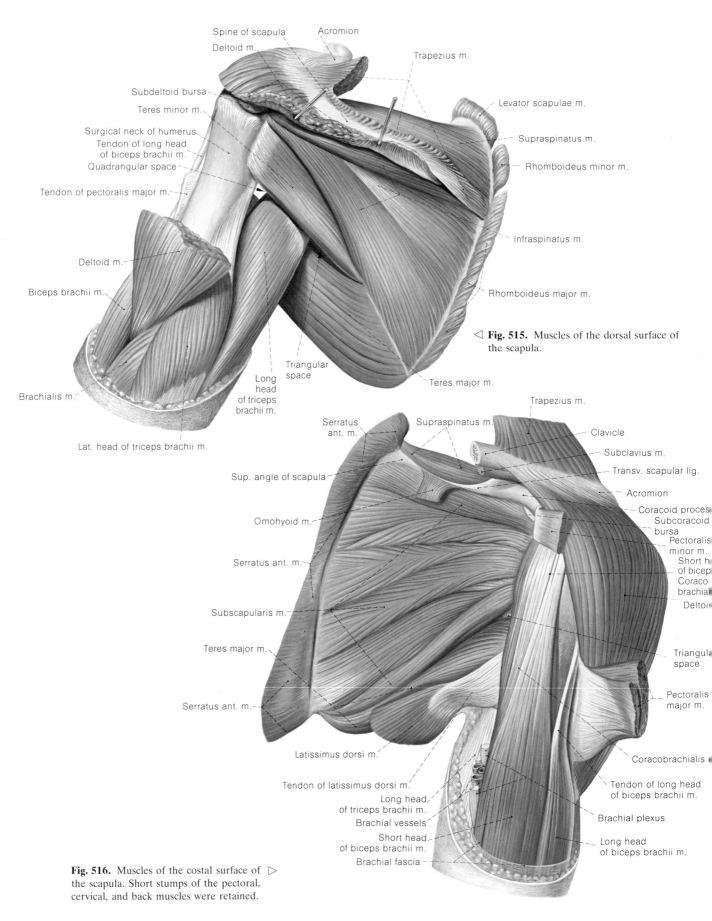

Spine of scapula
Acromion
Deltoid m.
Trapezius m.
Subdeltoid bursa
Teres minor m.
Levator scapulae m.
Surgical neck of humerus
Supraspinatus m.
Tendon of long head
of biceps brachii m.
Rhomboideus minor m.
Quadrangular space
Tendon of pectoralis major m.
Deltoid m.
Biceps brachii m.
Infraspinatus m.
Rhomboideus major m.
Brachialis m.
Triangular
space
Long
head
of triceps
brachii m.
Teres major m.
Lat. head of triceps brachii m.

**Fig. 515.** Muscles of the dorsal surface of the scapula.

Serratus
ant. m.
Supraspinatus m.
Trapezius m.
Clavicle
Sup. angle of scapula
Subclavius m.
Transv. scapular lig.
Omohyoid m.
Acromion
Coracoid proces
Subcoracoid
bursa
Serratus ant. m.
Pectoralis
minor m.
Short h
of bicep
Coraco
brachia
Subscapularis m.
Deltoi
Teres major m.
Triangula
space
Serratus ant. m.
Pectoralis
major m.
Latissimus dorsi m.
Coracobrachialis
Tendon of latissimus dorsi m.
Tendon of long head
of biceps brachii m.
Long head
of triceps brachii m.
Brachial vessels
Brachial plexus
Short head
of biceps brachii m.
Long head
of biceps brachii m.
Brachial fascia

**Fig. 516.** Muscles of the costal surface of the scapula. Short stumps of the pectoral, cervical, and back muscles were retained.

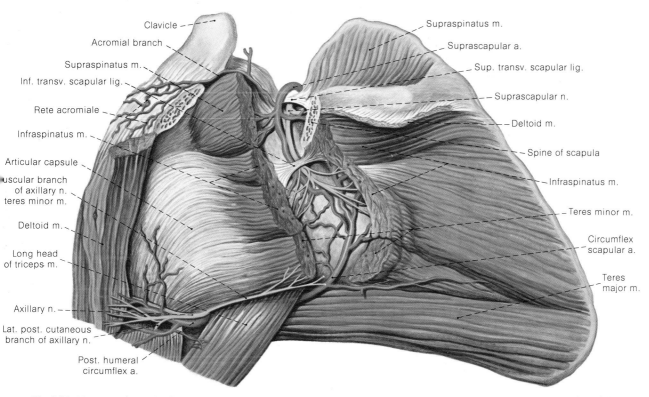

Clavicle
Acromial branch
Supraspinatus m.
Inf. transv. scapular lig.
Rete acromiale
Infraspinatus m.
Articular capsule
uscular branch
of axillary n.
teres minor m.
Deltoid m.
Long head
of triceps m.
Axillary n.
Lat. post. cutaneous
branch of axillary n.
Post. humeral
circumflex a.

Supraspinatus m.
Suprascapular a.
Sup. transv. scapular lig.
Suprascapular n.
Deltoid m.
Spine of scapula
Infraspinatus m.
Teres minor m.
Circumflex
scapular a.
Teres
major m.

**Fig. 517.** Nerves and vessels of the left shoulder region, dorsal view. Deltoid muscle partially removed and reflected. Portion of the acromion removed; supraspinatus, infraspinatus and teres minor muscles sectioned and somewhat pulled apart.

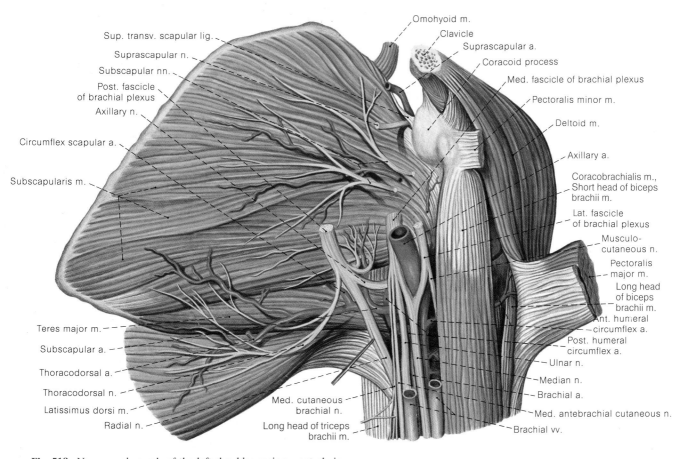

Sup. transv. scapular lig.
Suprascapular n.
Subscapular nn.
Post. fascicle
of brachial plexus
Axillary n.
Circumflex scapular a.
Subscapularis m.
Teres major m.
Subscapular a.
Thoracodorsal a.
Thoracodorsal n.
Latissimus dorsi m.
Radial n.

Omohyoid m.
Clavicle
Suprascapular a.
Coracoid process
Med. fascicle of brachial plexus
Pectoralis minor m.
Deltoid m.
Axillary a.
Coracobrachialis m.,
Short head of biceps
brachii m.
Lat. fascicle
of brachial plexus
Musculo-
cutaneous n.
Pectoralis
major m.
Long head
of biceps
brachii m.
Ant. humeral
circumflex a.
Post. humeral
circumflex a.
Ulnar n.
Median n.
Brachial a.
Med. antebrachial cutaneous n.
Brachial vv.

Med. cutaneous
brachial n.
Long head of triceps
brachii m.

**Fig. 518.** Nerves and vessels of the left shoulder region, ventral view.

309

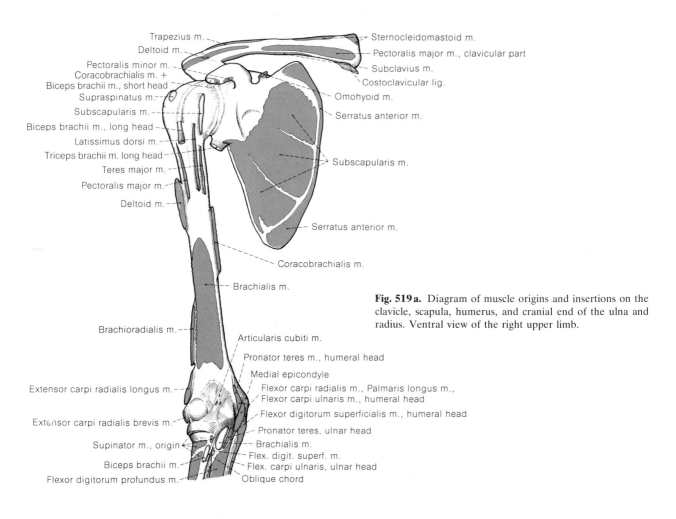

Trapezius m.
Deltoid m.
Pectoralis minor m.
Coracobrachialis m. +
Biceps brachii m., short head
Supraspinatus m.
Subscapularis m.
Biceps brachii m., long head
Latissimus dorsi m.
Triceps brachii m. long head
Teres major m.
Pectoralis major m.
Deltoid m.

Sternocleidomastoid m.
Pectoralis major m., clavicular part
Subclavius m.
Costoclavicular lig.
Omohyoid m.
Serratus anterior m.

Subscapularis m.

Serratus anterior m.

Coracobrachialis m.

Brachialis m.

Brachioradialis m.
Articularis cubiti m.
Pronator teres m., humeral head
Medial epicondyle
Flexor carpi radialis m., Palmaris longus m.,
Flexor carpi ulnaris m., humeral head
Extensor carpi radialis longus m.
Flexor digitorum superficialis m., humeral head
Extensor carpi radialis brevis m.
Pronator teres, ulnar head
Brachialis m.
Supinator m., origin
Flex. digit. superf. m.
Biceps brachii m.
Flex. carpi ulnaris, ulnar head
Flexor digitorum profundus m.
Oblique chord

**Fig. 519 a.** Diagram of muscle origins and insertions on the clavicle, scapula, humerus, and cranial end of the ulna and radius. Ventral view of the right upper limb.

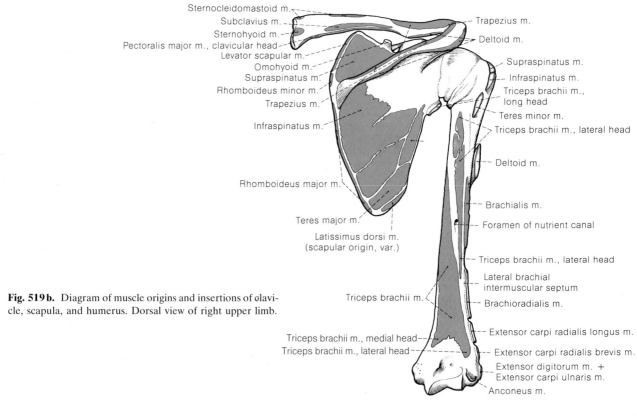

Sternocleidomastoid m.
Subclavius m.
Sternohyoid m.
Pectoralis major m., clavicular head
Levator scapular m.
Omohyoid m.
Supraspinatus m.
Rhomboideus minor m.
Trapezius m.
Infraspinatus m.

Trapezius m.
Deltoid m.
Supraspinatus m.
Infraspinatus m.
Triceps brachii m., long head
Teres minor m.
Triceps brachii m., lateral head

Deltoid m.

Rhomboideus major m.

Brachialis m.
Foramen of nutrient canal

Teres major m.
Latissimus dorsi m.
(scapular origin, var.)

Triceps brachii m., lateral head
Lateral brachial intermuscular septum
Brachioradialis m.

Triceps brachii m.

Extensor carpi radialis longus m.

Triceps brachii m., medial head
Triceps brachii m., lateral head
Extensor carpi radialis brevis m.
Extensor digitorum m. +
Extensor carpi ulnaris m.
Anconeus m.

**Fig. 519 b.** Diagram of muscle origins and insertions of clavicle, scapula, and humerus. Dorsal view of right upper limb.

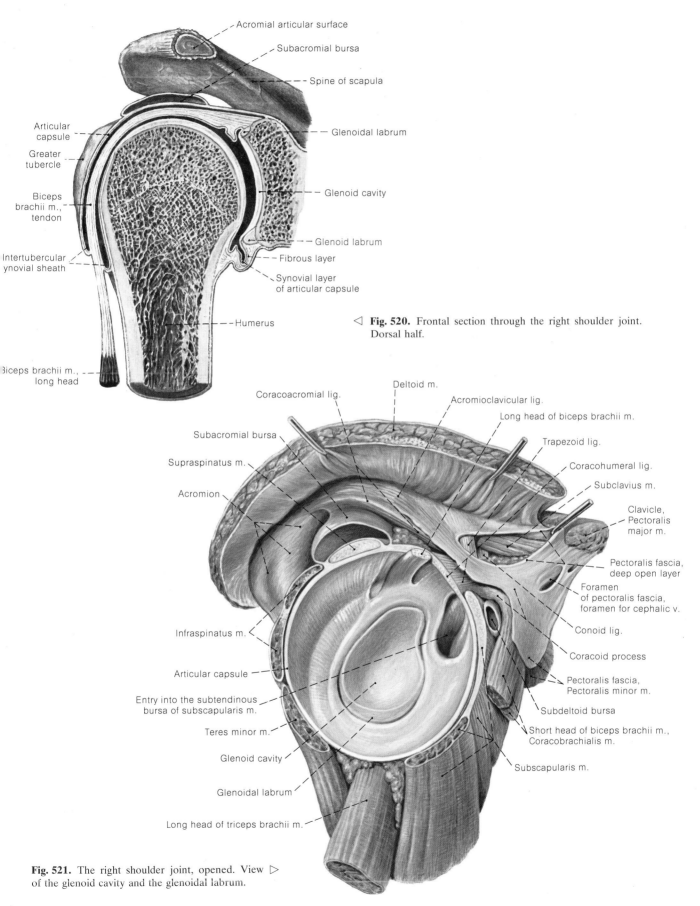

Acromial articular surface

Subacromial bursa

Spine of scapula

Articular capsule

Greater tubercle

Biceps brachii m., tendon

Intertubercular synovial sheath

Biceps brachii m., long head

Glenoidal labrum

Glenoid cavity

Glenoid labrum

Fibrous layer

Synovial layer of articular capsule

Humerus

◁ **Fig. 520.** Frontal section through the right shoulder joint. Dorsal half.

Coracoacromial lig.

Deltoid m.

Acromioclavicular lig.

Subacromial bursa

Supraspinatus m.

Acromion

Long head of biceps brachii m.

Trapezoid lig.

Coracohumeral lig.

Subclavius m.

Clavicle, Pectoralis major m.

Pectoralis fascia, deep open layer

Foramen of pectoralis fascia, foramen for cephalic v.

Conoid lig.

Coracoid process

Pectoralis fascia, Pectoralis minor m.

Subdeltoid bursa

Short head of biceps brachii m., Coracobrachialis m.

Subscapularis m.

Infraspinatus m.

Articular capsule

Entry into the subtendinous bursa of subscapularis m.

Teres minor m.

Glenoid cavity

Glenoidal labrum

Long head of triceps brachii m.

**Fig. 521.** The right shoulder joint, opened. View ▷ of the glenoid cavity and the glenoidal labrum.

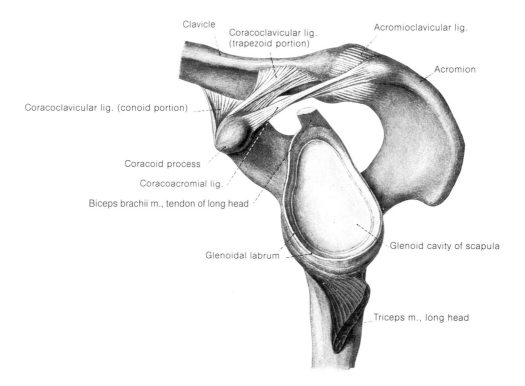

Clavicle

Coracoclavicular lig.
(trapezoid portion)

Acromioclavicular lig.

Acromion

Coracoclavicular lig. (conoid portion)

Coracoid process

Coracoacromial lig.

Biceps brachii m., tendon of long head

Glenoidal labrum

Glenoid cavity of scapula

Triceps m., long head

**Fig. 522.** Socket of the left shoulder joint. The joint capsule is cut off at the glenoidal labrum. The origin of the long head of the Triceps and the tendon of the long head of the Biceps is kept in place.

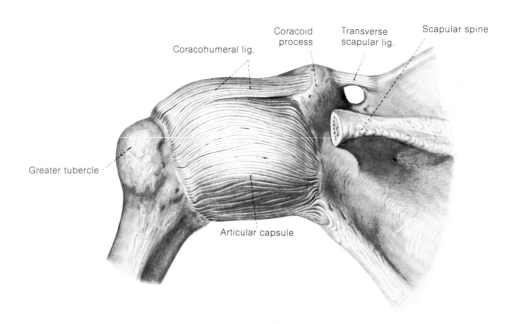

Coracoid
process

Transverse
scapular lig.

Scapular spine

Coracohumeral lig.

Greater tubercle

Articular capsule

**Fig. 523.** Left shoulder joint without muscle attachments. Dorsocranial view. The acromion is cut off with a saw.

**Fig. 524.** Left shoulder joint and acromioclavicular joint. Ventral ▷
view. * Communication point with the subacromial bursa.

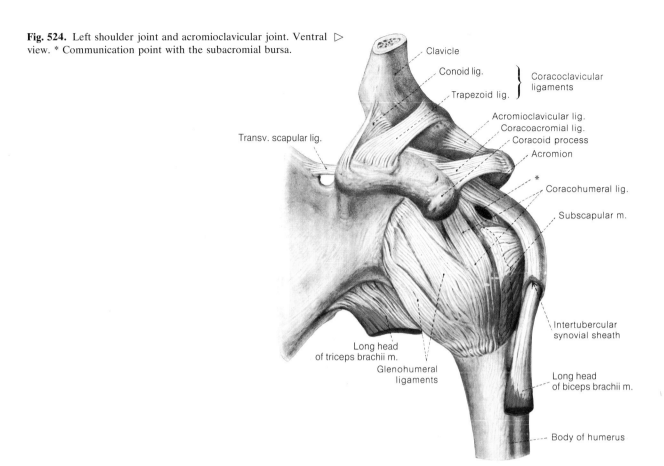

Clavicle

Conoid lig.

Trapezoid lig.

Coracoclavicular
ligaments

Acromioclavicular lig.
Coracoacromial lig.
Coracoid process
Acromion

Transv. scapular lig.

*

Coracohumeral lig.

Subscapular m.

Intertubercular
synovial sheath

Long head
of triceps brachii m.

Glenohumeral
ligaments

Long head
of biceps brachii m.

Body of humerus

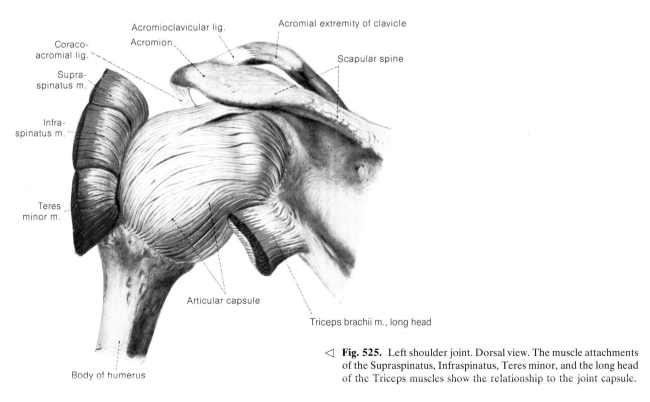

Coraco-
acromial lig.

Acromioclavicular lig.

Acromion

Acromial extremity of clavicle

Scapular spine

Supra-
spinatus m.

Infra-
spinatus m.

Teres
minor m.

Articular capsule

Triceps brachii m., long head

Body of humerus

◁ **Fig. 525.** Left shoulder joint. Dorsal view. The muscle attachments
of the Supraspinatus, Infraspinatus, Teres minor, and the long head
of the Triceps muscles show the relationship to the joint capsule.

313

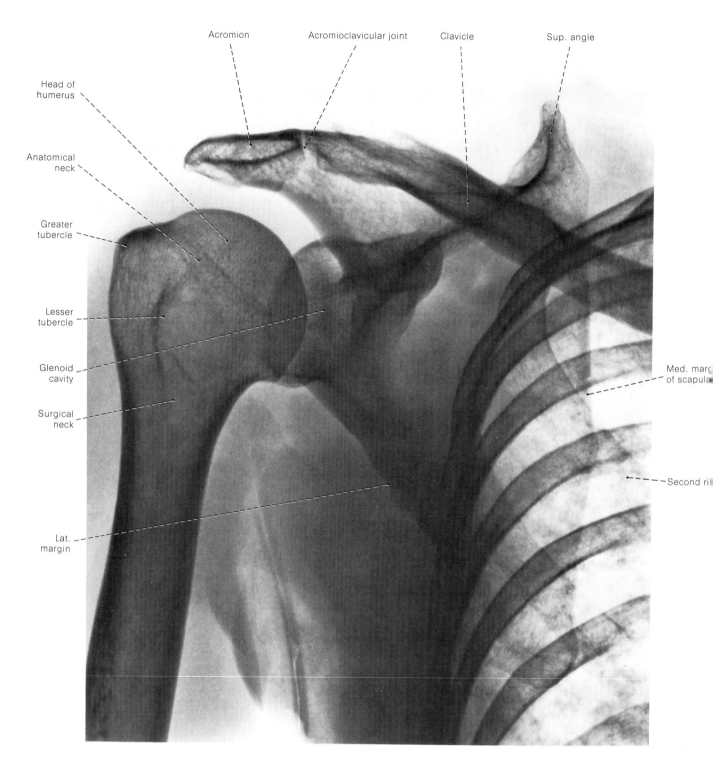

Acromion    Acromioclavicular joint    Clavicle    Sup. angle

Head of
humerus

Anatomical
neck

Greater
tubercle

Lesser
tubercle

Glenoid
cavity

Surgical
neck

Lat.
margin

Med. marg
of scapula

Second ri

**Fig. 526.** X-ray film of the right shoulder, sagittal projection. (From L. WICKE: Atlas der Röntgenanatomie, 2nd ed. Urban & Schwarzenberg, Munich–Vienna–Baltimore 1980.)

**Fig. 527.** Head of left humerus. Proximal view. Greater tubercle facets for: 1. the Supraspinatus muscle. 2. the Infraspinatus muscle. 3. the ▷ Teres minor muscle.

**Figs. 528–530.** Left scapula. Fig. 528 Dorsal view. Fig. 529 Ventral view. Fig. 530 Lateral view.

**Figs. 531 and 532.** Left clavicle. Fig. 531 Cranial view. Fig. 532 Caudal view.

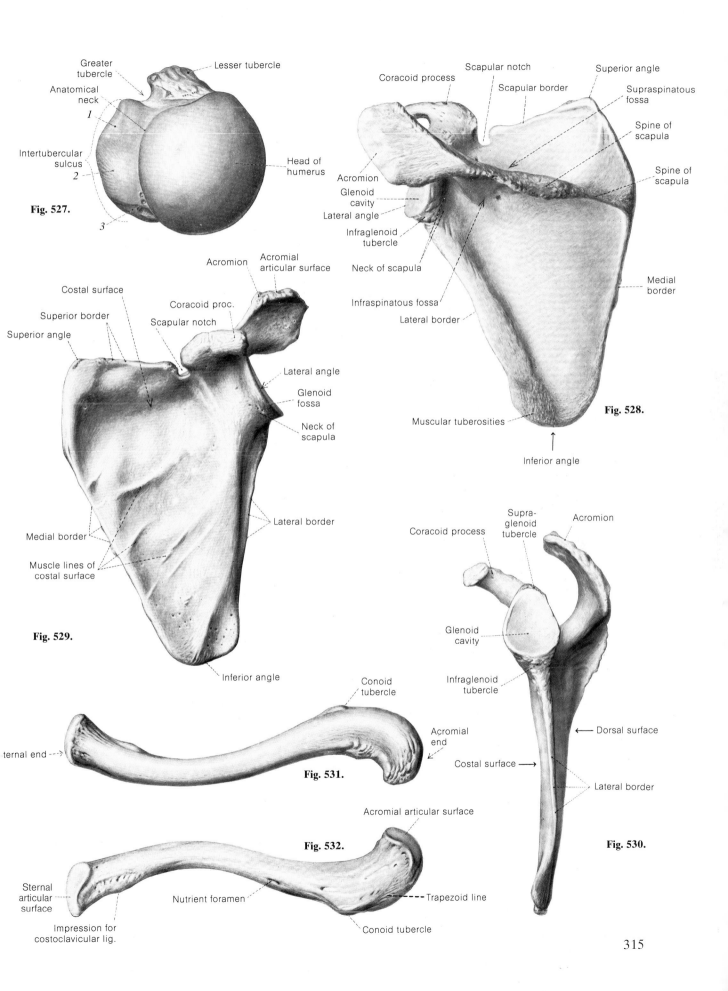

Fig. 527.

Greater tubercle
Lesser tubercle
Anatomical neck
1
Intertubercular sulcus
2
3
Head of humerus

Fig. 528.

Coracoid process
Scapular notch
Superior angle
Scapular border
Supraspinatous fossa
Spine of scapula
Spine of scapula
Acromion
Glenoid cavity
Lateral angle
Infraglenoid tubercle
Neck of scapula
Infraspinatous fossa
Lateral border
Medial border
Muscular tuberosities
Inferior angle

Fig. 529.

Costal surface
Acromion
Acromial articular surface
Superior border
Coracoid proc.
Superior angle
Scapular notch
Lateral angle
Glenoid fossa
Neck of scapula
Medial border
Lateral border
Muscle lines of costal surface
Inferior angle

Fig. 530.

Coracoid process
Supra-glenoid tubercle
Acromion
Glenoid cavity
Infraglenoid tubercle
Dorsal surface
Costal surface
Lateral border

Fig. 531.

Conoid tubercle
Acromial end
ternal end

Fig. 532.

Acromial articular surface
Sternal articular surface
Nutrient foramen
Trapezoid line
Impression for costoclavicular lig.
Conoid tubercle

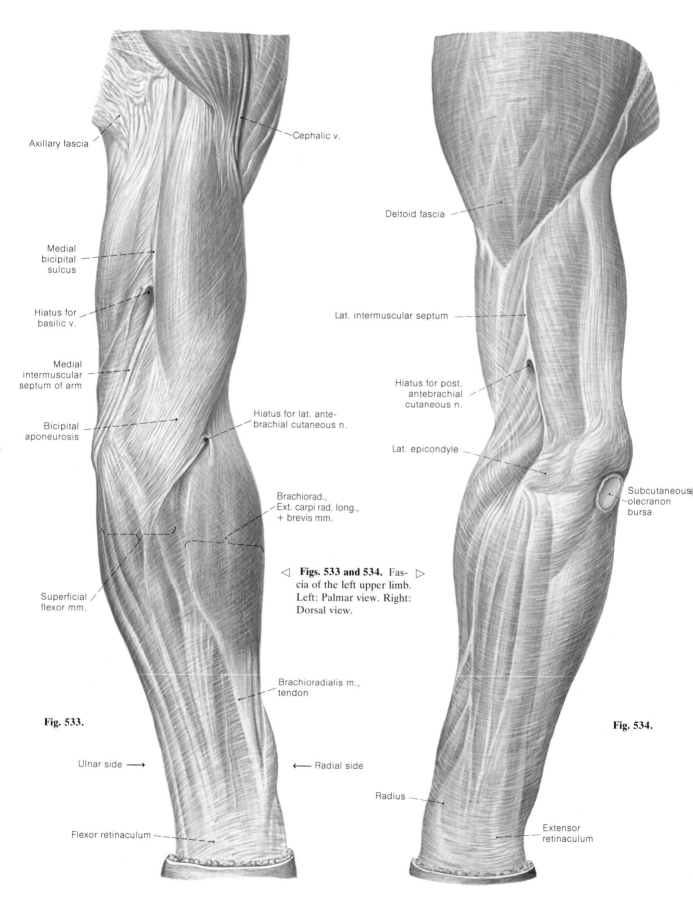

Axillary fascia

Cephalic v.

Deltoid fascia

Medial
bicipital
sulcus

Lat. intermuscular septum

Hiatus for
basilic v.

Medial
intermuscular
septum of arm

Hiatus for post.
antebrachial
cutaneous n.

Bicipital
aponeurosis

Hiatus for lat. ante-
brachial cutaneous n.

Lat. epicondyle

Brachiorad.,
Ext. carpi rad. long.,
+ brevis mm.

Subcutaneous
olecranon
bursa

◁ **Figs. 533 and 534.** Fas- ▷
cia of the left upper limb.
Left: Palmar view. Right:
Dorsal view.

Superficial
flexor mm.

**Fig. 533.**

**Fig. 534.**

Ulnar side ⟶

⟵ Radial side

Brachioradialis m.,
tendon

Radius

Flexor retinaculum

Extensor
retinaculum

## Extensor Muscle of the Upper Arm, Triceps brachii muscle

| Name | Origin | Insertion |
|---|---|---|
| **Triceps brachii muscle**<br>*Long head:*<br>(Operates 2 joints) | Infraglenoidal tubercle of scapula | Vertical muscle fibers running distalward to the olecranon |
| *Lateral head:*<br>(Operates 1 joint) | Lateral and dorsal side of humerus, lateral $^2/_3$ or lateral intermuscular septum | Joins the common tendon of insertion to the olecranon |
| *Medial head:*<br>(Operates 1 joint) | Dorsal side of humerus, lateral and distal to radial groove; medial and lateral intermuscular septa | Posterior aspect of olecranon and into deep fascia on both sides of the forearm |
| **Anconeus muscle**<br>(Situated in the forearm) | Lateral epicondyle of humerus. Developmentally, it appears to be a part of the Triceps brachii muscle | Posterior surface of ulna, slightly distal to olecranon |

*Nerve:*    Radial nerve (C 7, 8)

*Function:*    Extends forearm; adducts and extends arm, braces extended elbow joint (when pushing an object)

---

**Quandrangular and triangular spaces (Fig. 515):**
1. *Quandrangular Space:* Bounded by tendon of long head of Triceps brachii, medially; Teres major, inferiorly; the humerus, laterally; Teres minor and capsule of shoulder joint, superiorly.
   Transmits: Axillary nerve, posterior humeral circumflex vessels.
2. *Triangular space:* Bounded by Teres minor, superiorly; Teres major, inferiorly; long head of the Triceps, laterally.
   Transmits: Circumflex scapular artery.

---

## Flexor Muscles of the Upper Arm

| Name | | Origin | Insertion |
|---|---|---|---|
| **1. Biceps brachii muscle**<br>(Operates 2 joints) | *Long head:* | Tendon through shoulder joint to supraglenoid tubercle of scapula (long tendon) | Posterior half of radial tuberosity. Bicipital aponeurosis to antebrachial fascia |
| | *Short head:* | Short tendon from tip of coracoid processes of scapula | |

*Function:*    Flexes and supinates the forearm. Tenses antebrachial fascia. Long head aids in flexion of the shoulder joint and holds head of humerus in place

| | | | |
|---|---|---|---|
| **2. Coracobrachialis muscle**<br>(sometimes pierced by musculocutaneous nerve) | | Tip of the coracoid process (fused with short head of biceps) | Ventral and medial side of humerus near middle of shaft |

*Function:*    Flexes and adducts the arm

| | | | |
|---|---|---|---|
| **3. Brachialis muscle**<br>(Operates 1 joint) | | Distal half of anterior aspect of humerus and the medial and lateral intermuscular septa | Tuberosity of ulna (short tendon) and rough impression on anterior surface of coronoid process |

*Function:*    Primary flexor of forearm

*Nerve:*    Musculocutaneous nerve for all three muscles

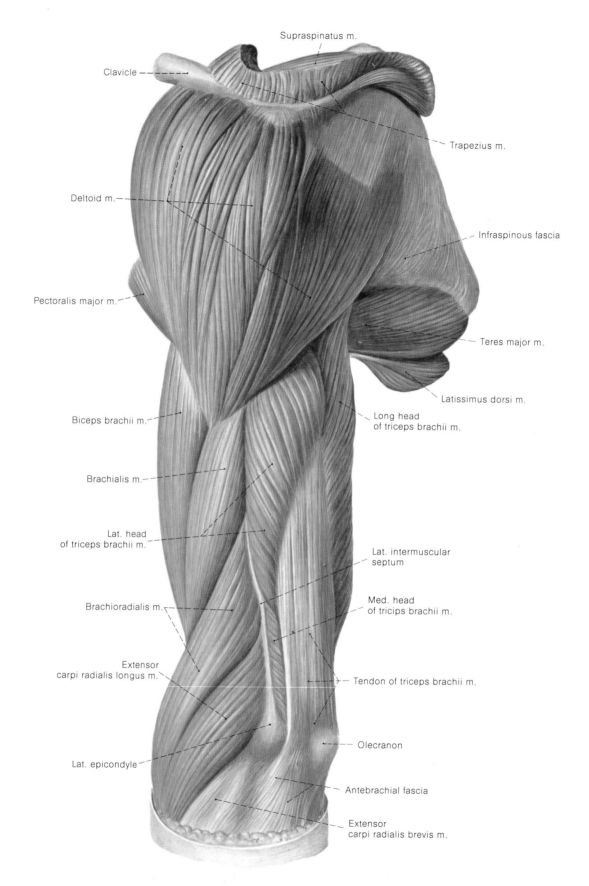

**Fig. 535.** The Deltoid muscle and muscles of the left upper arm. Dorsolateral view.

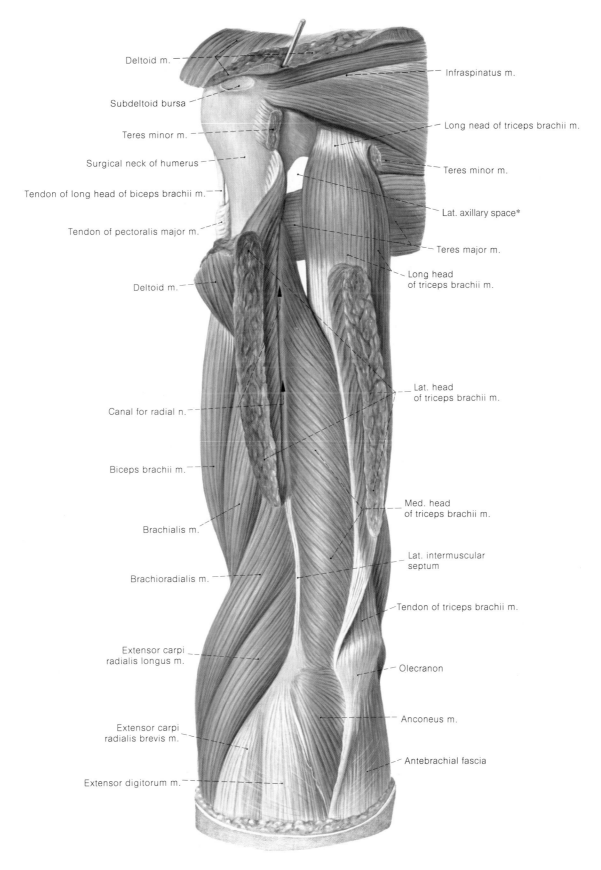

Deltoid m.

Subdeltoid bursa

Teres minor m.

Surgical neck of humerus

Tendon of long head of biceps brachii m.

Tendon of pectoralis major m.

Deltoid m.

Canal for radial n.

Biceps brachii m.

Brachialis m.

Brachioradialis m.

Extensor carpi radialis longus m.

Extensor carpi radialis brevis m.

Extensor digitorum m.

Infraspinatus m.

Long nead of triceps brachii m.

Teres minor m.

Lat. axillary space*

Teres major m.

Long head of triceps brachii m.

Lat. head of triceps brachii m.

Med. head of triceps brachii m.

Lat. intermuscular septum

Tendon of triceps brachii m.

Olecranon

Anconeus m.

Antebrachial fascia

**Fig. 536.** Muscles of the left upper arm, deeper layer. Dorsolateral view. The Deltoid muscle has been removed except for attachments. The antebrachial fascia was removed where it covered the Anconeus muscle; the Teres minor and lateral head of the Triceps brachii were cut and reflected. * the lateral (quadrangular) space.

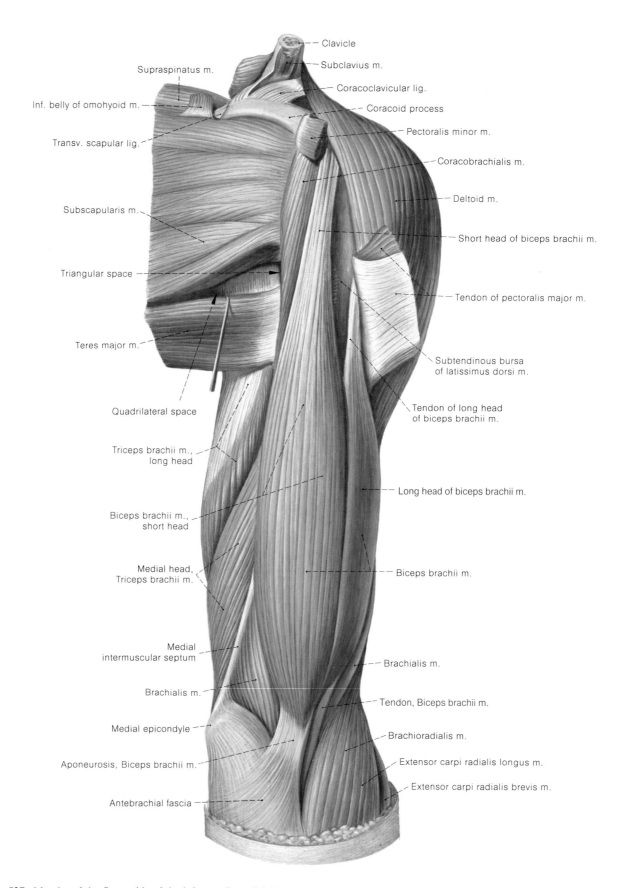

— Clavicle

Supraspinatus m. —

— Subclavius m.

— Coracoclavicular lig.

Inf. belly of omohyoid m. —

— Coracoid process

Transv. scapular lig. —

— Pectoralis minor m.

— Coracobrachialis m.

Subscapularis m. —

— Deltoid m.

— Short head of biceps brachii m.

Triangular space —

— Tendon of pectoralis major m.

Teres major m. —

— Subtendinous bursa of latissimus dorsi m.

Quadrilateral space —

Tendon of long head of biceps brachii m.

Triceps brachii m., long head —

— Long head of biceps brachii m.

Biceps brachii m., short head —

Medial head, Triceps brachii m. —

— Biceps brachii m.

Medial intermuscular septum —

— Brachialis m.

Brachialis m. —

— Tendon, Biceps brachii m.

Medial epicondyle —

— Brachioradialis m.

Aponeurosis, Biceps brachii m. —

— Extensor carpi radialis longus m.

— Extensor carpi radialis brevis m.

Antebrachial fascia —

**Fig. 537.** Muscles of the flexor side of the left arm. Superficial layer.

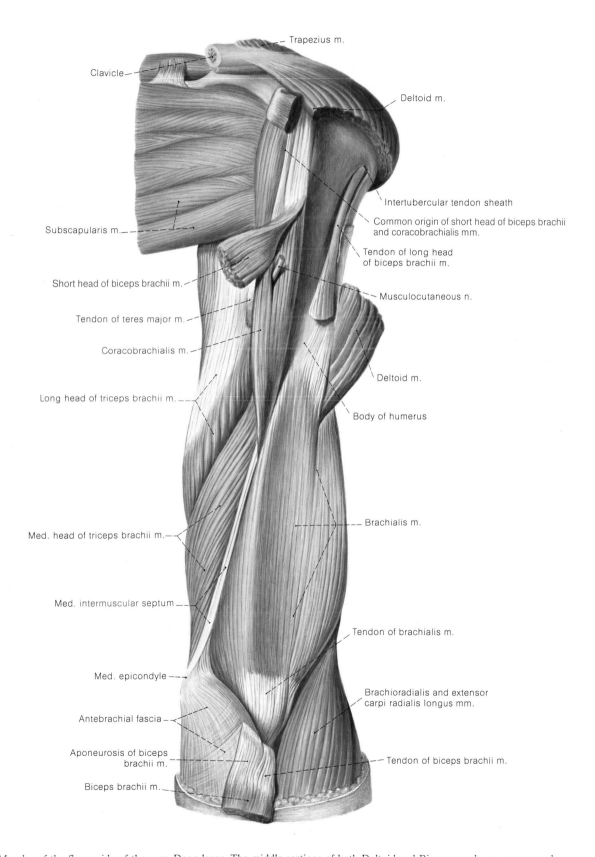

Trapezius m.

Clavicle

Deltoid m.

Intertubercular tendon sheath

Common origin of short head of biceps brachii and coracobrachialis mm.

Subscapularis m.

Tendon of long head of biceps brachii m.

Short head of biceps brachii m.

Musculocutaneous n.

Tendon of teres major m.

Coracobrachialis m.

Deltoid m.

Long head of triceps brachii m.

Body of humerus

Med. head of triceps brachii m.

Brachialis m.

Med. intermuscular septum

Tendon of brachialis m.

Med. epicondyle

Brachioradialis and extensor carpi radialis longus mm.

Antebrachial fascia

Aponeurosis of biceps brachii m.

Tendon of biceps brachii m.

Biceps brachii m.

**Fig. 538.** Muscles of the flexor side of the arm. Deep layer. The middle sections of both Deltoid and Biceps muscles were removed.

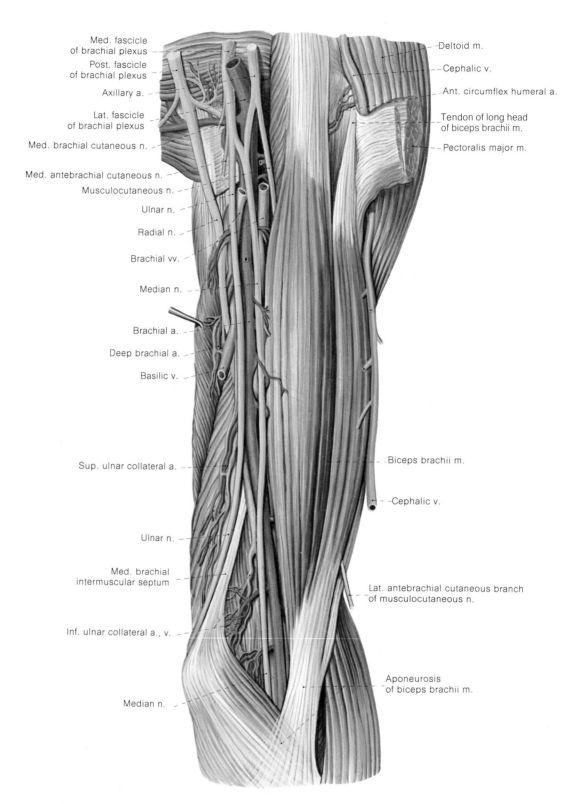

Med. fascicle
of brachial plexus

Post. fascicle
of brachial plexus

Axillary a.

Lat. fascicle
of brachial plexus

Med. brachial cutaneous n.

Med. antebrachial cutaneous n.

Musculocutaneous n.

Ulnar n.

Radial n.

Brachial vv.

Median n.

Brachial a.

Deep brachial a.

Basilic v.

Sup. ulnar collateral a.

Ulnar n.

Med. brachial
intermuscular septum

Inf. ulnar collateral a., v.

Median n.

Deltoid m.

Cephalic v.

Ant. circumflex humeral a.

Tendon of long head
of biceps brachii m.

Pectoralis major m.

Biceps brachii m.

Cephalic v.

Lat. antebrachial cutaneous branch
of musculocutaneous n.

Aponeurosis
of biceps brachii m.

**Fig. 539.** Nerves and vessels of flexor side of left arm.

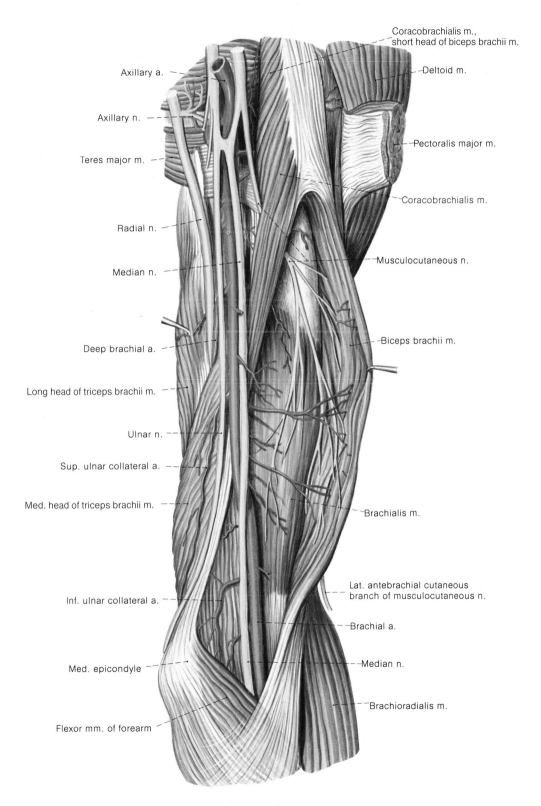

Coracobrachialis m.,
short head of biceps brachii m.

Axillary a.

Deltoid m.

Axillary n.

Pectoralis major m.

Teres major m.

Coracobrachialis m.

Radial n.

Median n.

Musculocutaneous n.

Biceps brachii m.

Deep brachial a.

Long head of triceps brachii m.

Ulnar n.

Sup. ulnar collateral a.

Med. head of triceps brachii m.

Brachialis m.

Lat. antebrachial cutaneous
branch of musculocutaneous n.

Inf. ulnar collateral a.

Brachial a.

Median n.

Med. epicondyle

Brachioradialis m.

Flexor mm. of forearm

**Fig. 540.** Same preparation as in Fig. 539. The biceps brachii muscle has been pulled sideward, the veins have been removed.

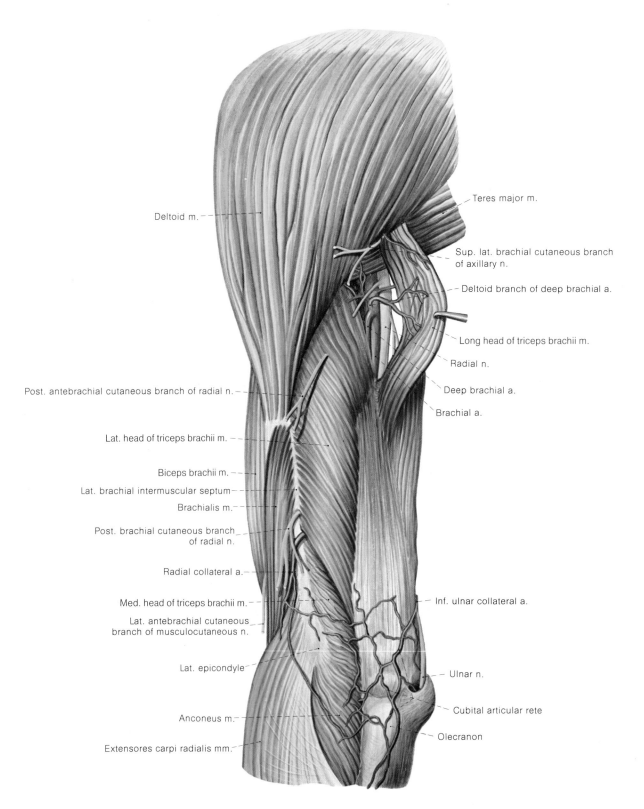

Teres major m.

Sup. lat. brachial cutaneous branch
of axillary n.

Deltoid branch of deep brachial a.

Long head of triceps brachii m.

Radial n.

Deep brachial a.

Brachial a.

Deltoid m.

Post. antebrachial cutaneous branch of radial n.

Lat. head of triceps brachii m.

Biceps brachii m.

Lat. brachial intermuscular septum

Brachialis m.

Post. brachial cutaneous branch
of radial n.

Radial collateral a.

Med. head of triceps brachii m.

Lat. antebrachial cutaneous
branch of musculocutaneous n.

Inf. ulnar collateral a.

Lat. epicondyle

Ulnar n.

Cubital articular rete

Anconeus m.

Olecranon

Extensores carpi radialis mm.

**Fig. 541.** Nerves and vessels of posterior aspect of left arm (superficial layer).

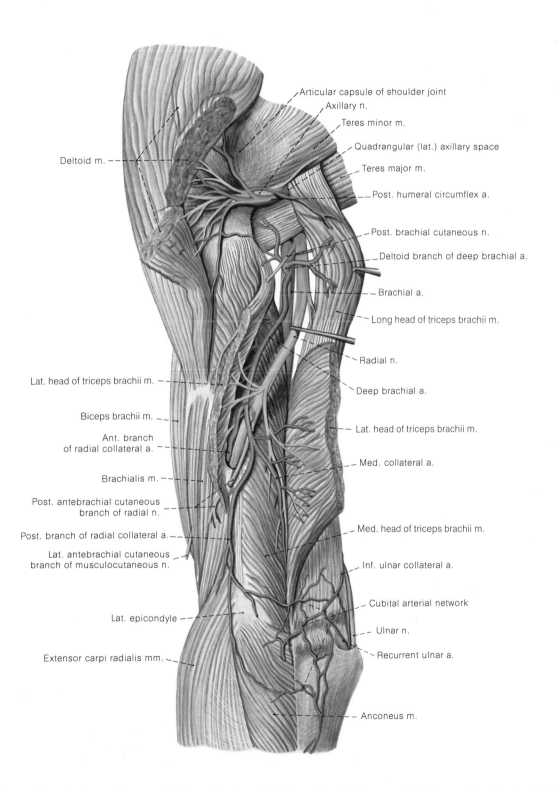

Articular capsule of shoulder joint

Axillary n.

Teres minor m.

Quadrangular (lat.) axillary space

Deltoid m.

Teres major m.

Post. humeral circumflex a.

Post. brachial cutaneous n.

Deltoid branch of deep brachial a.

Brachial a.

Long head of triceps brachii m.

Radial n.

Lat. head of triceps brachii m.

Deep brachial a.

Biceps brachii m.

Lat. head of triceps brachii m.

Ant. branch
of radial collateral a.

Med. collateral a.

Brachialis m.

Post. antebrachial cutaneous
branch of radial n.

Med. head of triceps brachii m.

Post. branch of radial collateral a.

Lat. antebrachial cutaneous
branch of musculocutaneous n.

Inf. ulnar collateral a.

Cubital arterial network

Lat. epicondyle

Ulnar n.

Recurrent ulnar a.

Extensor carpi radialis mm.

Anconeus m.

**Fig. 542.** Nerves and vessels of posterior aspect of left arm (deep layer). The lateral head of triceps muscle has been sectioned and reflected.

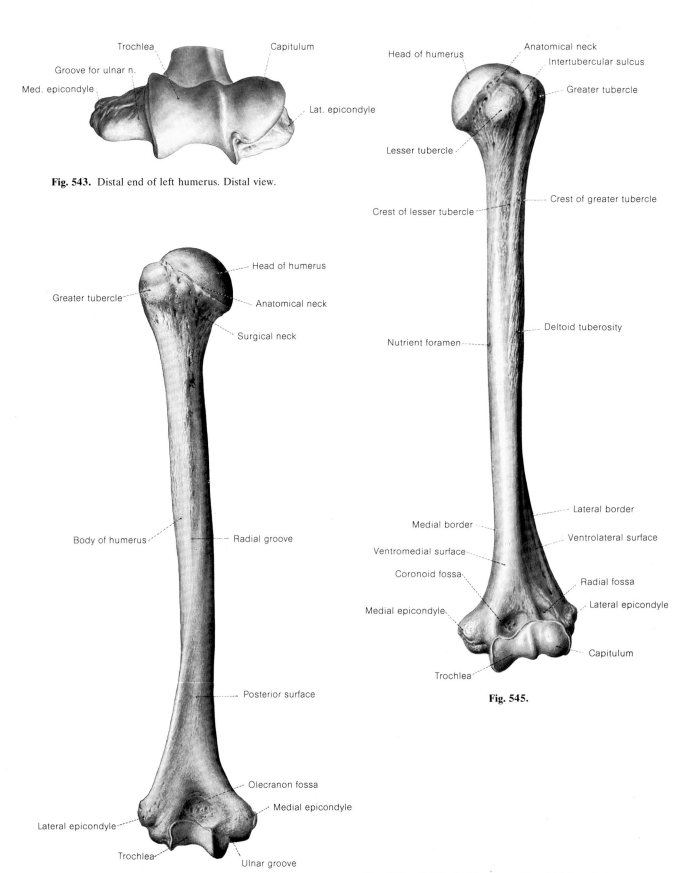

Fig. 543. Distal end of left humerus. Distal view.

Trochlea

Capitulum

Groove for ulnar n.

Med. epicondyle

Lat. epicondyle

Head of humerus

Anatomical neck

Intertubercular sulcus

Greater tubercle

Lesser tubercle

Crest of lesser tubercle

Crest of greater tubercle

Nutrient foramen

Deltoid tuberosity

Head of humerus

Greater tubercle

Anatomical neck

Surgical neck

Medial border

Lateral border

Ventromedial surface

Ventrolateral surface

Coronoid fossa

Radial fossa

Medial epicondyle

Lateral epicondyle

Body of humerus

Radial groove

Trochlea

Capitulum

Fig. 545.

Posterior surface

Olecranon fossa

Medial epicondyle

Lateral epicondyle

Trochlea

Ulnar groove

Fig. 544.

Figs. 544 and 545. Left humerus. Figs. 544 Dorsal view.
Fig. 545 Ventral view.

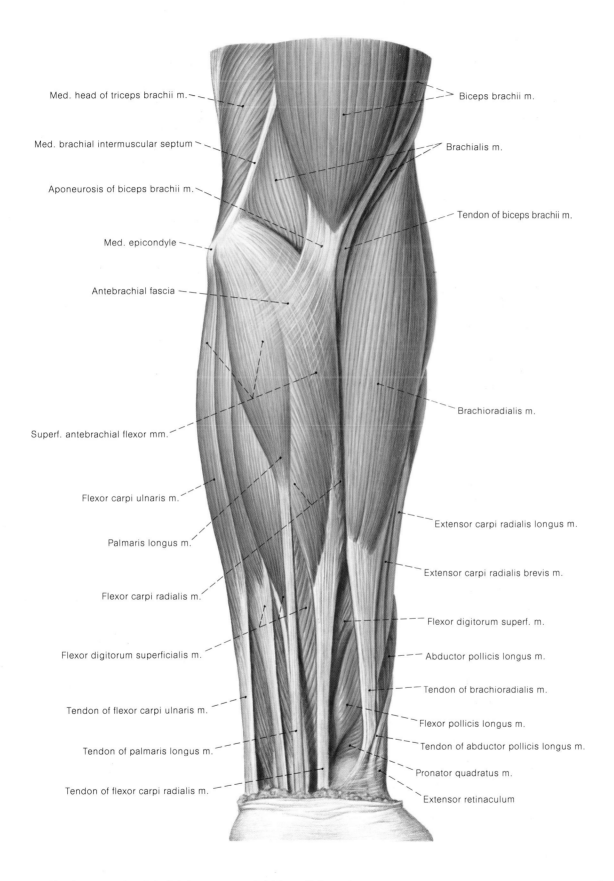

Med. head of triceps brachii m.

Med. brachial intermuscular septum

Aponeurosis of biceps brachii m.

Med. epicondyle

Antebrachial fascia

Superf. antebrachial flexor mm.

Flexor carpi ulnaris m.

Palmaris longus m.

Flexor carpi radialis m.

Flexor digitorum superficialis m.

Tendon of flexor carpi ulnaris m.

Tendon of palmaris longus m.

Tendon of flexor carpi radialis m.

Biceps brachii m.

Brachialis m.

Tendon of biceps brachii m.

Brachioradialis m.

Extensor carpi radialis longus m.

Extensor carpi radialis brevis m.

Flexor digitorum superf. m.

Abductor pollicis longus m.

Tendon of brachioradialis m.

Flexor pollicis longus m.

Tendon of abductor pollicis longus m.

Pronator quadratus m.

Extensor retinaculum

**Fig. 546.** Flexor muscles of the left forearm, superficial layer. Palmar view.

# Forearm

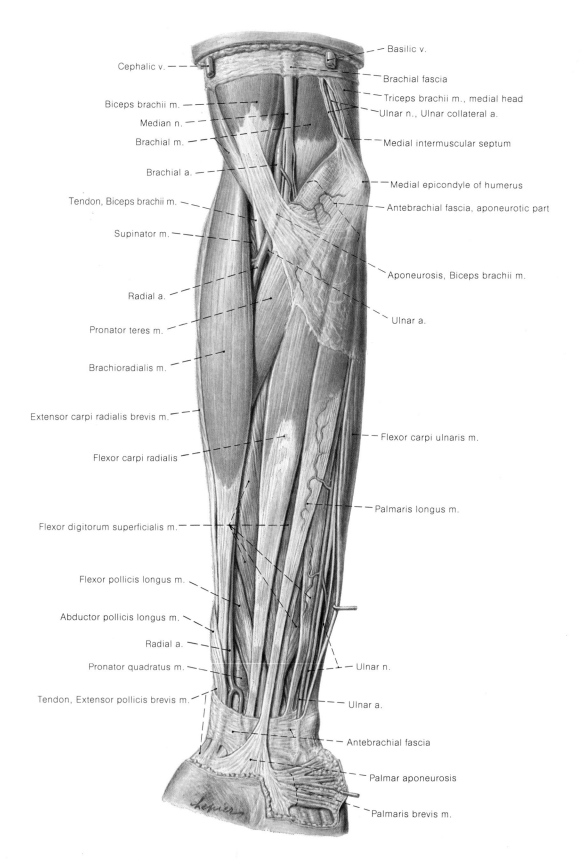

Cephalic v.

Biceps brachii m.

Median n.

Brachial m.

Brachial a.

Tendon, Biceps brachii m.

Supinator m.

Radial a.

Pronator teres m.

Brachioradialis m.

Extensor carpi radialis brevis m.

Flexor carpi radialis

Flexor digitorum superficialis m.

Flexor pollicis longus m.

Abductor pollicis longus m.

Radial a.

Pronator quadratus m.

Tendon, Extensor pollicis brevis m.

Basilic v.

Brachial fascia

Triceps brachii m., medial head

Ulnar n., Ulnar collateral a.

Medial intermuscular septum

Medial epicondyle of humerus

Antebrachial fascia, aponeurotic part

Aponeurosis, Biceps brachii m.

Ulnar a.

Flexor carpi ulnaris m.

Palmaris longus m.

Ulnar n.

Ulnar a.

Antebrachial fascia

Palmar aponeurosis

Palmaris brevis m.

**Fig. 547.** Muscles (superficial layers) of the flexor side of the forearm and the Brachioradialis muscle. Palmar view.

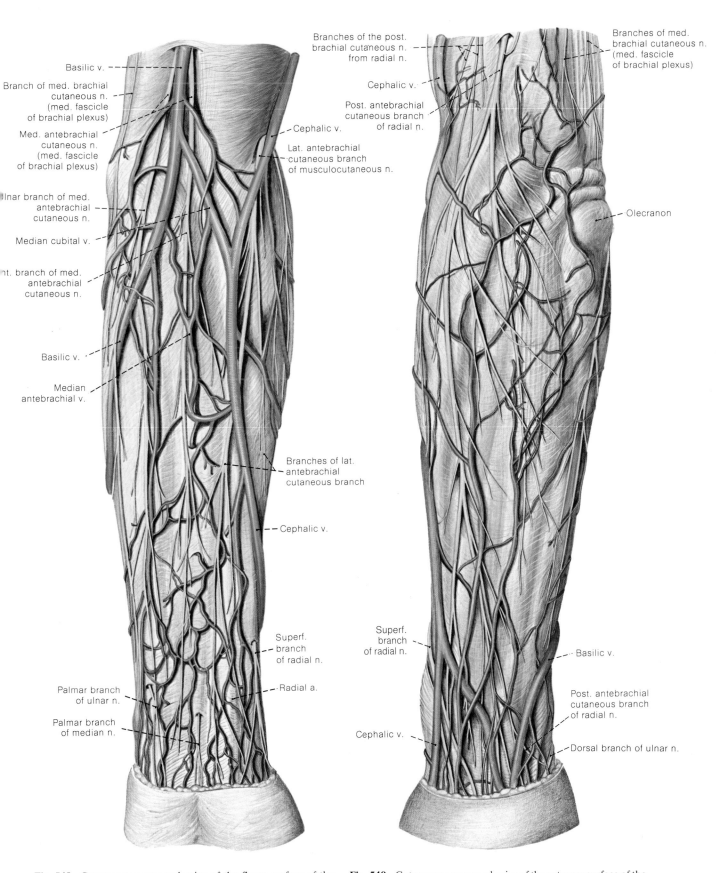

Basilic v.

Branch of med. brachial cutaneous n. (med. fascicle of brachial plexus)

Med. antebrachial cutaneous n. (med. fascicle of brachial plexus)

Ulnar branch of med. antebrachial cutaneous n.

Median cubital v.

nt. branch of med. antebrachial cutaneous n.

Basilic v.

Median antebrachial v.

Palmar branch of ulnar n.

Palmar branch of median n.

Branches of the post. brachial cutaneous n. from radial n.

Cephalic v.

Post. antebrachial cutaneous branch of radial n.

Cephalic v.

Lat. antebrachial cutaneous branch of musculocutaneous n.

Branches of lat. antebrachial cutaneous branch

Cephalic v.

Superf. branch of radial n.

Radial a.

Branches of med. brachial cutaneous n. (med. fascicle of brachial plexus)

Cephalic v.

Post. antebrachial cutaneous branch of radial n.

Olecranon

Superf. branch of radial n.

Basilic v.

Post. antebrachial cutaneous branch of radial n.

Cephalic v.

Dorsal branch of ulnar n.

**Fig. 548.** Cutaneous nerves and veins of the flexor surface of the left forearm.

**Fig. 549.** Cutaneous nerves and veins of the extensor surface of the left forearm.

329

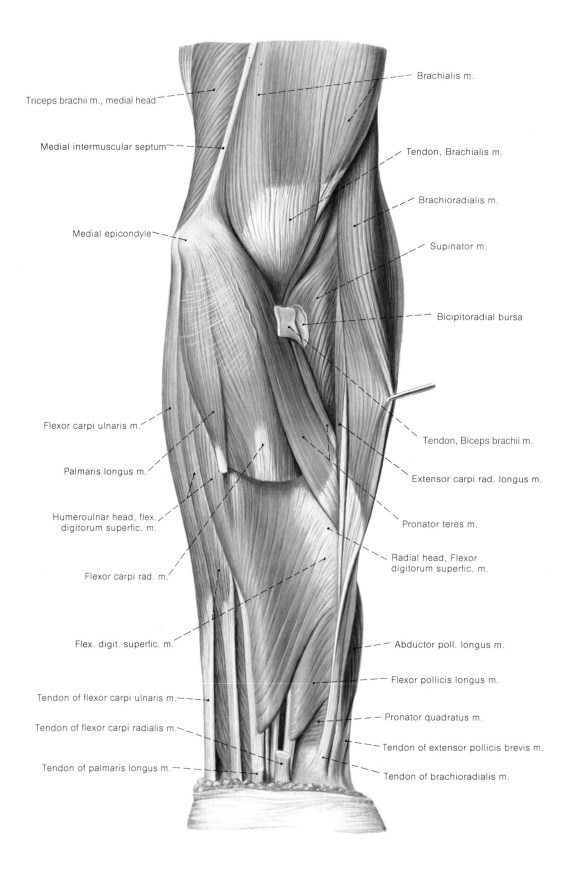

Triceps brachii m., medial head

Medial intermuscular septum

Medial epicondyle

Flexor carpi ulnaris m.

Palmaris longus m.

Humeroulnar head, flex. digitorum superfic. m.

Flexor carpi rad. m.

Flex. digit. superfic. m.

Tendon of flexor carpi ulnaris m.

Tendon of flexor carpi radialis m.

Tendon of palmaris longus m.

Brachialis m.

Tendon, Brachialis m.

Brachioradialis m.

Supinator m.

Bicipitoradial bursa

Tendon, Biceps brachii m.

Extensor carpi rad. longus m.

Pronator teres m.

Radial head, Flexor digitorum superfic. m.

Abductor poll. longus m.

Flexor pollicis longus m.

Pronator quadratus m.

Tendon of extensor pollicis brevis m.

Tendon of brachioradialis m.

**Fig. 550.** Flexor muscles of the left forearm after severing the Palmaris longus and Flexor carpi radialis muscles.

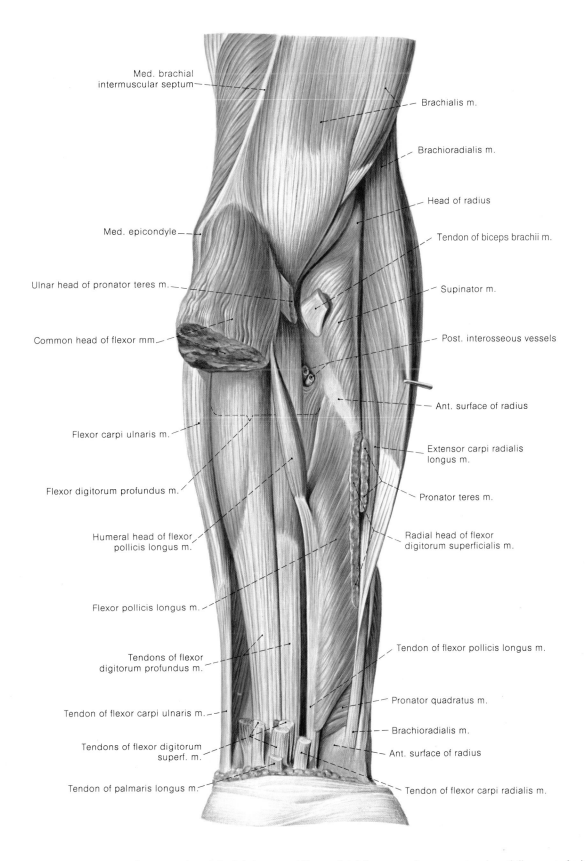

Med. brachial intermuscular septum

Brachialis m.

Brachioradialis m.

Head of radius

Med. epicondyle

Tendon of biceps brachii m.

Ulnar head of pronator teres m.

Supinator m.

Common head of flexor mm

Post. interosseous vessels

Ant. surface of radius

Flexor carpi ulnaris m.

Extensor carpi radialis longus m.

Flexor digitorum profundus m.

Pronator teres m.

Humeral head of flexor pollicis longus m.

Radial head of flexor digitorum superficialis m.

Flexor pollicis longus m.

Tendons of flexor digitorum profundus m.

Tendon of flexor pollicis longus m.

Pronator quadratus m.

Tendon of flexor carpi ulnaris m.

Brachioradialis m.

Tendons of flexor digitorum superf. m.

Ant. surface of radius

Tendon of palmaris longus m.

Tendon of flexor carpi radialis m.

**Fig. 551.** Deep layers of the flexor muscles of the left forearm. All superficial flexor muscles were cut and partially resected with the exception of the Flexor carpi ulnaris muscle.

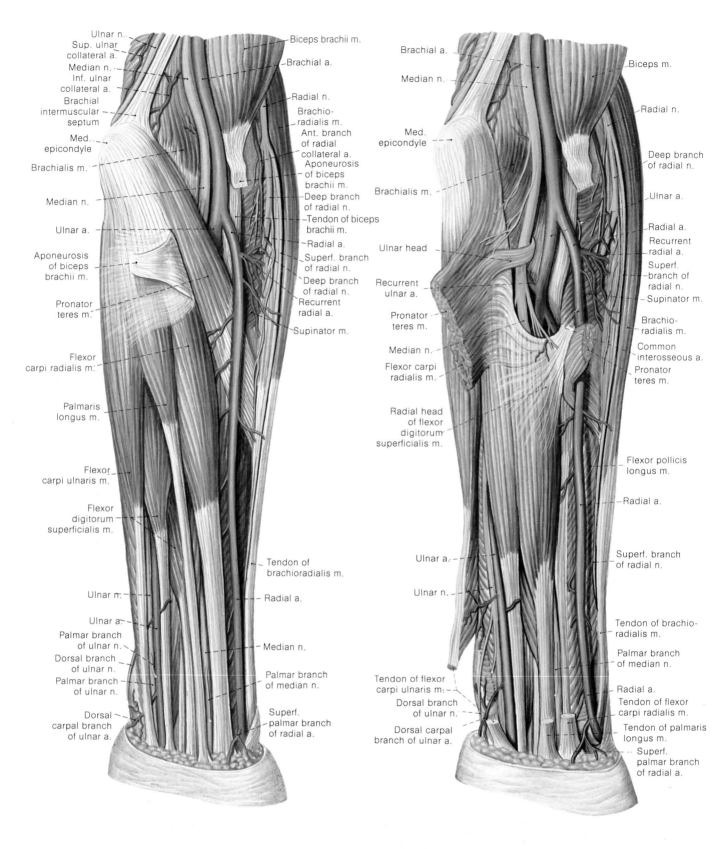

**Fig. 552.** Nerves and vessels of flexor side of left forearm (superficial layer). The aponeurosis of the biceps muscle has been sectioned, the brachioradialis muscle has been pushed backward.

**Fig. 553.** Nerves and vessels of flexor side of left forearm (deep layer). Pronator teres, palmaris longus, and flexor carpi radialis muscles have been partially removed.

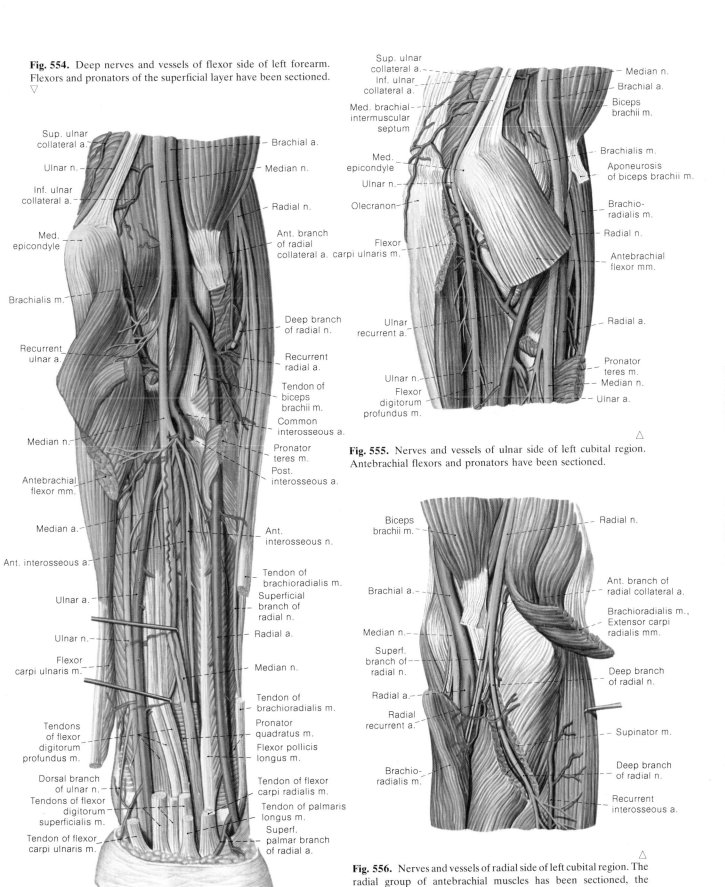

**Fig. 554.** Deep nerves and vessels of flexor side of left forearm. Flexors and pronators of the superficial layer have been sectioned.
▽

Sup. ulnar collateral a.

Ulnar n.

Inf. ulnar collateral a.

Med. epicondyle

Brachialis m.

Recurrent ulnar a.

Median n.

Antebrachial flexor mm.

Median a.

Ant. interosseous a.

Ulnar a.

Ulnar n.

Flexor carpi ulnaris m.

Tendons of flexor digitorum profundus m.

Dorsal branch of ulnar n.

Tendons of flexor digitorum superficialis m.

Tendon of flexor carpi ulnaris m.

Brachial a.

Median n.

Radial n.

Ant. branch of radial collateral a.

Deep branch of radial n.

Recurrent radial a.

Tendon of biceps brachii m.

Common interosseous a.

Pronator teres m.

Post. interosseous a.

Ant. interosseous n.

Tendon of brachioradialis m.

Superficial branch of radial n.

Radial a.

Median n.

Tendon of brachioradialis m.

Pronator quadratus m.

Flexor pollicis longus m.

Tendon of flexor carpi radialis m.

Tendon of palmaris longus m.

Superf. palmar branch of radial a.

Sup. ulnar collateral a.

Inf. ulnar collateral a.

Med. brachial intermuscular septum

Med. epicondyle

Ulnar n.

Olecranon

Flexor carpi ulnaris m.

Ulnar recurrent a.

Ulnar n.

Flexor digitorum profundus m.

Median n.

Brachial a.

Biceps brachii m.

Brachialis m.

Aponeurosis of biceps brachii m.

Brachioradialis m.

Radial n.

Antebrachial flexor mm.

Radial a.

Pronator teres m.

Median n.

Ulnar a.

**Fig. 555.** Nerves and vessels of ulnar side of left cubital region. Antebrachial flexors and pronators have been sectioned.
△

Biceps brachii m.

Brachial a.

Median n.

Superf. branch of radial n.

Radial a.

Radial recurrent a.

Brachioradialis m.

Radial n.

Ant. branch of radial collateral a.

Brachioradialis m., Extensor carpi radialis mm.

Deep branch of radial n.

Supinator m.

Deep branch of radial n.

Recurrent interosseous a.

△

**Fig. 556.** Nerves and vessels of radial side of left cubital region. The radial group of antebrachial muscles has been sectioned, the supinator muscle has been split along the deep branch of radial nerve.

333

# Forearm

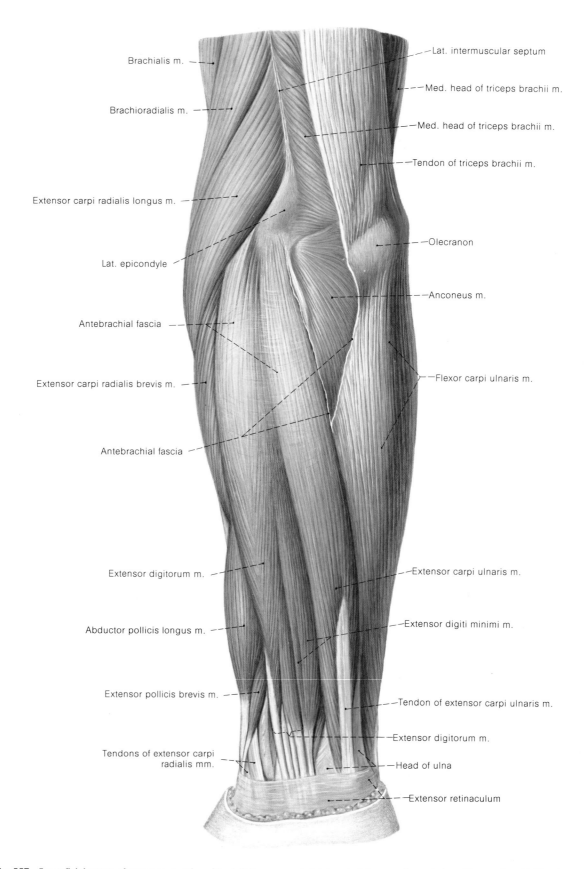

Brachialis m.

Brachioradialis m.

Extensor carpi radialis longus m.

Lat. epicondyle

Antebrachial fascia

Extensor carpi radialis brevis m.

Antebrachial fascia

Extensor digitorum m.

Abductor pollicis longus m.

Extensor pollicis brevis m.

Tendons of extensor carpi radialis mm.

Lat. intermuscular septum

Med. head of triceps brachii m.

Med. head of triceps brachii m.

Tendon of triceps brachii m.

Olecranon

Anconeus m.

Flexor carpi ulnaris m.

Extensor carpi ulnaris m.

Extensor digiti minimi m.

Tendon of extensor carpi ulnaris m.

Extensor digitorum m.

Head of ulna

Extensor retinaculum

**Fig. 557.** Superficial group of extensor muscles of the left forearm and distal part of the arm. Dorsal view. The antebrachial fascia over the anconeus muscle has been removed.

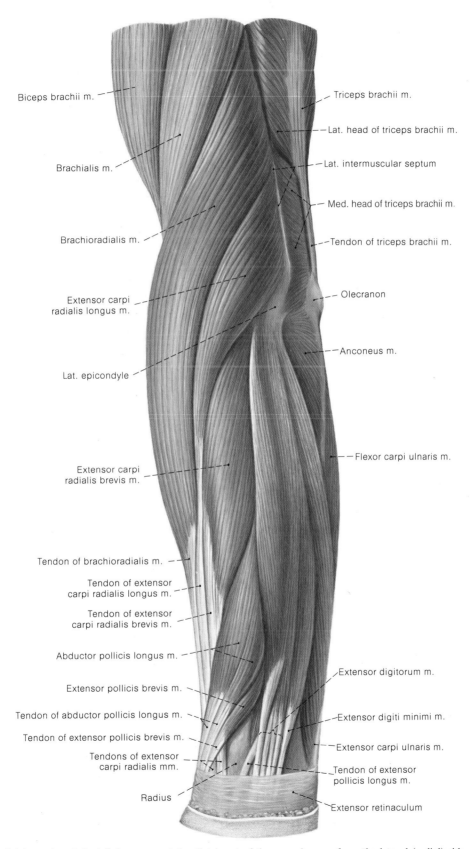

Biceps brachii m.

Brachialis m.

Brachioradialis m.

Extensor carpi
radialis longus m.

Lat. epicondyle

Extensor carpi
radialis brevis m.

Tendon of brachioradialis m.

Tendon of extensor
carpi radialis longus m.

Tendon of extensor
carpi radialis brevis m.

Abductor pollicis longus m.

Extensor pollicis brevis m.

Tendon of abductor pollicis longus m.

Tendon of extensor pollicis brevis m.

Tendons of extensor
carpi radialis mm.

Radius

Triceps brachii m.

Lat. head of triceps brachii m.

Lat. intermuscular septum

Med. head of triceps brachii m.

Tendon of triceps brachii m.

Olecranon

Anconeus m.

Flexor carpi ulnaris m.

Extensor digitorum m.

Extensor digiti minimi m.

Extensor carpi ulnaris m.

Tendon of extensor
pollicis longus m.

Extensor retinaculum

**Fig. 558.** Superficial muscles of the left forearm and the distal part of the arm. As seen from the lateral (radial) side.

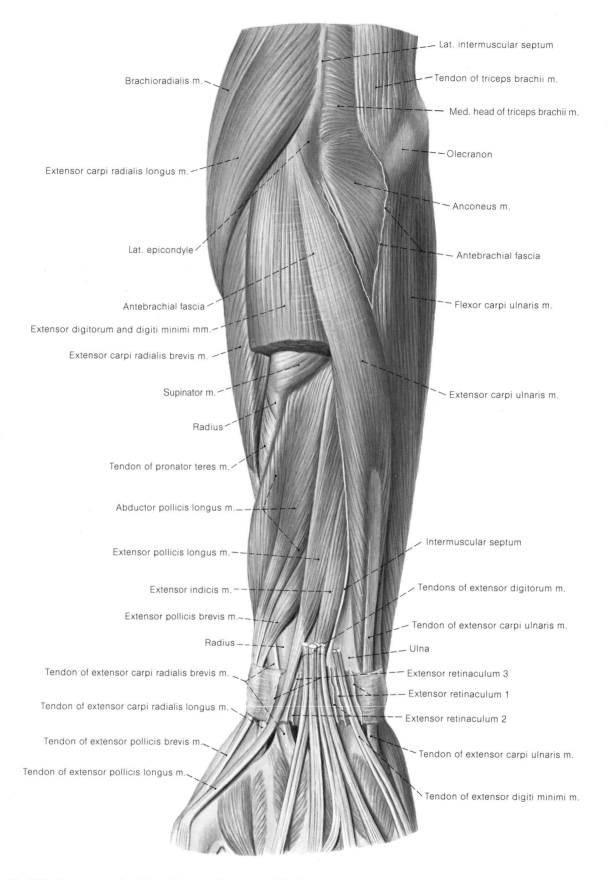

Lat. intermuscular septum

Tendon of triceps brachii m.

Med. head of triceps brachii m.

Olecranon

Anconeus m.

Antebrachial fascia

Flexor carpi ulnaris m.

Extensor carpi ulnaris m.

Intermuscular septum

Tendons of extensor digitorum m.

Tendon of extensor carpi ulnaris m.

Ulna

Extensor retinaculum 3

Extensor retinaculum 1

Extensor retinaculum 2

Tendon of extensor carpi ulnaris m.

Tendon of extensor digiti minimi m.

Brachioradialis m.

Extensor carpi radialis longus m.

Lat. epicondyle

Antebrachial fascia

Extensor digitorum and digiti minimi mm.

Extensor carpi radialis brevis m.

Supinator m.

Radius

Tendon of pronator teres m.

Abductor pollicis longus m.

Extensor pollicis longus m.

Extensor indicis m.

Extensor pollicis brevis m.

Radius

Tendon of extensor carpi radialis brevis m.

Tendon of extensor carpi radialis longus m.

Tendon of extensor pollicis brevis m.

Tendon of extensor pollicis longus m.

**Fig. 559.** Extensor muscles of the left forearm. Dorsal view. The Extensor digitorum and Digiti minimi were severed; the tendon compartments of the Extensor retinaculum were partly opened: 1. the Extensor digiti minimi; 2. Extensor digitorum and Extensor indicis; 3. the Extensor pollicis longus.

336

## Flexor Muscles of Forearm, Superficial Group (Figs. 546, 547, 550)

| Name | Origin | Insertion |
|---|---|---|
| **1. Pronator teres muscle** | | |
| *Humeral head* (strong) | Medial epicondyle of the humerus, antebrachial fascia | On the lateral and dorsal surface of radius (middle $^1/_3$) |
| *Ulnar head* (weak) | Coronoid process of ulna | |
| *Nerve:* Median nerve (passes through between the two heads) | | |
| *Function:* Pronates and flexes the forearm | | |
| **2. Flexor carpi radialis muscle** | Medial epicondyle of humerus and antebrachial fascia | Base of 2nd metacarpal bone, palmar surface |
| *Nerve:* Median nerve | | |
| *Function:* Flexes wrist and elbow; abducts wrist, pronates forearm | | |
| **3. Palmaris longus muscle** (inconstant) | Medial epicondyle of humerus; antebrachial fascia | Palmar aponeurosis |
| *Nerve:* Median nerve | | |
| *Function:* Tenses palmar aponeurosis; weak flexor of elbow and wrist | | |
| **4. Flexor digitorum superficialis muscle** | | |
| *Humeroulnar head:* | Medial epicondyle of humerus and coronoid process of ulna | 4 long tendons to the middle phalanges of fingers 2 to 5 |
| *Radial head:* | Upper half, anterior border of radius | |
| *Nerve:* Median nerve C 7, 8; T 1 | | |
| *Function:* Flexes middle phalanges of 4 medial fingers; assists in flexion of forearm; medial abduction of hand | | |
| **5. Flexor carpi ulnaris muscle** | | |
| *Humeral head:* | Medial epicondyle of the humerus | Pisiform bone and, by ligaments (Fig. 607), to 5th metacarpal and hamate bones |
| *Ulnar head:* | Olecranon and, via the antebrachial fascia, posterior border of ulna | |
| *Nerve:* Ulnar nerve (C 8, 8; T 1) | | |
| *Function:* Flexes and adducts wrist joint; flexor of elbow | | |

## Muscles of the Forearm, Deep, radial (oblique) Group of Extensors (Fig. 559)

| Name | Origin | Insertion |
|---|---|---|
| **1. Abductor pollicis longus muscle** | Posterior surface of ulna and radius; interosseous membrane | Base of 1st metacarpal of thumb, radial side |
| **2. Extensor pollicis brevis muscle** | Posterior surface of radius; interosseous membrane | Base of proximal phalanx of thumb |
| *Nerve:* Deep radial nerve | | |
| *Function:* Abducts thumb; extends 1st phalanx of thumb, and abducts hand | | |

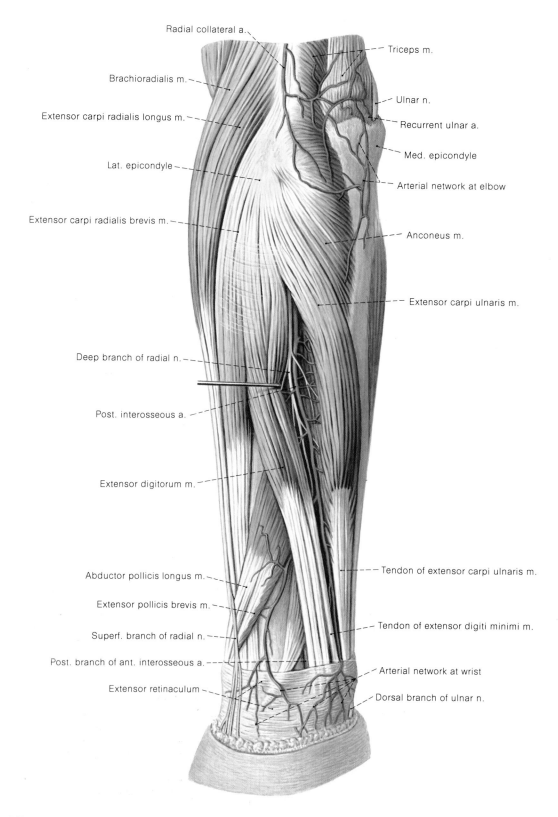

Radial collateral a.

Brachioradialis m.

Extensor carpi radialis longus m.

Lat. epicondyle

Extensor carpi radialis brevis m.

Deep branch of radial n.

Post. interosseous a.

Extensor digitorum m.

Abductor pollicis longus m.

Extensor pollicis brevis m.

Superf. branch of radial n.

Post. branch of ant. interosseous a.

Extensor retinaculum

Triceps m.

Ulnar n.

Recurrent ulnar a.

Med. epicondyle

Arterial network at elbow

Anconeus m.

Extensor carpi ulnaris m.

Tendon of extensor carpi ulnaris m.

Tendon of extensor digiti minimi m.

Arterial network at wrist

Dorsal branch of ulnar n.

**Fig. 560.** Superficial nerves and vessels of posterior aspect of left forearm.

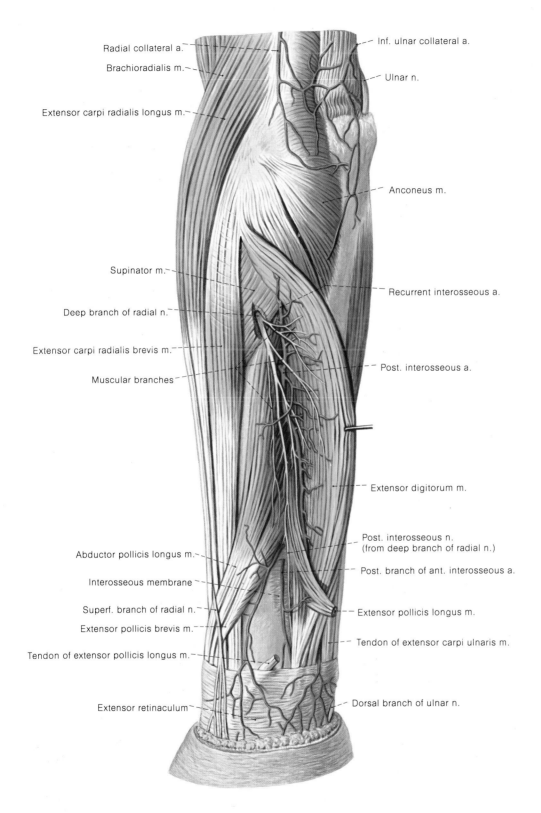

Radial collateral a.

Brachioradialis m.

Extensor carpi radialis longus m.

Inf. ulnar collateral a.

Ulnar n.

Anconeus m.

Supinator m.

Recurrent interosseous a.

Deep branch of radial n.

Extensor carpi radialis brevis m.

Muscular branches

Post. interosseous a.

Extensor digitorum m.

Abductor pollicis longus m.

Interosseous membrane

Superf. branch of radial n.

Extensor pollicis brevis m.

Tendon of extensor pollicis longus m.

Post. interosseous n.
(from deep branch of radial n.)

Post. branch of ant. interosseous a.

Extensor pollicis longus m.

Tendon of extensor carpi ulnaris m.

Extensor retinaculum

Dorsal branch of ulnar n.

**Fig. 561.** Deep nerves and vessels of posterior aspect of left forearm. Extensor digitorum and digiti minimi muscles have been pushed toward ulnar; extensor pollicis longus muscle has been cut; supinator muscle has been split along deep branch of radial nerve.

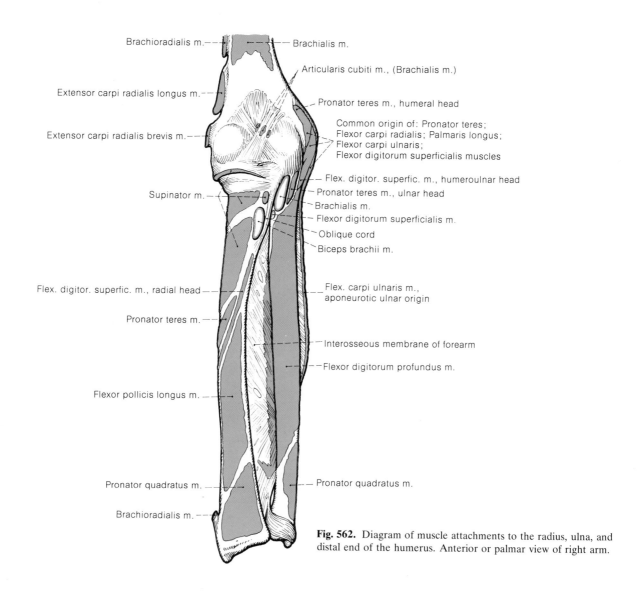

Fig. 562. Diagram of muscle attachments to the radius, ulna, and distal end of the humerus. Anterior or palmar view of right arm.

## Muscles of the Forearm, Radial Group

| Name | Origin | Insertion |
|---|---|---|
| **1. Brachioradialis muscle** | Lateral supracondylar ridge of humerus; lateral intermuscular septum | Proximal end of styloid process of radius |
| *Nerve:* Radial nerve (C 5, 6) | | |
| *Function:* Flexes forearm; pronates forearm if supinated; supinates, if forearm is pronated | | |
| **2. Extensor carpi radialis longus muscle** | Distal ⅓ of lateral supracondylar ridge of humerus and lateral intermuscular septum | Base of 2nd metacarpal bone |
| **3. Extensor carpi radialis brevis muscle** | Lateral epicondyle of humerus | Base of 3rd metacarpal bone |
| *Nerve:* Radial nerve (C 6, 7) | | |
| *Function:* Extends and abducts the hand | | |

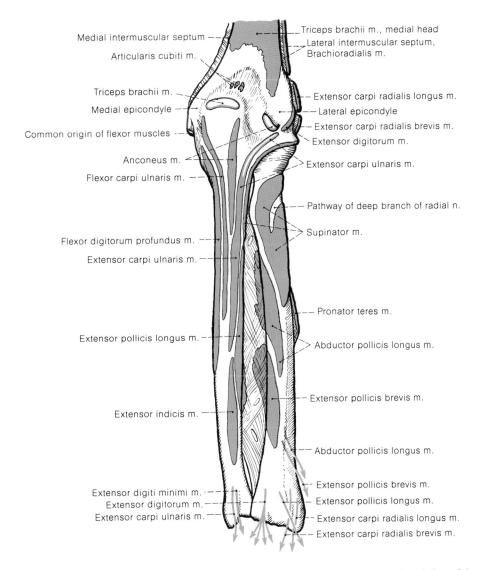

Medial intermuscular septum —
Articularis cubiti m. —
Triceps brachii m. —
Medial epicondyle —
Common origin of flexor muscles — -
Anconeus m. —
Flexor carpi ulnaris m. —
Flexor digitorum profundus m. — -
Extensor carpi ulnaris m. — -
Extensor pollicis longus m. —
Extensor indicis m. —
Extensor digiti minimi m. — -
Extensor digitorum m. — -
Extensor carpi ulnaris m. —

Triceps brachii m., medial head
Lateral intermuscular septum,
Brachioradialis m.
— Extensor carpi radialis longus m.
— Lateral epicondyle
— Extensor carpi radialis brevis m.
— Extensor digitorum m.
— Extensor carpi ulnaris m.
— Pathway of deep branch of radial n.
— Supinator m.
— Pronator teres m.
— Abductor pollicis longus m.
— Extensor pollicis brevis m.
— Abductor pollicis longus m.
— Extensor pollicis brevis m.
— Extensor pollicis longus m.
— Extensor carpi radialis longus m.
— Extensor carpi radialis brevis m.

**Fig. 563.** Muscle attachments mapped out on the radius, ulna, and distal end of the humerus. Posterior or dorsal view of the right arm. Arrows at distal end of the ulna and radius indicate the tendon compartments.

## Muscles of the Forearm, Superficial Layer of Extensors

| Name | Origin | Insertion |
|---|---|---|
| **1. Extensor digitorum muscle** | Lateral epicondyle of humerus; antebrachial fascia | By 4 tendons to middle and distal phalanges of the fingers |
| **2. Extensor digiti minimi muscle** | | Joins extensor tendon to little finger |
| *Nerve:* Deep radial nerve (C 6, 7, 8) | | |
| *Function:* Extends the little finger (proximal phalanges, in particular); indirectly the entire hand, also medial abduction | | |
| **3. Extensor carpi ulnaris muscle** Separated from above by an intermuscular septum | Lateral epicondyle of humerus; antebrachial fascia | Base of 5th metacarpal, dorsal surface |
| *Nerve:* Deep radial nerve (C 6, 7, 8) | | |
| *Function:* Extends (slightly) and adducts hand | | |

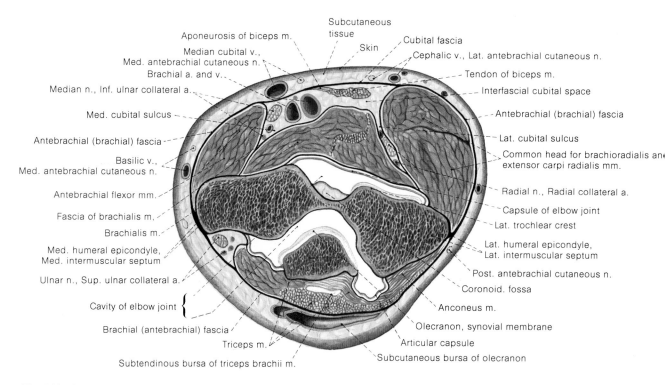

Subcutaneous tissue
Skin
Cubital fascia
Cephalic v., Lat. antebrachial cutaneous n.
Aponeurosis of biceps m.
Median cubital v.,
Med. antebrachial cutaneous n.
Brachial a. and v.
Tendon of biceps m.
Median n., Inf. ulnar collateral a.
Interfascial cubital space
Med. cubital sulcus
Antebrachial (brachial) fascia
Antebrachial (brachial) fascia
Lat. cubital sulcus
Basilic v.,
Med. antebrachial cutaneous n.
Common head for brachioradialis and extensor carpi radialis mm.
Antebrachial flexor mm.
Radial n., Radial collateral a.
Fascia of brachialis m,
Capsule of elbow joint
Brachialis m.
Lat. trochlear crest
Med. humeral epicondyle,
Med. intermuscular septum
Lat. humeral epicondyle,
Lat. intermuscular septum
Ulnar n., Sup. ulnar collateral a.
Post. antebrachial cutaneous n.
Coronoid. fossa
Cavity of elbow joint
Anconeus m.
Brachial (antebrachial) fascia
Olecranon, synovial membrane
Triceps m.
Articular capsule
Subtendinous bursa of triceps brachii m.
Subcutaneous bursa of olecranon

**Fig. 564.** Cross section through the right arm at the level of the elbow joint. (Figs. 464–567 after PERNKOPF: Atlas der topographischen und angewandten Anatomie des Menschen, Vol. 2, 2nd ed. [Ed. H. FERNER]. Urban & Schwarzenberg, Munich–Vienna–Baltimore 1980.)

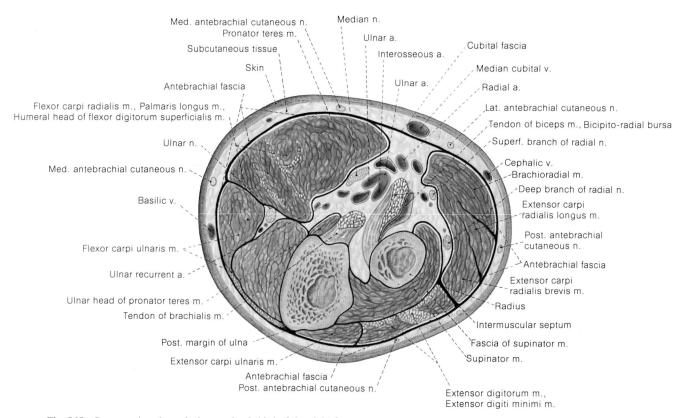

Med. antebrachial cutaneous n.
Median n.
Pronator teres m.
Ulnar a.
Cubital fascia
Subcutaneous tissue
Interosseous a.
Median cubital v.
Skin
Ulnar a.
Radial a.
Antebrachial fascia
Lat. antebrachial cutaneous n.
Flexor carpi radialis m., Palmaris longus m.,
Humeral head of flexor digitorum superficialis m.
Tendon of biceps m., Bicipito-radial bursa
Superf. branch of radial n.
Ulnar n.
Cephalic v.
Med. antebrachial cutaneous n.
Brachioradial m.
Deep branch of radial n.
Basilic v.
Extensor carpi radialis longus m.
Post. antebrachial cutaneous n.
Flexor carpi ulnaris m.
Antebrachial fascia
Ulnar recurrent a.
Extensor carpi radialis brevis m.
Ulnar head of pronator teres m.
Radius
Tendon of brachialis m.
Intermuscular septum
Post. margin of ulna
Fascia of supinator m.
Extensor carpi ulnaris m.
Supinator m.
Antebrachial fascia
Post. antebrachial cutaneous n.
Extensor digitorum m.,
Extensor digiti minimi m.

**Fig. 565.** Cross section through the proximal third of the right forearm.

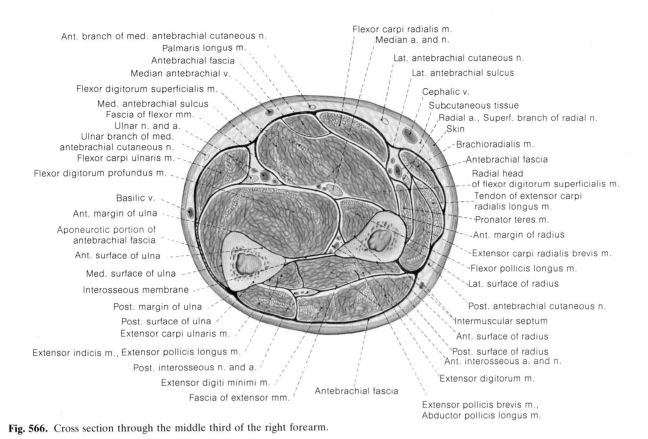

Ant. branch of med. antebrachial cutaneous n.
Palmaris longus m.
Antebrachial fascia
Median antebrachial v.
Flexor digitorum superficialis m.
Med. antebrachial sulcus
Fascia of flexor mm.
Ulnar n. and a.
Ulnar branch of med. antebrachial cutaneous n.
Flexor carpi ulnaris m.
Flexor digitorum profundus m.
Basilic v.
Ant. margin of ulna
Aponeurotic portion of antebrachial fascia
Ant. surface of ulna
Med. surface of ulna
Interosseous membrane
Post. margin of ulna
Post. surface of ulna
Extensor carpi ulnaris m.
Extensor indicis m., Extensor pollicis longus m.
Post. interosseous n. and a.
Extensor digiti minimi m.
Fascia of extensor mm.

Flexor carpi radialis m.
Median a. and n.
Lat. antebrachial cutaneous n.
Lat. antebrachial sulcus
Cephalic v.
Subcutaneous tissue
Radial a., Superf. branch of radial n.
Skin
Brachioradialis m.
Antebrachial fascia
Radial head of flexor digitorum superficialis m.
Tendon of extensor carpi radialis longus m.
Pronator teres m.
Ant. margin of radius
Extensor carpi radialis brevis m.
Flexor pollicis longus m.
Lat. surface of radius
Post. antebrachial cutaneous n.
Intermuscular septum
Ant. surface of radius
Post. surface of radius
Ant. interosseous a. and n.
Extensor digitorum m.

Antebrachial fascia

Extensor pollicis brevis m., Abductor pollicis longus m.

**Fig. 566.** Cross section through the middle third of the right forearm.

Subcutaneous tissue, Antebrachial subcutaneous v.
Antebrachial fascia
Flexor digitorum superficialis m.
Ulnar a. and n.
Flexor carpi ulnaris m.
Tendons of flexor digitorum profundus m.
Dorsal branch of ulnar n.
Pronator quadratus m.
Capsule of distal radio-ulnar joint
Antebrachial fascia
Ulna
Tendon of extensor carpi ulnaris m.
Distal radio-ulnar joint
Intervaginal septum
Subcutaneous v.
Tendon of extensor digiti minimi m.
Extensor indicis m.
Extensor digitorum m.
Extensor retinaculum

Skin
Tendon of palmaris longus m.
Tendons of flexor digitorum superficialis m.
Palmar branch of median n.
Median n.
Tendon of flexor carpi radialis m.
Tendon of flexor pollicis longus m.
Radial a.
Lat. antebrachial cutaneous n.
Intermuscular septum
Tendons of abductor pollicis longus m.
Tendon of extensor pollicis brevis m.
Cephalic v., Superf. branch of radial n.
Tendon of brachioradialis m.
Intervaginal septum
Tendons of extensor carpi radialis longus and brevis mm.
Radius
Antebrachial fascia
Subcutaneous tissue
Tendon of extensor pollicis longus m.
Cephalic v.

**Fig. 567.** Cross section through the distal end of the right forearm.

343

**Figs. 568 and 569.** Left elbow joint (articulatio cubiti). Fig. 568 Palmar view. Fig. 569 Dorsal view.

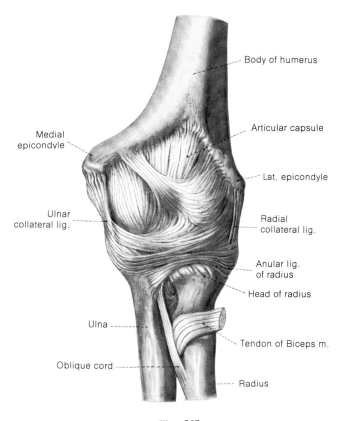

Body of humerus

Medial epicondyle

Articular capsule

Lat. epicondyle

Ulnar collateral lig.

Radial collateral lig.

Anular lig. of radius

Head of radius

Ulna

Tendon of Biceps m.

Oblique cord

Radius

**Figs. 568.**

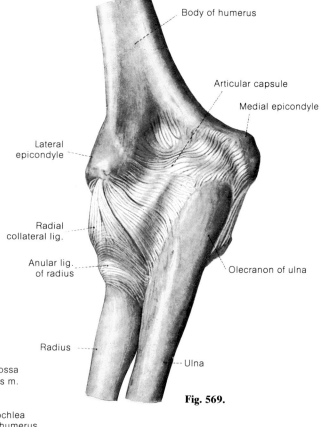

Body of humerus

Articular capsule

Medial epicondyle

Lateral epicondyle

Radial collateral lig.

Anular lig. of radius

Olecranon of ulna

Radius

Ulna

**Fig. 569.**

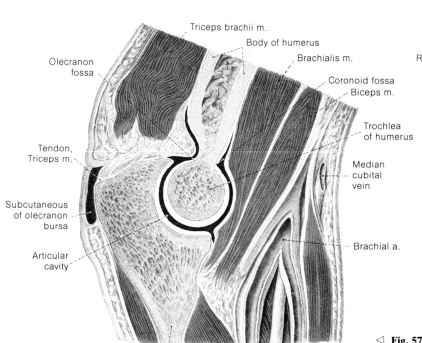

Triceps brachii m.

Body of humerus

Brachialis m.

Olecranon fossa

Coronoid fossa

Biceps m.

Tendon, Triceps m.

Trochlea of humerus

Median cubital vein

Subcutaneous of olecranon bursa

Articular cavity

Brachial a.

Ulna

◁ **Fig. 570.** Sagittal section through the left elbow joint.

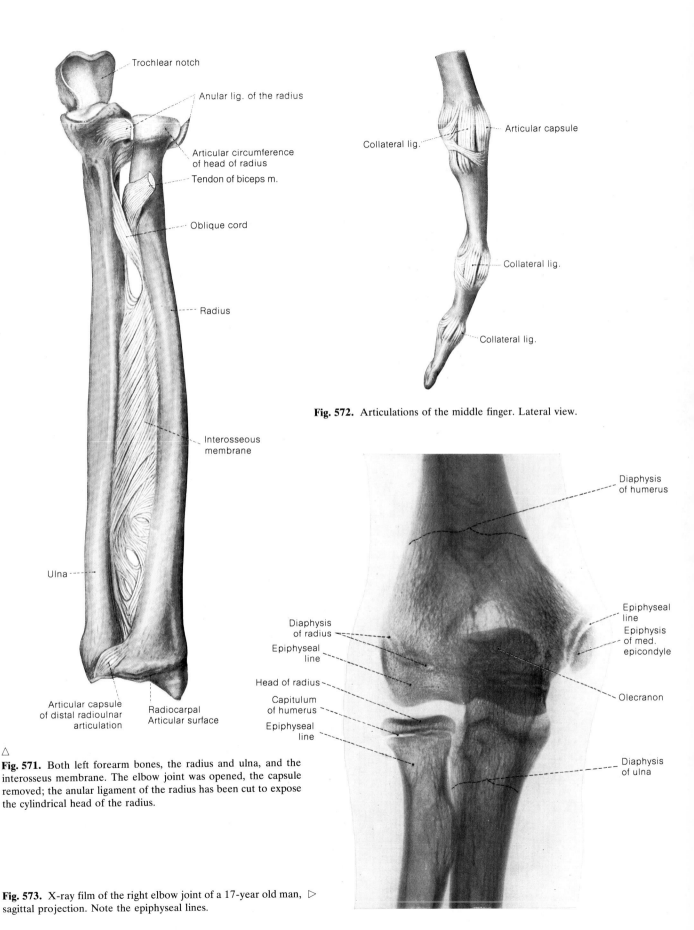

Trochlear notch

Anular lig. of the radius

Articular circumference of head of radius

Tendon of biceps m.

Oblique cord

Radius

Interosseous membrane

Ulna

Articular capsule of distal radioulnar articulation

Radiocarpal Articular surface

△

**Fig. 571.** Both left forearm bones, the radius and ulna, and the interosseus membrane. The elbow joint was opened, the capsule removed; the anular ligament of the radius has been cut to expose the cylindrical head of the radius.

Collateral lig.

Articular capsule

Collateral lig.

Collateral lig.

**Fig. 572.** Articulations of the middle finger. Lateral view.

Diaphysis of humerus

Diaphysis of radius

Epiphyseal line

Head of radius

Capitulum of humerus

Epiphyseal line

Epiphyseal line

Epiphysis of med. epicondyle

Olecranon

Diaphysis of ulna

**Fig. 573.** X-ray film of the right elbow joint of a 17-year old man, ▷ sagittal projection. Note the epiphyseal lines.

345

# Forearm

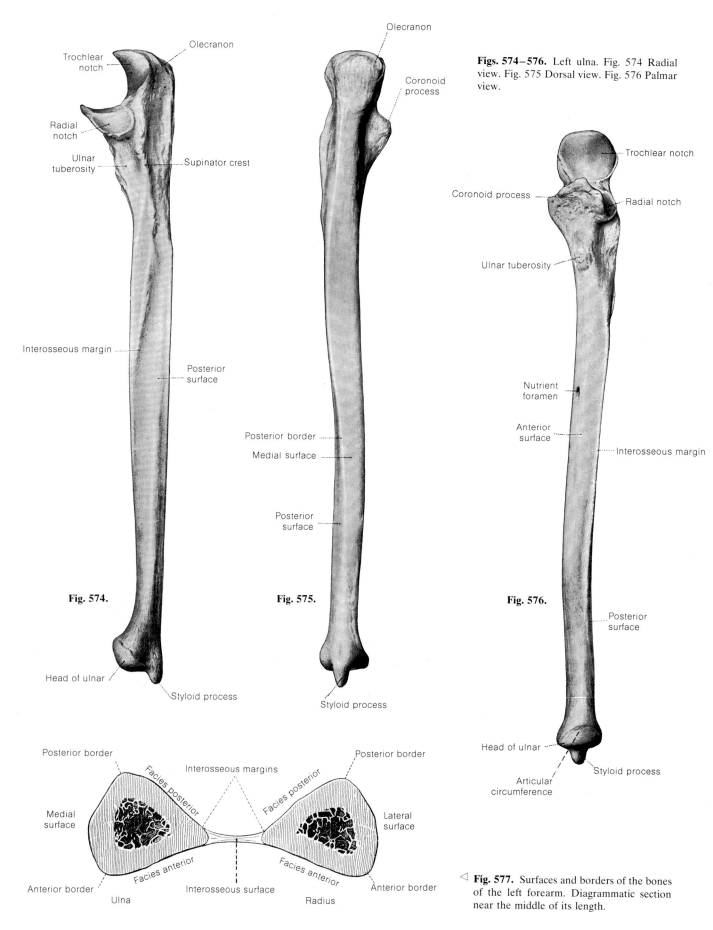

Trochlear notch

Olecranon

Radial notch

Ulnar tuberosity

Supinator crest

Interosseous margin

Posterior surface

**Fig. 574.**

Head of ulnar

Styloid process

Olecranon

Coronoid process

Posterior border

Medial surface

Posterior surface

**Fig. 575.**

Styloid process

**Figs. 574–576.** Left ulna. Fig. 574 Radial view. Fig. 575 Dorsal view. Fig. 576 Palmar view.

Trochlear notch

Coronoid process

Radial notch

Ulnar tuberosity

Nutrient foramen

Anterior surface

Interosseous margin

**Fig. 576.**

Posterior surface

Head of ulnar

Articular circumference

Styloid process

◁ **Fig. 577.** Surfaces and borders of the bones of the left forearm. Diagrammatic section near the middle of its length.

Posterior border

Interosseous margins

Facies posterior

Posterior border

Facies posterior

Medial surface

Lateral surface

Anterior border

Facies anterior

Interosseous surface

Facies anterior

Anterior border

Ulna

Radius

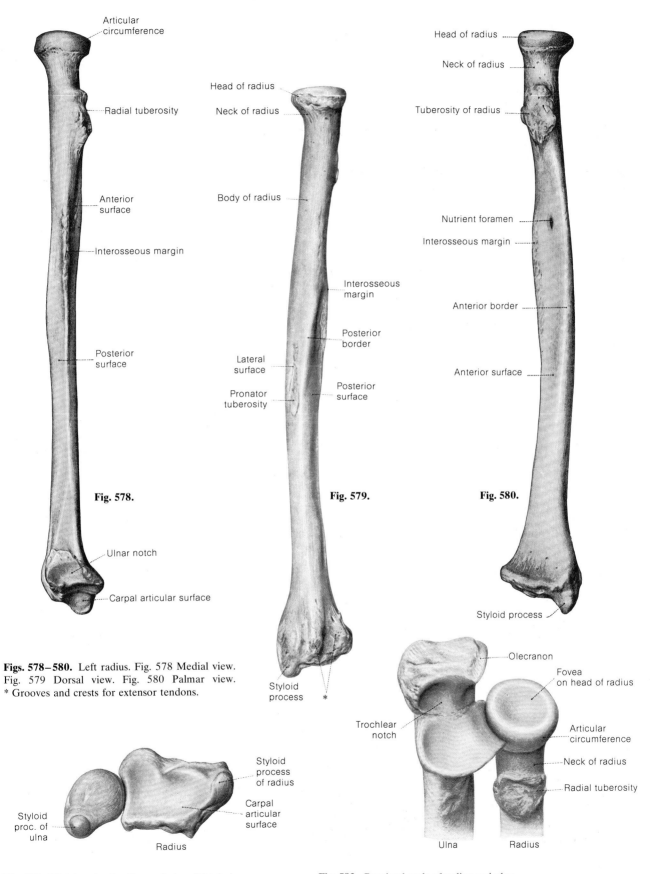

**Figs. 578–580.** Left radius. Fig. 578 Medial view.
Fig. 579 Dorsal view. Fig. 580 Palmar view.
* Grooves and crests for extensor tendons.

Fig. 578.

Fig. 579.

Fig. 580.

**Fig. 581.** Distal ends of radius and ulna. Distal view.

**Fig. 582.** Proximal ends of radius and ulna.

347

## Flexor Muscles of the Forearm, Deep Group (Fig. 551)

| Name | Origin | Insertion |
|---|---|---|
| **1. Flexor digitorum profundus muscle** | Anterior and medial surface of ulna; interosseous membrane | Distal phalanges of fingers 2 to 5 |
| *Nerve:* Ulnar nerve for ulnar side, median nerve for radial side (C 7, 8; T 1) | | |
| *Function:* Flexes joints of fingers 2 to 5 (especially the terminal phalanges but also the other phalanges) and wrist joint | | |
| **2. Flexor pollicis longus muscle** *Radial head* (the main part) | Anterior surface of radius; adjacent part of interosseous membrane | Terminal phalanx of thumb |
| *Humeral head* | Coronoid process of ulna or medial epicondyle of humerus | |
| *Nerve:* Anterior interosseous branch of median nerve (C 8; T 1) | | |
| *Function:* Flexes terminal phalanx of thumb; aids in flexion of proximal phalanx and adduction of metacarpal | | |
| **3. Pronator quadratus muscle** (Fig. 585) | Anterior surface of ulna, distal ¼ | Anterior surface of distal fourth of radius |
| *Nerve:* Anterior interosseous branch of median nerve (C 8; T 1) | | |
| *Function:* Pronates the hand | | |

## Muscles of the Forearm. Deep, ulnar (straight) Group of Extensors

| Name | Origin | Insertion |
|---|---|---|
| **1. Extensor pollicis longus muscle** | Posterior surface of ulna; interosseous membrane | Distal phalanx of thumb |
| **2. Extensor indicis muscle** | As the previous | Dorsal aponeurosis of the index finger |
| *Nerve:* Radial nerve | | |
| *Function:* Extend thumb and index finger; the former helps to extend the whole hand and to abduct the thumb | | |

## Muscles of the Forearm. Supinator Muscle (Figs. 551, 562, 563)

| Name | Origin | Insertion |
|---|---|---|
| **Supinator muscle** Two layers (superficial and deep) between which the deep branch of radial nerve lies | Lateral epicondyle of humerus; radial collateral ligament; anular ligament of radius; supinator crest of ulna | Lateral surface and posterior border of radius, proximal and distal to tuberosity of radius |
| *Nerve:* Deep radial nerve (C 6) | | |
| *Function:* Supinates hand and forearm | | |

# Hand

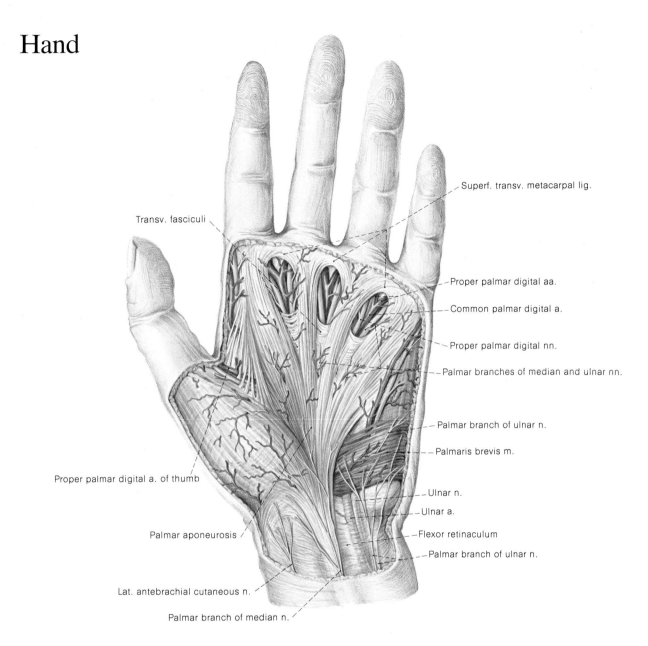

Transv. fasciculi

Superf. transv. metacarpal lig.

Proper palmar digital aa.

Common palmar digital a.

Proper palmar digital nn.

Palmar branches of median and ulnar nn.

Palmar branch of ulnar n.

Palmaris brevis m.

Ulnar n.

Ulnar a.

Flexor retinaculum

Palmar branch of ulnar n.

Proper palmar digital a. of thumb

Palmar aponeurosis

Lat. antebrachial cutaneous n.

Palmar branch of median n.

**Fig. 583.** Superficial nerves and arteries of palm of left hand.

| Name | Origin | Insertion |
|------|--------|-----------|
| **Palmaris brevis muscle** Cutaneous muscle, numerous separated fasciculi | Palmar aponeurosis, medial margin | Skin over medial border of palm |

| | |
|---|---|
| *Nerve:* | Ulnar nerve, superficial branch (C 8) |
| *Function:* | Tenses skin of medial side of palm |

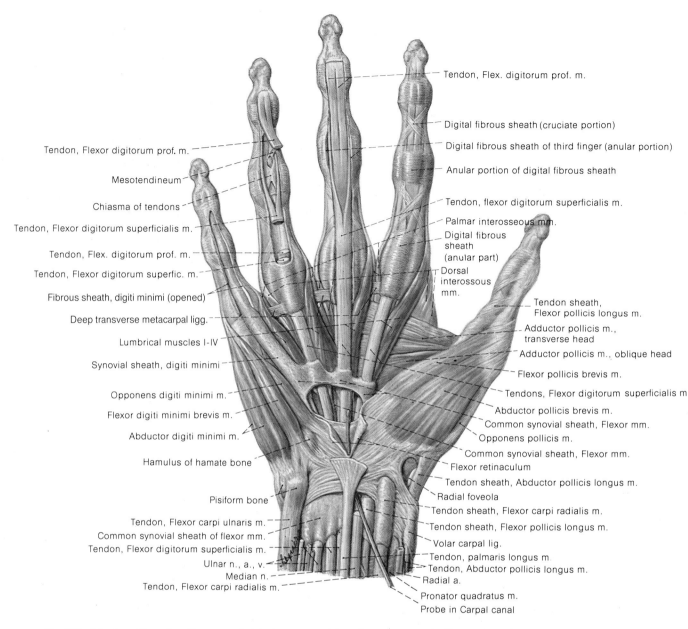

Tendon, Flex. digitorum prof. m.

Digital fibrous sheath (cruciate portion)

Digital fibrous sheath of third finger (anular portion)

Anular portion of digital fibrous sheath

Tendon, flexor digitorum superficialis m.

Palmar interosseous mm.

Digital fibrous sheath (anular part)

Dorsal interossous mm.

Tendon sheath, Flexor pollicis longus m.

Adductor pollicis m., transverse head

Adductor pollicis m., oblique head

Flexor pollicis brevis m.

Tendons, Flexor digitorum superficialis m

Abductor pollicis brevis m.

Common synovial sheath, Flexor mm.

Opponens pollicis m.

Common synovial sheath, Flexor mm.

Flexor retinaculum

Tendon sheath, Abductor pollicis longus m.

Radial foveola

Tendon sheath, Flexor carpi radialis m.

Tendon sheath, Flexor pollicis longus m.

Volar carpal lig.

Tendon, palmaris longus m.

Tendon, Abductor pollicis longus m.

Radial a.

Pronator quadratus m.

Probe in Carpal canal

Tendon, Flexor digitorum prof. m.

Mesotendineum

Chiasma of tendons

Tendon, Flexor digitorum superficialis m.

Tendon, Flex. digitorum prof. m.

Tendon, Flexor digitorum superfic. m.

Fibrous sheath, digiti minimi (opened)

Deep transverse metacarpal ligg.

Lumbrical muscles I-IV

Synovial sheath, digiti minimi

Opponens digiti minimi m.

Flexor digiti minimi brevis m.

Abductor digiti minimi m.

Hamulus of hamate bone

Pisiform bone

Tendon, Flexor carpi ulnaris m.

Common synovial sheath of flexor mm.

Tendon, Flexor digitorum superficialis m.

Ulnar n., a., v.

Median n.

Tendon, Flexor carpi radialis m.

**Fig. 584.** Muscles of the palm after removal of the larger part of the palmar aponeurosis. The tendon sheath of the middle finger was split along its entire length. The flexor retinaculum was partially opened.

**Dorsal and Palmar Interossei Muscles (Figs. 602, 603)**

| | |
|---|---|
| *Nerve:* | Ulnar nerve |
| *Function:* | Dorsal interossei muscles abduct; the Palmar interossei adduct the fingers |

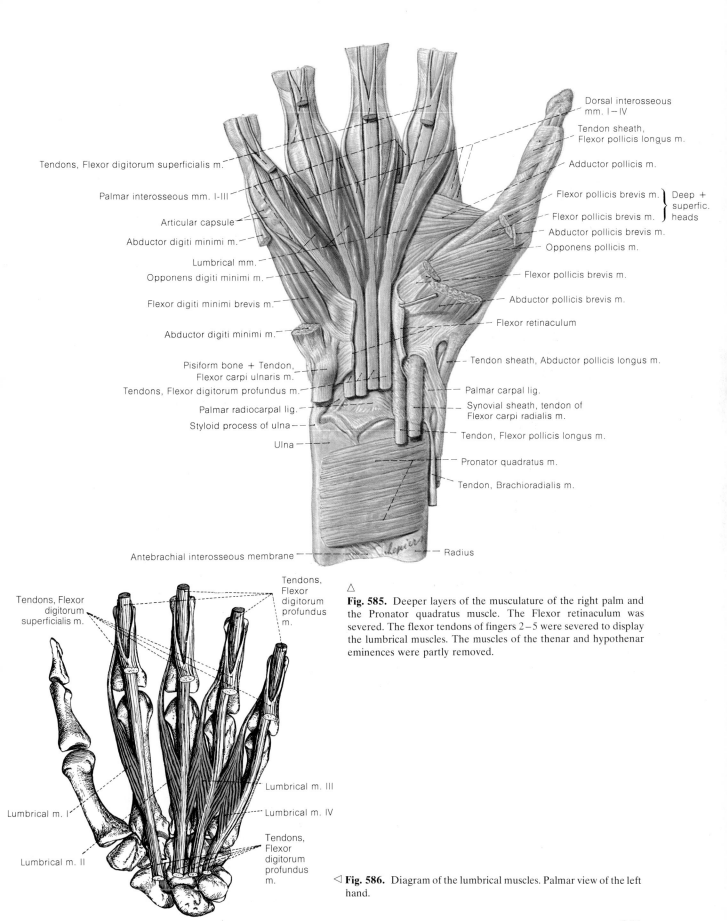

Dorsal interosseous mm. I–IV

Tendon sheath, Flexor pollicis longus m.

Adductor pollicis m.

Flexor pollicis brevis m. } Deep +
Flexor pollicis brevis m. } superfic. heads

Abductor pollicis brevis m.

Opponens pollicis m.

Flexor pollicis brevis m.

Abductor pollicis brevis m.

Flexor retinaculum

Tendon sheath, Abductor pollicis longus m.

Palmar carpal lig.

Synovial sheath, tendon of Flexor carpi radialis m.

Tendon, Flexor pollicis longus m.

Pronator quadratus m.

Tendon, Brachioradialis m.

Radius

Tendons, Flexor digitorum superficialis m.

Palmar interosseous mm. I–III

Articular capsule

Abductor digiti minimi m.

Lumbrical mm.

Opponens digiti minimi m.

Flexor digiti minimi brevis m.

Abductor digiti minimi m.

Pisiform bone + Tendon, Flexor carpi ulnaris m.

Tendons, Flexor digitorum profundus m.

Palmar radiocarpal lig.

Styloid process of ulna

Ulna

Antebrachial interosseous membrane

△
**Fig. 585.** Deeper layers of the musculature of the right palm and the Pronator quadratus muscle. The Flexor retinaculum was severed. The flexor tendons of fingers 2–5 were severed to display the lumbrical muscles. The muscles of the thenar and hypothenar eminences were partly removed.

Tendons, Flexor digitorum superficialis m.

Tendons, Flexor digitorum profundus m.

Lumbrical m. I

Lumbrical m. II

Lumbrical m. III

Lumbrical m. IV

Tendons, Flexor digitorum profundus m.

◁ **Fig. 586.** Diagram of the lumbrical muscles. Palmar view of the left hand.

351

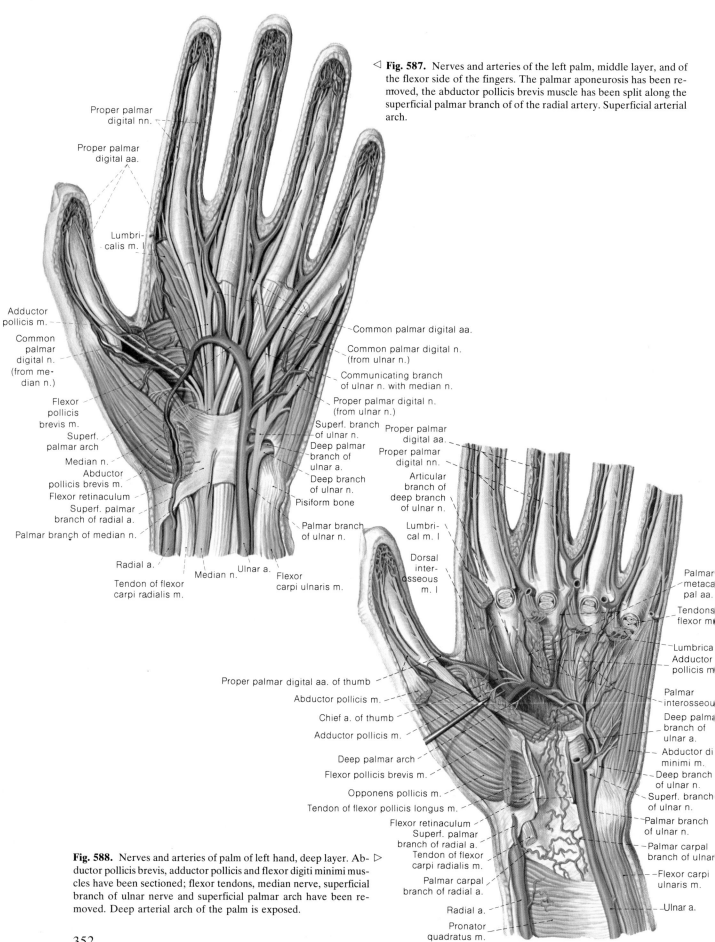

Proper palmar
digital nn.

Proper palmar
digital aa.

Lumbri-
calis m. I

Adductor
pollicis m.

Common
palmar
digital n.
(from me-
dian n.)

Flexor
pollicis
brevis m.

Superf.
palmar arch

Median n.

Abductor
pollicis brevis m.

Flexor retinaculum

Superf. palmar
branch of radial a.

Palmar branch of median n.

Radial a.

Tendon of flexor
carpi radialis m.

Median n.

Ulnar a.

Flexor
carpi ulnaris m.

◁ **Fig. 587.** Nerves and arteries of the left palm, middle layer, and of
the flexor side of the fingers. The palmar aponeurosis has been removed, the abductor pollicis brevis muscle has been split along the
superficial palmar branch of of the radial artery. Superficial arterial
arch.

Common palmar digital aa.

Common palmar digital n.
(from ulnar n.)

Communicating branch
of ulnar n. with median n.

Proper palmar digital n.
(from ulnar n.)

Superf. branch
of ulnar n.

Deep palmar
branch of
ulnar a.

Deep branch
of ulnar n.

Pisiform bone

Palmar branch
of ulnar n.

Proper palmar
digital aa.

Proper palmar
digital nn.

Articular
branch of
deep branch
of ulnar n.

Lumbri-
cal m. I

Dorsal
inter-
osseous
m. I

Palmar
metaca
pal aa.

Tendons
flexor m

Lumbrica
Adductor
pollicis m

Palmar
interosseou

Deep palma
branch of
ulnar a.

Abductor di
minimi m.

Deep branch
of ulnar n.

Superf. branch
of ulnar n.

Palmar branch
of ulnar n.

Palmar carpal
branch of ulnar

Flexor carpi
ulnaris m.

Ulnar a.

Proper palmar digital aa. of thumb

Abductor pollicis m.

Chief a. of thumb

Adductor pollicis m.

Deep palmar arch

Flexor pollicis brevis m.

Opponens pollicis m.

Tendon of flexor pollicis longus m.

Flexor retinaculum

Superf. palmar
branch of radial a.

Tendon of flexor
carpi radialis m.

Palmar carpal
branch of radial a.

Radial a.

Pronator
quadratus m.

**Fig. 588.** Nerves and arteries of palm of left hand, deep layer. Ab- ▷
ductor pollicis brevis, adductor pollicis and flexor digiti minimi muscles have been sectioned; flexor tendons, median nerve, superficial
branch of ulnar nerve and superficial palmar arch have been removed. Deep arterial arch of the palm is exposed.

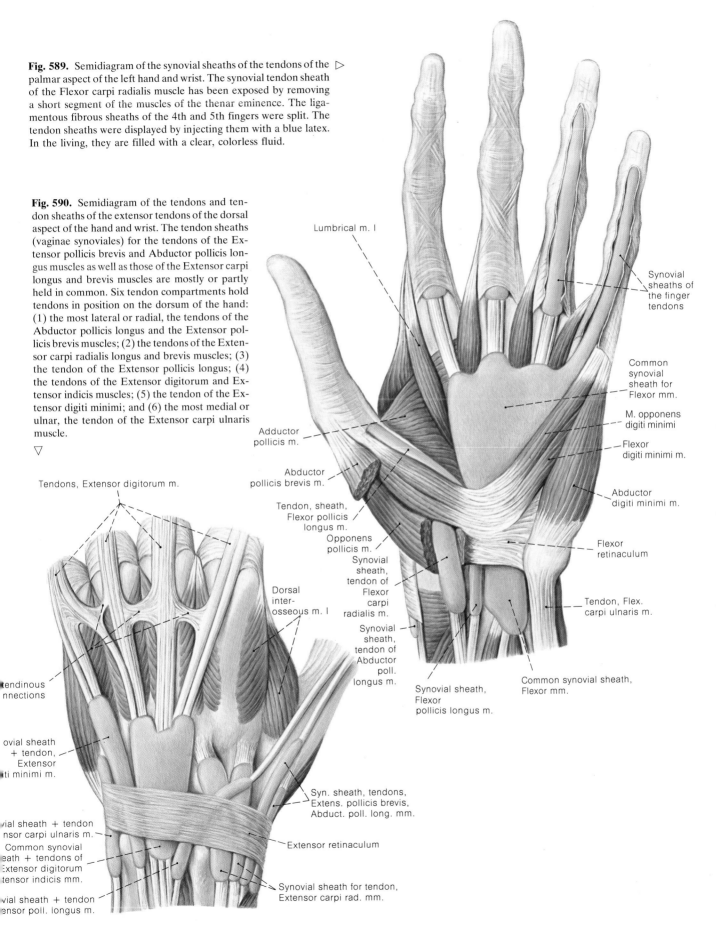

**Fig. 589.** Semidiagram of the synovial sheaths of the tendons of the ▷ palmar aspect of the left hand and wrist. The synovial tendon sheath of the Flexor carpi radialis muscle has been exposed by removing a short segment of the muscles of the thenar eminence. The ligamentous fibrous sheaths of the 4th and 5th fingers were split. The tendon sheaths were displayed by injecting them with a blue latex. In the living, they are filled with a clear, colorless fluid.

**Fig. 590.** Semidiagram of the tendons and tendon sheaths of the extensor tendons of the dorsal aspect of the hand and wrist. The tendon sheaths (vaginae synoviales) for the tendons of the Extensor pollicis brevis and Abductor pollicis longus muscles as well as those of the Extensor carpi longus and brevis muscles are mostly or partly held in common. Six tendon compartments hold tendons in position on the dorsum of the hand: (1) the most lateral or radial, the tendons of the Abductor pollicis longus and the Extensor pollicis brevis muscles; (2) the tendons of the Extensor carpi radialis longus and brevis muscles; (3) the tendon of the Extensor pollicis longus; (4) the tendons of the Extensor digitorum and Extensor indicis muscles; (5) the tendon of the Extensor digiti minimi; and (6) the most medial or ulnar, the tendon of the Extensor carpi ulnaris muscle.

▽

Lumbrical m. I

Synovial sheaths of the finger tendons

Common synovial sheath for Flexor mm.

M. opponens digiti minimi

Flexor digiti minimi m.

Abductor digiti minimi m.

Flexor retinaculum

Tendon, Flex. carpi ulnaris m.

Common synovial sheath, Flexor mm.

Adductor pollicis m.

Abductor pollicis brevis m.

Tendon, sheath, Flexor pollicis longus m.

Opponens pollicis m.

Synovial sheath, tendon of Flexor carpi radialis m.

Synovial sheath, tendon of Abductor poll. longus m.

Synovial sheath, Flexor pollicis longus m.

Tendons, Extensor digitorum m.

Dorsal interosseous m. I

tendinous nnections

ovial sheath + tendon, Extensor iti minimi m.

vial sheath + tendon nsor carpi ulnaris m.

Common synovial eath + tendons of Extensor digitorum tensor indicis mm.

vial sheath + tendon ensor poll. longus m.

Syn. sheath, tendons, Extens. pollicis brevis, Abduct. poll. long. mm.

Extensor retinaculum

Synovial sheath for tendon, Extensor carpi rad. mm.

353

**Muscles of the Thenar Eminence (Fig. 588)**

The superficial layer of the thenar eminence is formed by the Abductor pollicis brevis, Opponens pollicis muscles, and the superficial or lateral portion of the Flexor pollicis brevis muscle. The deep layers of the thenar eminence muscles are composed of the deep or medial portion of the Flexor pollicis brevis and the Adductor pollicis muscles.

| Name | Origin | Insertion |
|---|---|---|
| **1. Abductor pollicis brevis muscle** | Flexor retinaculum; tuberosity of scaphoid; ridge of trapezium | Radial side, proximal phalanx of thumb |
| *Nerve:* Median nerve | | |
| *Function:* Abducts thumb | | |
| **2. Opponens pollicis muscle** | Flexor retinaculum; ridge of trapezium | Entire length of radial border of 1st metacarpal of thumb |
| *Nerve:* Medial nerve (C 6, 7, [8, T 1]) | | |
| *Function:* Opposes thumb to other fingers, abducts, flexes, rotates first metacarpal | | |
| **3. Flexor pollicis brevis** | | |
|     *Superficial portion* | Flexor retinaculum | Radial side of proximal phalanx of thumb; lateral sesamoid bone |
|     *Deeper portion* | Ridge of trapezium | |
| *Nerve:* Lateral portion: Median nerve (C 6, 7). Deep or medial portion: Ulnar nerve, deep branch (C 8, T 1) | | |
| *Function:* Flexes proximal phalanx of thumb | | |
| **4. Adductor pollicis muscle** <br>     *a) Oblique head* | a) Capitate bone; bases of 2nd and 3rd metacarpals | Medial (ulnar) side of proximal phalanx of thumb, sesamoid bone |
|     *b) Transverse head* | b) Anterior surface of 3rd metacarpal | |
| *Nerve:* Ulnar nerve, deep palmar branch (C 8; T 1) | | |
| *Function:* Adducts the thumb; aids in opposition | | |

## Lumbrical Muscles

| | |
|---|---|
| *Origin:* | Tendons of Flexor digitorum profundus muscle |
| *Insertion:* | Dorsal aponeurosis of the proximal phalanx of fingers II to V |
| *Nerve:* | Two lateral lumbricals: Median nerve<br>Two medial lumbricals: Ulnar nerve |
| *Function:* | Flexes the metacarpophalangeal joints; extends the two distal phalanges |

## Muscles of the Hypothenar Eminence

| **Name** | *Origin* | *Insertion* |
|---|---|---|
| **1. Abductor digiti minimi muscle** | Pisiform bone and tendon of Flexor carpi ulnaris | Proximal phalanx of little finger, ulnar side |
| **2. Flexor digiti minimi brevis muscle** (variable) | Flexor retinaculum, hamalus of hamate bone | Ulnar side of proximal phalanx of little finger |
| **3. Opponens digiti minimi muscle** | Flexor retinaculum; hook of hamate bone | Ulnar margin of 5th metacarpal |

| | |
|---|---|
| *Nerve:* | Ulnar nerve, deep branch (C 8; T 1) |
| *Function:* | As their names indicate: Abducts and reflexes little finger; Opponens digiti minimi muscle also rotates 5th metacarpal and brings it out of plane of palm to meet the thumb and cup the hand |

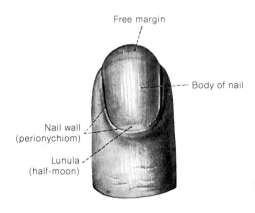

**Fig. 591.** Fingernail in its normal position, dorsal view.

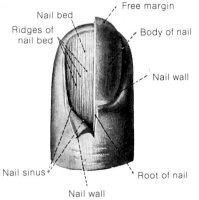

**Fig. 592.** Dorsal view of finger nail, sectioned longitudinally to expose the nail bed on the left side.

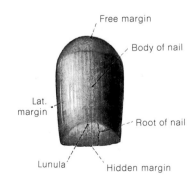

**Fig. 593.** Body of nail, removed from nail bed; dorsal view.

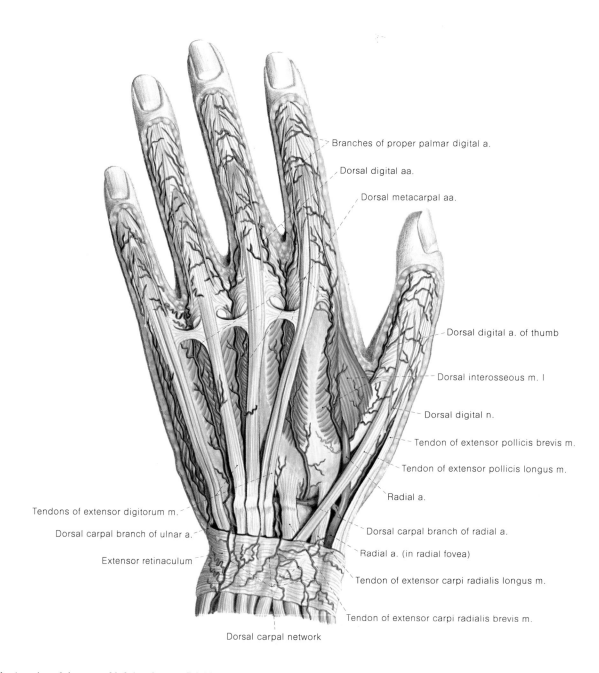

Branches of proper palmar digital a.

Dorsal digital aa.

Dorsal metacarpal aa.

Dorsal digital a. of thumb

Dorsal interosseous m. I

Dorsal digital n.

Tendon of extensor pollicis brevis m.

Tendon of extensor pollicis longus m.

Radial a.

Tendons of extensor digitorum m.

Dorsal carpal branch of ulnar a.

Dorsal carpal branch of radial a.

Extensor retinaculum

Radial a. (in radial fovea)

Tendon of extensor carpi radialis longus m.

Tendon of extensor carpi radialis brevis m.

Dorsal carpal network

**Fig. 594.** Arteries of dorsum of left hand, superficial layer.

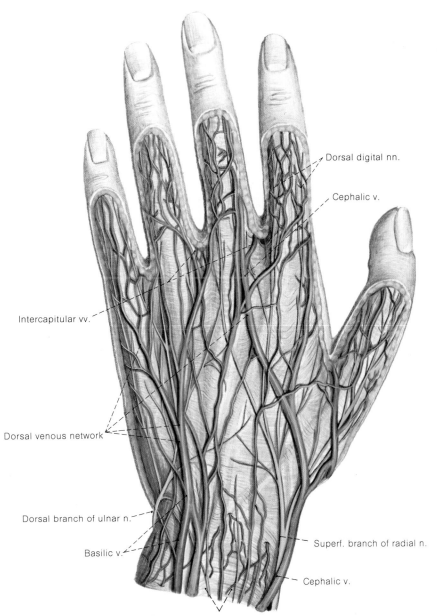

Dorsal digital nn.

Cephalic v.

Intercapitular vv.

Dorsal venous network

Dorsal branch of ulnar n.

Basilic v.

Superf. branch of radial n.

Cephalic v.

Post. antebrachial cutaneous branches of radial n.

**Fig. 595.** Superficial nerves and veins of dorsum of hand.

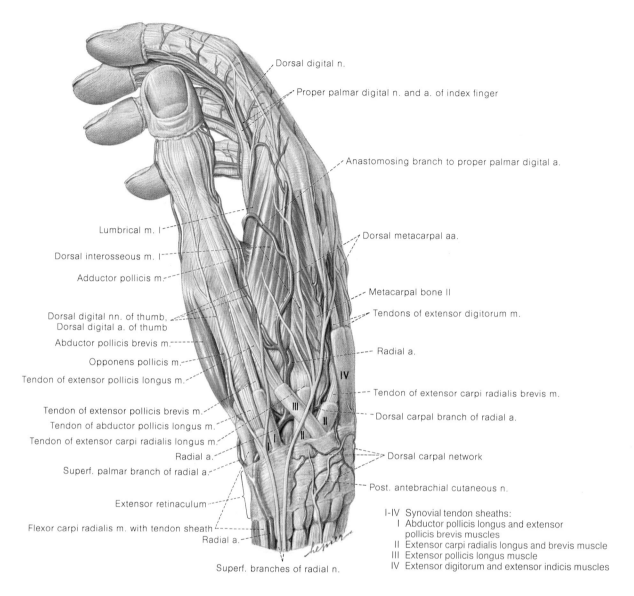

Dorsal digital n.

Proper palmar digital n. and a. of index finger

Anastomosing branch to proper palmar digital a.

Lumbrical m. I

Dorsal interosseous m. I

Adductor pollicis m.

Dorsal digital nn. of thumb, Dorsal digital a. of thumb

Abductor pollicis brevis m.

Opponens pollicis m.

Tendon of extensor pollicis longus m.

Tendon of extensor pollicis brevis m.

Tendon of abductor pollicis longus m.

Tendon of extensor carpi radialis longus m.

Radial a.

Superf. palmar branch of radial a.

Extensor retinaculum

Flexor carpi radialis m. with tendon sheath

Radial a.

Superf. branches of radial n.

Dorsal metacarpal aa.

Metacarpal bone II

Tendons of extensor digitorum m.

Radial a.

Tendon of extensor carpi radialis brevis m.

Dorsal carpal branch of radial a.

Dorsal carpal network

Post. antebrachial cutaneous n.

I-IV Synovial tendon sheaths:
  I Abductor pollicis longus and extensor pollicis brevis muscles
  II Extensor carpi radialis longus and brevis muscle
  III Extensor pollicis longus muscle
  IV Extensor digitorum and extensor indicis muscles

**Fig. 596.** Superficial arteries and nerves of the right hand, radial view. Skin, subcutaneous tissue and fascia have been removed. Note the radial artery in the radial fovea which is bordered by the tendons of the extensor pollicis brevis and longus muscles.

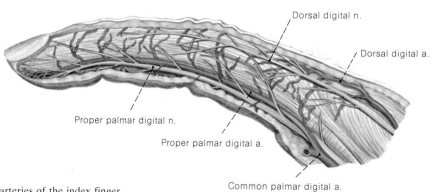

Dorsal digital n.

Dorsal digital a.

Proper palmar digital n.

Proper palmar digital a.

Common palmar digital a.

**Fig. 597.** Nerves and arteries of the index finger.

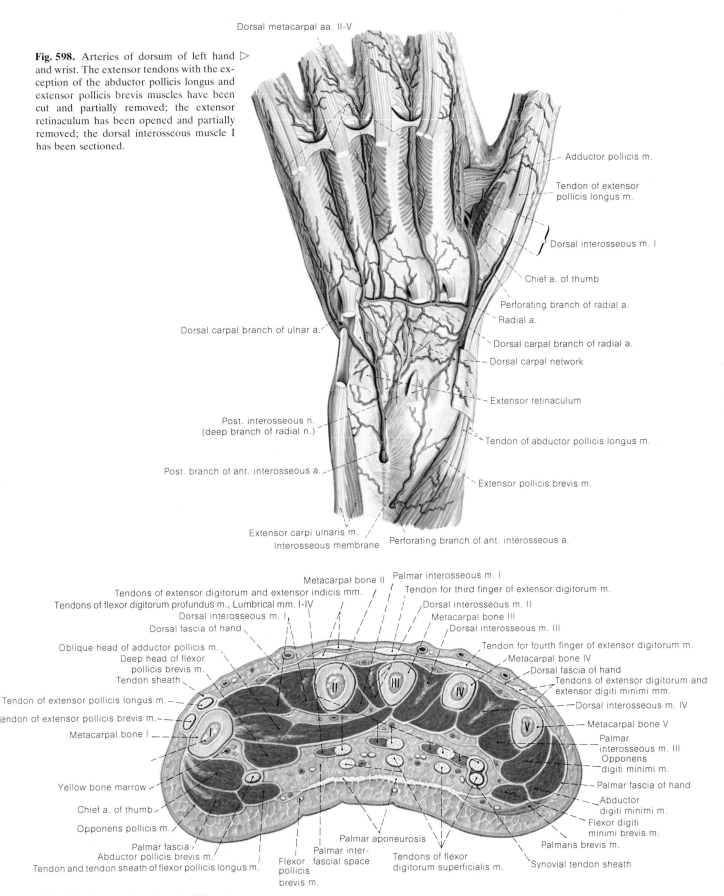

Dorsal metacarpal aa. II-V

**Fig. 598.** Arteries of dorsum of left hand ▷ and wrist. The extensor tendons with the exception of the abductor pollicis longus and extensor pollicis brevis muscles have been cut and partially removed; the extensor retinaculum has been opened and partially removed; the dorsal interosseous muscle I has been sectioned.

Adductor pollicis m.

Tendon of extensor pollicis longus m.

Dorsal interosseous m. I

Chief a. of thumb

Perforating branch of radial a.

Radial a.

Dorsal carpal branch of radial a.

Dorsal carpal network

Dorsal carpal branch of ulnar a.

Extensor retinaculum

Post. interosseous n. (deep branch of radial n.)

Tendon of abductor pollicis longus m.

Post. branch of ant. interosseous a.

Extensor pollicis brevis m.

Extensor carpi ulnaris m.
Interosseous membrane

Perforating branch of ant. interosseous a.

Metacarpal bone II · Palmar interosseous m. I
Tendons of extensor digitorum and extensor indicis mm. / Tendon for third finger of extensor digitorum m.
Tendons of flexor digitorum profundus m., Lumbrical mm. I-IV · Dorsal interosseous m. II
Dorsal interosseous m. I · Metacarpal bone III
Dorsal fascia of hand · Dorsal interosseous m. III

Oblique head of adductor pollicis m.
Deep head of flexor pollicis brevis m.
Tendon sheath

Tendon for fourth finger of extensor digitorum m.
Metacarpal bone IV
Dorsal fascia of hand
Tendons of extensor digitorum and extensor digiti minimi mm.

Tendon of extensor pollicis longus m.
Dorsal interosseous m. IV

Tendon of extensor pollicis brevis m.
Metacarpal bone V

Metacarpal bone I
Palmar interosseous m. III
Opponens digiti minimi m.

Yellow bone marrow
Palmar fascia of hand

Chief a. of thumb
Abductor digiti minimi m.

Opponens pollicis m.
Flexor digiti minimi brevis m.

Palmar fascia
Abductor pollicis brevis m.
Tendon and tendon sheath of flexor pollicis longus m.
Flexor pollicis brevis m.
Palmar inter-fascial space
Palmar aponeurosis
Tendons of flexor digitorum superficialis m.
Palmaris brevis m.
Synovial tendon sheath

**Fig. 599.** Cross section through right metacarpus.

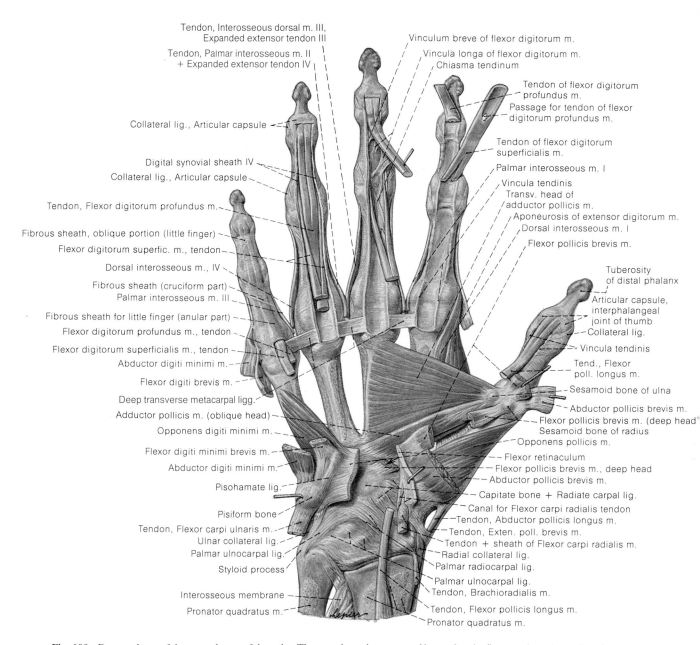

Tendon, Interosseous dorsal m. III,
Expanded extensor tendon III

Tendon, Palmar interosseous m. II
+ Expanded extensor tendon IV

Vinculum breve of flexor digitorum m.

Vincula longa of flexor digitorum m.

Chiasma tendinum

Collateral lig., Articular capsule

Tendon of flexor digitorum
profundus m.

Passage for tendon of flexor
digitorum profundus m.

Digital synovial sheath IV

Tendon of flexor digitorum
superficialis m.

Collateral lig., Articular capsule

Palmar interosseous m. I

Tendon, Flexor digitorum profundus m.

Vincula tendinis

Transv. head of
adductor pollicis m.

Fibrous sheath, oblique portion (little finger)

Aponeurosis of extensor digitorum m.

Flexor digitorum superfic. m., tendon

Dorsal interosseous m. I

Dorsal interosseous m., IV

Flexor pollicis brevis m.

Fibrous sheath (cruciform part)

Tuberosity
of distal phalanx

Palmar interosseous m. III

Articular capsule,
interphalangeal
joint of thumb

Fibrous sheath for little finger (anular part)

Collateral lig.

Flexor digitorum profundus m., tendon

Vincula tendinis

Flexor digitorum superficialis m., tendon

Tend., Flexor
poll. longus m.

Abductor digiti minimi m.

Sesamoid bone of ulna

Flexor digiti brevis m.

Abductor pollicis brevis m.

Deep transverse metacarpal ligg.

Flexor pollicis brevis m. (deep head)

Adductor pollicis m. (oblique head)

Sesamoid bone of radius

Opponens digiti minimi m.

Opponens pollicis m.

Flexor digiti minimi brevis m.

Flexor retinaculum

Abductor digiti minimi m.

Flexor pollicis brevis m., deep head

Pisohamate lig.

Abductor pollicis brevis m.

Capitate bone + Radiate carpal lig.

Pisiform bone

Canal for Flexor carpi radialis tendon

Tendon, Abductor pollicis longus m.

Tendon, Flexor carpi ulnaris m.

Tendon, Exten. poll. brevis m.

Ulnar collateral lig.

Tendon + sheath of Flexor carpi radialis m.

Palmar ulnocarpal lig.

Radial collateral lig.

Styloid process

Palmar radiocarpal lig.

Palmar ulnocarpal lig.

Interosseous membrane

Tendon, Brachioradialis m.

Pronator quadratus m.

Tendon, Flexor pollicis longus m.

Pronator quadratus m.

**Fig. 600.** Deepest layer of the musculature of the palm. The carpal canal was opened by cutting the flexor retinaculum. The origin and insertion of the Pronator quadratus muscle was severed at the distal end of the radius and ulna. The tendon of the Flexor pollicis longus was kept in place. The flexor tendons of the fingers (after opening the tendon sheaths) were dissected to their insertion.

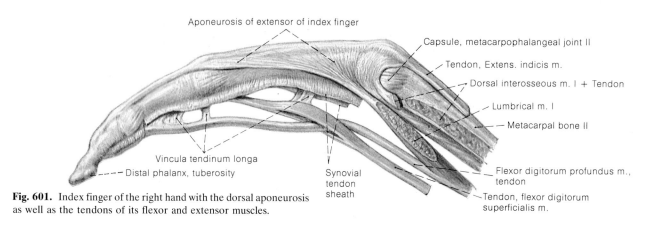

Aponeurosis of extensor of index finger

Capsule, metacarpophalangeal joint II

Tendon, Extens. indicis m.

Dorsal interosseous m. I + Tendon

Lumbrical m. I

Metacarpal bone II

Vincula tendinum longa

Distal phalanx, tuberosity

Synovial
tendon
sheath

Flexor digitorum profundus m.,
tendon

Tendon, flexor digitorum
superficialis m.

**Fig. 601.** Index finger of the right hand with the dorsal aponeurosis as well as the tendons of its flexor and extensor muscles.

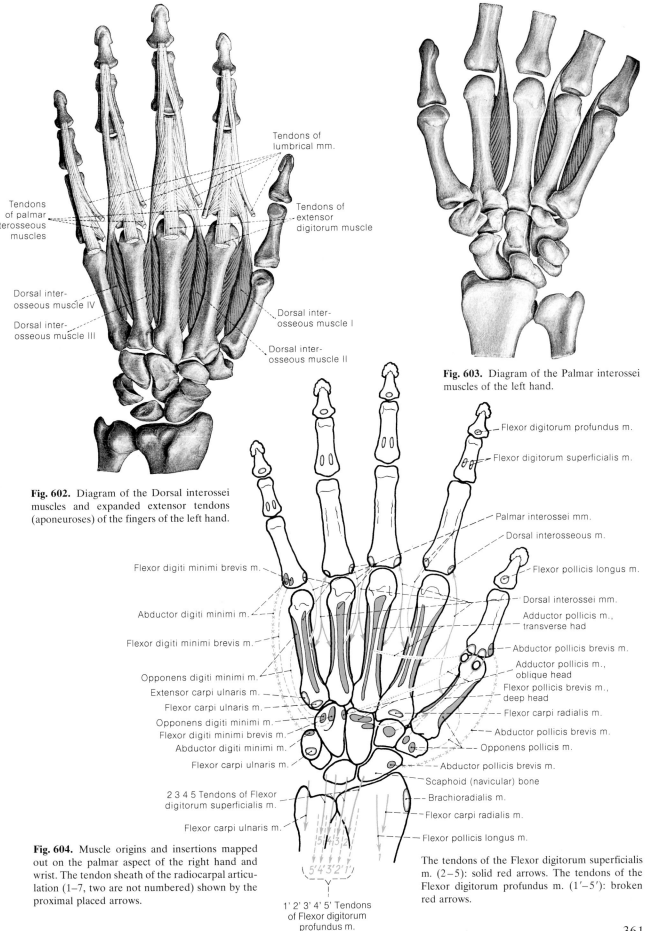

Tendons of lumbrical mm.

Tendons of palmar interosseous muscles

Tendons of extensor digitorum muscle

Dorsal interosseous muscle IV

Dorsal interosseous muscle III

Dorsal interosseous muscle I

Dorsal interosseous muscle II

**Fig. 602.** Diagram of the Dorsal interossei muscles and expanded extensor tendons (aponeuroses) of the fingers of the left hand.

**Fig. 603.** Diagram of the Palmar interossei muscles of the left hand.

Flexor digitorum profundus m.

Flexor digitorum superficialis m.

Palmar interossei mm.

Dorsal interosseous m.

Flexor pollicis longus m.

Dorsal interossei mm.

Adductor pollicis m., transverse had

Abductor pollicis brevis m.

Adductor pollicis m., oblique head

Flexor pollicis brevis m., deep head

Flexor carpi radialis m.

Abductor pollicis brevis m.

Opponens pollicis m.

Abductor pollicis brevis m.

Scaphoid (navicular) bone

Brachioradialis m.

Flexor carpi radialis m.

Flexor pollicis longus m.

Flexor digiti minimi brevis m.

Abductor digiti minimi m.

Flexor digiti minimi brevis m.

Opponens digiti minimi m.

Extensor carpi ulnaris m.

Flexor carpi ulnaris m.

Opponens digiti minimi m.

Flexor digiti minimi brevis m.

Abductor digiti minimi m.

Flexor carpi ulnaris m.

2 3 4 5 Tendons of Flexor digitorum superficialis m.

Flexor carpi ulnaris m.

**Fig. 604.** Muscle origins and insertions mapped out on the palmar aspect of the right hand and wrist. The tendon sheath of the radiocarpal articulation (1–7, two are not numbered) shown by the proximal placed arrows.

5 4 3 2

5' 4' 3' 2' 1'

1' 2' 3' 4' 5' Tendons of Flexor digitorum profundus m.

The tendons of the Flexor digitorum superficialis m. (2–5): solid red arrows. The tendons of the Flexor digitorum profundus m. (1'–5'): broken red arrows.

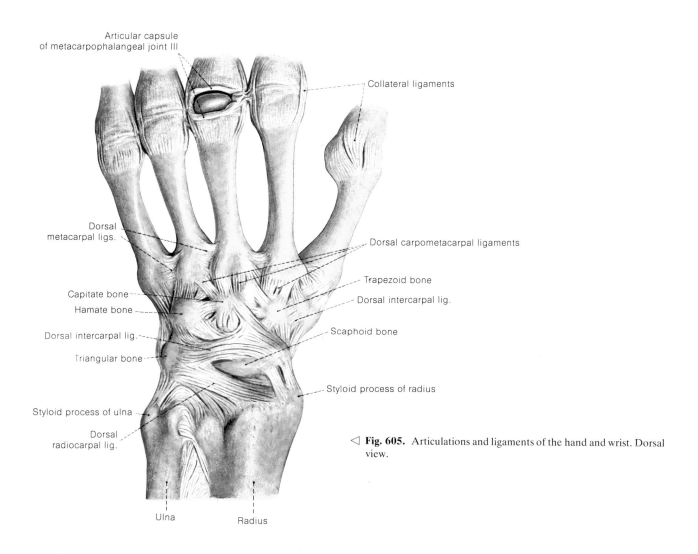

Articular capsule
of metacarpophalangeal joint III

Collateral ligaments

Dorsal
metacarpal ligs.

Dorsal carpometacarpal ligaments

Capitate bone

Trapezoid bone

Hamate bone

Dorsal intercarpal lig.

Dorsal intercarpal lig.

Scaphoid bone

Triangular bone

Styloid process of radius

Styloid process of ulna

Dorsal
radiocarpal lig.

◁ **Fig. 605.** Articulations and ligaments of the hand and wrist. Dorsal view.

Ulna

Radius

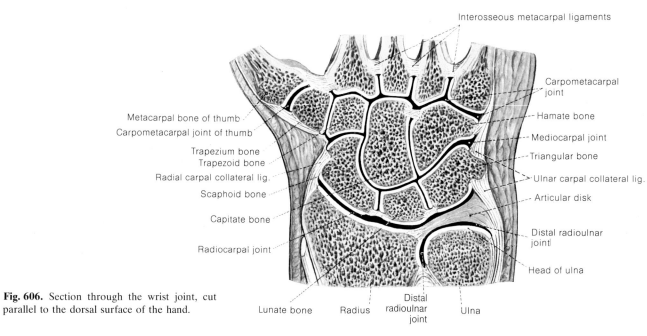

Interosseous metacarpal ligaments

Metacarpal bone of thumb

Carpometacarpal joint

Carpometacarpal joint of thumb

Hamate bone

Trapezium bone
Trapezoid bone

Mediocarpal joint

Radial carpal collateral lig.

Triangular bone

Scaphoid bone

Ulnar carpal collateral lig.

Capitate bone

Articular disk

Radiocarpal joint

Distal radioulnar jointl

Head of ulna

**Fig. 606.** Section through the wrist joint, cut parallel to the dorsal surface of the hand.

Lunate bone

Radius

Distal radioulnar joint

Ulna

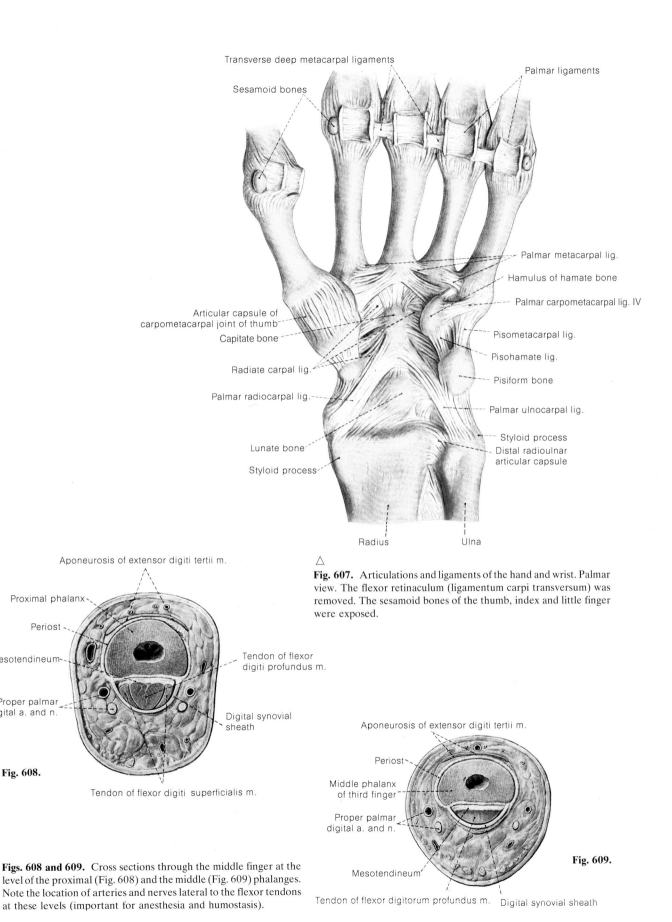

Transverse deep metacarpal ligaments

Palmar ligaments

Sesamoid bones

Palmar metacarpal lig.

Hamulus of hamate bone

Palmar carpometacarpal lig. IV

Articular capsule of
carpometacarpal joint of thumb

Capitate bone

Pisometacarpal lig.

Pisohamate lig.

Radiate carpal lig.

Pisiform bone

Palmar radiocarpal lig.

Palmar ulnocarpal lig.

Styloid process

Distal radioulnar
articular capsule

Lunate bone

Styloid process

Radius

Ulna

△

**Fig. 607.** Articulations and ligaments of the hand and wrist. Palmar view. The flexor retinaculum (ligamentum carpi transversum) was removed. The sesamoid bones of the thumb, index and little finger were exposed.

Aponeurosis of extensor digiti tertii m.

Proximal phalanx

Periost

Mesotendineum

Tendon of flexor
digiti profundus m.

Proper palmar
digital a. and n.

Digital synovial
sheath

**Fig. 608.**

Tendon of flexor digiti superficialis m.

Aponeurosis of extensor digiti tertii m.

Periost

Middle phalanx
of third finger

Proper palmar
digital a. and n.

Mesotendineum

**Fig. 609.**

Tendon of flexor digitorum profundus m.

Digital synovial sheath

**Figs. 608 and 609.** Cross sections through the middle finger at the level of the proximal (Fig. 608) and the middle (Fig. 609) phalanges. Note the location of arteries and nerves lateral to the flexor tendons at these levels (important for anesthesia and humostasis).

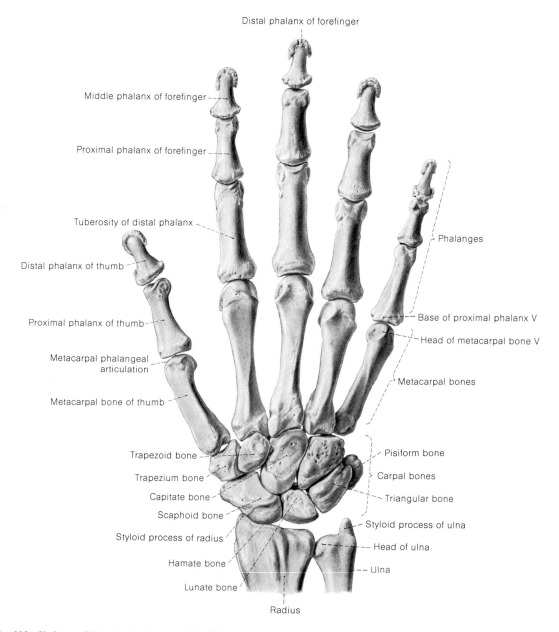

Distal phalanx of forefinger

Middle phalanx of forefinger

Proximal phalanx of forefinger

Tuberosity of distal phalanx

Distal phalanx of thumb

Proximal phalanx of thumb

Metacarpal phalangeal articulation

Metacarpal bone of thumb

Trapezoid bone

Trapezium bone

Capitate bone

Scaphoid bone

Styloid process of radius

Hamate bone

Lunate bone

Radius

Phalanges

Base of proximal phalanx V

Head of metacarpal bone V

Metacarpal bones

Pisiform bone

Carpal bones

Triangular bone

Styloid process of ulna

Head of ulna

Ulna

**Fig. 610.** Skeleton of right hand with extended, slightly spread fingers, and the distal end of the forearm with bones in their natural position. Dorsal view.

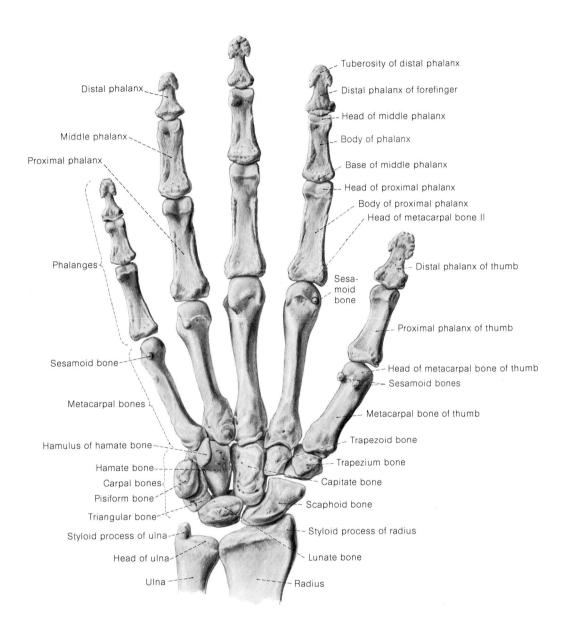

Distal phalanx

Middle phalanx

Proximal phalanx

Phalanges

Sesamoid bone

Metacarpal bones

Hamulus of hamate bone

Hamate bone
Carpal bones
Pisiform bone
Triangular bone
Styloid process of ulna

Head of ulna

Ulna

Tuberosity of distal phalanx

Distal phalanx of forefinger

Head of middle phalanx

Body of phalanx

Base of middle phalanx

Head of proximal phalanx

Body of proximal phalanx

Head of metacarpal bone II

Sesa-moid bone

Distal phalanx of thumb

Proximal phalanx of thumb

Head of metacarpal bone of thumb

Sesamoid bones

Metacarpal bone of thumb

Trapezoid bone

Trapezium bone

Capitate bone

Scaphoid bone

Styloid process of radius

Lunate bone

Radius

**Fig. 611.** Skeleton of right hand and wrist with bones in their natural position. (Same preparation as in Fig. 610.) Palmar view.

# Hand

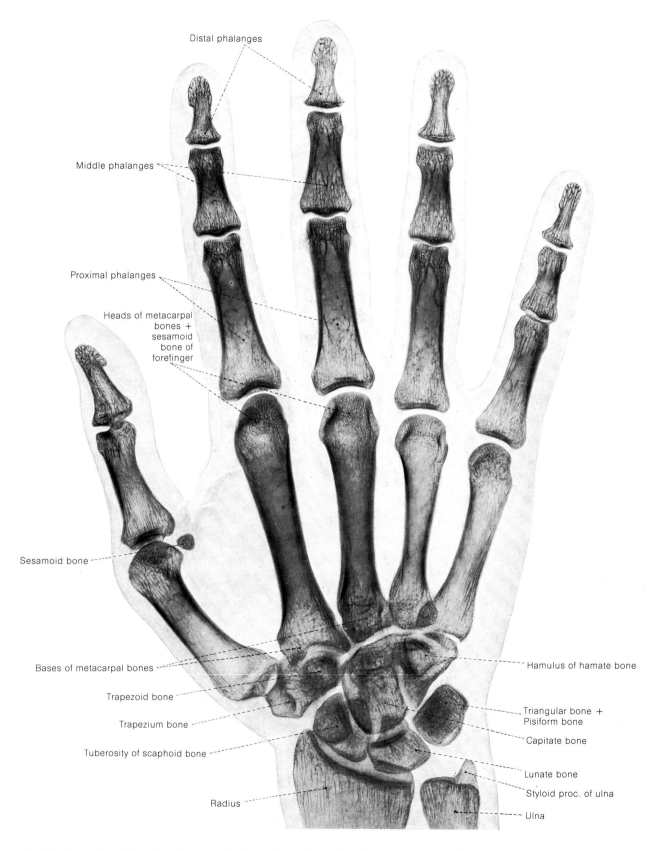

Distal phalanges

Middle phalanges

Proximal phalanges

Heads of metacarpal bones + sesamoid bone of forefinger

Sesamoid bone

Bases of metacarpal bones

Trapezoid bone

Trapezium bone

Tuberosity of scaphoid bone

Radius

Hamulus of hamate bone

Triangular bone + Pisiform bone

Capitate bone

Lunate bone

Styloid proc. of ulna

Ulna

**Fig. 612.** X-ray film of the left hand of an adult. The shadow of the pisiform bone is projected on that of the triangular. The soft parts are seen only as faint shadows. The thicker calcium-containing bones appear darker than the thin or calcium-deficient ones. The articular cartilages are not visible.

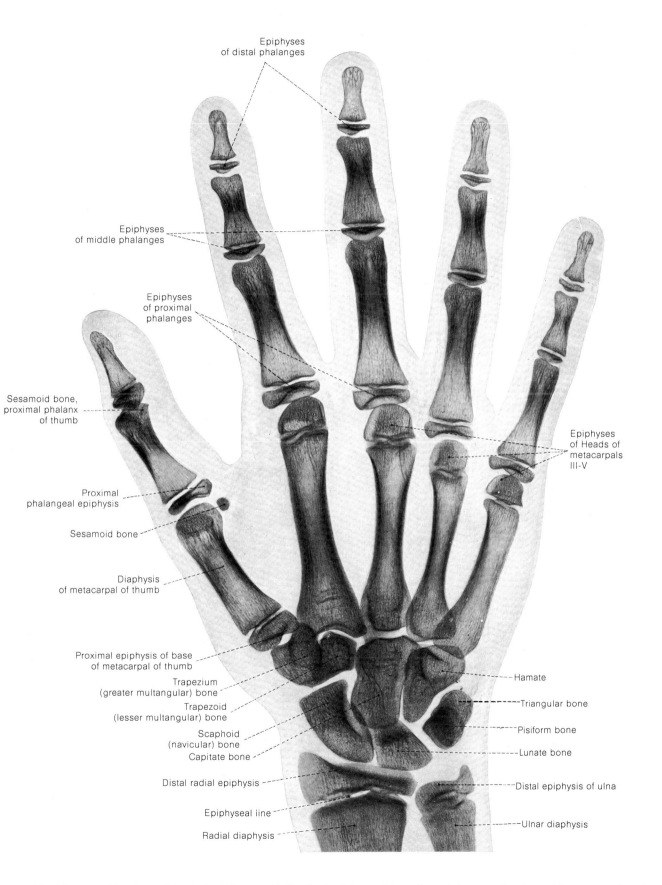

Epiphyses
of distal phalanges

Epiphyses
of middle phalanges

Epiphyses
of proximal
phalanges

Sesamoid bone,
proximal phalanx
of thumb

Epiphyses
of Heads of
metacarpals
III-V

Proximal
phalangeal epiphysis

Sesamoid bone

Diaphysis
of metacarpal of thumb

Proximal epiphysis of base
of metacarpal of thumb

Hamate

Trapezium
(greater multangular) bone

Triangular bone

Trapezoid
(lesser multangular) bone

Pisiform bone

Scaphoid
(navicular) bone

Lunate bone

Capitate bone

Distal radial epiphysis

Distal epiphysis of ulna

Epiphyseal line

Ulnar diaphysis

Radial diaphysis

**Fig. 613.** X-ray film of the left hand of a 15½-year old. The distal epiphyses of the radius and ulna, as well as those of the metacarpals ḟind phalanges, are ṇot yet united with their respective diaphyses. Note the definite epiphyseal lines.

367

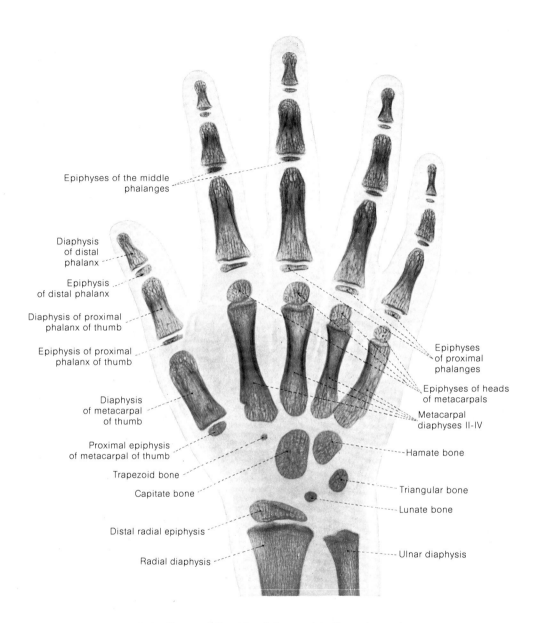

Epiphyses of the middle
phalanges

Diaphysis
of distal
phalanx

Epiphysis
of distal phalanx

Diaphysis of proximal
phalanx of thumb

Epiphysis of proximal
phalanx of thumb

Diaphysis
of metacarpal
of thumb

Proximal epiphysis
of metacarpal of thumb

Trapezoid bone

Capitate bone

Distal radial epiphysis

Radial diaphysis

Epiphyses
of proximal
phalanges

Epiphyses of heads
of metacarpals

Metacarpal
diaphyses II-IV

Hamate bone

Triangular bone

Lunate bone

Ulnar diaphysis

**Fig. 614.** X-ray film of the hand of a 5$^{1}$/$_{2}$-year old boy. The phalanges of the fingers have only one proximal epiphysis; the metacarpals II–V have only one distal. From this, one can see the metacarpal of the thumb as the proximal phalanx of the thumb. The center of ossification of the trapezoid and lunate bones are still very small; that of the scaphoid is absent. It is, therefore, possible to determine the age of children through investigation of the ossification.

# Etymology of Anatomical Terms*

L = from Latin; G = from Greek

## Rules employed in Naming the Joints and Ligaments

Most of the synarthrodial as well as diarthrodial joints are described by composite adjectives which consists of the names of the articulating bones as f. i. *articulatio sacroiliaca,* joint between sacrum and ilium. Similarly, ligaments receive adjectives which are composed of the names of the structures which they connect with each other. Only some of the larger joints have special names as f. i. *articulatio cubiti,* elbow joint; *articulatio coxae,* hip joint; likewise some ligaments have received special names as f. i. *lig. cruciforme atlantis, lig. cruciata* of the knee joint.

## Rules employed in Naming the Muscles

All muscles have the generic name *musculus,* only two muscles are excepted from this rule, *platysma* and *diaphragma.* In the selection of adjectives denoting the species of the muscle the following peculiarities are used.

1) **Shape** of the muscle as f. i. in *m. pyramidalis.* If there are several muscles of the same shape, further attributes are used to distinguish them; f. i. *m. rectus abdominis* and *m. rectus capitis.* Since, however, there are several straight muscles of the head, a differentiating adjective is added: *m. rectus capitis posterior* and *m. rectus capitis anterior;* again, there are two dorsal straight muscles of the head; these are distinguished from each other by a fourth attribute, *m. rectus posterior major* and *m. rectus capitis posterior minor.*

2) **Location** of the muscle as f. i. in *m. pectoralis;* again if there are several muscles of the same location, they are distinguished by addition of other adjectives as f. i. *m. pectoralis major* and *m. pectoralis minor.*

3) **Function** of the muscle, together with other criteria if there are several muscles of the same function: *m. abductor pollicis brevis* and *m. abductor pollicis longus; m. adductor brevis, m. adductor longus, m. adductor hallucis* and *m. adductor pollicis.*

4) **Attachments** (origin and insertion): f. i. *m. sternohyoideus, m. sternocleidomastoideus.*

---

* Literature:
  1. American Pocket Medical Dictionary. A dictionary of the principal terms used in medicine, nursing, pharmacy, dentistry, veterinary science and allied biological subjects. 19th Ed. B. Saunders Comp., Philadelphia-London 1953
  2. Dorland's Illustrated Medical Dictionary 26th Ed. W. B. Saunders, Philadelphia-London-Toronto 1982
  3. Nomina Anatomica. Third Ed. Prepared by the International Anatomical Nomenclature Committee appointed by the Fifth International Congress of Anatomists held at Oxford in 1950 and approved at the Sixth International Congress held at Paris in 1955, and including revisions approved at the Seventh and Eighth International Congresses of Anatomists held respectively at New York in 1960 and at Wiesbaden in 1960 and at Wiesbaden in 1965. Excerpta Medica Foundation, Amsterdam-New York-London-Paris-Milan-Tokyo-Buenos Aires 1968

**accessory:** L: *accedere; nervus accessorius* so called because it is accessory to the vagus nerve
**acetabulum:** L: *acetabulum* = small vessel to hold vinegar; cup-shaped socket of hipjoint
— L: *acetum* = vinegar
 *-bulum* = a small cup
Cup-shaped part of hip bone which resembles the Roman vinegar cruet.

**acromion:** G: *akron* = summit
 *ōmos* = shoulder
 Highest point of shoulder
**adipose:** L: *adeps* = fat
 *adiposus* = fatty
**ala:** L: a wing
**albicans albicantia (pl.):** L: *albicare* = to make white
**albuginea:** L: *albus* = white
 *albugo* = whiteness
 white spot
**alveolus:** L: dim. of *alveus* = a hollow, a cavity.
 Vesalius in 16th century called the tooth socket an *alveolus;* and Rossignol in 19th century applied the term to the minute parts of the lung.
**amnion:** G: dim. of *amnos* = lamb bowl, used to collect sacrificial blood. Galen was first to use this term.
**ampulla:** L: from Gr. *amphoreus* = flask or jug with globular body and two handles
**amygdaloid:** G: *amygdalē* = almond
**anconeus:** G: *ankon* = elbow
**angiogram:** G: *angeion* = vessel
 *gramma* = picture or writing
**angiography:** G: *angeion* = vessel
 *grapho* = I write
**antebrachium:** L: the forearm
**anularia:** L: relating to a signet ring
**anulus:** L: a small ring, *annulus* with two n's is a medieval misspelling
**anus:** L: a circular form, a ring (*anulus* a ring)
**apertura:** L: an opening, a hole
**aponeurosis:** G: *apo* = from
 *neuron* = any glistening fibrous structure. Later, Aristotle restricted use of *neuron* for nerves
**appendix:** L: *ad* = to
 *pendere* = to hang
 *appendere* = to hang upon, an appendage

**aqueduct:** L: water conduit
**arachnoid:** G: *arachnoidēs* from *ho arachnos* = the spider; spider web membrane covering brain and spinal cord
**arachnoidal:** G: *arachnē* = spider
 *eidos* = resemblance
 Applied in mid-17th century to the thin, cobweb-like structures.
**arcuate:** L: *arcus* = arch or bow
**artery:** Latinized Gr., etymology uncertain. Probably from *aggeia ta aera terenta* = air-containing vessels. The ancients thought that the arteries contained air.
**articulation:** L: *articulus* = dim. of *artus* = joint
 *-atio* = suffix, meaning action
**arytenoid:** G: *arytaina* = ladle
 *eidos* = resemblance
 Shaped like a pitcher
**aspera:** L: *asper, -era, -erum* = rough, *uneven*
**atlas:** Vesalius in 16th century gave this name to the 1st cervical vertebra which supported the head, naming it after the Greek god, who supported the heavens on his shoulders.
**atrium:** L: hall or entrance room
**auricle:** L: dim. of *auris* = ear
 The auricles are a part of the atria and resemble small ears; also outer ear
**azygos:** G: *a* negative, without
 *zygon* = yoke or pair
 unpaired

**biceps:** L: *bi* = double
 *caput* = head
**bile:** L: *bilis* = a yellowish-green fluid
**brachium:** L: arm
 G: *brachiōn* = arm
**brachycephalic:** G: *brachy* = wide
 *kephalē* = head
**bregma:** G: front of head
**brevis:** L: short

**bronchiole:** G: *bronchus* = windpipe
  L: *-olus* = dim. suffix
**bucca:** L: cheek
**buccinator:** L: *bucino* = to sound a trumpet
  *bucinator* = a trumpeter
  Buccinator muscles form the wall of the
  cheek.
**bulbus:** G: *bolbos*; L: *bulbus*
  a bulb (from the Gr. *ho bolbos* = onion)

**calcaneus:** L: *calx, calcis* = heel
**calcar avis:** L: the spur of the rooster
**calcarine:** Part of spur (from calcar)
**callosum:** L: *callum* = horny skin
**calvaria:** L: scalp without hair, roof of
  cranium
**calyx:** G: *kalyx* = cup or bud of a flower
**cancellus:** L: a grating, lattice, crisscross with
  lines, hence to disfigure. This gives rise to
  the term "to cancel" in modern usage.
**canine:** L: *caninus* = pertaining to dog, dog
  teeth, eye teeth. Canines are pointed teeth
  resembling those of a dog.
**capillary:** L: *capillus* = hair of the scalp
**capitate:** L: *capitatus* = having a head
  *caput* = head
**caput:** L: the head
**cardia:** G: *kardia* = heart
  Upper orifice of stomach nearest heart
**carina:** L: keel of a ship
**carneus:** L: from *carro* = flesh
**carpus:** G: *karpos* = root of the hand, wrist.
  Found in writings of Galen.
**cartilaget:** L: *cartilago* = gristle, cartilage
**caruncle:** L: *caruncula* = a little piece of
  flesh,
  dim. of *carro* = flesh. Applied to a small
  fleshy mass
**cauda:** L: tail or tail-like appendage
**cauda equina:** horse's tail (L. *cauda* = tail;
  *equina*, adj. from *equus* = horse); name
  applied to the roots of the lumbar and sacral
  spinal nerves which are arranged around
  the caudal end of the spinal cord like the
  hair of a horse's tail
**cava:** L: *cavus* = hollow *(venae cavae)*
**cavernosum:** L: full of hollows or cavities
**cavum:** L: *cavum* = hollow, cavity
**cecum:** L: *caecus* = blind, blind gut
**celiac:** G: *koilos* = hollow, referring to
  abdominal cavity
**cephalic:** G: *kephalikos* from
  *kephale* = head
**cerebellum:** L: diminutive of *cerebrum* = the
  small brain
**cerebrum:** L: brain; cerebral hemispheres
**cervix:** L: neck or nape
**chiasma:** G: crossing or intersecting in the
  manner of an X *(chi)*
**choana:** G: a funnel
**choledochus:** G: *chole* = bile
  *dochos* = receptacle, duct
**chorda tympani:** Cord of the middle ear
  cavity. Only nerve which is not called
  "*nervus*";
  it received its name at a time when its
  nervous nature was not known.
**chorioid:** G: *chorion* = a skin, membrane
**chorion:** G: membrane
**ciliary:** L: *cilium* = eyelash
**cingulum:** L: belt (from *cingere* = to gird or
  surround) Shingles is the common name for
  Herpes zoster. The vesicles encircle the
  body like a girdle, following the intercostal
  nerves. The word shingles is a corruption of
  *cingulum.*
**claustrum:** L: *claudere* = to close, bar
**clavicle:** L: *clavicula* = a small key,
  dim. of *clavis* = a key
**clitoris:** G: *kleitoris* from *klitorizein* = to
  tickle
**cluneal:** L: *clunis* = buttock
**coccyx (pl. coccyges):** G: *kokkyx* = cuckoo.
  An allusion to the resemblance to the
  cuckoo's bill. Herophilus applied this term
  about 300 B. C.

**cochlea:** shell of a snail (Lat., but perhaps
  originally Gr.)
**collum:** L: neck
**colon:** G: *kolon* = large bowel
  largest of the intestines
**commissure:** L: *committere* = to connect
**concha:** G: *konché* = shell of a mussel
  — L: *concha* = used for shell-shaped
  structures.
**condyle:** G: *kondylos;*
  L: *condylus* = knuckle
  Expanded parts of bones at joints.
**conjunctiva:** L: *conjungere* = to connect
**conoid:** G: *konos* = cone
  *eidos* = appearance, like
**conus:** G: *konos* = a cone, peg
  Used for tapered structures
**cor:** L: *cor*, genitive, *cordis* = heart
**coracoid:** G: *korakōdes*
  *korax* = raven
  *eidos* = resemblance
  Evidently the curved coracoid process was
  supposed to resemble a raven's beak.
  Actually, no crow or raven has a hooked
  beak.
**corium:** L., but originally Gr. = skin
**cornea:** L: *cornu* = horn
**corniculate:** L: *corniculatus* (dim. of *cornu*)
  Shaped like a small horn
**cornu (pl. cornua):** L: horn. Applied to
  hornshaped structures
**corona:** G: *korōnē*; L: *corona*
  a crown
**coronary:** L: *corona* = wreath, crown
**coronoid:** G: *korōnē* = crow
  *eidos* = resembling
  Shaped like the beak of a crow.
**corpus:** L: a body, mass or structure
**corrugator:** L: *con* (cor-) together
  *ruga* = wrinkle
  *corrugo* = to make wrinkles
**cortex (pl. cortices):** L: outer layer, bark,
  shell
**costal:** L: *costa* = rib, a side, a wall
**cotyledon:** G: *kotyle* = a cup
  *eidos* = resemblance
**cranium:** G: *kranion* = the skull
**cremaster:** G: *kremastēr* = a suspender
  Galen used this for muscle that suspends
  the testicle.
**cribriform:** L: *cribrum* = sieve
  *forma* = form
  A sieve-like structure; plate of ethmoid
**cricoid:** G: *krikos* = signet ring, or circle
  *eidos* = resemblance
**crista galli:** L: *crista* = a crest
  *gallus* = a cock
  A cock's comb
**cruciate:** L: *crux, cruris* = a cross,
  cross-shaped
**crus crura (pl.):** L: leg (adj. *cruralis*).
**cubital:** L: *cubitum* = elbow, cubit. An
  ancient measure, a cubit was equal to 18-22
  inches.
**culmen:** L: summit
**cuneiform:** L: *cuneus* = wedge
  *forma* = form
  Wedge-shaped bones in wrist and ankle.
**cuneus:** L: a wedge (adj. *cuneatus*)
**cupula:** L: *cupa* = cask
  dim.*-ula*
  Any cup- or dome-shaped structure
**cutaneous:** L: *cutis* = skin
**cysticus:** G: *kystis* = bladder

**deciduous:** L: *deciduus*, from *decidere* =
  falling off
**decussate:** L: *decussatio* = intersection of
  two lines
  *decussis* = ten was represented by X
  which is the intersection of two lines in the
  form of a cross.
**decussation:** L: *decussare* = to cross each
  other in the form of an X
**deferens:** L: *de* = away
  *ferre* = to carry

**deltoid:** G: *delta* = Greek letter Δ
  *eidos* = resembling
**dens:** L: tooth
**dentate:** L: *dens* = tooth
**diaphragm:** G: *dia* = across
  *phragma* = wall, fence
  a partition, wall
**diaphysis:** G: *dia* = between
  *physis* = growth
  separates growth areas
**diencephalon:** G: *dia* = between +
  encephalon
**digit:** L: *digitus* = finger
  Numbers are called digits because counting
  was first done on fingers.
**diploē:** G: fem. of *diplous* = double, folded.
  Ancient name for spongiosa of the bones of
  the *calvaria.*
**disc:** G: *diskos* = the flat disc between
  individual vertebrae
**diverticulum (pl. diverticula):**
  L: *divertere* = to turn aside
  (a small by-path)
**dolichocephalic:** G: *dolichos* = long
  *kephalē* = head
**dorsal:** L: *dorsum* = the back
**ductus deferens:** L: from *de* = away;
  *ferre* = to carry
**duodenum:** L: *duodeni* = twelve
  Twelve-finger gut, i. e. length of 12
  finger-widths.
**dura mater:** L: *durus* = hard;
  *mater* = mother, protection
**durum:** L: *durus* = hard

**ejaculatory:** L: *se ejaculari* = to expel
  suddenly
**emboliform:** L: from the Gr. *ho*
  *embolos* = plug
**encephalon:** G: from *he kēphalē* = the head,
  and *en* = in
**endocardium:** G: *endon* = within
  *kardia* = heart
**endometrium:** G: *endon* = within
  *metra* = uterus
**epicardium:** G: *epi* = upon
  *kardia* = heart
**epidermis:** G: *epi* = on top; and
  *derma* = skin
**epididymis:** G: *epi* = upon
  *didymos* = testes
**epigastric:** G: *epi* = above,
  *gaster* = stomach or belly
**epiglottis:** G: *epi* = on, upon
  *glottis* = larynx
**epiphysis:** G: *epi* = upon, on top
  *physis* = growth
  upon growth areas
**epiploicus:** G: *epiploon* = omentum
**epistropheus (BNA):** G: *epi* = upon
  *strephein* = to turn
  *ho epistropheys* = the turner, pivot, axis
  (second cervical vertebra)
**epoophoron:** G: *epi* = upon
  *oophoron* = ovary
  A rudiment of the mesonephric duct
**esophagus:** G: *oisophagos* = gullet
  *oiso* = to carry
  *phagein* = to feed
**ethmoid:** G: *ethmos* = a sieve
  *eidos* = resemblance
  — G: *ēthmos* = sieve
  *eidos* = resemblance

**facies:** L: a surface
**falx:** L: a sickle. A sickle or crescent-shaped
  structure, such as the falciform ligament
**fascia:** L: *fascia* = a band, girth
**fasciculus:** L: dim. of *fascis* = a small
  bundle
**fasciolar:** L: *fasciola* = a small band, dim.
  *fascia* = band
**fastigial:** L: *fastigium* = gable
**fauces (pl.):** L: *faucium* (gen) upper part of
  throat
**fellea:** L: *fel* = bile, gall

**femoral:** L: *femur, femoris* = the thigh

**fibula:** L: clasp, brooch, that which fastens two things together. The tibia and fibula resemble a bar-pin. (see also *peroneal*)

**filiform:** L: *filum* = thread
*forma* = shape

**fimbria:** L: *fimbria* = fringe
Any structure with many fine processes

**flaccid:** L: *flaccidus* = flabby, soft
— L: *flaccus* = flabby

**flava:** L: *flavus* = golden yellow

**flexure:** L: *flectere* = to bend

**flocculus:** L: dim. *floccus* = a flock or tuft (of wool)

**foliatus:** L: *folium* = leaf

**fontanel:** L: *fons, fontis* = spring, fountain
Fr.*fontanelle* = dim. of *fontaine* = fountain. The fontanels in the infant skull are probably so-called because the rhythmical pulsation, which is visible, resembles a small bubbling fountain.

**foramen:** L: a hole, an opening

**fornix (pl. fornices):** L: arch of a vault
"In ancient Rome, prostitutes plied their trade in the vaulted arches opening on the street - - - the term *fornication* came from this meaning and not from the word *fornix* as used medically."

**fossa:** L: a ditch; in anatomy, a depressed area

**fovea:** L: a pit; in anatomy, a shallow depression

**foveola:** L: dim. *fovea* = a small pit

**frenulum:** L: dim. of *frenum* = bridle or check rein

**frondosum:** L: *frondosus* = leafy

**frontal:** L: *frons, frontis* = forehead

**fungiform:** L: *fungus* = mushroom

**funiculus:** L: dim. of *funis* = a little cord

**gall:** Anglo-Saxon, *gealla* = bile

**ganglion:** G: swelling, node

**gastric:** G: *gaster* = stomach, belly

**gastrocnemius:** G: *gaster* = belly
*kneme* = lower leg
A muscle belly resting upon the shin-bone (the bulging belly of the calf) Spigelius, in 17th century, coined the term.

**gastroepiploic:** G: *gaster* = stomach;
G: *epiploon* = greater omentum

**gemellus:** L: dim. *geminus* = double, twins paired

**geniculate:** L: *geniculum* = a small knee

**genioglossus:** G: *geneion* = chin,
*glossa* = tongue

**genu:** L: knee (genitive, *genus*)
Used for bent structures.

**gingiva:** L: gum

**ginglymus:** G: *ginglymos* = a hinge-joint

**glabella:** L: *glaber* = beardless, smooth, bald.
A smooth prominence more pronounced in the male.

**gladiolus:** L: dim. of *gladius* = a sword.
Middle portion or body of the sternum was formerly called gladiolus because of its swordshape.

**glans:** L: acorn (the shape of the head of the penis)

**glomerulus:** L: dim. of *glomus* = a ball of yarn

**glossus:** G: *glossa* = tongue

**glottis:** G: of a flute, mouthpiece, voice box, larynx

**gluteus:** G: *gloutos* = buttocks
— G: *gloutos* = rump,
pl., the buttocks

**gonad:** G: *gone* = a seed or generation

**gracilis:** L: slender, thin, strap-like

**griseus:** L: gray

**gyrus:** G: *gyros* = a convolution

**habenula:** L: diminutive of *habena* = bridle, strap

**hallux:** L: *hallex* = great toe
*allex* = an older Latin term for thumb or great toe

**hamate:** L: *hamus* = hook, curved

**hamulus:** L: dim. of *hamus* = a small hook

**haustrum (pl. haustra):** L: machine for drawing water
The *haustrum* was derived from the verb: *haurio, hausi, haustum* = to drain or drink up. When these were named, it is doubtful that the function of the large intestine was fully appreciated.

**helicine:** G: *helix* = a coil or screw

**helicotrema:** G: *helix* = snail, and
*trema* = hole

**hemorrhoidal:** G: *haima* = blood
*rhein* = to flow

**hepar:** G: liver

**hiatus:** L: *hiare* = to gape, an opening
— L: *hiatus* = an opening, a yawn, aperture, cleft

**hilus:** L: *hilum* = a small thing
Point of attachment of a seed. In anatomy, where vessels and nerves enter and leave a structure.

**hippocampus:** G: from *hippos* = horse; and *kamptein* = to bend. Refers to the shape of the foot *(pes hippocampi)* of a legendary animal and is one of the fantastic names of the old nomenclature.

**hirci:** L: *hircus* = buck or he-goat.
Hair of the axilla

**humerus:** L: shoulder

**hyaloid:** G: *hyaloeidēs* = like glass

**hymen:** G: membrane, skin

**hyoid:** G: *hy* = Gr. letter upsilon.
*eidos* = resemblance
Hyoid bone resembles a Greek upsilon.
— G: *hyoeides*
*hy* = the Gr. letter U
*eidos* = resemblance

**hypoglossus:** G: *hypo* = beneath, and
*glossa* = tongue

**hypophysis:** G: *hypo* = below, under
*physis* = growth, origin
This gland grows under the brain.

**hypothalamus:** G: *hypo* = beneath. The part of the brain located beneath the thalamus

**hystera:** G: the womb, uterus

**ileum:** G: *eilos*from eilein, to roll up or twist
L: *ilia* = groin or flank, entrails of animals

**ilium:** L: *ilia* = groin, flank

**Inca bone:** Occasionally exists as a separate bone, separated from the rest of the occipital by the *sutura mendosa* (INA). Observed especially in the ancient Peruvian skulls among the Incas. (PNA, interparietal bone)

**incisivus:** L: *incidere* = to cut into

**incisura:** L: *in* = into
*caedere* = to cut
*incido* = an incision, to cut into

**incus:** L: *cudere* = to beat; anvil, one of the ossicles of the ear
— L: *cudere* = to beat
*incus (incudis)* = an anvil.
Galen first noted the resemblance of the ossicle to an anvil.

**index:** L: *indico* = to point out, inform, betray
*index, -icis* = a discoverer, an informer

**infundibulum:** L: funnel
— L: *infundere* = to pour into, to wet, moisten
*-bulum* = the vessels, small cup, funnel. A funnel-shaped passage.

**inguinal:** L: *inguen* = groin, front part of body
between the hips

**integument:** L: *integere* = to cover; clothe

**iris:** G: *iris*. Gen. *iridis* = rainbow

**ischium:** G: *ischion* = hip

**isthmus:** G: *isthmos* = narrow passage

**jejunum:** L: *jejunus* = fasting, or empty
Galen thought that this part of the small intestine was always empty after death and called ist *nestis* which was translated into Latin as *jejuneus*.

**juga (cerebralia):** L: *jugo* = to bind, to join
(A crossbeam or rail fastened horizontally to perpendicular poles)

**labium (labia pl.):** L: lip. Applied to other liplike structures besides the mouth.

**labium (pl. labia):** L: lip

**lacrimal:** L: *lacrima* = a tear

**lacuna:** L: *lacus* = lake

**laeve:** L: *levis* (also erroneously written *laevis*) smooth, not rough, soft

**lambdoidal:** G: *lambda* = Gr. letter λ
*eidos* = resemblance
Applied to suture shaped like the Gr. lambda λ.

**lanugo:** L: *lana* = wool; the fine primary hair

**larynx:** G: voice box. First used in English in 16th century.

**latum:** L: *latus, -a, -um* = broad, wide

**latus:** L: broad, wide, extended, side or flank

**lenticular:** L: from *lens*, Gen. *lentis* = lentil

**leptomeninx:** G: *leptos* = soft, delicate

**levator:** L.*levere* = to raise
*levator, -oris* = a lifter, a thief

**lien:** L: spleen

**lingua:** L: tongue

**lingula:** L: dim. of *lingua* = applied to small, tongue-shaped structures

**lumbar:** L: *lumbus* = loin

**lumbrical:** L: *lumbricus* = intestinal worm, earthworm-shaped

**lunate:** L: *luna* = the moon
*lunatus* = crescent-shaped

**luteum:** L: *luteus* = yellow pigment of egg yolk, from *lutum* = a yellow weed used for dyeing yellow

**luteus:** L: yellow

**lymph:** L: *lympha* = a clear liquid

**malar:** L: *mala* = cheek bone, jaw

**malleolar:** L: *malleolus*, dim. *malleus* = a small hammer. The "little hammers" of the foot are much larger than those of the ear.

**malleus:** L: *malleus* = a hammer, mallet, maul.

**mamilla:** L: dim. from *mamma* = female, breast, nipple

**mandible:** L: *mandere* = to chew
*mandibula* = lower jaw

**mandibula:** L: *mando, -onis* = a glutton
*mandere* = to chew
lower jaw

**manubrium:** L: handle, from *manus* = a hand.
Handle of a sword.

**manus:** L: the hand

**masseter:** G: *masētēr* = the chewer
One of the few muscles named by Galen.

**mastoid:** G: *mastos* = breast
*eidos* = resembling
Mastoid process resembles the nipple.

**maxilla:** L: dim. of *mala* = jaw bone
Now restricted to upper jaw.

**meatus:** L: a channel or way

**mediastinum:** L: intermediate; originally a servant

**medulla (pl. medullas or medullae):** L: inside, kernel, innermost part, marrow of bones, pith of plants

**meninges:** G: (sing. *meninx*) = membrane

**meniscus:** G: *meniskos* = a crescent
L: *menis* = a little half-moon

**mentalis:** L: *mentum* = chin

**mentum:** L: chin

**mesaticephalic:** G: *mesatius* = medium
*kephalē* = head

**mesenterium:** G: *mesos* = middle
*enteron* = intestine

**metacarpus:** G: *meta* = after, between, over
*karpos* = the wrist

**metatarsus:** G: *meta* = after, between
*tarsos* = the flat of the foot

**metra:** G: *metrā* = womb or uterus

**molar:** L: *mola* = millstone
A grinding tooth.

**mollis:** L: *molle* = soft
**multangulum:** L: *multus* = many
  *angulus* = corner
  having many angles
**multifidus:** L: *multus* = many
  *findo* = to split, to divide,
  cleft into many parts, diverse, manifold
**musculus:** L: dim. of *mus* = mouse; in old
  German texts actually called "Mäuslein."
  A muscle resembles a little mouse running
  under the skin.
**myenteric:** G: *mys* = muscle, *enteron* = gut.
  Nerve plexus in muscle layer of gut
**mylohyoid:** G: *myle* = a mill, for posterior
  teeth meaning grinders
  *hy* = ancient Gr. Y
  *eidos* = resemblance
**mylohyoideus:** G: *myle* = a millstone
  *hyoid* = U-shaped letter
**myocardium:** G: *mys* = muscle
  *kardia* = heart
**myology:** G: *mys* = mouse or muscle
  *logus* = word or study
  The study or knowledge of muscles.
**myometrium:** G: *mys* = muscle
  *metrā* = uterus

**nares (pl.):** L: *naris*(sing.) nostril
**navicular:** L: *navis* = boat
  *-cula* = dim.
  This bone resembles a small boat.
**nephros:** G: kidney
**nerve:** Latinized Gr. from *to neyron* = (at
  first)tendon; later, nerve
**nucha(l):** Latinized from the Arabic, means
  nape or dorsal region of the neck.
**nucleus:** L: *nux* = nut, literally a kernel,
  designates an aggregation of nerve cells

**obturator:** L: *obturare* = to stop up. The
  membrane and muscles close the obturator
  foramen.
— L: *obturo* = to stop up, close
  Applied to muscles, a fascia, a nerve, a
  foramen, and a membrane.
**occipital:** L: *occipitium*
  *ob* = back
  *caput* = head
  Back part of head.
**occlusal:** L: *ob (oc)* = against
  *claudere* = to close
**olecranon:** G: *olēnē* = elbow
  *kranion* = skull or head
  Head of the elbow.
**olfactory:** L: *olfacere* = to smell
  *odere* = to have a smell
  *facere* = to make
**omentum:** L: the fat skin, adipose membrane
  Any skin or membrane which envelops an
  internal part of the body.
**omphalus:** G: *omphalos* = the navel
**oophoros:** G: *oon* = egg
  *-pherein* = bearing, carry
**operculum:** L: *operire* = to cover; lid or
  cover
**ophthalmic:** G: *ophthalmikos* = pertaining
  to the eye
**optic:** L: *opticus*
  G: *optikos*
  relating to the eye
**orbicular:** L: *orbiculus*, dim. *orbis* = circle or
  orb
**orbital:** L: *orbita* = wheel-rut, a circuit,
  orbit, but used since ancient times for the
  eye socket.
**os:** L: *os, oris* = mouth
— L: *os, ossis* = bone
— L: *ossa* = (pl.) bone
  L: *oris* (gen.), *ora* (pl.)
  mouth
**osteology:** G: *osteon* = bone
  *logos* = study
  The study of bones.
**ostium (pl. ostia):** L: opening, entrance
**ovary:** L: *ovūm* = egg
  *ovarius* = an egg-keeper
  (one who took charge of newly aid eggs)

**pachymeninx:** G: *pachys* = thick, firm;
  *meninx* = membrane
**pallidus:** L: pale
**palpebra:** L: eyelid
**palpebral:** L: *palpebra* = eyelid
**pampiniform:** L: *pampinus* = shoot of any
  climbing plant, as in connection with plexus
  pampiniformis in spermatic cord
  *forma* = form
  interwoven tendrils
**pancreas:** G: *pan* = all
  *kreas* = flesh
  abdominal sweetbread
**papilla:** L: small nipple-shaped elevation
**papyracea:** G: *papyrus* = paper made from
  the bark of tree
  L: *papyraceus* = made of papyrus, papery
**parathyroid:** G: *para* = next to, beside (the
  thyroid)
**paries:** L: wall
**parietal:** L: *paries* = wall
**parotid:** G: *para* = beside
  *ous (ot)* = ear
  Parotid gland lies just in front of ear.
**patella:** L: dim. *patina* = a small pan, little
  plate, knee cap (an ancient word)
**pecten:** L: *pecten, -inis* = comb, weaving.
  Anatomical structures with comb-like
  projections.
**pectoral:** L: *pectus, -oris* = chest,
  brey breast
**pedes (pl.):**
**peduncle:** L: diminutive of *pes* = foot
**pellucidus:** L: *pellucere* = to shine through
**pelvis (pl. pelves):** L: basin, basin-like
  structure
**penis:** L: male sex organ
  The word meant a tail, originally.
**pericardium:** G: *peri* = all around, about
  *kardia* = heart
**perimetrium:** G: *peri* = all around, about
  *metra* = uterus
**perineum:** G: *perinaion* = perineum
  *peri* = around
  *naiein* = to dwell
  "The space between the sexual parts and the
  fundament" (anus) (Andrew's Latin-English
  Lexicon, 1850)
**peritoneum:** G: *peri* = around
  *teinein* = to stretch
  over or around
**peroneal:** G: *perone* = brooch, the fibula,
  small bone of leg
**pes:** L: *pes, pedis* = foot
**petros:** L: *petrosus* = rocky, stony
  G: *petra* = stony
  Hard as a rock
  Petrous portion of temporal bone is most
  dense bone in the body.
**petrosal:** G: *petra* = rock; as applied to pars
  petrosa (hardest portion) of temporal bone
**phalanx (pl. phalanges):** L: Because of their
  arrangement in rows, the bones of the fingers
  are compared with the Greek battle
  formation.
**pharynx:** G: *pharynx* = throat
**philtrum:** G: *philtron* = love potion
**phrenic:** G: *phrēn, phrenos* = the diaphragm,
  the mind
**pia mater:** L: *pius* = soft; *mater* = mother,
  in the sense of protection
**pineal:** L: *pinus* = pine tree
**piriform:** L: *pirum* = a pear
  *forma* = form
  pear-shaped
**piriformis:** L: *pirum* = pear
  *forma* = shape
**pisiform:** L: *pisum* = a pea
  *forma* = shape
**pituitary:** L: *pituita* = phlegm
  The nasal glutinous mucus was once
  thought to come from the hypophysis or
  brain.
**placenta:** L: a cake, from the
  G: *plakous* = a flat cake
**plantar:** L: *planta* = sole of the foot

**platysma:** G: *platys* = a plate, broad, flat,
  Galen first called it the *platysma myoides*,
  because it resembled a muscle.
  (*mys* = muscle, and *eidos* = resemblance)
**pleura:** G: a rib, or the side of chest. It now
  means the covering of ribs and lungs.
**plexus:** L: *plectere* = to interweave
**plica:** L: *plicare* = to fold, to double up, plait
  *plicatura* = a folding, doubling
**pneumo:** G: *pnein* = to breathe, to blow
  *pneuma* = wind, air, breath
  *pneumon* = lung
**pollex:** L: *pollex, pollicis* = thumb
**pons:** L: bridge
**popliteal:** L: *poples, -itis* = ham of the knee
**prepuce:** L: *prae* = before
  G: *posthion* = penis
  foreskin
**profundus:** L: deep bottomless, boundless
**promontory:** L: *promineo* = to jut out
  *promontorium* = highest part of mountain
  ridge, a headland
**pronate:** L: *pronare* = to bend forward, to
  bow.
  To turn palm or face downward.
**prostate:** G: *pro* = before
  *sta* = stand
  The term *prostate* meant a guard in ancient
  Greece – one who stood in front. The
  prostate gland is in front of the bladder.
**psoas:** G: *psoa* = a muscle of the loin
**pterygoid:** G: *pteryx* = wing
  *eidos* = resemblance
  The pterygoid process resembles a wing in
  shape.
**pubis (pl. pubes):** L: *pubis* = the pubic bone
  (pl.) *pubes* = evidence of maturity. Hair in
  the pubic region was considered to be
  evidence of being grown up, therefore,
  called *pubes*.
**pudendal:** L: *pudere* = to be ashamed
  *pudendum* = external genitalia
**pudendalis:** L: *pudenda* = the parts of
  shame, the private parts
**pulmo:** L: lung
  *pulmonis*(pl.) = of the lung
  *pulmones*(pl.) = lungs
**pulp:** L: *pulpa* = flesh. The softer part of a
  tooth. Cicero used the word for the soft
  flesh of the breasts and buttocks of young
  girls.
**pupil:** L: a little girl, a small doll; this name
  for the pupil is very ancient and refers to
  the diminutive mirror image which the
  observer sees of himself in the cornea of a
  (female) person confronting him. The pupil
  of the eye.
**pyelogram:** G: *pyelos* = pelvis
  *gramma* = mark
**pylorus:** G: *pyle* = gate
  *ouros* = a guard
  keeper of the gate
**pyramid:** L: *pyramis, -idis*
  G: *pyramis, -idos*
  Egypt.*pi-mar* = the pyramid

**quadriceps:** L: *quadri-quattuor*
  *caput* = head four
**quadrigeminal:** L: *quadri* = combining form
  of *quattuor*, four, and *geminus* = twin or
  alike

**radius:** L: spoke of a wheel. Galen used this
  term.
**ramus:** L: branch
**raphe:** G: *rhaphe* = a seamlike juncture or
  suture
**rectum:** L: *rectus* = straight, so-called by
  Galen because he observed it to be straight
  in animals.
**rectus:** L: *rego, rexi, rectum* = to keep
  straight
  *rectus, -a, -um* = straight, upright
**ren:** L: kidney
  *renalis* = of, or pertaining to the kidney

**rete:** L: network
**retinaculum:** L: *retineo* = to hold back, to restrain
*retinaculum* = that which holds back or binds.
**rostral:** L: *rostrum* = beak, bill, mouth; located towards the front end of the body
The curved end of a ship's prow.
**ruga:** L: wrinkle

**sacculus:** L: a small sack, dim. from *saccus* = a sack or bag
**sacrum:** L: *sacer* = sacred. An ancient anatomical term. Applied to the pelvic keystone because it was thought this bone survived after death and became part of the body after resurrection.
**sagittal:** L: *sagitta* = shaft, arrow, arrow-shaped, such as the fontanelles on child's head
**salpinx (pl. salpinges):** G: a trumpet, used for sounding signals
**saphenous:** Hebrew or Aramaic, hidden; *vena saphena* = the hidden vein of lower extremity, so called because it does not show through the skin
**sartorius:** L: *sartor* = a patcher, tailor
The sartorius muscle is the only muscle that flexes both knee and hip joints. It is used in crossing the legs in the tailor's position.
**scala:** L: staircase
**scalene:** G: *skalēnos* = uneven, triangular with uneven sides. These muscles were named by Riolan in the mid-17th century.
**scapha:** G: *skaphē* = boat; a boat-shaped depression
**scaphoid:** G: *skaphe* = boat
*eidos* = resemblance
The scaphoid bone is of this shape.
**scapula:** L: *scapula* = shoulder blade. In ancient times it was used in the plural to mean the back. This term was adopted in the 17th century from the Gr.
*skaptein* = to dig, because the bone resembles a spade.
**sciatic:** L: *sciaticus* = corruption of *ischiadikos* = the hip
**sclera:** G: *skleros* = hard
**scrotum:** L: *scrotum* = leather
**sella turcica:** L: *sella* = saddle
*turcica* = of the Turks
A saddle-shaped depression on the sphenoid bone, lodging the hypophysis.
**seminal:** L: *seminalis* = of or pertaining to seed from *semen, seminis* = seed
**serratus:** L: *serra* = saw
— L: *serratus* = notched
**sesamoid:** G: *sesame* = an herb
*eidos* = resemblance
Galen used this name for the little bones because they resembled sesame seeds.
**sigmoid:** G: *sigma* = letter S
*eidos* = resemblance
Originally, the Greek wrote *sigma*, with a curve like our letter C. The sigmoid colon resembles *sigma*.
— L: *sigma* = a semi-circular couch for reclining at meals.
**sinus:** L: a cavity, a hollow, roundish recess
— L: *sinum* = a large round drinking vessel with bulged out sides
*sinus* = a hollow, a cavity
**soleus:** L: *solum* = lowest part of a thing, sole of foot or sandal. The soleus muscle moves the sole of the foot.
**spermatic:** L: *spermaticus* = of, or relating to seed (seminal)
**sphenoid:** G: *sphen* = wedge
*eidos* = resembling
Wedge-shaped from any view, but it resembles a butterfly.
**spinalis:** L: *spinalis* = of or belonging to the spine or vertebral column.
— L: *spina* = thorn; used in the sense of belonging to the spinal column

**splanchnic:** G: *splanchnon* = an entrail. Used to indicate connection with, or relation to, the viscera
**splenius:** G: *splēnion* = plaster, bandage Applied to any structure resembling a bandage.
**spongiosum:** G: *spongia* = sponge
L: *spongiosus* = spongy, porous
**squama:** L: a fish scale
**stapes:** A late L. word from *stare* = to stand, and *pes* = foot; stirrup, one of the ossicles of the ear
— L: *stirrup* = Smallest ossicle ressembles a stirrup. It is thought that the ancients used no stirrups, and that the term was adopted into Medieval Latin from Old High German, *stapf*, a step.
**sternum:** G: *sternon* = the male chest, until Galen limited the meaning to breast bone.
**stratum:** L: *(sterno, stravi, stratum)* a layer, to spread out flat, to smooth, to cover over anything by spreading something out.
**striatus:** L: *stria* = stripe
**sulcus:** L: groove, ditch, furrow made by a plow.
**supercilium:** L: *super* = above
*cilium* = eyelash
eyebrow
**supinate:** L: *supinus, -a, -um* = bent backward, thrown backward, lying on the back, supine
**sura:** L: calf of the leg
**suralis:** L: *sura* = calf of the leg
**sustentaculum:** L: *sub* = under
*teneo* = to hold
*sustento* = to hold upright, support
**suture:** L: *suo, sui, sutum* = to sew or stitch together
*sutura* = a seam, a suture
**sympathetic:** A division of the autonomic nervous system. Gr. *syn* = with and *pathos* = suffering, compassion
**symphysis (pl. symphyses):** G: *syn. (sym-)* = together with
*phyein* = to grow
*physis* = growth
Grown together, not a true joint.
**synchondrosis:** G: *syn* = with, together
*chondros* = cartilage
**synovial:** G: *syn* = with
L *ovum* = egg
Modern Latin word invented by Paracelsus in the 16th century. He evidently thought the joint synovial fluid resembled egg white.

**talus:** L: ankle or one of a set of dice. The Romans carved the heelbone or talus of horses for dice.
**tapetum:** L: carpet, curtain
**tarsus:** G: *tarsos* = a wickerwork frame. In the anatomy of the eye, it designates the cartilage of the eyelid; in the skeleton, the anklebones of the foot
— G: *tarsos* = the flat of the foot (also edge of eyelid)
**tegmen:** L: *tego* = to cover, to shelter, protect
*tegumen* = a covering, a roof
**tela:** L: a web, spider web
Some Roman gladiators used a *tela* to entangle their adversaries.
**telencephalon:** G: *telos* = end + encephalon,
endbrain or cerebral hemispheres
**temporal:** L: *tempus, time*
*temporalis* = lasting but for a time, of or belonging to the temples of the head. The temporal region was so named because human hair first turns gray at temples, and this is one of the indications of the passage of time.
**tenia:** L: band, stripe
— L: *taenia* = A band or ribbon *(taenia solium,* commonest form of tape worm)

**tentorium:** L: a tent, something stretched out from *tendere* = to stretch
**teres:** L: round
**testis (pl. testes):** L: *testis* = testicle witness, i. e. to manhood
**thalamus:** G: chamber; does not designate a cavity as the word would suggest, but two massive bodies forming the walls of the third ventricle.
**thorax:** G: *thōrax* = chest, breast plate
**thymus:** G: *thymos* = (the throat sweetbread of lambs and calves). Derivation uncertain; a warty outgrowth, thyme, or soul.
**thyroid:** G: *thyreos* = a large oblong shield used by Greeks
*eidos* = resemblance
Named by Wharton in the 17th century. However, Vesalius was the first person to accurately describe the thyroid.
**tibia:** L: an ancient flute, originally made from an animal's leg bone.
**torus:** L: bulge, prominence
**trabeculae:** L: dim. of *trabs* = a beam
**trachea:** G: *tracheia* = rough, rugged
L: *trachia* = windpipe
Aristotle called the windpipe a rough artery in contrast to smooth arteries. The ancients believed arteries contained air. *Trachea* should actually be spelled *trachia*.
**tractus:** L: *trahere* = to drag or conduct; in neuroanatomy a large bundle of nerve fibers (larger than a fasciculus)
**tragus:** G: *tragos* = a buck or he-goat; so named from the longer and thicker hair growing on that part of the outer ear and carrying the same name
**triceps:** L: *tri* = three
*caput* = head
**trigone:** G: *tri* = three
*gonia* = angle, corner
L: *trigonum* = a triangle or triangular area
**triquetrum:** L: *triquetrus* = having 3 corners, angles, or edges; triangular
**triticea:** L: *triticeus* = wheat
Relating to size and shape of a grain of wheat.
**trochanter:** G: *trechein* = to run
*trochantēr* = runner
*trochos* = a wheel
Muscles used for running are attached to the trochanter.
**trochlea:** L: pulley
**tuba:** L: a straight trumpet
**tubarius:** L: *tuba* = trumpet
**tuber:** L: a hump, a knot, or swelling (eminence)
L: *tumeo, -ere* = to swell
**tuberculum:** L: dim. *tuber* = a small swelling or protuberance
**tuberosity:** L: dim. *tuber*
*-osity* = condition
*tuberosus* = full of lumps
Prominence for attachment of muscles.
**tunica:** L: an undergarment of the Romans. A coating, skin, membrane, or husk
**tympanum:** G: *tympanon* = drum; the cavity of the middle ear
— L: *tympanum* = tambourine
The eardrum.

**ulna:** L: elbow, forearm. Now limited to the larger bone of the forearm.
**umbilicus:** L: the navel, the middle, center
**uncinate:** L: *uncus* = hooks
*uncinatus* = furnished with hooks or barbs.
**unguis:** L: nail of a finger or toe
**urachus:** G: *ourachos*
*ouron* = urine
*achos* from echein, to hold
A fetal canal connecting bladder with allantois
**ureter:** G: *ourētēr* = urinary canal
**urethra:** G: *ourethra* from *ourein* = to urinate

**uterus:** L: *uter* = bag (goat skin) for wine, oil, etc., womb

**utricle:** L: *utriculus* = small skin or leather bottle dim. of *uterus* = bag bottle

**uvula:** L: *uva* = a grape
*-ula* = dim. "little grape"

**vagina:** L: a sheath, scabbard

**vagus:** L: wandering, roving; *nervus vagus* = so called because its branches extend as far as the abdomen although the nerve takes origin from the brain

**vallatae:** L: *vallatus* = walled
Having a rim or wall

**vallecula:** L: dim. of *valles*, depression or valley

**vas:** L: a vessel (pl. = *vasa;* gen.pl. = *vasorum*)

**vastus:** L: huge, immense

**velamentous:** L: *velamen velamentum* veil, curtain, covering

**velum:** L: a veil or covering, curtain

**ventricle:** L: ventriculus = the belly; used to designate the cavities of the brain, and also the two great chambers of the heart

**ventriculus:** L: dim. of *venter* = belly, stomach

**vermiform:** L: *vermis* = worm
*forma* = form
worm-like

**vertebra:** L: *vertero* = to turn
*vertebra* = joint
This term adopted in early 17th century.

**vesica:** L: bladder or blister

**vesicalis:** L: *vesica* = bladder

**vestibular:** L: *vestibulum* = an entrance, opening

**vibrissa:** L: *vibrare* = to tremble or vibrate; hair of the nostril

**vibrissae:** L: (pl.) hairs in nostrils

**villus:** L: (pl. *ville*) shaggy hair, tuft of hair

**viscus (pl. viscera):** L: inner parts of body. "The nobler parts, hearts, lungs, liver, as well as the ignobler, the stomach, entrails, etc."
(Andrew's Latin-English Lexicon 1850)

**vitreus:** L: *vitrum* = glass; translucent like glass

**vocalis:** L: *vox* = voice
*vocalis* = vocal, sound

**vomer:** L: ploughshare, name suggested by shape of the vomer bone, because the nasal septum usually deviates.

**vorticose:** L: *vortex* = whirl

**Wormian:** Small irregularly shaped bones sometimes found along the cranial sutures. These were named for Ole Worm, Danish anatomist, 1599-1654. They are now called sutural bones.

**xiphoid:** G: *xiphos* = sword
*eidos* = resemblance
The name for the tip of the sternum, due to its swordshape.

**zygomatic:** G: *zygon* = yoke
*zygoma* = bolt or bar
Cheek bone yokes or joins several bones together.

# Index

All numbers refer to the numbers of figures

acromion 459, 505–506, 513, 515–516, 520–522, 524–526, 528–530
adenohypophysis 58
adhesion, interthalamic 75, 78, 102–103, 111, 117–118, 127, 129, 144, 177
ala central lobule 171
– cinerea 154
– nasi 248
alveolus, dental 268, 292
ampulla anterior semicircular canal 450–452
– anterior semicircular duct 429, 454, 456–457
– lacrimal canaliculus 349–350
– lateral semicircular canal 451–452
– lateral semicircular duct 454, 457
– posterior semicircular canal 450–453
– posterior semicircular duct 454, 456
amygdala 104, 118–119
angle frontal 50–51
– inferior scapular 528–529
– iridocorneal 383–384, 396
– lateral ocular 344, 346, 355–356
– lateral scapular 528–529
– mandible 2, 4, 277–280, 282, 291, 300–301, 500, 502, 505
– mastoid 50–51
– medial ocular 344–345, 355–356
– occipital 50–51
– sphenoidal 3, 50–51
– superior of scapula 505, 516, 526, 528–529
– venous 477
ansa cervicalis 223, 464–466, 468, 472–474, 476–477, 480
– lenticularis 118
– peduncularis 117
– subclavia 207, 209, 481
– thyroid 209
anthelix 412–413
antitragus 413
antrum, mastoid 430, 432–433, 435
aorta ascending 477
– thoracic 192
aperture external of cochlear canaliculus 45
– external of vestibular aqueduct 43
– lateral of fourth ventricle 127, 140, 143
– median of fourth ventricle 57, 78, 127, 140
– piriform 2, 9, 12, 282
– tympanic of canaliculus of chorda tympani 428
apex nasi 248
– petrous bone 11, 43, 45, 502
– posterior horn 193, 200–201
– tongue 254, 293
aponeurosis biceps brachii muscle 154, 533, 537–539, 546–547, 552, 555, 564
– epicranial 210
– palatine 251, 502
– palmar 547, 583, 599
– tongue 255
aqueduct, cerebral 57, 71, 75, 101, 127, 129, 141, 157, 166–168, 177
arbor vitae 57, 178

arch alveolar mandibular 278
– anterior of atlas 4, 302, 486, 500
– aorta 302, 313, 478, 481
– axis 487–489, 495
– cricoid cartilage 302, 309, 312, 321–322, 324, 326–328, 475
– deep palmar 511, 588
– inferior dental 259
– palatoglossal 250–251, 253–254, 258
– palatopharyngeal 250–252, 258, 302, 306, 313
– posterior of atlas 486–487, 497, 500, 504
– superciliar 48, 242, 248
– superficial palmar 511, 587
– superior dental 256, 258
– venous jugular 302, 310, 463, 476
– zygomatic 4, 7–8, 23, 219–220, 222–223, 264, 299–300, 308, 505
area(-ae) cochlear 447, 450
– cribriform of sclera 383, 396, 398
– facial nerve 447
– inferior vestibular 139, 447
– striata 395
– subcallosal 75, 77, 85, 107, 121, 177
– superior vestibular 139, 447
arteriole inferior macular 394
– inferior nasal retinal 394
– inferior temporal retinal 394
– medial retinal 394
– superior macular 394
– superior temporal retinal 394
artery(-ies) angular 87, 212, 214–215, 221–224
– angular gyrus 81
– anterior cerebral 54, 79–81, 84–87, 95, 120, 133
– anterior choroidal 85–88, 99, 106, 109–110, 112, 130
– anterior ciliary 346, 380, 386–388
– anterior circumflex humeral 511, 518, 539
– anterior communicans 79, 85
– anterior ethmoidal 19, 234, 236, 295, 358, 378, 380, 382
– anterior interosseous 511, 554, 560–561, 566, 598
– anterior meningeal 19, 236, 295, 378, 380, 382
– anterior recurrent 84
– anterior spinal 79, 85, 191–192, 205–206, 209
– anterior tympanic 222–223, 235
– ascending cervical 465–466, 479–480
– ascending palatine 212, 223, 234, 296, 304
– ascending pharyngeal 212, 304
– axillary 466, 475, 479–480, 511, 518, 539–540
– basilar 54, 57, 63, 79, 85, 88, 179–180, 205
– brachial 511, 516, 518, 539–542, 547, 552–556, 564, 570
– buccal 212, 221–224, 358
– callosomarginal 79, 81, 83, 87
– central retinal 382, 386, 396–398
– ciliary body 386
– circumflex scapular 517–518

*artery(-ies)*
– common carotid 207, 212, 220, 223, 313, 459, 464–467, 471–472, 474–481, 483
– common iliac 205
– common interosseous 511, 553–554, 565
– common palmar digital 583, 587, 597
– conjunctival 386
– deep auricular 222–223, 235
– deep brachial 511, 539–542
– deep cervical 479, 481, 504
– deep lingual 295, 471
– deep temporal 87, 212, 222–223, 358
– descending palatine 212, 234
– descending scapular 479
– dorsal digital of hand 594, 596–597
– dorsal metacarpal 594, 596, 598
– dorsal nasal 221, 224, 380
– episcleral 386
– external carotid 212, 217, 220–222, 224, 234, 253, 304, 464–467, 471, 473–474, 480
– external nasal 236
– facial 212, 214–215, 221–224, 253, 298, 304, 466, 468–469, 473–477, 480
– frontopolar 81, 83, 87
– greater palatine 234, 236, 251, 296
– inferior alveolar 212, 221–224, 234–235, 253
– inferior anterior cerebellar 79, 81, 85, 180
– inferior labial 212
– inferior laryngeal 314
– inferior posterior cerebellar 79, 85, 88, 179–180
– inferior temporal 389, 391
– inferior thyroid 209, 304, 306, 313–314, 466, 472, 479–480
– inferior ulnar collateral 511, 539–542, 552, 554–555, 561, 564
– infraorbital 212, 222–223, 358, 367, 382
– internal carotid 19, 63, 65, 80–81, 84–85, 87, 94–95, 130–133, 221, 224, 233–235, 253, 289, 304, 313, 358, 374, 378–380, 395, 429, 439–440, 448, 466–467, 480
– internal thoracic 466, 476, 478–481
– labyrinthine 19, 85, 180, 448
– lacrimal 356, 378–381
– lateral posterior nasal and septal 234, 236, 295–296, 358
– lateral thoracic 480
– lesser palatine 234, 251
– lingual 212, 221, 223–224, 253, 295, 304, 464–465, 469–471, 473
– masseteric 221–222, 224
– maxillary 212, 222–224, 234–235, 358
– medial collateral 511, 542
– median 511, 554, 566
– mental 212, 221–222, 224
– middle cerebral 81, 83–87, 120
– middle meningeal 19, 65, 94, 130, 212, 222–223, 235, 358
– middle temporal 81, 212, 221–224
– nasopalatine 236, 296

*artery(-ies)*
– occipital 19, 61, 212, 215, 221–224, 313, 462–464, 466, 480, 501, 504
– ophthalmic 19, 81, 87, 132–133, 233, 378–380, 382
– palmar metacarpal 588
– pericallosal 81, 83, 87
– posterior auricular 212, 214, 217, 221–224, 462, 465, 501
– posterior cerebral 61, 79–81, 83, 85–86, 88, 130
– posterior circumflex humeral 511, 517–518, 542
– posterior communicans 79–81, 85, 130
– posterior ethmoidal 295, 358, 380, 382
– posterior intercostal 479
– posterior interosseous 511, 551, 554, 560–561, 566
– posterior long ciliary 386–388
– posterior meningeal 304
– posterior short ciliary 386–388
– posterior spinal 79, 191, 206
– prerolandic 81
– principal of thumb 588, 598–599
– proper palmar digital 583, 587–588, 594, 596–597, 608–609
– pterygoid canal 234, 358
– radial 511, 547–548, 552–556, 565–567, 584, 587–588, 594, 596, 598
– radial collateral 511, 541–542, 552, 554, 556, 560–561, 564
– radial recurrent 511, 552–554, 556
– recurrent interosseous 511, 556, 561
– renal 205, 209
– rolandic 81
– sphenopalatine 212, 223, 234, 296, 358
– sternocleidomastoid 212
– stylomastoid 212, 222, 224
– subcentral 87
– subclavian 205, 209, 313, 464–467, 477–481
– sublingual 223, 253, 295, 470–471
– submental 212, 222–224, 465–466, 468–469, 474, 480
– subscapular 518
– superficial cervical 464–466, 479–480
– superficial temporal 211, 214–217, 221, 223–224
– superior cerebellar 61, 79, 81, 85, 88, 100, 130, 180
– superior labial 212, 236
– superior laryngeal 293, 308, 313–314, 335–336, 464–466, 468, 470–471, 473–474
– superior mesenteric 209
– superior posterior alveolar 212, 358
– superior temporal 389, 391
– superior thyroid 212, 223, 342, 464–466, 468, 471, 473–474, 480
– superior tympanic 19
– superior ulnar collateral 511, 539–540, 547, 552, 554–555, 564
– supramarginal 87
– supraorbital 221, 367, 378–380
– suprascapular 464, 466, 479–480, 517–518
– supratrochlear 221–222, 380
– supreme intercostal 209, 479

artery(-ies)
– thoracoacromial 464–466, 480
– thoracodorsal 518
– transverse cervical 464–465, 477, 480, 501, 504
– transverse facial 212, 215, 217, 222
– triangular 81
– ulnar 511, 547, 552–555, 565–567, 583–584, 587–588
– ulnar recurrent 511, 542, 553–555, 560, 565
– vertebral 19, 63, 79, 81, 85, 88, 95, 176, 180, 205, 209, 466, 472, 479–481, 503–504
– zygomaticoorbital 212, 221–222
articulation(-s) (see also joint) lateral atlantoaxial 4, 494–496
– median atlantoaxial 302–303, 499
atlas 231, 484–486, 492, 494–497
axis 231, 487–489, 494–498, 500, 505
– eyeball 383
– lens 401
– optic 383

base cochlea 451
– external of skull 22–23
– internal of skull 17–18
– mandible 8, 305, 475, 502
– stapes 425, 434
bifurcation, trachea 309
body(-ies) ciliary 383, 396, 403, 405
– corpus callosum 75, 77, 105, 108, 110, 114, 118, 144, 177
– fornix 61, 75, 78, 104, 108, 112, 117–118, 144, 177
– hyoid bone 311, 327
– incus 426
– lateral geniculate 101, 121, 124, 128, 140–142, 160, 395
– mammillary 71, 75–76, 78, 104, 108, 117–118, 121, 141, 143–144, 177–178
– mandible 2–3, 8
– maxilla 2
– medial geniculate 128, 140–142, 166, 458
– phalanx 611
– pineal 54, 56–57, 75, 79, 102–103, 111, 129, 140, 177–178, 458
– restiform 153–155, 175
– sphenoid bone 29–31, 58, 301–302
– tongue 244
– trapezoid 162–163, 458
bone(-s) capitate 600, 605–607, 610–614
– carpal 610–611
– ethmoid 32–34, 237, 239, 359, 361–362
– frontal 3, 8–9, 18, 24, 48–49, 54, 237, 242, 352, 359, 362, 364–365, 367, 376, 381
– hamate 605–606, 610–611, 613–614
– hyoid 9, 54, 56, 220, 223, 255, 281, 283, 291–292, 294, 298, 302–303, 310–312, 315–318, 329, 331–332, 334, 342, 459, 470–471, 473–475, 477
– interparietal 26
– lacrimal 3, 8, 360–361
– lunate 606–607, 610–614
– metacarpal 596, 599, 601, 610–611
– nasal 3, 8, 11, 226, 229, 237, 239–241, 302–303, 347, 361–362
– occipital 12–13, 18, 26–29, 99, 240, 409, 495–496, 498, 500
– palatine 39–41, 256, 285–286
– parietal 3, 8, 13, 18, 20, 23, 25–26, 50–51, 53, 363

bone(-s)
– piriform 584–585, 587, 600, 607, 610–613
– scaphoid 604–606, 610–611, 613
– sesamoid of hand 600, 607, 611–613
– sphenoid 18, 29–31, 131, 239–240, 286, 359, 361–365
– sutural 26
– temporal 8, 11–13, 18, 26, 42–45, 60, 304, 359, 409, 411, 429, 438
– trapezium 606, 610–613
– trapezoid 605–606, 610–614
– triangular 605–606, 610–614
– zygomatic 3, 8, 12, 35–36, 52–53, 222–224, 238, 247, 300, 347, 351–352, 359–361, 366
brachium conjunctivum 128, 156–157, 164, 167, 175, 458
– inferior collide 128, 139–140, 142
– pontis 114, 156, 162–163, 458
– superior collicle 128, 140, 142
branch(-es) acromial of suprascapular artery 517
– acromial of thoracoacromial artery 480
– anterior meningeal of spinal nerve 191–192
– anterior of medial antebrachial cutaneous nerve 508
– anterior superior alveolar 289–290
– auricular of vagus nerve 214, 221–224, 304, 440
– buccal of facial nerve 214–217
– carpal of ulnar artery 511, 552–553, 594, 598
– cervical of facial nerve 215, 217, 463–464, 468
– communicating of hypoglossal nerve with lingual nerve 477
– communicating of ulnar nerve with median nerve 587
– communicating with ciliary ganglion 380
– cricohyoid of superior thyroid artery 302
– cutaneous of medial brachial nerve 548
– cutaneous of posterior circumflex humeral artery 507
– deep of transverse cervical artery 465
– deep of ulnar nerve 587
– deep palmar of ulnar artery 587–588
– deltoid of deep brachial artery 541, 542
– deltoid of thoracoacromial artery 464
– dental of posterior superior alveolar artery 222
– digastric of facial nerve 221, 223, 439
– dorsal carpal of radial artery 594, 598
– dorsal of spinal nerve 183, 192
– esophageal of recurrent laryngeal nerve 192, 314
– external nasal of anterior ethmoidal nerve 221–224, 236
– femoral of genitofemoral nerve 207
– frontal of middle meningeal artery 19
– frontal of superficial temporal artery 212, 216, 221, 224
– genital of genitofemoral nerve 207
– inferior palpebral of infraorbital nerve 221
– infrahyoid of superior thyroid artery 464
– interganglionic 182

branch(-es)
– internal nasal of anterior ethmoidal nerve 295
– lateral cutaneous of dorsal branches 501
– lateral nasal of anterior ethmoidal nerve 234, 296
– lateral of supraorbital nerve 214, 216
– lingual of glossopharyngeal nerve 296, 314
– mandibular 3, 220–221, 253, 277–279, 282, 291, 297, 301, 303–304
– marginal mandibular 214–215, 474
– mastoid of occipital artery 212, 489, 501, 504
– medial of supraorbital nerve 214
– meningeal of mandibular nerve 65, 378
– meningeal of maxillary nerve 65, 378
– meningeal of occipital artery 19
– meningeal of ophthalmic nerve 65
– meningeal of spinal nerve 183
– meningeal of vertebral artery 19
– middle superior alveolar 289–290, 358
– muscular of axillary nerve 517
– muscular of brachial plexus 480
– muscular of cervical plexus 463
– muscular of mandibular nerve 290
– muscular of medial pterygoid nerve 444
– muscular of oculomotor nerve 380
– muscular of radial nerve 561
– muscular of vertebral artery 504
– mylohyoid of inferior alveolar artery 222, 234–235
– nasal of anterior ethmoidal artery 234, 295–296
– nasal posterior superior and inferior lateral 235, 296, 358
– occipital of occipital artery 212, 501, 504
– occipital of posterior auricular artery 212, 462, 465, 501
– palmar carpal of radial artery 511, 588
– palmar carpal of ulnar artery 511
– palmar of median nerve 548, 552–553, 567, 583, 587, 599
– palmar of ulnar nerve 548, 552, 583, 587–588
– parietal of middle cerebral artery 64
– parietal of superficial temporal artery 212, 216, 221–224
– perforating of internal thoracic artery 476
– perforating of internal thoracic vein 476
– petrous of middle meningeal artery 19
– pharyngeal of glossopharyngeal nerve 304
– pharyngeal of inferior thyroid artery 304
– pharyngeal of maxillary nerve 358
– pharyngeal of superior thyroid artery 304
– pharyngeal of vagus nerve 304
– posterior choroid 86
– posterior meningeal of spinal nerve 191–192

branch(-es)
– posterior superior alveolar 223, 289–290, 358
– spinal of intercostal artery 191–192, 205
– spinal of intercostal vein 191
– spinal of thyrocervical trunk 205
– sternocleidomastoid of occipital artery 212, 465–466
– sternocleidomastoid of superior thyroid artery 464
– stylohyoid of facial nerve 439
– superficial of anterior spinal artery 206
– superficial of transverse cervical artery 465
– superficial palmar of radial artery 511, 552–554, 587–588
– superior cervical cardiac 304, 313, 472, 480
– superior of oculomotor nerve 380
– suprahyoid of lingual artery 464
– sympathetic for ciliary ganglion 380
– temporal of facial nerve 215–217
– tentorial of ophthalmic nerve 378
– thyrohyoid of ansa cervicalis 465, 468
– tonsillar of ascending palatine artery 314
– tonsillar of glossopharyngeal nerve 296, 314
– tracheal of inferior thyroid artery 314
– ulnar of medial antebrachial cutaneous nerve 508, 548
– upper lip 221
– ventral of spinal nerve 183, 190, 192
– zygomatic of facial nerve 214–217
– zygomaticofacial 214, 221
– zygomaticotemporal 221
bronchus(-i) anterior basal segmental 309
– anterior segmental 309
– apical segmental 309
– inferior lingular 309
– lateral basal segmental 309
– lateral segmental 309
– left inferior lobar 309
– left main 309
– left superior lobar 309
– medial basal segmental (cardiac) 309
– medial segmental 309
– posterior basal segmental 309
– posterior segmental 309
– right inferior lobar 309
– right main 309
– right middle lobar 309
– right superior lobar 309
– superior lingular 309
– superior segmental 309
bulb inferior of jugular vein 304, 313, 465, 477
– olfactory 76, 85, 104, 108, 143, 229, 232, 236
– posterior horn 109, 112, 116
– superior of jugular vein 93, 97, 304, 313, 409
bulla, ethmoidal 231
bursa(-ae) bicipitoradial 550, 565
– mucous subhyoid 312
– pectoralis major muscle 514
– pharyngeal 236, 302
– retrohyoid 302
– subacromial 520–521
– subcoracoid 514, 516
– subcutaneous of olecranon 534, 564, 570
– subdeltoid 514–515, 521, 536
– subhyoid 317–318

*bursa(-ae)*
– subtendinous of latissimus dorsi muscle 537
– subtendinous of subscapularis muscle 521
– subtendinous of triceps brachii muscle 564

calamus scriptorius 139
calcar avis 98, 109–112, 116
calvarium 2, 24–25, 99
canal(-s) anterior semicircular 429, 446, 450–453, 457
– carotid 23, 44–45, 87, 426, 431–433, 437, 442, 478, 502
– carpal 584
– central 57, 75, 127, 149–152, 177, 200
– condylar 18, 23, 27–28, 502
– facial 138, 432, 435–436, 438–439, 445
– greater palatine 52, 290, 303
– hypoglossal 11, 18, 22–23, 27–29, 301, 478, 497
– incisive 11, 228, 234, 239–241, 296
– infraorbital 238, 359, 363
– lateral semicircular 429, 437–438, 445–446, 450–453, 457
– longitudinal of modiolus 449
– mandibular 9, 261, 262a, 262b, 263–264
– musculotubar 44–45, 436, 444, 478
– nasolacrimal 287, 350
– optic 18, 29, 361–362, 374, 378, 382
– posterior semicircular 429, 446, 450–453, 456
– pterygoid 30–31, 363
– root of tooth 269
– spiral of cochlea 429, 449, 452
– vertebral 209
– vertebral artery 485
canaliculus, mastoid 23
capitulum of humurus 543, 545, 573
capsule articular of carpometacarpal joint of thumb 607
– articular of lateral atlantoaxial joint 478, 495–496, 498
– articular of lateral atlantooccipital joint 494, 497–498
– cricoarytenoid joint 330
– cricothyroid joint 329–331
– dentate nucleus 174
– distal radioulnar joint 567, 571, 607
– elbow joint 564, 569
– external 99–100, 102, 107, 114–115, 117, 119–120
– extreme 99, 102, 120
– internal 99, 101–102, 114–115, 117, 119–120, 144
– interphalangeal joints 600
– intervertebral joints 503
– lens 399a, 400
– metacarpophalangeal joint of index finger 601
– metacarpophalangeal joints 572, 585, 605
– shoulder joint 520–521, 523, 525, 542, 568
– temporomandibular joint 219–220, 299–300, 308, 401, 502
– thyroid gland 472
cartilage accessory nasal 226
– acoustic meatus 220, 412, 416, 419
– apical of nose 303
– arytenoid 317, 321–322, 324, 327–328, 330, 332, 335–336
– auditory tube 236, 307, 313, 429
– auricular 409
– corniculate 324–326, 328, 330, 332

*cartilage*
– cricoid 56, 310, 315–318, 321, 324, 328–329, 331–332, 336, 342, 470
– cuneiform 332–333
– epiglottic 255, 302, 315–318, 323, 330, 342
– greater alar 226–228, 236
– lateral nasal 226–228, 303
– nasal septal 226–229, 236, 245, 302
– thyroid 255, 302, 309–312, 314–320, 327–332, 336, 342, 345, 470–471, 475
– trachael 293, 308–309, 315–316, 318, 327, 329–331, 342, 472
– triticea 312, 329–331, 334
caruncle lacrimal 248, 344–346, 348–350, 377
– sublingual 249, 253, 294, 302–303, 470
cauda equina 181, 186, 188, 196
cavity elbow joint 564, 570
– glenoid 520–522, 526, 528–530
– nasal 232–233, 263–264, 301, 366–367, 374
– oral 9, 244, 250–251
– pulp 269
– tympanic 289, 410, 426–427, 430, 437–438, 445, 448, 457
cavum conchae 413
– septum pellucidum 98, 100–101, 103, 106–107, 110–112
cecum ampullare 456
– vestibulare 456–457
cell(-s) ethmoidal 4, 9, 32–41, 225, 233, 238, 243–244, 247, 358–360, 366–367, 374, 376
– mastoid 4, 61, 289, 305–306, 409–410, 432–433, 435–436, 438
– pneumatic of auditory tube 444, 448
– supraorbital 247
– tympanic 433
cementum 269
center medullary 105, 113
– tendinous 192
cerebellum 59–61, 63, 76, 100, 106, 125, 138, 169–174, 177, 186
chamber anterior of eye 383–384, 396, 403
– posterior of eye 223, 383, 396
cheek 250
chiasm optic 56, 71, 75–81, 113, 118–121, 127, 133, 141, 143, 177–178, 233–234, 375, 395
– tendinous 584, 600
chin 248
choanae 13, 229, 230b, 256, 295, 306
chord, oblique 519a, 562, 568, 571
chorda tympani 223, 234–235, 289–290, 409, 426–431, 439–440
choroid membrane 383–384, 386, 393, 396, 398, 407
circle arterial of brain 85
– major iridial arterial 386, 388
– minor iridial arterial 386, 388
circumference articular of radius 571, 578, 582
– articular of ulna 576
cistern(-s) ambiens 63, 175
– cerebellomedullary 54, 56–57, 61, 63, 146, 175
– chiasmatic 57, 63, 146
– corpus callosum 146
– great cerebral vein 112, 146
cistern interpeduncular 57, 63
– lateral cerebral fissure 63, 146
– pontine 136a, 146
– sagittal cerebellar 146
– trigeminal 130, 134–136, 136a, 146
claustrum 99–102, 107, 114–115, 117, 119–120, 126

clavicle 459–461, 464, 475, 477, 513, 518, 521–522, 524, 526, 531–532, 535, 538
clivus 18, 87, 228, 301, 305–306
cochlea 429, 446, 450, 458
colliculus facial 139, 163
– inferior 103, 121, 139–140, 142, 175
– superior 17, 100–103, 139–140, 142, 160
collum dentis 269
column anterior 148–152, 193–194, 200
– cervical vertebral 492–493, 500
– fornix 75, 77–79, 98–104, 106, 108, 110–112, 114–115, 119, 140, 177
– lateral 193
– posterior 148, 152, 193–194, 199–200
commissure anterior 57, 75, 77–78, 101, 108, 113, 115, 119, 127, 140, 177
– anterior white 193, 200
– fornix 104, 110
– habenular 111, 140
– hippocampal 109
– inferior 103, 111
– lateral of eyelids 344, 377
– medial of eyelids 377
– posterior 57, 75, 78, 101, 128, 177–178
concha ear 413
– inferior nasal 3–4, 230a, 231–232, 234, 238, 240, 244–245, 247, 296, 306–307, 348, 359, 367
– medial nasal 3, 33, 230a, 231–232, 234, 238, 240–241, 244–245, 296, 306–307, 348, 359
– superior nasal 230a, 231, 234, 240, 296, 306–307
condyle, occipital 8, 23, 27–28, 441, 502, 505
confluens, sinuses 54, 56, 59, 91, 93–95, 97, 179, 213
conjunctiva bulbar 344–346, 348, 352, 368, 383
– palpebral 345–346, 348, 354, 356
connections, intertendinous 590
conus elasticus 318, 327–328, 334, 342
– medullary 186, 189, 196
cord, spinal 56, 75–76, 114, 142–143, 175, 177, 181, 186–189, 195–196, 209
cornea 233, 364, 368, 383–384, 386–387, 396
cornu greater 281, 283, 291–293, 295, 303, 305, 308, 311, 314, 329–331
– lesser 281, 283, 291, 303, 311, 329–331
– mouth 248
– superior of thyroid cartilage 311, 314, 328–331
corpus callosum 67, 79, 100, 104–106, 109, 111, 115, 119–120, 122, 140, 145, 178
– striatum 84, 107
cortex cerebellar 162
– insular 126
– lens 400
crest anterior lacrimal 284, 361–362
– buccinator 505
– cochlear window 453
– conchal 41, 285
– ethmoidal 41, 240–241, 285
– external occipital 26–27, 505
– frontal 4, 18, 24, 49, 244
– greater tubercle 545
– inframtemporal 23, 30, 299
– infrazygomatic 505
– internal occipital 18, 28–29
– lateral trochlear 564
– lesser tubercle 545

*crest*
– nasal 11, 245, 287
– orbital 30
– posterior lacrimal 361–362
– pyramidal 4, 247
– sphenoidal 30, 239
– supinator 574
– transverse 447, 450
– vestibular 452–453
crista arcuata 324
– galli 4, 11, 18, 32–34, 54, 228–229, 238–240, 244, 359, 375
crown, tooth 269
crus anterior of internal capsule 98–100, 126
– anterior of stapes 425, 430, 434
– cerebral 71, 114, 141, 165–168
– lateral of greater alar cartilage 226–227
– medial of greater alar cartilage 226–229, 302
– posterior of internal capsule 98–100
– simplex 454
crypts, tonsillar 254
culmen 169, 171, 177
cuneus 67, 71, 75, 77, 108, 121, 395
cupula, cochlea 451–452, 456–457
cymba cochleae 413

declive 169, 171, 177
decussation lemniscus 151–153
– pyramids 76, 114, 143, 148–150, 179, 189
– superior cerebellar peduncles 167, 174, 177
– tegmental 168
– trochlear nerves 157
dentine 268–269
diaphragm, oral 291
– sellae 15, 58
diaphysis humerus 573
– radius 573, 613–614
– ulnar 573, 613–614
diencephalon 143
digitations, hippocampus 111, 116, 123
diploe 9, 20, 24, 57
disk distal articular radioulnar 606
– intervertebral 191, 481, 494
– optic 366, 383, 388–389, 391, 393–394
– temporomandibular 297, 299
dorsum nose 248
– sella 9, 11, 18, 31, 229, 243, 301, 305
– tongue 250–251, 254, 296
duct anterior semicircular 429, 448, 454, 457
– cochlear 409, 411, 448, 454–457
– endolymphatic 429, 448, 454, 456
– greater sublingual 294, 470
– lacrimal 225, 348–350
– lateral semicircular 445, 448, 454, 456–457
– lesser sublingual 294, 470
– nasolacrimal 225, 244, 348–350
– parotid 210, 215, 217, 219–220, 252, 298, 308, 459, 469
– posterior semicircular 448, 454, 456
– submandibular 223, 253, 294, 469–470
– thoracic 192
– utriculosaccular 456
ductules, excretory of lacrimal gland 347–348, 356
ductus reuniens 456–457
dura mater brain 19–20, 53, 57, 60–61, 99, 179
– spinal 56, 95, 187–192, 195–196, 198, 209, 302–303

ear external 409, 411–413, 416

*ear*
- internal 409, 411
- middle 409–411, 448
edge, cutaneous of mouth 248
eminence arcuate 11, 43–44, 435–436
- collateral 109, 111–112, 116
- concha 416
- frontal 12, 48
- medial 139, 164
- parietal 12–14, 25, 50
- pyramidal 427, 430, 433, 435, 445
- triangular fossa 416
enamel 268–269
encephalon 186
enlargement cervical 186, 189
- lumbar 186, 189, 199
epicondyle lateral humeral 507, 513, 534–535, 541–545, 557–560, 563–564, 568–569
- medial humeral 506, 514, 519a, 537–538, 540, 543–547, 550–555, 560, 563–564, 568–569
epidural adipose tissue 192
epiglottis 231, 254, 306–307, 312–314, 327, 329, 332–334, 337, 339–340
epiphysis 56
epithelium, lens 399a
equator of eyeball 383
- of lens 385, 399, 401
esophagus 192, 293, 302, 304, 307–308, 472
- muscular coat 305, 313
eyeball 19, 344, 364–365, 369, 375, 380, 383, 396
- vascular coat 407
eyebrow 248, 344, 377
eyelashes 377
eyelid lower 344, 346, 349–350, 357–358, 381
- upper 344, 346, 349–350, 354, 381

facet inferior articular 486–487
- radial head 582
- superior articular 484–485, 487, 499
falx cerebellar 54, 56, 94, 179
- cerebral 15, 19, 54, 56–57, 59–61, 86, 94–95, 99, 303
fascia(-ae) antebrachial 533, 535–538, 546–547, 557, 559, 564–567
- axillary 533
- brachial 460, 516, 533–534, 547, 564
- buccinator 253
- cervical 298, 303, 461, 469
- cervical, angular band 298, 461, 468–469
- cervical, pretracheal lamina 461, 472, 475
- cervical, prevertebral lamina 472
- cervical, superficial lamina 210–211, 219, 298, 460–461, 468–469, 472
- clavipectoral 475
- cubital 564–565
- deltoid 534
- dorsal of hand 599
- endothoracic 192
- infraspinous 501, 513, 535
- masseteric 253, 298, 461, 468
- muscular 353
- palmar of hand 599
- paralingual 461
- parotid 211, 298, 460
- pectoral 460, 521
- pharyngeal 253
- pharyngobasilar 302, 305, 307–308, 313
- pterygoid 253
- submandibular 461
- temporal 219, 221, 224
- tonsillar 253

fascicle lateral of brachial plexus 518, 539
- longitudinal of pons 114, 163–164, 177
- mammillothalamic 108, 114, 117
- medial longitudinal 152, 154–157, 163–164, 166–168, 174, 177, 458
- medial of brachial plexus 518, 539
- posterior of brachial plexus 518, 539
- thalamocortical 126
fasciculus cuneate 139, 148, 150, 178, 200, 202
- gracilis 139–140, 148, 150, 200, 202
fastigium 61, 127, 129, 177, 179
fat pad buccal 210, 219, 244, 250, 253, 298, 459
- laryngeal 302, 315–318, 330, 333
- orbital 53, 233, 244, 351, 353, 366–367, 374–375, 377–378
fibers external arcuate 153–155
- internal arcuate 153
- olivocerebellar 161
- transverse pontine 143, 156, 162–164, 167
- zonular 384, 403, 405
fibrocartilage, in foramen lacerum 502
filum(-a) lateral pontine 140, 142
- radicular 76, 142, 192, 197–201
- spinal dura mater 187–189
- terminal 3, 189, 196
fimbria, of hippocampus 101, 104, 108, 111–112, 116–117, 122–123, 147, 175
finger pad 506
fissure anterior median 148, 152, 155, 189, 191, 193–196, 199–200
- antitragohelicine 412–413
- calcarine 80
- cerebellar 174
- cerebrocerebellar 75
- hippocampal 101
- horizontal cerebellar 170–172
- inferior orbital 3, 23, 52, 238, 359–361, 364–365, 367, 381
- lateral cerebral 72, 102, 107, 114–115, 117, 119–120, 129
- longitudinal cerebral 62, 70–71, 76, 98–100, 105–106, 109–115, 117–120, 143, 145
- parietooccipital 80
- petrooccipital 18
- petrosquamous 18, 44, 46–47
- petrotympanic 42, 45, 438
- primary 169
- sphenopetrous 442
- superior orbital 3–4, 18, 29–31, 52, 238, 359, 376
- transverse cerebral 106
- tympanomastoid 42, 438
flocculus 76, 113–114, 140, 143, 162, 170–172, 180
fold(-s) anterior axillary 506
- anterior mallear 414, 426–429, 431
- anterior petroclinoidal 133
- aryepiglottic 306–307, 313, 318, 334, 337, 339
- chorda tympani 427
- ciliary 405–406
- interarytenoid 338, 340
- iridial 405–408
- lacrimal 231
- lateral glossoepiglottic 254
- median glossoepiglottic 254, 353
- pharyngoepiglottic 306–307, 313
- posterior axillary 506
- posterior mallear 414, 428, 431
- salpingopalatine 231, 302, 306

*fold(-s)*
- salpingopharyngeal 302, 306, 313
- semilunar of conjunctiva 345–346, 348–349
- sublingual 249, 253, 470
- superior laryngeal nerve 306–307, 313
- transverse palatine 258
- triangular 254
- vestibular 302, 334–335, 337–340, 342–343
- vocal 54, 56, 302, 318, 334–335, 337–338, 340, 342–343
folium, of vermis 169–170, 177, 179
follicles, lingual 254, 296, 307
fontanelle anterior 14
- posterior 14
- sphenoidal 12
foramen(-ina) alveolar 7, 284
- anterior ethmoidal 361–362
- anterior jugular vein 461
- apical dental 269
- cecum 11, 18, 49, 143, 243
- cecum of tongue 231, 254–255, 302, 307
- condylar 505
- greater palatine 23, 41, 286
- incisive 11, 23, 52, 286–287
- infraorbital 3, 284, 352
- interventricular 57, 75, 78, 88, 91, 96, 98–100, 106, 108–112, 115, 127, 129, 140, 177
- intervertebral 191
- jugular 18–19, 23, 304, 502
- lacerum 18, 23
- lesser palatine 256, 286
- Luschkae 127
- Magendie 127
- magnum 13, 18, 23, 27, 29, 94
- mandibular 259, 264, 280, 282, 291, 505
- mastoid 11, 18, 23, 42–45, 505
- mental 3, 8, 210, 259, 261, 262a, 262b, 264, 277–279, 292
- optic 52
- ovale 7, 18, 23, 29, 441, 443
- parietal 25–26, 50–51
- posterior ethmoidal 242, 361–362
- pterygospinal 301
- rotundum 4, 18, 29–31, 52, 362–363
- singular 447
- sphenopalatine 52, 240–241, 362
- spinous 18, 23, 29
- stylomastoid 23, 45, 138, 289, 305–306, 432, 435–436, 439
- supraorbital 3, 48
- transverse of atlas 484–486
- transverse of axis 487, 489
- transverse of cervical vertebra 409, 493
- vertebral of atlas 484, 486
- vertebral of axis 489
- vertebral of cervical vertebra 490
- vertebral of vertebra prominens 491
- zygomaticofacial 7, 35, 361
- zygomaticoorbital 35–36, 363, 381
- zygomaticotemporal 36
forceps major 98
formation, reticular 149, 152–157, 161–164, 202
fornix 54, 56–57, 78, 95, 106, 108, 145, 178
- inferior conjunctival 345, 348, 351, 353
- lacrimal sac 348–349
- superior conjunctival 348, 351, 353–354, 356
fossa anterior cranial 17–18, 375
- anthelix 416
- axillary 506

*fossa*
- canine 284
- condylar 27
- coronoid 545, 564, 570
- cubital 506
- digastric 280, 282, 292
- greater supraclavicular 460–461
- hypophyseal 4, 9, 17–18, 29, 58, 243, 247, 301, 303, 448
- incus 431, 433
- infraclavicular 460, 476, 508
- infraspinous 528
- infratemporal 7, 364
- interpeduncular 76, 114, 143, 167–168, 177
- jugular 23, 45, 460, 478
- lacrimal gland 237
- lacrimal sac 360
- lateral cerebral 66, 71, 105, 143
- lesser supraclavicular 460–461, 475
- mandibular 23, 42, 45, 308
- middle cranial 15, 17–18, 52
- occipital cerebellar 28–29
- olecrani 544, 570
- posterior cranial 17–18
- pterygoid 11, 31, 228
- pterygopalatine 7, 363
- radial 545
- rhomboid 60, 128, 139–140, 142, 153–155, 163, 174, 177, 187
- scaphoid 31
- subarcuata 18, 43–44
- submandibular 461
- subtonsillar 250
- supraspinous 505, 528
- temporal 8
- triangular 413
fossula(-ae) cochlear window 414, 427, 432–433, 437, 453
- petrosa 23, 45
- tonsillar 254
- vestibular window 432
fovea centralis 383, 389, 391, 393–394, 396, 398
- dentis 484–487, 499
- inferior 139
- oblong 324
- pterygoid 278
- sublingual 280, 282
- submandibular 280, 282
- superior 139
- triangular 324
- trochlear 242
foveola ethmoidal 242
- granular 4, 24, 49, 57
frenulum lower lip 250
- superior medullary velum 139, 173
- tongue 249, 253
- upper lip 250
fundus, of internal acoustic meatus 447, 449
funiculus anterolateral 202
- dorsal 151, 193, 200
- lateral 193, 200–201
- lateral of medulla oblongata 143
- ventral 148, 193, 200–201

galea aponeurotica 20, 59, 210–211, 214–215, 219–220
ganglion(-ia) celiac 182, 209
- ciliary 379–380, 395
- coccygeal 182
- geniculate 289–290, 429, 439, 448
- geniculate of facial nerve 430, 445
- impar 182, 207
- inferior cervical 207, 209, 304, 313, 481
- inferior mesenteric 182
- inferior of glossopharyngeal nerve 289–290, 304, 440
- inferior of vagus nerve 182, 235, 304, 313

*ganglion(-ia)*
- lumbar 182, 186
- middle cervical 182, 207, 209, 304, 313, 480–481
- optic 235, 290
- pterygopalatine 234–235, 289–290, 358
- sacral 182, 186, 207
- semilunar 130, 133
- spinal 182–183, 185–188, 190–192, 195–197
- spiral of cochlea 455
- splanchnic 207, 209
- stellate 182, 207, 472
- submandibular 223, 290, 469–470
- superior cervical 182, 207, 234–235, 253, 304, 313, 395, 480
- superior mesenteric 182
- superior of vagus nerve 161, 235, 304
- sympathetic trunk 182–183, 185, 209
- thoracic 182, 207, 209, 313
- trigeminal 19, 76, 130, 133–135, 136a, 137, 156, 235, 288–289, 358, 378–379, 439, 443
genu corpus callosum 75, 77–78, 95, 98, 101–103, 105–106, 108–109, 112, 121, 177
- facial nerve 162–163
- internal capsule 98–100
gingiva 250, 259, 268–269
glabella 48, 242, 248
gland(-s) accessory parotid 217, 219, 298, 459, 469
- anterior lingual 470
- buccal 252–253
- ceruminous 419
- inferior parathyroid 305–307, 313, 342
- labial 252–253, 303
- lacrimal 347, 351–352, 356, 366, 375, 378–381
- laryngeal 318, 334–335
- palatine 236, 244, 251, 303
- parotid 210, 214, 216, 219, 253, 298, 305–306, 459, 462, 467–469, 473–477
- pharyngeal 305
- sebaceous 303, 419
- sublingual 53, 223, 253, 294, 303, 469–471
- submandibular 219, 222–223, 294, 305–306, 459, 464–470, 473–476
- superior parathyroid 305–307, 313
- tarsal 345–346, 354–355, 377
- thyroid 304–305, 307, 311–314, 342, 459, 465–466, 470–472, 475, 477
- trachael 317, 330, 333, 472
globus pallidus 99–102, 114–115, 117, 119, 126, 144
glomus, choroid 106, 109–110, 112
granulations, arachnoid 20, 57, 62, 64
gyrus(-i) angular 66, 70, 72
- cerebellar 100
- cingular 67, 71, 75, 78–79, 119, 121
- dentate 104, 108, 116, 122–123
- fasciolar 77, 122
- inferior frontal 66, 72, 107
- inferior temporal 66–68, 71–72, 77
- insular 98–100, 102, 114–115
- lateral occipitotemporal 67–68, 71, 76–77, 147
- long insular 73
- medial occipitotemporal 67–68, 71, 75, 77, 121
- medial temporal 66, 72
- middle frontal 66, 70, 107
- occipital 70, 72, 99, 109
- orbital 66, 68, 71, 76, 107

*gyrus(-i)*
- parahippocampal 67–68, 71, 76–77, 104, 111, 116–118, 122–123, 147, 175
- paraterminal 67, 75, 119, 177
- postcentral 66, 70, 72
- precentral 66, 70, 72, 125
- rectus 68, 71
- short insular 73
- superior frontal 66–67, 70, 72, 75, 77, 107, 112, 114, 121
- superior temporal 60, 66, 72
- supramarginal 66, 70, 72
- transverse temporal 105, 458

habenula 102
hamulus(-i) hamate bone 584, 607, 611–612
- pterygoid 7, 11, 23, 30–31, 228, 239–241, 251, 301, 303, 307–308, 362–363, 502
- spiral lamina 453
head caudate nucleus 98–103, 106–107, 109–112, 114–115, 119–120, 124, 126, 140
- deep of flexor pollicis brevis muscle 599–600, 604
- humeral of flexor carpi ulnaris muscle 519a
- humeral of flexor digitorum superficialis muscle 519a, 565
- humeral of flexor pollicis longus muscle 551
- humeral of pronator teres muscle 519a, 562
- humeroulnar of flexor digitorum superficialis muscle 550, 562
- humerus 526–527, 544–545
- lateral of triceps brachii muscle 513–515, 519b, 535–536, 541–542, 558
- long of biceps brachii muscle 514, 516, 518, 519a, 520–521, 524, 537
- long of triceps brachii muscle 513–518, 519a, 519b, 521–522, 524–525, 535–538, 540–542
- malleus 409, 420–422, 426, 429, 431, 434, 436
- mandible 278, 280, 282, 297, 299
- medial of triceps brachii muscle 513–514, 519b, 535–538, 540–542, 546–547, 550, 557–559, 563
- metacarpal bone 610–612
- oblique of adductor pollicis muscle 584, 599–600, 604
- phalanx 61
- radial of flexor digitorum superficialis muscle 550–551, 553, 562, 566
- radius 573, 579–580
- short of biceps brachii muscle 514, 516, 518, 519a, 521, 537–538, 540
- stapes 425, 429–430, 437, 445
- transverse of adductor pollicis muscle 584, 600, 604
- ulna 574, 576, 606, 610–611
- ulnar of flexor carpi ulnaris muscle 519a, 562
- ulnar of pronator teres muscle 519a, 551, 553, 562, 565
helix 412–413, 461
hemisphere cerebellar 75, 103, 113–114, 177
- telencephalic 374
hiatus aortic 207
- canal for greater petrosal nerve 44
- facial canal 433
- maxillary 240–241
- semilunar 231
hilus dentate nucleus 173–174
- olivary nucleus 153–155

hippocampus 61, 78, 101, 109, 116, 118, 175
horn anterior 201
- anterior of lateral ventricle 98–102, 106–107, 109–112
- inferior of lateral ventricle 147, 175
- posterior 201
- posterior of lateral ventricle 98–101, 106, 109, 111–112, 116, 127
humerus 514, 520, 524–525, 538, 544–545, 568–570
hypopharynx 307
hypophysis 19, 54, 57–58, 63, 75–76, 94, 129, 131, 177, 231, 395
hypothalamus 54, 56, 144, 178
hypothenar 506

impression(-s) costoclavicular ligament 532
- digitate 11, 18, 127, 243, 436
- facial collicle 127
- petrous bone 69, 436
- trigeminal 432–433, 443
incus 423–424, 429, 431, 434, 436
indentation, optic disk 398
indusium griseum 104, 145
infundibulum 15, 58, 75–76, 115, 119, 141, 143, 177
- ethmoidal 225
insula 73–74, 85, 105, 119
iris 233, 344, 383, 387–388, 396, 403, 407–408
isthmus cingulate gyrus 71, 77
- ear cartilage 416
- fauces 250–251, 307
- posterior column 200
- thyroid gland 302, 311–312, 318, 472, 476

joints(-s) (see also articulation) acromioclavicular 505, 524, 526
- atlantooccipital 4, 409, 494–496
- carpometacarpal 606
- carpometacarpal of thumb 606
- cricoarytenoid 336
- cricothyroid 328
- cubital 564, 568, 573
- distal radioulnar 567, 606
- elbow 564, 568, 573
- humeroulnar 570
- incudomallear 429, 434, 436
- incudostapedial 434
- interphalangeal of hand 572
- intervertebral 505
- lateral atlantoaxial 4, 494–496
- median atlantoaxial 302–303, 499
- mediocarpal 606
- metacarpophalangeal of thumb 610
- radiocarpal 606
- shoulder 520–524
- sternoclavicular 475, 505
- temporomandibular 297, 299–301
juga alveolaria 277, 284
- cerebralia 11

labrum, glenoidal 520–522
labyrinth bony 451–453
- ethmoidal 32, 34, 233, 237–238, 241, 359
- membranous
- 411 454, 456–457
lacunae, lateral 20, 64
lake, lacrimal 345, 349
lamina(-ae) affixa 103, 106, 109–110, 112, 140, 144–145
- anterior limiting 383
- basilar 455
- bony spiral 449, 452–453, 455, 457
- choriocapillary 386

*lamina(-ae)*
- cribrosa 9, 11, 18, 32, 228, 237, 239–241, 295
- cricoid cartilage 302, 321–322, 326–327, 333
- horizontal of palatine bone 13, 23, 40–41, 239–240, 286, 441
- lateral medullary 100
- lateral of cartilage of auditory tube 441, 443
- lateral of pterygoid process 11, 30–31, 229, 286, 308, 362, 441
- medial medullary 100
- medial of cartilage of auditory tube 441, 443
- medial of pterygoid process 11, 30–31, 239–240, 286, 303, 441, 502
- medullary of thalamus 144
- membranous of auditory tube 443
- modiolus 449, 453
- orbital 8, 32–33, 360–362
- perpendicular of ethmoid bone 11, 32–33, 228, 237–239, 301, 359
- perpendicular of palatine bone 40–41, 240, 285
- posterior limiting 383–384
- pretracheal of cervical fascia 302
- prevertebral of cervical fascia 302
- quadrigemina 128, 167–168
- secondary spiral 449, 453
- superficial of cervical fascia 302
- suprachoroid 386
- tectum 75, 95, 111, 128, 139–140, 167, 177–178, 395
- terminal 56, 75, 104, 108, 121, 143, 177
- thyroid cartilage 308, 319
- tragus 216, 412, 461
- white 174
larynx 309, 313, 315, 318, 327, 329, 331–332, 334–336, 342
layer fibrous 520
- granular of cerebellum 174
- molecular 174
- pigment of ciliary body 383
- pigment of retina 383, 398
- white of cortex 122
lemniscus acoustic 164
- lateral 156–157, 164, 167, 458
- medial 151, 154–157, 161, 163–164, 166–168, 178
lens 233, 386–387, 396, 401, 403, 407–408
leptomeninx, of brain 62–63
ligament(-s) acromioclavicular 521–522, 524–525
- alar 497–498
- anterior auricular 461
- anterior longitudinal 192, 302, 481, 494
- anular radial 568–569, 571
- anular trachael 309, 317, 330, 333, 342
- apical of odontoid process 179, 303, 498
- conoid 514, 521–522, 524
- coracoacromial 521–522, 524–525
- coracoclavicular 514, 522, 524, 537
- coracohumeral 521, 523–524
- costoclavicular 475, 519a
- cricopharyngeal 317, 327, 330
- cricothyroid 302, 309, 311–312, 317–318, 327, 329, 331, 333–334, 471, 475
- cricotracheal 293, 329–330, 342
- cruciform of atlas 302, 497
- cubital radial collateral 568–569
- deep transverse metacarpal 584, 600, 607

*ligament(-s)*
- denticulate 95, 190–192, 195, 197, 209
- dorsal carpometacarpal 605
- dorsal intercarpal 605
- dorsal metacarpal 605
- dorsal radiocarpal 605
- glenohumeral 524
- hyoepiglottic 302, 315–318, 333
- iliolumbar 207
- inferior transverse of scapula 517
- interclavicular 302, 459, 475
- interosseous metacarpal 606
- interphalangeal collateral of hand 572, 600
- lateral 300, 502
- lateral mallear 426
- medial palpebral 210, 219, 347, 349–351, 459
- median thyrohyoid 302, 312, 315–316, 318, 327, 329, 331, 470, 475
- metacarpophalangeal collateral 572, 605
- nuchae 467
- palmar carpal 585
- palmar carpometacarpal 607
- palmar metacarpal 607
- palmar metacarpophalangeal 607
- palmar radiocarpal 585, 600, 607
- palmar ulnocarpal 600, 607
- pectinate 383–384, 387, 403, 407–408
- pisohamate 600, 607
- pisometacarpeal 607
- posterior cricoarytenoid 325, 328, 330
- posterior longitudinal 191–192, 302
- posterior of incus 429, 431
- pterygospinal 301, 502
- radial carpal collateral 600, 606
- radiate carpal 600, 607
- sphenomandibular 224, 301, 303, 305, 307, 505
- spiral of cochlea 455
- stylohyoid 292–293, 303, 305, 308, 461, 502, 505
- stylomandibular 253, 300–301, 303, 306, 461, 502, 505
- stylopharyngeal 253
- superficial transverse metacarpal 583
- superior auricular 461
- superior mallear 409, 426, 429, 431
- superior of incus 431
- superior transverse of scapula 514, 516–518, 523–524, 537
- temporomandibular 298, 308
- thyroepiglottic 302, 315–318, 327
- thyrohyoid 317, 329–331, 334
- transverse of atlas 179, 302–303, 499
- trapezoid 514, 521–522, 524
- ulnar carpal collateral 600, 606
- vestibular 317, 342
- vocal 317, 324, 326–328, 336, 342
- volar carpal 584
*limb(-s)* anthelix 413
- common of anterior and posterior semicircular ducts 429, 454, 456
- long of incus 414, 423, 427, 429, 431, 434, 436
- posterior of stapes 414, 425, 430, 434
- short of incus 423–424, 429, 431, 434
- single of lateral semicircular canal 450

*limbus* anterior palpebral 344–345, 356, 377
- osseous of spiral lamina 455
- posterior palpebral 344–345, 354, 356, 377
*limen* insula 143
- nasi 231–232
*line* anterior median 1
- cephalic 506
- inferior nuchal 23, 26–27, 505
- inferior temporal 8, 25, 42, 48, 50
- mensal 506
- mylohoid 280, 282, 292, 301, 505
- oblique of mandible 277–279
- oblique of thyroid cartilage 331
- stomachic (fortune) 506
- superior nuchal 23, 26–27, 505
- superior temporal 8, 25–26, 50
- supreme nuchal 27, 505
- trapezoid 532
- vital 506
*lingula* cerebellar 140, 169, 171, 173–174, 177, 179
- mandible 280, 282, 301
- sphenoidal 18, 29, 31
*lip* lower 248–249, 255
- tympanic limbus 455
- upper 248–249
*lobe* frontal 53, 68–70, 74, 99, 105, 107, 119–120
- occipital 69, 74, 105, 108, 395
- parietal 69, 72, 74, 105, 114
- pyramidal 312, 470
- temporal 68–69, 74, 105, 107, 114, 117, 119–120, 175
*lobule* biventral 170, 172
- central 169, 171, 177
- ear 413, 416
- inferior parietal 66, 70
- inferior semilunar 169–170
- paracentral 67, 75, 77, 121
- quadrangular 169
- simplex 169
- superior parietal 66, 70
- superior semilunar 169–170
*locus* ceruleus 139, 164
*lunula,* of nail 591, 593
*lymph node(-s)* buccal 482–483
- deep inferior cervical 483
- deep superior cervical 482–483
- jugulodigastric 483
- juguloomohyoid 483
- mandibular 482
- maxillary 482
- occipital 482–483
- paratracheal 302
- retroauricular 482–483
- submandibular 468–469, 482–483
- submental 482–483
- superficial cervical 482–483
- superficial paraotid 216, 482–483

*macula* 393–394
- flava 318
- medial cribrose 450, 453
- superior cribrose 450
*malleus* 420–422, 434, 439
*mandible* 2–4, 8, 12–13, 53, 255, 259, 261, 277–280, 282, 291–293, 295–296, 302–303, 305
*manubrium* malleus 414, 420–422, 426–429, 431, 434, 436
- sternum 302, 505
*margin* anterior of radius 577, 580
- anterior of ulna 577
- ciliary 403, 407–408
- corneal 383
- free of nail 591–593
- frontal of parietal bone 50–51
- frontal of sphenoid bone 29–30
- hidden of nail 593

*margin*
- infraorbital 3, 35, 247, 284, 352, 364
- interosseous of radius 577–580
- interosseous of ulna 574, 576–577
- lacrimal 284
- lambdoid 27–29
- lateral of humerus 545
- lateral of nail 593
- lateral of scapula 526, 528–530
- mastoid 28–29
- medial of humerus 545
- medial of scapula 526, 528–529
- occipital of parietal bone 25, 50–51
- occipital of temporal bone 42–43, 45
- orbital 9
- parietal of frontal bone 43, 48–49
- parietal of sphenoid bone 29, 31
- parietal of temporal bone 42
- posterior of radius 577, 579
- posterior of ulna 565, 575, 577
- pupillary 396, 405, 407–408
- sagittal 50
- sphenoid 42–45, 49
- squamous of parietal bone 50–51
- squamous of sphenoid bone 29, 31
- superior of petrous bone 9, 15, 17, 43
- superior of scapula 505, 528–529
- supraorbital 3–4, 242, 365
- supraorbital of frontal bone 48
- tongue 249, 254
- vestibular window 453
- zygomatic 30
*mass,* lateral of atlas 484–486
*massa* intermedia 75, 78, 102–103, 111, 117–118, 127, 129, 144, 177
*matrix,* of nail 592
*matter,* gray of superior colliculus 102, 166, 168
*maxilla* 3–4, 8, 261, 284–286, 295, 302, 362, 364–365
*meatus* common nasal 52, 225, 245
- external acoustic 8, 300, 308, 409
- inferior nasal 52–53, 225, 238, 240, 348, 359
- internal acoustic 9, 11, 18, 43, 440, 446–447, 449
- middle nasal 53, 225, 240
- nasopharyngeal 302
- superior nasal 225, 240
*medulla* oblongata 19, 61, 63, 75–76, 113, 125, 140, 142–143, 173, 175, 177, 186, 189
- vermis 75, 173–175, 177
*membrane* antebrachial interosseous 561–562, 566, 571, 577, 585, 598, 600
- anterior atlantooccipital 179, 302–303, 478, 494
- arachnoid of brain 20, 62–63, 99, 145
- arachnoid of spinal cord 190–192, 195, 209
- mucous of auditory tube 429, 444
- mucous of conus elasticus 336
- mucous of isthmus of fauces 307
- mucous of mouth 259, 293–294
- mucous of nasal septum 302
- mucous of nose 245, 303
- mucous of pharynx 317–318
- mucous of tongue 255, 314
- mucous of trachea 472
- posterior atlantooccipital 179, 303, 495, 503

*membrane*
- quadrangular 342
- stapedial 430, 445
- tectorial 179, 496
- thyrohyoid 293, 303, 308, 311–312, 317, 327, 329–331, 333, 342, 470–471, 475
- tympanic 409, 414, 426, 428–431
- vestibular 455
*meninges* 20
*mesencephalon* 54, 95, 128, 130, 143
*mesopharynx* 307
*modiolus* 449
*monticuli* 506
*muscle* abductor digiti minimi 584–585, 588–589, 599–600, 604
- abductor pollicis brevis 584–585, 587–589, 599–600, 604
- abductor pollicis longus 513, 546–547, 550, 557–561, 563, 566
- adductor pollicis 513, 584–585, 587–588, 596, 598–600, 604
- anconeus 513, 519a, 536, 541–542, 557–561, 563–564
- antebrachial flexor 506, 533, 540, 546, 554–555
- anterior auricular 459
- anterior intertransversarii cervicis 478, 503
- antitragicus 417
- arrectores pilorum 20
- articularis cubiti 519a, 562–563
- aryepiglotticus 307, 313, 332–333, 342
- biceps brachii 506, 513–516, 518, 519a, 521, 524, 535, 542, 546–547, 552–553, 555–556, 558, 562, 570
- brachialis 513–515, 519a, 519b, 535–538, 540–542, 546–547, 550–555, 557–558, 562, 564, 570
- brachioradialis 513, 519a, 519b, 533, 535–538, 540, 546–547, 550–553, 555–566, 604
- buccinator 53, 210, 214, 219–224, 244, 250–253, 298, 303, 308, 459
- buccopharyngeal 253
- ciliary 383–384, 387, 396, 407
- compressor naris 308
- coracobrachialis 506, 514, 516, 518, 519a, 521, 537–538, 540
- cricothyroid 293, 308, 311–312, 333–334, 342, 470–471, 475
- deltoid 459, 465–466, 475, 480, 501, 506, 513–518, 519a, 519b, 521, 535–542
- depressor anguli oris 210–211, 219–220, 298, 308, 459–460, 468
- depressor labii inferioris 210–211, 219–220, 252, 459
- depressor septi 210, 227
- depressor supercilii 210–211, 219–220
- digastric 292, 294, 303, 439, 461, 465, 475, 503
- digastric, anterior belly 53, 219–221, 223–224, 234, 292, 308, 459, 461, 464, 466–470, 473, 475–477, 483, 502
- digastric, posterior belly 217, 220–221, 223–224, 292, 304–308, 313, 459, 467–469, 474, 478, 502
- dilator pupillae 384
- dorsal interosseous of hand 513, 584–585, 588, 596, 598–602, 604
- epicranial 210–211, 219–220, 459
- extensor carpi radialis brevis 513, 519a, 519b, 533, 535–537, 546–547, 556–563, 565–566

*muscle*
- extensor carpi radialis longus 513, 519a, 519b, 533, 535–538, 546, 550–551, 556–563, 565–566, 598, 604
- extensor digiti minimi 557–559, 563, 565–566
- extensor digitorum manus 513, 519b, 536, 557–561, 563, 565–567
- extensor indicis 559, 563, 566–567
- extensor pollicis brevis 513, 557–561, 563, 566, 598
- extensor pollicis longus 559, 561, 563, 566
- external intercostal 192, 467, 475
- flexor carpi radialis 513–514, 519a, 546–547, 550, 552–553, 562, 565–566, 604
- flexor carpi ulnaris 519a, 546–547, 550–552, 554–555, 557–559, 562–563, 565–567, 587–588, 604
- flexor digiti minimi brevis 584–585, 599–600, 604
- flexor digitorum profundus 519a, 551, 555, 562–563, 566, 604
- flexor digitorum superficialis 519a, 546–547, 550, 552–553, 562, 565–567, 604
- flexor pollicis brevis 584–585, 587–588, 599–600, 604
- flexor pollicis longus 513, 546–547, 550–551, 553–554, 562, 566, 604
- genioglossus 53, 234–235, 253, 255, 291, 293–295, 302–303, 469–471, 502
- geniohyoid 53, 56, 234–235, 255, 291, 293–295, 302–303, 469–471, 502
- greater of helix 417, 461
- hyoglossus 223, 253, 293, 295, 303, 459, 469–471, 473–477
- hyothyroid 315–316
- iliocostalis cervicis 467
- iliocostalis thoracis 467
- inferior oblique 349–353, 358, 364–366, 368–371, 372a, 372c, 372d, 373, 377, 382
- inferior oblique capitis 503–504
- inferior pharyngeal constrictor 220, 304–305, 335–336, 459, 468, 470, 475
- infraspinatus 515, 517, 519a, 521, 525, 536
- internal intercostal 192, 467
- interspinales cervicis 503
- laryngeal 332–333
- lateral cricoarytenoid 333–334, 342
- lateral pterygoid 222–223, 297, 299, 303, 305, 307, 502
- latissimus dorsi 501, 513–514, 516, 518, 519a, 519b, 535
- lesser of helix 417, 461
- levator anguli oris 210, 219–220, 252, 308, 459
- levator labii superioris 210–211, 219–221, 252, 308, 459
- levator labii superioris alaeque nasi 210–211, 219–220, 227, 308, 357, 459
- levator palpebrae superioris 19, 351–353, 364–367, 373, 375–376, 378–380, 382
- levator scapulae 220, 459–460, 462, 467, 475, 478, 483, 501, 513–515, 519e
- levator veli palatini 303, 305–308, 442–443, 502
- levatores pharyngis 335–336
- longissimus capitis 467, 478, 501–504

*muscle*
- longissimus cervicis 467
- longitudinalis inferior linguae 253, 293
- longitudinalis superior linguae 255
- longus capitis 303, 475, 478, 481, 502
- longus colli 472, 478, 481
- lumbricalis 584–589, 596, 599, 601
- masseter 53, 210, 217, 219–222, 224, 244, 253, 459, 461, 468–469, 475, 502
- medial pterygoid 222–224, 234–235, 253, 289, 294, 299, 303, 305–307, 469, 475, 502
- mentalis 210–211, 219–220, 252, 308, 459
- middle pharyngeal constrictor 304–305, 307–308
- multifidus 503–504
- mylohyoid 53, 223, 234–235, 255, 291–292, 294–295, 302–303, 308, 459, 461, 465–466, 468–470, 473–477, 502
- nasalis 210–211, 219–220, 227, 459
- oblique arytenoid 307, 313–314, 332–335
- oblique auricular 418
- oblique externus abdominis 513
- occipitofrontal 210–211, 219–221, 224, 459, 462, 476, 501, 504, 537
- omohyoid 220, 303, 308, 459–461, 463–468, 470, 475–477, 480, 483, 513–514, 516, 518, 519a, 519b, 537
- opponens digiti minimi 584–585, 589, 599–600, 604
- opponens pollicis 584–585, 588–589, 596, 599–600, 604
- orbicularis oculi 210–211, 216–217, 219–220, 224, 348–350, 354, 357, 459
- orbicularis oris 210–211, 219–221, 224, 227, 236, 252–253, 303, 308, 459
- orbitalis 376
- palatoglossus 251, 253–254, 293, 295
- palatopharyngeus 236, 251, 253–254, 307, 313
- palmar interosseous 584–585, 588, 599–600, 603–604
- palmaris brevis 547, 583, 599
- palmaris longus 519a, 546–547, 550, 552, 562, 565–566
- pectoralis major 459, 464–467, 475–477, 480, 513–514, 516, 518, 519a, 519b, 521, 535, 539–540
- pectoralis minor 465–466, 475, 480, 514, 516, 518, 519a, 521, 537
- pharyngoepiglotticus 313
- posterior auricular 211, 217, 418, 459
- posterior cricoarytenoid 307, 313–314, 332–334, 336
- posterior intertransversarii cervicis 478, 503
- process 210–211, 219, 303, 308
- pronator quadratus 546–547, 550–551, 554, 562, 567, 584–585, 588, 600
- pronator teres 513–514, 519a, 547, 550–555, 562–563, 565–566
- psoas major 207
- rectus capitis anterior 478, 502
- rectus capitis lateralis 478, 502–503
- rectus capitis posterior major 502–504
- rectus capitis posterior minor 502–503

*muscle*
- rectus inferior 353, 358, 364, 366–371, 372b, 372c, 372d, 373, 376–377, 382
- rectus lateralis 53, 233, 364–371, 372a, 372c, 372d, 373–382, 386
- rectus medialis 233, 358, 365–371, 372a, 372b, 372c, 373–377, 380, 382–383
- rectus superior 19, 353, 364–371, 372a, 372b, 372d, 373, 375–380, 382
- rhomboides major 501, 504, 514–515, 519b
- risorius 210–211, 219, 252, 298, 460
- salpingopharyngeus 236, 307, 313
- scalenus anterior 220, 459, 465, 467, 472, 475, 477–478, 480–481, 483, 513
- scalenus medius 220, 459–460, 467, 472, 475, 481, 483, 503, 513
- scalenus posterior 220, 478, 481, 483, 503, 513
- semispinalis capitis 211, 220, 459, 467, 501–504
- semispinalis cervicis 503–504
- serratus anterior 467, 475, 513–514, 516, 519a
- serratus posterior superior 467
- sphincter pupillae 383–384
- splenius capitis 211, 220, 459–460, 466–467, 478, 483, 501–504
- splenius cervicis 467, 475, 503, 513
- stapedius 289, 437
- sternocleidomastoideus 210–211, 217, 219–221, 298, 303, 459–466, 469, 472–478, 483, 501–502, 513, 519a, 519b
- sternohyoid 220, 303, 308, 459, 461, 464, 467–470, 472, 475, 477, 480, 513, 519b
- sternothyroid 220, 302, 342, 459, 464, 467, 470, 472, 475, 477, 480
- styloglossus 220, 223, 253, 293, 295, 303, 305, 308, 461, 469, 471, 502
- stylohyoid 220–221, 223–224, 292–293, 303, 305, 307–308, 439, 459, 461, 465, 467–470, 473–476, 502
- stylopharyngeus 253, 293, 303–305, 307–308, 502
- subclavius 475, 514, 516, 519a, 519b, 521, 537
- subscapularis 514, 516, 518, 519a, 521, 524, 537–538
- superior auricular 418, 461
- superior oblique 365–367, 370, 372a, 372b, 372d, 373, 375–376, 378–380, 382
- superior oblique capitis 502–504
- superior pharyngeal constrictor 236, 251, 304–305, 307, 313
- supinator 519a, 547, 550–553, 556, 559, 561–563, 565
- supraspinatus 514–517, 519a, 519b, 521, 525, 535, 537
- temporalis 53, 220–224, 233, 374, 502
- temporoparietalis 210–211, 216, 219, 221, 459
- tensor tympani 289, 409, 426–427, 429–431, 437, 444–445
- tensor veli palatini 235, 303, 307–308, 313, 442–443, 502
- teres major 501, 513–518, 519a, 519b, 535–537, 540–542
- teres minor 513, 515, 517, 519b, 521, 525, 536, 542
- thyroarytenoid 333, 335–336

*muscle*
- thyrohyoid 220, 293, 303, 308, 342, 459, 468, 470, 475
- tragicus 417, 461
- transverse arytenoid 302, 307, 313, 318, 332–335
- transverse auricular 418
- transverse linguae 255
- trapezius 211, 220–221, 459–460, 462, 465, 475–476, 483, 501, 504, 513, 515–516, 519a, 519b, 535, 538
- triceps brachii 506, 513, 519b, 558, 560, 563–564, 570
- triceps brachii, lateral head 513–515, 519b, 535–536, 558
- triceps brachii, long head 513–518, 519a, 519b, 521–522, 524, 535–536, 538
- triceps brachii, medial head 513–514, 519b, 535–536, 538, 540, 546–547, 557–559, 563
- uvular 236, 251, 307, 313
- vocalis 334–336, 342
- zygomaticus major 210–211, 216–217, 219, 221, 252, 298, 308, 459
- zygomaticus minor 210–211, 219, 308, 459

nail 591–593
neck anatomical of humerus 526–527, 544–545
- malleus 420–422, 427
- mandible 280, 299, 502
- radius 579–580, 582
- scapula 528–529
- surgical of humerus 515, 526, 536, 544

nerve(-s) abducent 19, 63, 76, 85, 95, 131–133, 162–163, 378–380, 382, 439
- accessory 19, 76, 85, 95, 138, 142–143, 149, 151, 154, 189, 217, 304, 313, 439, 462–466, 473–474, 480, 501, 504
- accessory phrenic 481
- anterior ampullary 454, 457
- anterior auricular 216
- anterior ethmoidal 221, 223–224, 234, 290, 295
- anterior interosseous 554, 566
- anterior supraclavicular 463
- auriculotemporal 214–217, 221–224, 235, 290
- axillary 197, 506, 517–518, 540, 542
- buccal 214, 221–224, 253, 358
- caroticotympanic 289, 440
- cervical 61, 150, 187, 207, 465–466, 504
- ciliary 380, 387, 403, 407
- coccygeal 187, 196, 207
- common digital palmar of median nerve 587
- common palmar digital of ulnar nerve 587
- deep petrosal 234, 289–290
- deep temporal 222–223
- dorsal digital 595–596
- dorsal digital of radial nerve 596–597
- dorsal digital proper 583, 587–588, 597
- dorsal digital proper of median nerve 596, 608–609
- dorsal digital proper of ulnar nerve 587
- dorsal scapular 501, 504
- external acoustic meatus 222–224
- facial 19, 76, 85, 114, 133, 138, 142–143, 163, 214, 217–218, 221–224, 235, 289–290, 357, 429, 431, 437, 439–440, 445, 448, 463, 468
- femoral 207
- frontal 221, 224, 290, 367, 378

*nerve(-s)*
- genitofemoral 207
- glossopharyngeal 19, 76, 85, 95, 114, 138, 142–143, 155, 187, 290, 295–296, 304, 313–314, 439–440
- great auricular 214–215, 217, 460, 462–463, 501
- greater occipital 215, 221, 462–464, 480, 501, 504
- greater palatine 234–235, 251, 290, 296
- greater petrosal 19, 234–235, 289–290, 429–430, 437, 439–440, 445, 448
- greater splanchnic 182–183, 192, 207, 209
- hypoglossal 19, 76, 85, 94–95, 138, 143, 153–154, 161, 187, 189, 220, 223, 253, 295, 304, 313, 465–466, 468–471, 473–474, 476–477, 480
- iliohypogastric 207
- ilioinguinal 207
- incisive 236
- inferior alveolar 221–224, 234–235, 253, 288, 290, 358
- inferior cervical cardiac 182, 207, 209
- inferior laryngeal 314
- infraorbital 214, 220–224, 235, 288–290, 336–337, 348, 357, 376, 381–382
- infratrochlear 221–224, 357–358, 380, 382
- intercostal 184a, 185–186, 207, 209, 476
- intercostobrachial 480, 508
- intermedius 19, 76, 114, 138, 143, 289, 429, 439
- internal carotid 289, 304, 313
- jugular 304
- lacrimal 290, 356–357, 367, 378–381
- lateral ampullary 454, 457
- lateral antebrachial cutaneous 508, 539–542, 548, 564–567, 583
- lateral femoral cutaneous 207
- lateral pterygoid 223
- lateral supraclavicular 507
- lesser occipital 215–216, 221, 462–465, 480, 501
- lesser palatine 234, 251, 290, 296
- lesser petrosal 19, 289–290, 440
- lesser splanchnic 182, 207, 209
- lingual 222–224, 234–235, 251, 253, 288, 290, 295, 358, 469–471, 477
- lumbar 187, 196, 207
- lumbar splanchnic 182
- mandibular 76, 130, 133, 135, 223, 235, 288–290, 358, 378, 382, 443
- masseteric 221–224
- maxillary 19, 76, 131, 133, 135, 235, 288–290, 358, 378–379, 382, 439
- medial antebrachial cutaneous 508, 518, 539, 548, 564–565
- medial lateral brachial cutaneous 507–508, 518, 539, 549
- medial pterygoid 235
- medial supraclavicular 463
- median 197, 518, 539–540, 547–548, 552–556, 564–567, 583–584, 587, 599
- mental 214, 221–222, 224, 288, 290
- middle cervical cardiac 182, 207, 304, 480
- musculocutaneous 197, 518, 538–540
- mylohyoid 222–224, 234–235, 253, 290, 465–466, 474, 480
- nasociliary 290, 358, 378–380
- nasopalatine 234–236, 295–296
- obturator 207

*nerve(-s)*
- oculomotor 19, 63, 75–76, 79, 85, 95, 113, 131–133, 165–166, 168, 358, 376, 378–380, 382, 395, 439
- olfactory 229, 232, 236, 295–296
- ophthalmic 19, 76, 131, 133, 135, 235, 288–290, 358, 378–380, 439
- optic 19, 53, 58, 63, 75–76, 79, 84, 94–95, 108, 120, 130–132, 141, 178, 233–235, 289, 353, 364–365, 367, 369, 371, 374–382, 387, 396–398
- phrenic 192, 207, 465–466, 477, 480–481
- posterior ampullary 429, 454, 457
- posterior antebrachial cutaneous 507–508, 541–542, 549, 564–566, 595–596
- posterior auricular 217–218, 221, 223–224, 440, 462, 465
- posterior ethmoidal 358, 380, 382
- posterior interosseous 561, 566, 598
- posterior lateral brachial cutaneous 507, 541–542, 549
- posterior supraclavicular 463, 507–508
- pterygoid canal 234–235, 289–290, 358, 440
- pterygopalatine 235, 289
- radial 197, 518, 539–542, 548, 552–556, 560–561, 565–567, 595–596
- recurrent laryngeal 182, 313–314, 472, 477, 480
- saccular 454, 457
- sacral 187, 207
- spinal 183, 185, 190–192, 197, 209
- sublingual 290, 470–471
- suboccipital 504
- subscapular 518
- superior alveolar 222, 288
- superior brachial cutaneous 507, 517, 541
- superior cervical cardiac 182, 207, 304, 472, 480
- superior recurrent laryngeal 253, 293, 304, 308, 313–314, 335–336, 466, 468, 470–471, 473–474
- supraclavicular 462
- supraorbital 222, 224, 357, 378–379
- suprascapular 480, 517–518
- supratrochlear 221–224, 290, 357, 378–379
- tensor tympani muscle 235
- tensor veli palatini muscle 235
- tentorial 65
- thoracic 185–187, 209, 504
- thoracic, long 480
- thoracodorsal 480, 518
- transverse cervical 462–463
- trigeminal 19, 63, 76, 85, 94–95, 113, 121, 130, 132, 136, 142–143, 156, 166, 234–235, 288–290, 378–380, 382, 439
- trochlear 19, 76, 79, 95, 121, 128, 130–133, 139–140, 142–143, 157, 378–380, 458
- tympani 289–290, 430, 437, 440, 445
- ulnar 197, 518, 539–542, 547–549, 552–555, 560–561, 564–567, 583–584, 587–588, 595
- utricular 454, 457
- utriculoampullary 429, 454
- vagus 19, 76, 85, 95, 114, 138, 142–143, 153–154, 187, 192, 220–221, 223–224, 235, 289, 304, 313, 439–440, 465–466, 472–474, 477, 480

*nerve(-s)*
- vertebral 209
- vestibulocochlear 19, 76, 85, 95, 114, 121, 133, 138, 142–143, 154–155, 235, 429, 439, 446, 457–458
- zygomatic 216, 221, 289–290, 358, 381–382
network arterial of elbow 511, 541–542, 560
- arterial of nasal septum 236
- arterial of wrist 560, 594, 596, 598
- venous of dorsum of hand 595
neurocranium 8, 23, 54, 59–61
neurohypophysis 58
nidus avis 172
nodule 61, 170–173, 177, 179
nose, external 226
nostrils 248, 302
notch anterior cerebellar 170
- anterior of ear 413
- cartilage of acoustic meatus 412
- ethmoidal 242
- frontal 48, 361
- inferior thyroid 320
- interarytenoid 306–307, 313–314, 337, 340
- intertragic 412–413
- jugular 29
- lacrimal 284
- mandibular 278, 282
- mastoid 23, 26, 42, 45, 505
- nasal 284
- parietal 42–44
- posterior cerebellar 170–172, 174
- pterygoid 11, 30–31
- radial 574, 576
- scapular 528–529
- sphenopalatine 39, 41, 285
- superior thyroid 319–320, 328–329, 331
- supraorbital 237, 242, 351
- tentorial 15
- trochlear 571, 574, 576, 582
- tympanic 427–428
- ulnar 578
nucleus abducent 158, 160, 162–163, 458
- accessory 158, 160, 166
- ambiguus 148–149, 153–155, 158, 160–161
- anterior thalamic 114, 126, 144
- arcuate 152, 154–155
- caudate 61, 102–103, 106, 110, 112, 124, 140, 144–145
- central thalamic 126
- centralis caudalis 158, 160
- cuneate 149, 151–153, 178
- dentate 162, 173–174
- dorsal accessory olivary 154
- dorsal cochlear 154, 160, 458
- dorsal longitudinal fascicle 161
- dorsal of trapezoid body 162
- dorsal of vagus 152–154, 158–161
- dorsolateral 158, 160, 166
- emboliform 174
- facial 158, 160, 163, 458
- fastigial 174
- globose 174
- gracilis 149–152, 159
- hypoglossal 158, 160–161
- inferior collicle 167, 458
- inferior olivary 153–154
- inferior salivatory 153, 158, 160
- inferior vestibular 160
- intercalatus 154
- interpeduncular 168
- lateral geniculate body 100, 102
- lateral lemniisues 156, 164, 458
- lateral thalamic 114, 126, 144
- lateral vestibular 155, 160
- lens 400

*nucleus*
- lentiform 99–100, 102, 107, 114–115, 117, 119
- mammillary body 114, 117, 144
- medial accessory olivary 152–154
- medial thalamic 114, 126, 144
- medial vestibular 154–155, 160, 162
- mesencephalic tract of trigeminal nerve 159–160, 166
- metencephalic olivary 458
- motor of trigeminal nerve 156, 158, 160, 458
- oculomotor 168
- olivary 114, 151, 154–155, 161, 178
- parasympathetic of trigeminal nerve 158, 160
- pontine 156–157, 162–164, 178
- posterior thalamic 126
- principal sensory of trigeminal nerve 156, 159–160
- rostral thalamic 118
- ruber 102, 133, 141, 166, 168
- solitary tract 153–154, 159–161
- spinal of accessory nerve 148–149, 158, 160
- spinal of trigeminal nerve 148–152, 154–155, 159–163
- subthalamic 102, 114
- superior salivatory 158, 160
- superior vestibular 160, 163
- tegmental 164
- thalamic 100, 114
- trochlear 157–158, 160, 167
- ventral cochlear 155, 160, 458
- ventral of trapezoid body 163
- ventral thalamic 118
- ventromedial 158, 160

obex 75, 139, 188
olecranon 507, 513, 535–536, 541, 549, 555, 557–559, 564, 569, 573–575, 582
olive 76, 121, 142–143
opening nasofrontal canal 241
- pharyngeal of auditory tube 54, 229, 231–232, 295, 302, 306, 313
- tympanic of auditory tube 428–433, 437
operculum frontal 69, 74, 84
- frontoparietal 69, 72
- parietal 74
- temporal 69, 74, 84
ora serrata 374, 383–384, 386, 396, 406
orbiculus ciliaris 383, 403, 405–406
orbit 4, 233, 238, 264, 361, 366–367, 374
organ spiral 455
- vomeronasal 229
ossicles, auditory 411, 434

palate hard 9, 52, 229, 231, 236, 244, 250, 258, 286–287, 303
- panniculus adiposus of cheek 211
- soft 231, 250, 258, 306
papilla(-ae) conical 254
- filiform 254
- foliate 254, 293
- fungiform 254
- incisive 258
- lacrimal 345, 348–349, 377
- optic nerve 233, 383
- vallate 254, 296, 306–307, 314
peduncle cerebral 76, 79, 121, 130, 140–144, 165, 177
- flocculus 140, 171–172
- inferior cerebellar 139, 142, 153–155, 163, 175
- mammillary body 143

*peduncle*
- middle cerebellar 114, 121, 128, 139–140, 142, 156–157, 162–163, 171, 458
- superior cerebellar 61, 128, 139–140, 142, 156–157, 164, 171–175, 458
periodontium 269
periorbit 358, 364–366, 376
pes of hippocampus 100, 111, 114, 116–117, 123, 143, 147
petiolus of epiglottis 317, 323, 327, 330, 337, 340
phalanx(-ges) distal of hand 601, 610, 612
- middle of hand 609–612
- proximal of hand 608, 610–612
pharynx 295–296, 306–307, 335–336, 500
- muscular coat 253
philtrum 248
pia mater brain 20, 60, 63, 99, 144–145, 147
- spinal 190–191, 200–201
plane nuchal 4, 26–27, 247
- occipital 11, 27
- sphenoid 4, 247
- temporal 2, 8, 26
platysma 53, 210–211, 217, 220, 250, 298, 308, 460–463, 466, 468–469, 472, 475
pleura, costal 192
plexus aortic abdominal 192, 209
- basilar 19, 97
- brachial 197, 207, 220, 459, 464–467, 475, 477, 480–481, 483, 516, 518, 539
- cardiac 182
- celiac 182
- cervical 462–464
- choroid of fourth ventricle 57, 60, 76, 85, 114, 140, 143, 161, 173, 177, 179–180
- choroid of lateral ventricle 60, 86, 99–100, 106, 109–110, 112, 117, 143–145, 147, 175
- choroid of third ventricle 57, 60, 117, 144–145, 177
- common carotid 304, 313
- esophageal of vagus 192
- inferior dental 224, 288
- inferior hypogastric 182
- internal carotid 19, 234, 395, 440
- internal carotid venous 443
- internal vertebral venous 190, 192, 209
- parotid of facial nerve 214, 217–218
- pelvic 182
- pharyngeal 304, 335
- pterygoid 93, 213, 224
- renal 182
- subclavian 207
- superior hypogastric 182
- superior mesenteric 182
- superior thyroid artery 207
- unpaired thyroid 477
- venous of foramen ovale 93, 97
- venous suboccipital 504
- vertebral artery 207
plica fimbriata 249, 470–471
pole anterior of eyeball 383
- anterior of lens 383, 385, 401, 403, 407
- frontal 70–72, 75–77, 108, 244
- occipital 70–72, 75–77, 108, 395
- posterior of eyeball 383
- posterior of lens 383, 385, 401
- temporal 71–72, 76–77, 116
pons 54, 56, 75–76, 113, 125, 138, 142–143, 167, 172, 177, 189
portion, anular of digital fibrous sheath 584, 600
porus trigemini 95, 134, 136, 136a, 138
precuneus 67, 75, 77, 121

process alveolar of mandible 251, 277–279
- alveolar of maxilla 3, 238, 247, 256, 284, 359, 362
- anterior clinoid 18, 29, 31
- ciliary 384, 396, 403, 405–406
- cochleariform 426, 431–433, 437, 445
- condylar 8–9, 263–264, 277–278, 280, 282, 292, 300, 500
- coracoid 475, 505, 514, 516, 518, 521–524, 528–530, 537
- coronoid of mandible 8–9, 263–264, 277–278, 282, 291–292, 300, 505
- coronoid of ulna 575–576
- ethmoidal of inferior nasal concha 241
- frontal of maxilla 3, 226, 239, 284–285, 347, 349–350
- frontal of zygomatic bone 35–36
- inferior articular of axis 487–489
- inferior articular of cervical vertebra 500, 505
- intrajugular of occipital bone 29
- intrajugular of temporal bone 11, 43, 45
- jugular 18, 27–29
- lenticular 424, 427, 429, 431
- mastoid 4, 8–9, 23, 26, 42, 44–45, 221, 304, 306, 308, 313, 412, 433, 435–436, 438–439, 478, 505
- maxillary 36, 39, 41
- medial clinoid 29
- muscular of arytenoid cartilage 328, 333
- odontoid of axis 4, 9, 54, 487–489, 492, 498–500, 505
- orbital 39–41, 360, 362
- palatine of maxilla 13, 23, 228, 238–240, 256, 285–286, 359
- posterior clinoid 18, 29, 31
- pterygoid 7, 13, 23, 287, 300–301, 363, 502, 505
- pyramidal 7, 23, 39–41, 256, 286
- sphenoidal 39–41
- spinous of axis 487–489, 499–500, 504
- spinous of cervical vertebra 490, 505
- styloid of radius 507, 579–581, 605, 607, 610–611
- styloid of temporal bone 4, 8, 11, 23, 26, 42–43, 45, 253, 290, 293, 300–301, 303–308, 412, 433, 436, 438, 478, 503, 505
- styloid of ulna 506, 574–576, 581, 585, 600, 605, 607, 610–612
- superior articular of cervical vertebra 490, 500, 505
- temporal 35–36
- transverse of atlas 4, 478, 484, 486, 495–496, 503, 505
- transverse of axis 487–489, 500, 503
- transverse of cervical vertebra 493, 500, 505
- uncinate 33, 241
- vaginalis 31
- vocal 326–328, 336–340
- zygomatic of frontal bone 3, 48–49, 237, 242, 352
- zygomatic of maxilla 23, 284, 286, 362
- zygomatic of temporal bone 23, 42, 44–45, 300
prominence facial canal 430, 433, 437
- laryngeal 311, 319–320, 459–460, 476–477
- lateral semicircular canal 430, 433
- mallear 414

*prominence*
- spiral 455
promontory, of tympanic cavity 414, 426–427, 430, 432–433, 435, 437, 445
protuberance external occipital 11, 23, 26–27, 138, 502, 504–505
- internal occipital 9, 18, 28–29
- mental 4, 8, 277–278, 292
pulp cavity of tooth 268–269
pulvinar of thalamus 61, 92, 103, 121, 124, 128, 140–142
punctum, lacrimal 345–346, 348–349, 356, 358
pupil 344, 368, 388, 405
putamen 98–102, 114–115, 117–120, 124, 126
pyramid 76, 121, 142–143, 149, 152–154
- vermis 170, 172, 177

radiation acoustic 125–126, 458
- corpus callosum 107, 114–115, 117
- optic 98, 124–126, 395
- tegmental 166
radius 513, 565–569, 571, 577–581, 585
rami communicantes of spinal nerves 183, 185, 309, 504
- communicantes of sympathetic trunk 183, 209, 480
- dorsal of spinal nerve 183, 192
- ventral of spinal nerve 183, 190, 192
raphe lateral palpebral 347, 351
- mylohyoid 292
- palatine 250–251, 258
- pharyngeal 305
- pons 163–164
- pterygomandibular 251, 253, 303, 308
rays of lens 399, 401–403
recess cochlear 453
- elliptical 453
- epitympanic 409, 426, 428–429, 431, 436
- infundibular 57, 75, 127, 129, 177
- lateal of fourth ventricle 127, 139–140, 171
- optic 57, 75, 127, 129, 140, 177
- pharyngeal 231–232, 302, 306–307, 443
- pineal 57, 75, 129, 139, 142, 177
- piriform 306–307, 313–314, 335–336, 343
- sphenoethmoidal 231
- spherical 453
- superior of tympanic membrane 426
- suprapineal 57, 128–129, 177
- triangular 101, 127
region anterior cervical 1
- axillary 506
- buccal 1
- clavicular 506
- deltoid 1, 506
- frontal 1
- infraclavicular 1, 506
- infraorbital 1
- lateral cervical 1
- lateral thoracic 506
- mammary 506
- medial antebrachial 506
- medial brachial 506
- mental 1
- nasal 1
- occipital 1
- olfactory 230a, 230b
- oral 1
- orbital 1
- palmar cubital 506
- palmar digital 506
- parietal 1
- parotideomasseteric 1, 298
- radial 506

*region*
- radial brachial 506
- radial cubital 506
- respiratory 230a, 230b
- sternal 1
- sternocleidomastoid 1
- sublingual 469
- submandibular 469
- temporal 1
- zygomatic 1
rete acromiale 507, 517
retina 374, 386, 393, 396, 398
retinaculum extensor 513, 534, 546, 557–561, 567, 590, 594, 596, 598
- flexor 533, 583–585, 587–589, 600
rhombencephalon 175, 180
ribs 467, 505, 526
ridges cerebral 18, 49, 243
- nail bed 592
rima glottidis 335–340, 342–343
ring common tendinous 364, 373, 375–376
- fibrocartilaginous 414, 426–428, 431
- greater (major) iridial 407–408
- lesser iridial 407–408
- tympanic 12–13, 414, 436
root(-s) dorsal of spinal nerve 183, 186, 188, 190–191
- inferior of ansa cervicalis 465
- motor of trigeminal nerve 76, 133, 135, 137–138, 142, 235, 289
- nail 592–593
- nose 248
- oculomotor of ciliary ganglion 380
- sensory of trigeminal nerve 134–136, 138, 235, 380
- superior of ansa cervicalis 465
- tongue 254–255, 306–307, 313, 315–316
- tooth 269
- ventral of spinal nerve 183, 190–192
rostrum corpus callosum 54, 75, 77, 107–108, 177
- sphenoidal 31

sac conjunctival 233
- dural 136a
- endolymphatic 448, 456
- lacrimal 225, 349–351
- trigeminal 134
saccule 454, 456–457
- larynx 335
scala tympani 449, 452–453, 455–457
- vestibuli 452–453, 455–457
scapha 412–413
scapula 505, 528
sclera 233, 344, 346, 366, 374, 383–384, 386–387, 393, 396, 398
segment, spinal cord 181, 184
sella turcica 17, 129, 231–233
semicanal auditory tube 436, 444–445
- tensor tympani muscle 433, 436, 444–445
septum antebrachial intermuscular 559, 565–567
- bony nasal 3, 38, 228, 239, 301, 306
- lateral brachial intermuscular 513, 519b, 534–536, 541, 557–559, 563–564
- lingual 255
- medial brachial intermuscular 514, 533, 537–539, 546–547, 550–552, 555, 563–564
- musculotubar canal 430–431, 433, 437, 444–445
- nasal 4, 56, 229, 230b, 233, 244, 247–248, 263–264, 296, 303, 307, 366–367, 374
- orbital 347, 353, 357

*septum*
- pellucidum 54, 75, 77, 98–100, 102–103, 106–112, 114–115, 117, 119–120, 140, 177
- sphenoidal sinus 52
- spinal arachnoid 179

sheath common synovial of flexor muscles 584, 589, 599, 601
- external of optic nerve 353, 367, 374, 376, 382–383, 396–398
- eyeball 353, 358, 366, 374, 377
- fibrous of fingers 584
- fibrous of little finger 600
- internal of optic nerve 397–398
- rectus abdominus muscle 513
- styloid process 23, 42, 45, 348
- synovial intertubercular 514, 520, 524, 538
- synovial of extensor digitorum muscle 590, 596
- synovial of fingers 596, 600, 608–609
- synovial of little finger 584
- synovial of tendon of abductor pollicis longus muscle 584–585, 589–590, 596
- synovial of tendon of extensor carpi radialis brevis muscle 596
- synovial of tendon of extensor carpi radialis longus muscle 596
- synovial of tendon of extensor carpi radialis muscles 590
- synovial of tendon of extensor carpi ulnaris muscle 590
- synovial of tendon of extensor digiti minimi muscle 590
- synovial of tendon of extensor indicis muscle 590, 596
- synovial of tendon of extensor pollicis brevis muscle 590, 596
- synovial of tendon of extensor pollicis longus muscle 590, 596, 599
- synovial of tendon of flexor carpi radialis muscle 584–585, 589, 596, 599–600
- synovial of tendon of flexor pollicis longus muscle 584–585, 589, 599

sinus cavernous 19, 87, 93–94, 97, 131, 213
- ethmoidal 53, 225
- frontal 4, 9, 11, 49, 54, 99, 225, 228–229, 230b, 231–232, 236, 238–239, 241, 243–244, 247, 303, 358–359
- inferior petrosal 94, 97, 213
- inferior sagittal 19, 56–57, 86, 90–91, 93–94, 99, 213
- intercavernous 19, 97
- marginal 97
- maxillary 4, 9, 52–53, 225, 238, 244, 247, 263–264, 287, 289, 350, 359, 363–366
- nail 592
- occipital 94, 97
- posterior of tympanic cavity 433
- rectus 19, 54, 57, 90–91, 93–94, 179, 213
- sigmoid 9, 19, 61, 90, 93–94, 97, 138, 175, 213, 304, 313, 438
- sphenoidal 11, 30, 34, 52, 54, 58, 131, 228–229, 230a, 230b, 231–232, 234, 236, 239–241, 243, 295, 301–303, 363, 374
- sphenoparietal 19, 93–94, 97
- superior petrosal 19, 90, 94, 97, 130, 136a, 213
- superior sagittal 9, 19–20, 56–57, 59–61, 64, 84, 86, 90–91, 93–94, 97, 99, 213
- transverse 19, 59–60, 91, 97, 138, 213, 304, 313, 439
- tympanic 433, 445

*sinus*
- venous of sclera 383–384, 386, 396

skull 2–4, 8–9, 12–13
space between sheaths of optic nerve 353, 383, 397–398
- cranial pharyngeal 253
- craniovertebral 505
- epidural 61, 179, 190, 302
- esophagotracheal 302, 318, 472
- infraglottic 318, 342–343
- interarcual 505
- interfascial of elbow 564
- interfascial palmar 599
- lateral axillary (quadrangular) 515, 536–537, 542
- medial axillary (triangular) 515–516, 537
- perichoroidal 383
- pretracheal 475
- retroesophageal 302, 472
- subarachnoid 20, 57, 60, 190–192
- subdural 191–192
- zonular 384

spine anterior nasal 3, 8–9, 228, 240–241, 284
- ethmoidal 29
- genioglossus muscle 280, 291
- greater tympanic 427–428
- helix 412, 416
- lesser tympanic 427–428
- mental 280, 282
- nasal 48–49, 242
- palatine 286
- posterior nasal 23, 40–41, 239, 241, 285–287
- rectus lateralis muscle 363
- scapular 505, 513, 515, 517, 520, 523, 525, 528
- sphenoid bone 7, 18, 23, 30–31, 301, 441
- suprameatal 42
- trochlear 242

splenium, corpus callosum 54, 61, 71, 77–78, 98–99, 104–106, 108–109, 122, 177, 395
squama frontal 3, 8, 48–49, 239, 363
- occipital 8–9, 12–14, 25, 27–28, 505

stapes 425–427, 434–435, 439, 445, 456
sternum 475
stratum zonale of thalamus 144–145, 147
stria(-ae) lateral longitudinal 105, 109, 144
- mallear 414
- medial longitudinal 105, 109, 144
- medullary of fourth ventricle 127, 139, 142, 155, 458
- medullary of thalamus 103, 140, 178
- olfactory 76, 143
- terminalis 103, 106, 112, 128, 140

stroma, of iris 384
subiculum, of promontory 433
substance anterior perforate 71, 76, 78, 141, 143
- central gelatinous 199
- central gray 20, 141, 147, 164, 167–168
- intermedial central 152, 193–194, 199–201
- posterior perforate 75, 85, 141, 143, 167
- white 122, 147

substantia gelatinosa 200–202
- nigra 71, 114, 141, 165–168
- reticularis alba 104, 147

sulcus(-i) anterior lateral 142, 189, 200
- anterior paraolfactory 75, 77, 177
- arterial 11, 16, 18, 24, 31, 54

*sulcus(-i)*
- auditory tube 31
- basilar of pons 143, 163
- calcarine 68, 71, 75, 77, 79, 98, 106, 108–109, 116, 121, 395
- carotid 18, 29, 31, 132
- central 66, 69–70, 72, 74–75, 77, 125, 129
- cingulate 70, 75, 77, 108, 121
- cingulate of insula 73, 105
- collateral 71, 77, 121, 123, 147
- corpus callosum 75, 77, 121, 144
- deltoideopectoral 506
- fimbriodentate 147
- greater palatine 39–40
- greater petrosal nerve 18, 44
- hippocampal 71, 116, 123, 147
- hypothalamic 75, 177
- inferior frontal 70
- inferior palpebral 248
- inferior petrosal sinus 18, 43
- inferior temporal 71–72, 76
- infraorbital 284, 360–362
- intermediate antebrachial 506
- intertubercular 527, 545
- intraparietal 66, 70, 72
- lacrimal of maxilla 285
- lateral antebrachial 566
- lateral of mesencephalon 128, 141, 167
- lesser petrosal nerve 18, 44
- limb of helix 416
- limitans 139
- medial antebrachial 506, 566
- medial bicipital 506, 514, 533
- median of rhomboid fossa 127, 139
- median of tongue 254
- mentolabial 248
- middle temporal artery 42
- mylohyoid 280, 282, 301
- nasal alar 248
- nasolabial 248
- occipital artery 45, 505
- occipitotemporal 71, 77
- oculomotor nerve 143
- olfactory 71, 76, 107, 143
- palatine 256, 286
- palpebromalar 248
- parietooccipital 66, 68–72, 75, 77, 79, 108, 121, 395
- postcentral 70, 72
- posterior intermediate 139, 142, 200
- posterior lateral 69, 139, 142, 188, 195, 200
- posterior of tongue 139, 149, 152–153, 188, 193–195, 199–200
- posterior paraolfactory 75, 177
- precentral 70, 72, 77
- promontory 433
- pterygopalatine 30
- radial antebrachial 506
- radial nerve 544
- sigmoid sinus 11, 18, 28–29, 43–44, 51, 497
- spinal nerve 490, 493
- subparietal 75, 77
- superior frontal 70
- superior palpebral 210, 248, 344
- superior petrosal sinus 11, 18
- superior sagittal sinus 18, 24, 28, 49, 51
- superior temporal 70, 72
- terminal of tongue 254, 307
- transverse anthelical 416
- transverse occipital 72
- transverse sinus 11, 18, 28–29
- transverse temporal 105
- tympanic 433
- ulnar nerve 543–544
- vertebral artery 484, 495

suture coronal 3, 8, 11–12, 14, 24–25
- frontal 14
- frontoethmoidal 18

*suture*
- frontolacrimal 3
- frontomaxillary 3, 226, 361
- frontonasal 3, 226, 228, 239
- frontozygomatic 4, 8
- incisive 23, 286
- infraorbital 361
- internasal 3
- lacrimoethmoidal 362
- lacrimomaxillary 8
- lambdoid 4, 8–9, 11–12, 23–26
- median palatine 23, 286
- nasomaxillary 3, 8, 226
- occipitomastoid 8, 18, 23, 26
- parietomastoid 8, 26
- sagittal 4, 14, 20–21, 24–26
- sphenofrontal 3, 8, 18, 363
- sphenoparietal 3
- sphenosquamous 8, 18
- sphenozygomatic 3, 8, 381
- squamous 8, 11, 26
- temporozygomatic 8
- transverse occipital 12–13, 26
- transverse palatine 23, 228, 285–287
- vomeromaxillary 228
- zygomatico maxillary 3, 238, 359–361

synchondrosis petrooccipital 305–307, 502
- sphenooccipital 18, 29, 240
- sphenopetrosal 429

syndesmosis, arycorniculate 332

table external 9, 24
- internal 4, 9, 24
tail caudate nucleus 98–102, 114, 118, 124, 140
- helix 412, 417
tapetum 116
tarsus inferior 347, 351, 353, 355–356, 377
- superior 347, 351, 353–357
tectum 128, 165
tegmen fourth ventricle 171
- tympani 44
tegmentum 141, 165–168, 179
- pons 178
tela choroid of fourth ventricle 75, 140, 161, 179
- choroid of prosencephalon 57, 86
- choroid of third ventricle 54, 75, 79, 98, 110, 112, 144–146
telencephalon 186
tendon abductor pollicis longus muscle 513, 546, 558, 567, 596, 598, 600
- biceps brachii muscle 515–516, 520, 522, 536–539, 546–547, 550–552, 554, 564–565, 568, 571
- brachialis muscle 538, 550, 565
- brachioradialis muscle 533, 546, 550, 552–554, 558, 567, 585, 600
- cricoesophageal 307
- digastric muscle 473
- extensor carpi radialis brevis muscle 557–559, 567, 594, 596
- extensor carpi radialis longus muscle 557–559, 566–567, 594, 596
- extensor carpi ulnaris muscle 557, 559–561, 567
- extensor digiti minimi muscle 559–560, 567, 599
- extensor digitorum muscle 559, 590, 594, 596, 599, 602
- extensor indicis muscle 599
- extensor pollicis brevis muscle 513, 547, 550, 558–559, 567, 594, 596, 599–600
- extensor pollicis longus muscle 513, 558–559, 561, 567, 594, 596, 598–599
- flexor carpi radialis muscle 506, 546, 550–551, 553–554, 567, 584, 587–588, 600

*tendon*
- flexor carpi ulnaris muscle 546, 550–551, 553–554, 584–585, 589, 600
- flexor digitorum profundus muscle 551, 554, 567, 584–586, 599–601, 604, 608–609
- flexor digitorum superficialis muscle 551, 554, 567, 584–586, 599–600, 604, 608
- flexor pollicis longus muscle 551, 567, 585, 588, 599–600
- inferior oblique muscle 352
- latissimus dorsi muscle 514, 516
- levator palpebrae superioris muscle 347, 353
- omohyoid muscle 475
- palmaris longus muscle 506, 546, 550–551, 553–554, 567, 584
- pectoralis major muscle 515, 536–537
- pronator teres muscle 559
- rectus inferior muscle 353, 358
- rectus lateralis muscle 352, 374, 383, 396
- rectus medialis muscle 352, 374
- rectus superior muscle 352
- serratus posterior superior muscle 467
- stapedius muscle 427, 430, 445
- stylohyoid muscle 461
- superior oblique muscle 351–352, 365, 368–369, 371, 375, 377, 380, 382
- tensor tympani muscle 409, 426–427, 429–431, 445
- teres major muscle 514, 538
- trapezius muscle 467, 502
- triceps brachii muscle 514, 535–536, 557–559, 570
tenia choroid 106, 128, 140
- fornix 106, 144
- fourth ventricle 139, 153
- thalamus 144
tentorium cerebelli 15, 19, 59–61, 86, 94, 130, 136a, 138, 175, 231, 303
thalamus 54, 56, 75, 78, 96, 98–99, 101–103, 106, 108, 126, 128, 145, 177–178
thenar 506
thymus 302
tongue 223, 249–251, 253–254
tonsil cerebellar 76, 170, 172–173, 176, 179
- lingual 254, 296, 307
- palatine 250–251, 253–254, 293, 296, 302, 306–307, 313–314
- pharyngeal 229, 231–232, 236, 302–303, 306–307, 313
tooth(teeth) canine 256–259, 261, 264, 270
- deciduous 262a, 262b, 263, 265, 267–268
- incisor 256–259, 264
- molar 256–259, 261, 264, 271–272
- permanent molar 262a, 262b, 263, 266, 273–276
- premolar 256–259, 261, 264
torus levatorius 302, 306
- tubarius 231, 236, 302–303, 306, 313
trachea 302, 305, 309–312, 314, 318, 334, 338, 342, 461, 471–472, 475, 500
tract anterior corticospinal 202, 204
- anterior spinocerebellar 148, 150–152, 156, 161–162, 164, 202, 204
- central tegmental 150–157, 161–162
- corticocerebellar 125
- corticonuclear (corticobulbar) 125, 156–157, 162, 166

*tract*
- corticopontine 125, 156–157, 162, 166
- corticospinal 114, 121, 151, 156–157, 161–162, 166, 178, 458
- corticotectal 125
- frontopontine 125–126, 157
- frontothalamic 125
- geniculotectal 395
- lateral corticospinal 148, 202, 204
- mammillothalamic 118
- mesencephalic of trigeminal nerve 156, 164
- occipitopontine 125–126, 157, 166
- olfactory 76, 85, 95, 104, 107–108, 143, 229, 232, 236
- olivocerebellar 153–155, 161
- olivospinal 148, 150–151, 161, 204
- optic 114–115, 117–119, 121, 124, 130, 141–144, 233, 395
- parietopontine 157
- posterior spinocerebellar 148, 150–152, 161, 202, 204
- pyramidal 121, 148, 151, 156–157, 161–164, 166, 458
- reticulospinal 204
- rubrospinal 150–151, 156–157, 161–162, 204
- solitary 153–155, 161
- spinal spinocerebellar 447, 449
- spinal of trigeminal nerve 148–153, 156, 161–162
- spinobulbar 204
- spinocortical 125
- spinoolivary 204
- spinotectal 204
- spinothalamic 150–151, 161–162, 204
- tectospinal 168, 204
- temporopontine 125–126, 157, 166
- thalamoolivary 153, 155, 164, 167–168
- vestibulospinal 204
tragus 409, 413, 419
triangle, deltopectoral 460
trigone collateral 110, 123
- habenular 111, 128, 140, 177
- hypoglossal 139
- lemniscus 95, 128, 142, 458
- lingual 469, 473
- olfactory 71, 104, 141, 143
- omoclavicular 1, 461
- retromandibular 259
- retromolar 2, 253, 282
- submandibular 1, 468, 473–474
- vagus 139, 155
trochlea humerus 543–545, 570
- superior oblique muscle 358, 365, 373, 375, 382
trunk anterior vagal 182
- brachiocephalic 302, 313, 477–479, 481
- costocervical 205, 209, 479
- inferior of brachial plexus 481
- jugular lymphatic 472
- lumbrosacral 207
- medial of brachial plexus 481
- posterior vagal 182
- superior of brachial plexus 464
- sympathetic 182–183, 192, 207–209, 304, 313, 480–481
- thyrocervical 205, 313, 466, 479–481
tube, auditory 289, 410, 429–431, 443–444
tuber, cinereum 71, 76, 141, 143, 177
- vermis 169–170, 177
tubercle anterior of atlas 478, 484, 486
- anterior of axis 488
- anterior of cervical vertebra 490, 493

*tubercle*
- anterior of thalamus 103, 111, 140
- articular of temporal bone 23, 42, 45, 264, 299, 500
- auricular 413
- Carabelli's 272
- carotid 478
- conoid 531–532
- corniculate 302, 306–307, 313, 315–316, 318, 333–334, 337–338
- cuneate nucleus 95, 139, 142, 152
- cuneiform 302, 306–307, 313, 315–316, 318, 333–334, 337–338
- epiglottic 332, 334
- greater of humerus 520, 523, 526–527, 544–545
- inferior thyroid 293, 319–320
- infraglenoidal 528, 530
- jugular 18, 28–29
- lesser of humerus 526–527, 545
- mental 277, 292
- nucleus gracilis 139, 142, 152
- pharyngeal 23, 306
- posterior of atlas 9, 484, 486
- posterior of axis 488
- posterior of cervical vertebra 490, 493
- rib 505
- superior labial 248
- superior thyroid 319–320
- supraglenoidal 530
tuberculum cinereum 139, 142
- sellae 18, 29
tuberosity deltoid 545
- distal phalanx 600–601, 610–611
- masseteric 278, 300
- maxillary 52
- pronator of radius 579
- pterygoid 280, 282, 299, 301
- radius 578, 580, 582
- scaphoid bone 612
- ulna 574, 576

ulna 566–571, 574–577, 581, 585, 605, 607, 610–612
umbo, tympanic membrane 414, 426
uncus 67–68, 71, 76–77, 104, 108, 111, 116, 121, 123
utricle 454, 456–457
uvula palatine 234, 250, 258, 295–296, 306–307
- vermis 170–172, 177

vallecula cerebellar 171
- epiglottic 231, 254–255, 314–316, 318, 343
valves, venous 509b
vein(-s) accessory cephalic 510
- angular 93, 213, 215
- antebrachial basilic 510
- antebrachial cephalic 510
- antebrachial cubital 508, 510, 548, 564–565, 570
- anterior ciliary 386
- anterior jugular 310, 460, 463, 472, 476–477
- anterior spinal 192, 209
- anterior temporal diploic 21, 213
- apex linguae 253
- axillary 466, 475–476, 480
- azygos 192, 209
- basal 90–93
- basilic 508, 510, 539, 547–549, 564–566, 595
- basivertebral 191
- brachial 516, 518, 539, 564
- brachiocephalic 302, 313, 465–466, 477–478, 480–481
- central retinal 382, 386, 396–398
- cephalic 459, 464–466, 475–477, 480, 507–508, 510, 533, 539, 547–549, 564–567, 595

*vein(-s)*
- choroid 86, 96, 110
- ciliary 19
- ciliary body 386
- comitant of hypoglossal nerve 213, 253, 469–470, 476–477
- condylar emissary 213
- conjunctival 386
- deep cervical 213, 481, 504
- deep facial 221, 224
- deep lingual 471
- deep medial cerebral 84
- diploic 9, 20
- episcleral 386
- esophageal 192
- external jugular 213–214, 217, 460–466, 468–469, 473–474, 476–477, 480, 501
- facial 93, 213–215, 221, 224, 253, 298, 463–465, 468–469, 473–477
- frontal diploic 21, 213
- frontal emissary 93
- great cerebral 15, 19, 54, 57, 79–80, 90–96, 110, 112
- hemiazygos 192
- hepatic 192
- inferior anastomotic 90, 93, 97
- inferior cerebral 15, 94
- inferior labial 213
- inferior ophthalmic 213, 233
- inferior temporal 389, 391
- inferior thyroid 306, 476–477, 480
- inferior ulnar collateral 539
- infraorbital 93
- intercapital 595
- intercostal 209
- internal cerebral 61, 79, 86, 90–93, 96, 98, 110
- internal jugular 65, 93, 213, 217, 220–221, 224, 304, 459, 464–467, 472–477, 480, 483
- internal thoracic 476–478, 481
- intervertebral 209
- lacrimal 19
- lateral thoracic 480
- lingual 471
- mastoid emissary 93, 213
- maxillary 213
- median antebrachial 508, 510, 548, 566
- middle meningeal 94, 97, 213
- middle temporal 221, 224
- middle thyroid 477
- nasofrontal 19, 213
- occipital 61, 93, 96, 213, 215, 462–464, 476–477, 501, 504
- occipital diploic 21, 213
- parietal emissary 20, 213
- petrosal 130
- pharyngeal 213, 304
- posterior auricular 217, 462–464, 501, 504
- posterior interosseous 551
- posterior temporal diploic 21, 213
- retromandibular 93, 213–215, 217, 221, 224, 253, 463–466, 469, 473, 476–477
- septum pellucidum 86, 96, 98, 110
- subclavian 313, 465, 467, 477–478
- sublingual 469–471, 477
- submental 213, 221, 224, 465, 469, 476
- superficial cervical 476–477
- superficial temporal 211, 213–217, 224
- superior anastomotic 90
- superior cerebral 15, 59–60, 62, 64, 90–91, 93–94
- superior labial 213
- superior laryngeal 293, 308, 313, 335–336, 468, 470
- superior ophthalmic 19, 93, 213

*vein(-s)*
– superior temporal  389, 391
– superior thyroid  213, 342, 465,
  476–477, 480
– supratrochlear  213
– terminal  86, 90, 96, 98
– thalamostriate  86, 90, 93, 96,
  98, 103, 110, 112, 117–118,
  144–145
– thoracoacromial  465, 476
– thoracoepigastric  480
– thymic  477
– thyroid ima  302, 472
– transverse cervical  463,
  476–477, 501
– ulnar  584
– vertebral  209, 472, 480–481,
  504
– vorticose  19, 386–388
velum anterior medullary  128,
  179
– inferior medullary  171–173

*vein(-s)*
– superior medullary  75,
  139–140, 164, 171–174, 177
vena cava inferior  192
– superior  313, 477–478, 481
ventricle fourth  57, 75, 78, 127,
  129, 156, 161–164, 173,
  177, 179
– laryngeal  54, 56, 231, 235, 302,
  318, 334–335, 342–343
– lateral  109–112, 127, 129, 144
– third  57, 60, 75, 99–101, 103,
  111, 114–115, 117, 119,
  127–129, 139–140, 144–145,
  177, 458
venule inferior macular  394
– inferior nasal retinal  394
– inferior temporal retinal  394
– medial retinal  394
– superior macular  394
– superior nasal retinal  394
– superior temporal retinal  394

vermis, cerebellar  75–76,
  101–103, 106, 111, 170–172,
  174, 177
vertebra(-ae) cervical  9, 479, 481,
  490, 492–493, 500, 505
– prominens  491, 500
– thoracic  505
vertex, cornea  383
vestibule larynx  307, 318, 337,
  342–343
– mouth  225, 236, 244, 250, 253,
  255
– nose  230a, 231–232, 236, 302
– osseous labyrinth  450–452
vibrissae  600
vinculum breve  600
– lingual  171
– longum  600–601
– tendinis of hand  600
viscerocranium  23
vomer  3, 11, 13, 23, 37–38, 228,
  238–239, 245, 301, 306, 359

wall inferior orbital  244
– labyrinthine  432
– mastoid  433
– membranous  436
– membranous of trachea  313,
  317–318, 330, 333, 472
– nail  591–592
– tegmental  448
– vestibular of cochlea duct  455
window cochlear  432, 435,
  450–452, 456
– vestibular  46, 432–433, 435,
  438, 451–452, 456
wing(-s) crista galli  18, 32, 34
– greater  3, 8, 12, 23, 29–30, 233,
  360, 367, 374–376, 381
– lesser  3–4, 17–18, 29–31, 52,
  243, 247, 363
– vomer  37–38, 239, 302

zona incerta  118
zonula, ciliary  383, 396, 403

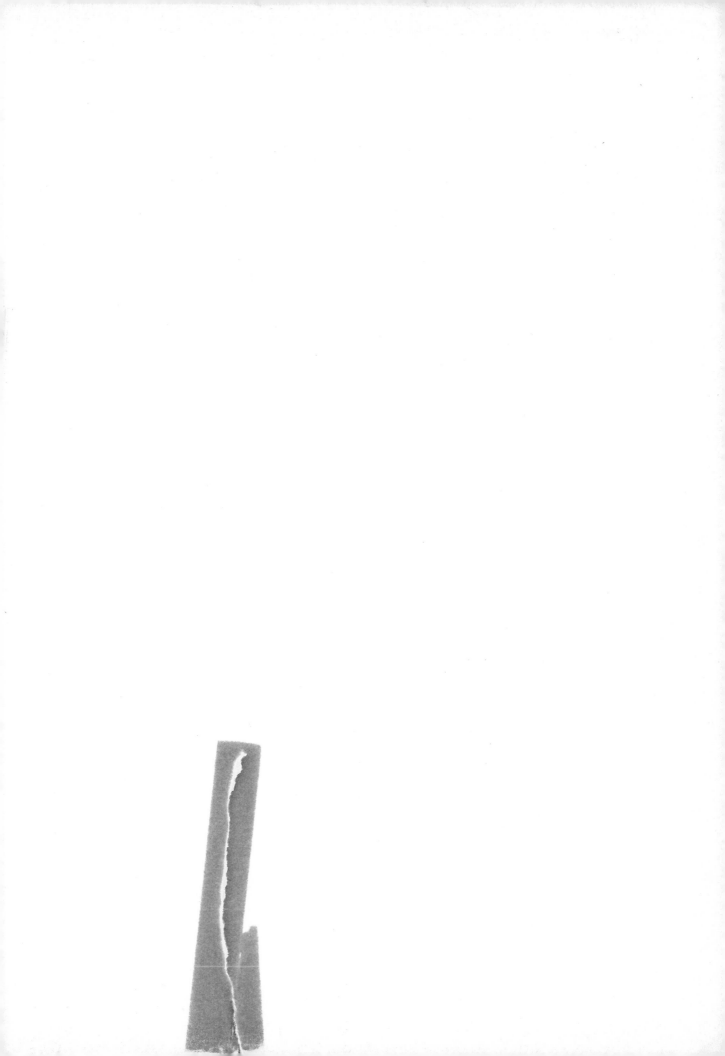

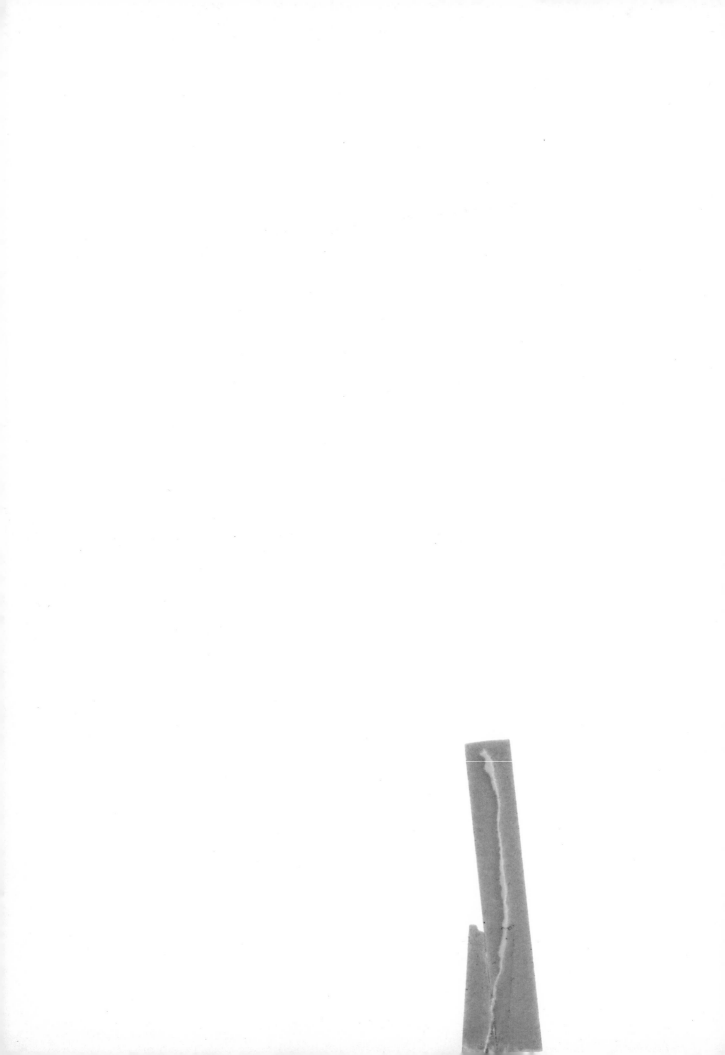